T0189118

H. Michael Dreher, PhD, RN, FAAN, is the Elizabeth Bell LeVaca dean and professor, School of Nursing & Healthcare Professions, The College of New Rochelle, New Rochelle, New York. He has worked in the field of nursing for 32 years and was associate director of BSN programs, director of MSN programs, and founding chair of the Doctoral Nursing Department at Drexel University College of Nursing and Health Professions, Philadelphia, Pennsylvania. He developed the first MSN in Nursing Innovation in 2007 and one of the first Doctor of Nursing Practice programs in the country in 2005. This program included the first mandatory doctoral nursing study abroad program in the United States. He regularly contributes to scholarly publications on legal issues in nursing education and advanced practice doctoral nursing education and has coauthored four books, including *Philosophy of Science for Nursing Practice: Concepts and Applications* (2011, 2016, with Michael D. Dahnke, PhD), which received a 5-Star Doody Review in 2011 and was selected as a Core Doody Title 2011 to 2013; and two first-place *American Journal of Nursing* Books of the Year: *Role Development for Doctoral Advanced Nursing Practice* (2011, with Mary Ellen Smith Glasgow) and *Legal Issues Confronting Today's Nursing Faculty: A Case Study Approach* (2012, with Mary Ellen Smith Glasgow and Toby Oxholm III, JD). He is the former associate editor for *Clinical Scholars Review: The Journal of Doctoral Nursing Practice* (where he edited a column on practice evidence) and *Holistic Nursing Practice* (where he edited a column on innovation in health and healing). He was a recent scholar in residence at the University of Connecticut School of Nursing in Storrs, Connecticut. He is well known as an innovator, an architect of forward-thinking nursing curricula, and a national and international scholar on the professional/practice doctorate. He was inducted as a fellow in the American Academy of Nursing (AAN) in 2012.

Mary Ellen Smith Glasgow, PhD, RN, ACNS-BC, ANEF, FAAN, is dean and professor, Duquesne University School of Nursing, Pittsburgh, Pennsylvania. An early driver and adopter of innovation, she has developed many innovative academic programs; incorporated the cooperative education model; envisioned and implemented the use of online courses and standardized patients, simulation, and various technologies in the nursing and undergraduate health profession curricula. She advanced online pedagogy, developing one of the largest online nursing programs in the country, utilizing asynchronous and synchronous creative teaching strategies. She recently developed the first dual undergraduate-degree program in nursing and biomedical engineering in the nation at Duquesne University. She was honored with the Villanova University College of Nursing Alumni Medallion for Distinguished Contribution to Nursing Education. She was the former associate editor for Oncology Nursing Forum, where she was responsible for the leadership and professional development feature. She was a trustee of Princeton HealthCare System and was selected as a 2009 Robert Wood Johnson Foundation Executive Nurse Fellow. She has more than 70 publications, 135 national and international presentations, and recently coauthored two books: *Role Development for Doctoral Advanced Nursing Practice* (2011, first edition), the recipient of the 2011 *American Journal of Nursing Book-of-the-Year Award*, and *Legal Issues Confronting Today's Nursing Faculty: A Case Study Approach* (2012), the recipient of the 2012 *AJN* Book-of-the-Year Award. Her research interests include safety and interprofessional simulation and leadership development in nursing, for which she secured $2 million in funding. She was elected as a fellow of the American Academy of Nursing and the National League for Nursing Academy of Nursing Education.

DNP Role Development for Doctoral Advanced Nursing Practice

Second Edition

H. Michael Dreher, PhD, RN, FAAN

Mary Ellen Smith Glasgow, PhD, RN, ACNS-BC, ANEF, FAAN

Editors

SPRINGER PUBLISHING COMPANY

NEW YORK

Springer Publishing Company, LLC
11 West 42nd Street
New York, NY 10036
www.springerpub.com

Acquisitions Editor: Margaret Zuccarini
Compositor: Newgen KnowledgeWorks

ISBN: 978-0-8261-7173-3
e-book ISBN: 978-0-8261-7174-0
Instructor's PowerPoints ISBN: 978-0-8261-9486-2

Instructors materials: Qualified instructors may request supplements by e-mailing textbook@springerpub.com.

16 17 18 19 20 / 5 4 3 2 1

The author and the publisher of this Work have made every effort to use sources believed to be reliable to provide information that is accurate and compatible with the standards generally accepted at the time of publication. Because medical science is continually advancing, our knowledge base continues to expand. Therefore, as new information becomes available, changes in procedures become necessary. We recommend that the reader always consult current research and specific institutional policies before performing any clinical procedure. The author and publisher shall not be liable for any special, consequential, or exemplary damages resulting, in whole or in part, from the readers' use of, or reliance on, the information contained in this book. The publisher has no responsibility for the persistence or accuracy of URLs for external or third-party Internet websites referred to in this publication and does not guarantee that any content on such websites is, or will remain, accurate or appropriate.

Library of Congress Cataloging-in-Publication Data
Names: Dreher, Heyward Michael, editor. | Glasgow, Mary Ellen Smith, editor.
Title: DNP role development for doctoral advanced nursing practice / H. Michael Dreher,
    Mary Ellen Smith Glasgow, editors.
Other titles: Role development for doctoral advanced nursing practice.
Description: Second edition. | New York, NY: Springer Publishing Company, LLC, [2017] | Preceded
    by Role development for doctoral advanced nursing practice / [edited by] H. Michael Dreher,
    Mary Ellen Smith Glasgow. c2011. | Includes bibliographical references and index.
Identifiers: LCCN 2016040605 | ISBN 9780826171733 (paperback)
Subjects: | MESH: Advanced Practice Nursing–trends | Advanced Practice Nursing–education |
    Education, Nursing, Graduate–trends | Nurse's Role | Career Choice
Classification: LCC RT75 | NLM WY 128 | DDC 610.73071/1–dc23
LC record available at https://lccn.loc.gov/2016040605

Printed in the United States of America by Bradford & Bigelow.

To Morris Traube and Albert S. Jung, who really saved my life, and Michael D. Dahnke, who enriches it every day. I am so sad to hear of the passing away of Miss Helen Burke, my dear, dear teacher. If she had not poked my head with science in high school at Hillcrest of Dalzell, South Carolina, I know I would not have become a registered nurse and had my wonderful career. She always beat her own drum, to hell if you didn't like it, but with love. I beat my own drum with you dear teacher . . . rest in peace.

—HMD

To my husband, Thomas W. Glasgow, my partner in life, for making everything possible; and Kathy Smith Pickup, Frank Smith, and Mike Smith, who are great siblings and even better friends.

—MEG

Contents

Contributors   *xi*
Reviewers   *xix*
Foreword   Linda Roussel, PhD, RN, NEA-BC, CNL, FAAN   *xxi*
Preface   *xxiii*

SECTION I: HISTORICAL AND THEORETICAL FOUNDATIONS FOR ROLE DELINEATION IN DOCTORAL ADVANCED NURSING PRACTICE

Introduction   *3*
H. Michael Dreher and Mary Ellen Smith Glasgow

1. **The Historical and Political Path of Doctoral Nursing Education to the Doctor of Nursing Practice Degree**   *9*
   H. Michael Dreher
   Reflective Response—*Lynne M. Dunphy*   *52*

2. **Role Theory and the Evolution of Professional Roles in Nursing**   *55*
   H. Michael Dreher and Jeannine Uribe
   Reflective Response—*Sheila P. Davis*   *75*

3. **The Evolution of Advanced Practice Nursing Roles**   *77*
   Marcia R. Gardner, Bobbie Posmontier, Michael E. Conti, and Mary Ellen Roberts
   Reflective Response 1—*Ann L. O'Sullivan*   *101*
   Reflective Response 2—*Patti Rager Zuzelo*   *108*

4. **How Doctoral-Level Advanced Practice Roles Differ From Master's-Level Advanced Practice Nursing Roles**   *113*
   Kym A. Montgomery and Sharon K. Byrne
   Reflective Response 1—*Connie L. Zak*   *133*
   Reflective Response 2—*Karen Kaufman*   *136*

SECTION II: PRIMARY AND SECONDARY CONTEMPORARY ROLES FOR DOCTORAL ADVANCED NURSING PRACTICE

5. **The Role of the Practitioner**   *141*
    Sandra Bellini and Regina M. Cusson
    Reflective Response—*Lucy N. Marion*   *157*

6. **The Role of the Clinical Executive**   *161*
    Barbara Wadsworth, Tukea L. Talbert, and Robin Donohoe Dennison
    Reflective Response—*Patricia S. Yoder-Wise and Karen A. Esquibel*   *178*

7. **The Role of the Educator**   *181*
    Ruth A. Wittmann-Price, Roberta Waite, and Debra L. Woda
    Reflective Response—*Theresa "Terry" M. Valiga*   *198*

8. **The Role of the DNP in Quality Improvement and Patient Safety Initiatives**   *203*
    Catherine Johnson
    Reflective Response—*Susan Baseman*   *214*

9. **The Clinical Scholar Role in Doctoral Advanced Nursing Practice**   *217*
    Elizabeth W. Gonzalez and M. Christina R. Esperat
    Reflective Response 1—*Bernadette Mazurek Melnyk*   *226*
    Reflective Response 2—*DeAnne Zwicker*   *229*
    Reflective Response 3—*Lydia D. Rotondo*   *231*

SECTION III: OPERATIONALIZING ROLE FUNCTIONS OF DOCTORAL ADVANCED NURSING PRACTICE

10. **Role Strain in the Doctorally Prepared Advanced Practice Nurse: The Experiences of Doctor of Nursing Practice Graduates in Their Current Professional Positions—An Updated and Current View**   *237*
    Mary Ellen Smith Glasgow, Rick Zoucha, and Catherine Johnson
    Reflective Response—*Rita K. Adeniran*   *251*

11. **The 2016 Report on a National Study of Doctoral Nursing Faculty: A Quantitative Replication Study**   *255*
    Mary Ellen Smith Glasgow, Frances H. Cornelius, Anand Bhattacharya, and H. Michael Dreher
    Reflective Response—*Nancy C. Sharts-Hopko*   *280*

12. **The DNP and Academic–Service Partnerships**   *285*
    Sandra Rader, Sandra J. Engberg, and Jacqueline Dunbar-Jacob
    Reflective Response—*Judy A. Beal*   *294*

13. **Executive Coaching to Support Doctoral Role Transitions and Promote Leadership Consciousness** 297
    Beth Weinstock and Mary Ellen Smith Glasgow

    Reflective Response 1—*Margo A. Karsten* 316

    Reflective Response 2—*Diane S. Hupp* 319

14. **Leveraging Technology to Support Doctoral Advanced Nursing Practice** 323
    Frances H. Cornelius, Gary M. Childs, and Linda Wilson

    Reflective Response 1—*Victoria M. Bradley* 348

    Reflective Response 2—*Cecilia Kennedy Page* 353

15. **Negotiation Skills for the Doctoral Advanced Practice Nurse** 357
    Vicki D. Lachman and Cheryl M. Vermey

    Reflective Response—*Jared D. Simmer* 371

16. **Seeking Lifelong Mentorship and Menteeship in the Doctoral Advanced Nursing Practice Role** 375
    Roberta Waite and Deena Nardi

    Reflective Response 1—*Marlene Rosenkoetter* 391

    Reflective Response 2—*Debra A. Simons* 394

17. **Interdisciplinary and Interprofessional Collaboration: Essential for the Doctoral Advanced Practice Nurse** 397
    Julie Cowan Novak

    Reflective Response 1—*Grant Charles* 406

    Reflective Response 2—*Jihane Hajj* 412

18. **The DNP-Prepared Nurse's Role in Health Policy and Advocacy** 415
    Sr. Rosemary Donley and Carmen Kiraly

    Reflective Response—*Irene C. Felsman* 427

19. **Enhancing the Doctoral Advanced Practice Nursing Role With Reflective Practice** 429
    Graham Stew

    Reflective Response—*Rosalie O. Mainous* 439

20. **Enhancing the Doctor of Nursing Practice Degree With a Mandatory Study-Abroad Program** 443
    H. Michael Dreher, Mary Ellen Smith Glasgow, Vicki D. Lachman, Rick Zoucha, Melanie T. Turk, Scott Oldfield, Cynthia Gifford-Hollingsworth, and Margie Molloy

    Reflective Response—*Joyce J. Fitzpatrick* 463

21. **The DNP Certification Examination: Yes? No? You Decide**   *467*
   Bobbie Posmontier and Sandra N. Cayo
   Reflective Response 1—*Michael Clark*   *477*
   Reflective Response 2—*Geraldine M. Budd*   *479*

22. **Advising Doctor of Nursing Practice "Clinicians" and How Their Role Will Evolve With a Practice Doctorate: Perspectives From a 35-Year Nurse Practitioner**   *483*
   Joan Rosen Bloch
   Reflective Response 1—*Carol Savrin*   *499*
   Reflective Response 2—*Ann B. Townsend*   *502*

23. **When the DNP Chair Is a DNP Graduate: The DNP in the Academic Role**   *505*
   Susan DeNisco and Sandra Bellini
   Reflective Response 1—*Anne Marie Hranchook*   *521*
   Reflective Response 2—*Lisa A. Johnson*   *524*

24. **A Critique of the 2006** *Essentials of Doctoral Education for Advanced Nursing Practice*: **Do They Guide Practice?**   *527*
   David G. Campbell-O'Dell and H. Michael Dreher
   Reflective Response—*Joy Elwell*   *549*

25. **Today, Tomorrow, and in the Future: What Roles Are Next for Nurses Engaged in Doctoral Advanced Nursing Practice?**   *553*
   H. Michael Dreher and Mary Ellen Smith Glasgow
   Reflective Response 1—*Suzanne S. Prevost*   *570*
   Reflective Response 2—*Margaret Slota*   *573*

Index   *577*

Contributors

Rita K. Adeniran, DrNP, RN, CMAC, NEA-BC, FAAN
President and CEO
Innovative and Inclusive Global Solutions (IIGS)
Drexel Hill, Pennsylvania

Susan Baseman, DrNP, APRN, NEA-BC
Managing Director and Practice Area Director
American Institutes for Research
Washington, DC

Judy A. Beal, DNSc, RN, FAAN
Dean and Professor
Simmons School of Nursing and Health Sciences
Boston, Massachusetts

Sandra Bellini, DNP, APRN, NNP-BC, CNE
Associate Clinical Professor, Coordinator, DNP Program
University of Connecticut School of Nursing
Storrs, Connecticut
Neonatal Nurse Practitioner
Connecticut Children's Medical Center
Hartford, Connecticut

Anand Bhattacharya, MS
Independent Statistical Consultant and Adjunct Professor
Villanova University College of Nursing
Villanova, Pennsylvania

Joan Rosen Bloch, PhD, CRNP
Associate Professor
Doctoral Nursing Department
College of Nursing and Health Professions and Joint Appointment
Department of Epidemiology and Biostatistics
School of Public Health, Drexel University
Philadelphia, Pennsylvania

Victoria M. Bradley, DNP, RN, FHIMSS
Principal
Bradley HIT Consulting, LLC
Lexington, Kentucky
Standards and Content Consultant
Applied Clinical Informatics, Tenet Healthcare
Dallas, Texas

Geraldine M. Budd, PhD, CRNP, FNP-BC, FAANP
Associate Professor and Assistant Dean
Harrisburg Campus
Widener University School of Nursing
Chester, Pennsylvania

Sharon K. Byrne, DrNP, CRNP, NP-C, AOCNP, CNE
Co-Chair and Associate Professor
The College of New Jersey School of Nursing, Health, and Exercise Science
Trenton, New Jersey
Advanced Practice Nurse
Cancer Screening Project, Cancer Institute of New Jersey at Cooper University Hospital
Camden, New Jersey

David G. Campbell-O'Dell, ARNP, FNP-BC, FAANP
President
Doctors of Nursing Practice, Inc.
Key West, Florida

Sandra N. Cayo, DNP, FNP-BC
Northeast Medical Group APRN
Assistant Clinical Professor
New York University Rory Meyers College of Nursing
New York, New York

Grant Charles, PhD
Associate Professor
School of Social Work, University of British Columbia
Affiliated Associate Professor
Division of Adolescent Health and Medicine, British Columbia Children's Hospital
Vancouver, BC, Canada

Gary M. Childs, MS
Education/Reference Librarian
Drexel University Libraries
Philadelphia, Pennsylvania

Michael Clark, DrNP, APN, AGPCNP, DCC
Director, DNP Program—Adult Gerontology and Clinical Assistant Professor
Rutgers University School of Nursing
Camden, New Jersey

Michael E. Conti, CRNA, MSN
Assistant Professor and Assistant Center Director
Albany Medical College
Nurse Anesthesiology Program
Albany, New York
PhD student
Villanova University
Villanova, Pennsylvania

Frances H. Cornelius, PhD, MSN, RN-BC, CNE
Clinical Professor, Chair
MSN Advanced Role Department and Coordinator of Informatics Projects
Drexel University College of Nursing and Health Professions
Philadelphia, Pennsylvania

Regina M. Cusson, PhD, NNP-BC, APRN, FAAN
Dean and Professor
University of Connecticut School of Nursing
Storrs, Connecticut

Sheila P. Davis, PhD, RN, FAAN
Professor of Nursing
University of Southern Mississippi School of Nursing
Hattiesburg, Mississippi

Susan DeNisco, DNP, APRN, FNP-BC, CNE, CNL
Director, DNP Program and Professor, Director, Doctor of Nursing Program, Executive Director
College of Health Professions Center for Community Health and Wellness
Sacred Heart University College of Nursing
Fairfield, Connecticut

Robin Donohoe Dennison, DNP, APRN, CCNS, CEN, CNE
Associate Professor of Clinical Nursing
University of Cincinnati College of
  Nursing
Cincinnati, Ohio

Sr Rosemary Donley, PhD, APRN-BC, FAAN
Donley Professor
Jacques Laval Endowed Chair for Justice
  for Vulnerable Populations
Duquesne University School of Nursing
Pittsburgh, Pennsylvania

H. Michael Dreher, PhD, RN, FAAN
Elizabeth Bell LeVaca Dean
  and Professor
School of Nursing & Healthcare
  Professions
The College of New Rochelle
New Rochelle, New York

Jacqueline Dunbar-Jacob, PhD, RN, FAAN
Dean and Distinguished Service Professor
  of Nursing, Professor of Psychology,
  Epidemiology, and Occupational
  Therapy
University of Pittsburgh School of
  Nursing
Pittsburgh, Pennsylvania

Lynne M. Dunphy, PhD, FNP-BC, FAAN
Professor and Associate Dean for Practice
  and Community Engagement
Florida Atlantic University Christine
  E. Lynn College of Nursing
Boca Raton, Florida

Joy Elwell, DNP, FNP-BC, CNE, FAANP
Associate Clinical Professor and Director
DNP Program
University of Connecticut School of
  Nursing
Storrs, Connecticut

Sandra J. Engberg, PhD, RN, CRNP, FAAN
Professor and Associate Dean
  for Graduate Clinical Education,
  Health Promotion & Development
University of Pittsburgh School
  of Nursing
Pittsburgh, Pennsylvania

M. Christina R. Esperat, PhD, RN
Associate Dean for Clinical Services and
  Community Engagement
Texas Tech Health Sciences Center School
  of Nursing
Lubbock, Texas

Karen A. Esquibel, PhD, DPS, APRN, RN, CPNP
Director, Pediatric Nurse
  Practitioner Program
Associate Professor
Texas Tech University Health Sciences
  Center
Lubbock, Texas

Irene C. Felsman, DNP, MPH, RN
Clinical Nurse Educator
Duke University School of Nursing
Durham, North Carolina

Joyce J. Fitzpatrick, PhD, MBA, RN, FAAN
Elizabeth Brooks Ford Professor of
  Nursing at the Frances Payne Bolton
  School of Nursing
Case Western Reserve University
Cleveland, Ohio

Marcia R. Gardner, PhD, RN, CPNP, CPN
Associate Professor and Associate Dean
  for Undergraduate Programs and
  Assessment
Seton Hall University College
  of Nursing
South Orange, New Jersey

Cynthia Gifford-Hollingsworth, DrNP, MSN, CRNP, CPNP
Surgical Research Nurse Supervisor
Department of Surgery, College of Medicine
Drexel University
Philadelphia, Pennsylvania

Mary Ellen Smith Glasgow, PhD, RN, ACNS-BC, ANEF, FAAN
Dean and Professor
Duquesne University School of Nursing
Pittsburgh, Pennsylvania

Elizabeth W. Gonzalez, PhD, APRN-BC
Associate Professor and Chair of the Doctoral Nursing Department
College of Nursing and Health Professions
Drexel University
Philadelphia, Pennsylvania

Jihane Hajj, DrNP, ACNP-BC
Assistant Professor
Widener University School of Nursing
Chester, Pennsylvania

Anne Marie Hranchook, CRNA, DNP
Assistant Professor and Director of the Nurse Anesthesia Program, Beaumont Graduate Program of Nurse Anesthesia
Oakland University
Rochester, Michigan

Diane S. Hupp, DNP, RN, NEA-BC
Chief Nursing Officer and Vice President of Patient Care Services
University of Pittsburgh Medical Center (UPMC) Children's Hospital of Pittsburgh
Pittsburgh, Pennsylvania

Catherine Johnson, PhD, FNP, PNP
Assistant Professor
Duquesne University School of Nursing
Pittsburgh, Pennsylvania

Lisa A. Johnson, DrNP, CRNP, ACNP-BC
Director, Adult Gerontology Acute Care Nurse Practitioner Program and Assistant Professor
De Sales University
Department of Nursing & Health
Center Valley, Pennsylvania

Margo A. Karsten, PhD, MSN, RN
Chief Executive Officer
Cheyenne Regional Medical Center
Cheyenne, Wyoming

Karen Kaufman, MS
President and Co-Founding Principal
The Kaufman Partnership, Ltd,
Organizational Dynamics
Philadelphia, Pennsylvania

Carmen Kiraly, MSN, CRNP-BC
Associate Professor of Nursing
Suffolk Community College
Long Island, New York
PhD Candidate
Duquesne University
Pittsburgh, Pennsylvania

Vicki D. Lachman, PhD, MBE, APRN
President of V. L. Associates
Avalon, New Jersey

Rosalie O. Mainous, PhD, ARNP, NNP-BC, FAANP
Dean and Professor
Wright State University College of Nursing and Health Administration
Dayton, Ohio

Lucy N. Marion, PhD, RN, FAAN, FAANP
Professor and Dean
Kellett Distinguished Chair of Nursing
Augusta University School of Nursing
Augusta, Georgia

Bernadette Mazurek Melnyk, PhD, RN, CPNP, PMHNP, FNAP, FAAN
Dean, Associate Vice President
    for Health Promotion,
    Chief Wellness Officer
The Ohio State University
Columbus, Ohio

Margie Molloy, DNP, RN, CNE, CHSE
Director, Center for Nursing Discovery
Duke University School of Nursing
Durham, South Carolina

Kym A. Montgomery, DrNP, WHNP-BC, FAANP
Associate Clinical Professor and Chair
    of MSN Nurse Practitioner
    Department
Drexel University, College of Nursing
    and Health Professions
Philadelphia, Pennsylvania

Deena Nardi, PhD, PMHCNS-BC, FAAN
Professor and Director, Doctor
    of Nursing Practice Program
University of St. Francis Leach
    College of Nursing
Joliet, Illinois

Julie Cowan Novak, DNSc, RN, CPNP, FAANP, FAAN
Nancy B. Willerson Distinguished
    Professor Associate Dean, Practice and
    Engagement, Chief Wellness Officer,
    Director
UT Health Science Center School of
    Nursing at Houston (UT Health)
Houston, Texas

Scott Oldfield, MSN, CRNP
Nurse Practitioner
Geisinger Medical Center
Danville, Pennsylvania

Ann L. O'Sullivan, PhD, FAAN, CRNP
Dr. Hildegarde Reynolds Endowed
    Term Professor of Primary Care Nursing
University of Pennsylvania School of
    Nursing
Philadelphia, Pennsylvania

Cecilia Kennedy Page, DNP, RN-BC, CPHIMS, CHCIO, PMP, FACHE, FAAN
Chief Information Officer
University of Kentucky HealthCare
Lexington, Kentucky

Bobbie Posmontier, PhD, CNM, PMHNP-BC
Associate Professor, Professor
Doctoral Nursing Department
Drexel University
College of Nursing and Health Professions
Philadelphia, Pennsylvania

Suzanne S. Prevost, PhD, RN, FAAN
Dean and Professor
The University of Alabama
Capstone College of Nursing
Tuscaloosa, Alabama

Sandra Rader, DNP, RN, NEA-BC
Chief Nursing Officer and Vice President
    of Patient Care Services
University of Pittsburgh Medical Center
    UPMC Shadyside and Presbyterian
    Hospitals
Pittsburgh, Pennsylvania

Mary Ellen Roberts, DNP, APN-C, FNAP, FAANP, FAAN
Assistant Professor
Graduate Programs
Seton Hall University College of Nursing
South Orange, New Jersey

Marlene Rosenkoetter, RN, PhD, FAAN
Professor
Department of Biobehavioral Nursing
Augusta University College of Nursing
    and College of Graduate Studies
Augusta, Georgia

Lydia D. Rotondo, DNP, RN, CNS
Interim Associate Dean for Education &
    Student Affairs
Director, Doctor of Nursing Practice
    Program
Assistant Professor of Clinical Nursing
Deputy Title IX Coordinator
University of Rochester School of Nursing
Rochester, New York

Carol Savrin, DNP, CPNP-PC,
  FNP-BC, FAANP
Associate Professor, and Director of MSN
  Programs
Frances Payne Bolton School of Nursing
Case Western Reserve University
Cleveland, Ohio

Nancy C. Sharts-Hopko, PhD, RN, FAAN
Director, PhD Program and Professor
Villanova University College of Nursing
Villanova, Pennsylvania

Jared D. Simmer, JD, MLIR, EdD
Executive Director of the Piedmont Private
  Adjudication Center and Faculty
Carnegie Mellon University's Heinz
  Graduate School of Public Policy and
  Information Systems Management and
  University of Pittsburgh's Katz School
  of Business
Pittsburgh, Pennsylvania

Debra A. Simons, PhD, RN, CNE,
  CHSE, CCM
Associate Professor and Associate Dean
  of Nursing
The College of New Rochelle School
  of Nursing
New Rochelle, New York

Margaret Slota, DNP, RN, FAAN
Associate Professor and Director, Doctor
  of Nursing Practice (DNP) Program
Georgetown University, School
  of Nursing and Health Studies
Washington, DC

Graham Stew, DPhil, MA, RGN, RMN,
  RNT, FHEA
Principal Lecturer
Professional Doctorate in Health
  and Social Care
University of Brighton
Brighton, United Kingdom

Tukea L. Talbert, DNP, RN
Assistant Hospital Director
UK HealthCare
Lexington, Kentucky

Ann B. Townsend, DrNP, RN,
  ANP-C, CNS-C, CEN
Assistant Professor
LaSalle University School of Nursing
  and Health Sciences
Philadelphia, Pennsylvania

Melanie T. Turk, PhD, MSN, RN
Associate Professor
PhD and MSN Advanced Role
  Programs
Duquesne University School
  of Nursing
Pittsburgh, Pennsylvania

Jeannine Uribe, PhD, RN
Assistant Professor
LaSalle University School
  of Nursing and
  Health Sciences
Philadelphia, Pennsylvania

Theresa "Terry" M. Valiga, EdD,
  RN, CNE, ANEF, FAAN
Professor and Director
Institute for Educational
  Excellence, and Chair,
  Clinical Health Systems & Analytics
  Division
Duke University School
  of Nursing
Durham, North Carolina

Cheryl M. Vermey, EdD, RN,
  CPCC, ACC
President and CEO
EnVision Coaching, Inc.
West Chester, Pennsylvania

Barbara Wadsworth,
  DNP, RN, MBA, NEA-BC,
  FACHE, FAAN
Senior Vice President of Patient
  Services and the Chief Nursing
  Officer (CNO) of Main Line
  Health (MLH)
Bryn Mawr, Pennsylvania

**Roberta Waite, EdD, RN,
PMHCNS-BC, ANEF, FAAN**
Professor and Assistant Dean of
  Academic Integration and Evaluation
  of Community Programs
Doctoral Nursing Department
Drexel University College of Nursing and
  Health Professions
Philadelphia, Pennsylvania

Beth Weinstock, PhD
Independent Consultant
Philadelphia, Pennsylvania

**Linda Wilson, PhD, RN, CPAN,
CAPA, BC, CNE, CHSE,
CHSE-A, ANEF, FAAN**
Associate Clinical Professor
  and Assistant Dean for Special
  Projects, Simulation, and CNE
  Accreditation
Drexel University
Philadelphia, Pennsylvania

**Ruth A. Wittmann-Price, PhD, RN, CNE,
CHSE, ANEF, FAAN**
Dean of Health Sciences and
  Professor of Nursing, Department
  of Nursing Healthcare Administration
  Director
Frances Marion University
Florence, South Carolina

Debra L. Woda, DNP, CNM
Midwife
University of South Carolina Children
  and Family Healthcare
Columbia, South Carolina

**Patricia S. Yoder-Wise, RN, EdD,
NEA-BC, ANEF, FAAN**
President, The Wise Group, Professor,
  Editor-in-Chief, *The Journal of
  Continuing Education in Nursing*, Editor
  in Chief, Nursing Forum, Faculty
Texas Tech University Health Sciences
  Center School of Nursing
Lubbock, Texas

Connie L. Zak, DNP, MBA, FNP-BC
Vice President of Healthcare
  Management at Community Care
  Alliance of Illinois
Chicago, Illinois

**Rick Zoucha, PhD, PMHCNS-BC,
CTN-A, FAAN**
Professor and Chair of PhD and MSN
  Advanced Role Programs
Duquesne University School of Nursing
Pittsburgh, Pennsylvania

**Patti Rager Zuzelo, EdD, RN, ACNS-BC,
ANP-BC, FAAN**
Clinical Professor
Doctor of Nursing Practice Department
College of Nursing and Health
  Professions
Drexel University
Philadelphia, Pennsylvania

**DeAnne Zwicker, DrNP, MSN, ANP/
GNP-BC**
Geriatric Consultant and Faculty
George Mason University, Fairfax School
  of Nursing
Washington, DC

Reviewers

Linda Bellmare, DNP, RN
Clinical Assistant Professor
College of New Rochelle School of
  Nursing
New Rochelle, New York

Mark C. Crider, PhD, RN
Assistant Dean for Administration and
  Special Projects
Duquesne University School
  of Nursing
Pittsburgh, Pennsylvania

Manjulata Evatt, DNP, RN, CMSRN
Assistant Professor
Duquesne University School of Nursing
Pittsburgh, Pennsylvania

Dory Ferraro, DNP, RN
Assistant Professor
College of New Rochelle School
  of Nursing
New Rochelle, New York

Linda S. Koharchik, DNP, RN, CNE
Assistant Professor and Director
Adjunct Faculty and Clinical Affairs
Duquesne University School of Nursing
Pittsburgh, Pennsylvania

Frank Kosnosky, Jr., DNP, RNC, CRNP,
  NNP-BC, FNP-BC
Assistant Professor
Duquesne University School of Nursing
Pittsburgh, Pennsylvania

Ann Kriebel-Gasparro, DrNP, CRNP,
  FNP-BC, GNP-BC
Assistant Professor of Instruction in
  Nursing, AGNP-DNP Program
  Coordinator
Temple University
College of Public Health
Philadelphia, Pennsylvania

Rose Marie E. Kunaszuk, DrNP, CNM
Owner/Midwife at Woman's Wellness
  Center of Conshohocken
Conshohocken, Pennsylvania
Adjunct Nursing Faculty
Duquesne University
Pittsburgh, Pennsylvania

Mary Kay Loughran, DNP, MHA, RN
Assistant Professor
Duquesne University School of Nursing
Pittsburgh, Pennsylvania

Michael Neft, DNP, MHA, CRNA, FAAN
Associate Professor, Vice Chair for
  Administration, Assistant Program
  Director, Nurse Anesthesia
University of Pittsburgh School
  of Nursing
Pittsburgh, Pennsylvania

Cecilia Kennedy Page, DNP, RN-BC,
  CPHIMS, CHCIO, PMP, FACHE,
  FAAN
Chief Information Officer at University of
  Kentucky HealthCare
Lexington, Kentucky

Salwa Paige, DNP, RN
Assistant Professor
College of New Rochelle School
   of Nursing
New Rochelle, New York

Maggie Richardson, DrNP
Nurse Practitioner
Take Care Health Systems
Conshohocken, Pennsylvania

**M. Elizabeth Teixeira, DrNP, RN, APN,
  AGPCNP-BC**
Assistant Professor
The College of New Jersey
  School of Nursing and Exercise
  Science
Ewing, New Jersey

Cynthia A. Walters, DNP, RN
Assistant Professor and RN-BSN Program
  Coordinator
Duquesne University School of Nursing
Pittsburgh, Pennsylvania

Yvonne L. Weideman, DNP, MBA, RN
Assistant Professor and Second Degree
  BSN Program Coordinator
Duquesne University School of Nursing
Pittsburgh, Pennsylvania

Missi Willmarth-Stec, DNP, APRN, CNM
Associate Professor of Clinical Nursing
Director, DNP Program
University of Cincinnati
College of Nursing
Cincinnati, Ohio

Foreword

I am most impressed with this second edition of *DNP Role Development for Doctoral Advanced Nursing Practice*, a notable winner of the *American Journal of Nursing* first-place award in the Advanced Practice Education category in its first edition. Drs. Dreher and Glasgow continue to provide insights in their work toward advancing the role of advanced practice nurses (APNs) by presenting a rich historical perspective on the evolution of the Doctor of Nursing Practice (DNP) degree and critical content on role development, and by promoting the progression of doctoral nursing roles within our complex health care system. When writing a foreword, it is important to respond to the following: distinguishing the credibility of the authors; determining the importance of the book relative to others; and describing the value of the book to the reader. Drs. Dreher and Glasgow are well-qualified authors who are educating and mentoring DNP students working in leadership and academic roles. Their involvement in the DNP degree and advancing nursing practice has been from the beginning very prominent in the national discourse, with their first text paving the way to greater discoveries and innovative insights. In this second edition, the many diverse contributors provide important perspectives that are unique and worth reading, given their extensive backgrounds in doctoral nursing education and advanced practice nursing.

As our health care systems become more complex (high-reliability organizations), we are charged with greater accountability to provide safe, quality value-added care. To not do so would be irresponsible. In September 2010, the American Association of Colleges of Nursing (AACN) reported 121 DNP programs and one DrNP program. In 2015, the AACN noted 264 DNP programs and 60 or more in development. The tipping point toward the DNP-degree model has been quick, with the National Organization of Nurse Practitioner Faculties (NONPF) supporting the position of the "DNP by 2015." Although this position has yet to be realized, the NONPF continues to advance the notion, with other primary nursing specialty organizations (nurse anesthetists, nurse-midwives, and clinical nurse specialists), that the profession advance the DNP discussion as a replacement for the master's degree for advanced practice registered nurses (APRNs). We know that by the year 2025, educating nurse anesthesia students will be done at the doctoral level. However, we still have far to go, as there have been no regulatory actions in any state that is requiring the DNP degree as a replacement for the master's degree for APRNs. Although we struggle for consensus—and it is a slow process of modifying 50 individual State Nurse Practice Acts, changing regulatory requirements on the federal, state, accrediting organizational, and specialty practice levels—the passion for the DNP degree continues, particularly among nurse educators and DNP graduates. The true "proof of success" will be the DNPs' influence in health systems as well as the value-added, data-driven outcomes of these graduates. Those working side by side with these expert clinicians and clinical executives may be puzzled as to why seeking advanced education is necessary. We are, however, noting less discussion on the need and reasons for DNP education and greater attention focused on refinement of the degree and future implications and expectations. Specifically, the nature of the final project, initially recommended to be called a capstone project by the AACN (2006) and now a DNP project (2015) by the AACN in a new white paper, *The Doctor of Nursing Practice: Current Issues and Clarifying Recommendations*, remains a centerpiece for discussion with the degree.

Purposeful and intentional conversations about knowledge development occurring as the DNP degree evolves are critical, especially as many senior nurse scientists are retiring and PhD enrollments are remaining flat. This second edition is a "must read" and adds value to evolving DNP programs and education for APNs. The concept of DNPs generating practice-based evidence, although in many discussions it was related to what "deliverables" the degree should encompass, was not always first and foremost as an end goal. It is more evident now this was (and is) a critical concern, and that the profession was missing opportunities for practice-generated knowledge. The recent white paper (AACN, 2015) has made advances in this area, recognizing "that practice-focused graduates are prepared to generate new knowledge" (p. 2) and noting that "new knowledge generated through practice innovation, for example, could be of value to other practice settings" (pp. 2–3). We are at a critical juncture to discuss future considerations given our 10-year history with DNP education. The profession must not be complacent and lose precious time toward seeking understanding on what we agree on regarding outcomes and what might not be value-added in this still-new degree. The editors, contributors, and reflective commentators in this second edition provide ongoing discussions that are essential to the future development of DNP education. This is particularly important as the literature does not provide overwhelming evidence that the degree is "superior" and focuses more on what the role of the DNP graduate is with regard to knowledge development and how DNP graduates will be socialized to be more engaged stewards of the discipline than master's graduates. Notable inclusions in this text focus on why doctorally educated clinicians and practitioners in particular need to enhance their emphasis on reflective practice; a distinctive way in which the delivery of patient-centered care cannot be overwhelmed by the forces of population-based care (Chapter 19) and important data from a very large comparative study on the state of doctoral nursing faculty (Chapter 11). One or more Reflective Responses accompany each chapter as commentaries on the content; these are written by recognized DNP leaders from diverse roles and reflect the experiences of educators, practitioners, and administrators from different DNP programs. Thought-provoking discussions are anticipated as faculty and students address the reflections of DNP leaders. The beauty of this second edition is the provocative nature of the content relevant to DNP education and unfolding role development. It will be a wonderful resource in DNP role development courses and courses covering contemporary DNP-degree issues.

Linda Roussel, PhD, RN, NEA-BC, CNL, FAAN
DNP Program Director
School of Nursing
University of Alabama at Birmingham
Birmingham, Alabama

■ REFERENCE

American Association of Colleges of Nursing. (2015). *The doctor of nursing practice: Current issues and clarifying recommendations*. Washington, DC: Author.

Preface

Functioning as both a graduate textbook and a professional resource, *DNP Role Development for Doctoral Advanced Nursing Practice* explores the historical and evolving role of the doctoral advanced practice registered nurse, as well as describes Doctor of Nursing Practice (DNP)-educated nurse practitioners, nurse-midwives, nurse anesthetists, and clinical nurse specialists. Similarly, this text addresses roles for nurses engaged in doctoral advanced nursing practice, which describes the role of the clinical executive, faculty member with a clinical focus, quality officer, and the other diverse roles that the DNP graduate may assume. There is a growing literature on the domain of practice "beyond the MSN," and this text specifically focuses on this emerging discussion. Because the role of the DNP graduate is still evolving, the primary authors and contributing authors of this text present positions and Reflective Responses that represent a wide range of current views on the DNP role and the diverse "ideals" of what the role of this graduate should be. This text also exclusively examines the evolving and expanding role functions of the DNP graduate.

Too often, nursing texts offer the sole view of the author. This text uniquely offers the views of many diverse faculty, executives, practitioners, and scholars. The distinctive feature of this text is the two-part chapter organization that presents the chapter content followed by one or more Reflective Responses, which provide commentaries that may counter or support the opinions of each chapter author or authors. Each Reflective Response is written by a well-known DNP leader or leaders representing the diverse roles and experiences of academics, administrators, and practitioners, including graduates from different DNP programs. This innovative chapter presentation is bound to enhance classroom discussion. The work in its entirety is hopefully stimulating and provocative, and a well-rounded presentation of issues germane to DNP education, core competencies, and unfolding role development. We believe this is a "must have" text in DNP role development courses and courses covering contemporary DNP-degree issues.

Each of the textbook's sections thoroughly covers important aspects of role development:

- Section I provides background information on the evolution of the DNP degree, essential content on role theory, what nursing "roles" are and how they evolved, and a discussion of how master's- versus doctoral-level advanced nursing practices differ.
- Section II focuses on the three basic roles of the DNP graduate that currently predominate: practitioner, clinical executive, and faculty member with a clinical focus. This section also addresses the role of the clinical scholar, something each graduate is expected to embrace as a steward of the discipline.

- Section III covers the diverse skills that comprise the doctoral advanced practice registered nurse (APRN) and doctoral advanced practice nurse (APN) role, including leadership content, negotiation skills, quality improvement, and leveraging technology to support doctoral advanced level practice; it includes doctoral global health competencies with mandatory study abroad and how the doctoral APRN or the DNP engaged in doctoral advanced practice nursing can use these new competencies to function at a higher level.

There always has been debate in nursing about the direction of the profession. We have witnessed the evolution of our practice-focused disciplinary trajectory from our earliest nursing curricula in the 19th century, to the predominance of the diploma-educated nurse, and now to current forces attempting to supplant the master of science in nursing (MSN) in favor of the DNP for entry-level advanced practice. Throughout the text, authors raise important questions about the current state of doctoral education, DNP outcomes, role satisfaction, and contributions to nursing practice and health. This text aims to honor our history of diverse discourse and add to the growing literature about the evolution of nursing "practice" emerging at the doctoral level. **Qualified instructors may access a PowerPoint presentation that details the important aspects of this book by e-mailing testbook@springerpub.com.**

H. Michael Dreher
Mary Ellen Smith Glasgow

Historical and Theoretical Foundations for Role Delineation in Doctoral Advanced Nursing Practice

Introduction

H. Michael Dreher and Mary Ellen Smith Glasgow

Although the Doctor of Nursing Practice (DNP) degree was introduced by one pioneering program in 2001, the degree first came into prominence in 2005 when a group of schools implemented several diverse models of DNP degree curricula (American Association of Colleges of Nursing [AACN], 2010; Fulton & Lyon, 2005). In the first edition of this book we reported that there were 121 DNP programs and one DrNP program (as of September 2010). In 2015, the AACN reported an astounding 264 DNP programs and 60 or more in development. The momentum toward the DNP degree model has been swift. However, in this early wave of momentum, aside from the National Organization of Nurse Practitioner Faculties (NONPF), the other primary nursing specialty organizations (representing nurse anesthetists, nurse-midwives, and clinical nurse specialists) were on the periphery of the substantive discussion. Over time, there has been considerable outreach to the specialty advanced practice organizations regarding the 2015 goal of endorsing the DNP degree as the entry-level degree for advanced practice nursing. And although the 2015 date has come and passed, there have been no regulatory actions in any state that have in any way inscribed the DNP degree as a required replacement for the master's degree for advanced practice registered nursing (APRN). Nevertheless, what has changed, rather enormously, is the health care marketplace. In 2005, there was no indication of a pending global recession. Additionally, there was also no indication that a young senator from Illinois, in his first term, would become president and pass historic health care reform, resulting in the signage into law on March 23, 2010, of The Patient Protection and Affordable Care Act (PPACA), commonly called the Affordable Care Act (ACA, 2010). In 2010, we saw extensive dialogue and discussion about the still relatively new DNP degree. Today, in 2016, the debate has waned considerably, and contemporary thought leaders in doctoral nursing education are more focused on how to reengineer the DNP curriculum more consistently across programs.

In early 2010, the American Nurses Association (ANA) published a draft of its position statement on the DNP degree. It was thought that the ANA would offer a policy stand after a period of public comment, but as of the writing of this second edition, the ANA has been silent on the DNP. Despite the reluctance to formalize doctoral entry into advanced practice nursing and begin the slow process of modifying 50 individual State Nurse Practice Acts, changing regulatory requirements on the federal, state, accrediting organizational, and specialty practice levels, there is enormous enthusiasm for this degree among nurse educators and DNP graduates who have graduated from the earliest founded programs. The primary authors of this text nevertheless believe that the ultimate success of this degree will be largely affected by the marketplace as well as the data-driven outcomes of these graduates. Therefore, it is critical, especially in a time of health care upheaval and an economy with limited resources still recovering from the Great Recession, that DNP degree outcome research be conducted and data disseminated (Krugman, 2009; Rhodes, 2011).

This text explores the intricately complex historical trajectory of the discipline toward the nursing "practice doctorate" with an emphasis on the evolution of doctoral nursing practice roles. This new quest to prepare nurse clinicians (the four traditional APRN roles) and the nurse executives at the doctoral level is progressive, to some exhilarating, and still to others, regressive and not necessarily welcome. Mainly, the real opposition to the DNP degree has waned, and the discussion now is, "what is the future of the doctor of nursing practice degree?" and "how does the degree need to be refined?" The nature of the final scholarly project, initially recommended to be called a capstone project by the AACN (2006) and now a scholarly project (2015b) by the AACN in a new white paper *The Doctor of Nursing Practice: Current Issues and Clarifying Recommendations*, remains a central issue with the degree. These authors hope that a more meaningful discussion about knowledge development occurs as the DNP degree evolves, especially because many senior nurse scientists are retiring and PhD enrollments are remaining flat. In the first edition of this text, it was worrisome that the profession was missing an opportunity to embrace DNP-generated "practice knowledge development." But again the new white paper (AACN, 2015b) has made advances in this area recognizing "that practice-focused graduates are prepared to generate new knowledge" (p. 2) and recognizing that "new knowledge generated through practice innovation, for example, could be of value to other practice settings" (pp. 2–3). However, we must continue to be diligent in promoting the different aspects of knowledge development that are critical to the evidence base of the scientific basis of our discipline. More than ever, clinicians need to practice safely and expertly and for a degree in its seminal stages of maturation, the doctoral nursing community needs to continue to debate and discuss the vision and essential competencies of this degree.

The first doctoral degree in nursing was a professional doctorate (EdD) in nursing education at Teachers College, Columbia University, in 1933 (Roy, 2007). Remarkably, despite its innovation, this degree model was never replicated in the profession until recently with the emergence of programs at Southern Connecticut State University, the University of West Georgia, University of Alabama, Capstone College of Nursing, and Western Connecticut State University (EdD programs housed in Schools of Education with some form of concentration in nursing education were excluded from this review). The first PhD in nursing was founded at New York University in 1934, and yet it was 20 years before the next PhD at the University of Pittsburgh was founded in 1954 (AACN, 2009). This text actually may be the first to declare that the first doctorate in nursing, the EdD, was actually *a practice doctorate*. Because the EdD degree is classified globally as a professional doctorate (Maxwell, 2003; Townsend, 2002) and the term "professional doctorate" has become mostly synonymous with "practice doctorate"[1] (the influential Carnegie Project on the Education Doctorate [n.d.] calls the EdD a "professional practice doctorate"), the DNP may actually be a doctoral degree that returns us to the practice roots of our profession and discipline. Thus, some may even consider the DNP degree "an awakening" and a welcome departure from our recent emphasis on the science of nursing at the expense of its art of practice. Alas, even the often used term *the practice of medicine* is still defined and described as both "art" and "science" (Tucker, 1999). The DNP degree will certainly undergo further metamorphosis and we have no idea what it will ultimately look like in 20 years. The anticipated transformation of the DNP degree is actually what makes graduate and doctoral nursing education so fascinating today.

We embrace debate, discourse, and difference in this text. The concept "difference" in many ways is naturally associated with "innovation" and indeed the statement made by Collinge, Burfitt, and MacNeill (2006) that " 'Innovation' is the process of bringing 'novelty' into being, but to analyse this a little further it is useful to recognise that novelty is a kind of 'difference' " (p. 4). For this reason, as this degree moves beyond its first real decade, differences in DNP programs ought not be the focus. Premature conformity in any industry (including education) can stamp out innovation and that is why "disruptive innovators" like Uber (founded in 2009) and Twitter (founded in 2006) generally burst onto the scene with success (Christensen, 1997). In higher education, both online and digital learning remain disrupted innovations that many (including academics) still bemoan and malign for different reasons (Horn, 2014). But simply choosing to ignore the impact of digital learning and its penetration into most aspects of higher education is really not a realistic option. What may be the better focus for the DNP and the current dialogue on doctoral preparation for APRNs may be to examine what curricular areas require strengthening or refocusing? This might allow the discipline to spend less time on issues with the practice doctorate, such as "whether we should have this degree" or whether "doctoral nursing practice is better than master's practice" (we contend it is more advanced, but the literature does not yet support it is better) and focus more on "what is the role of the DNP graduate with regard to knowledge development" and "how will DNP graduates be socialized to be more engaged stewards of the discipline than master's graduates?" We aver that DNP graduates *must* advance the discipline, even if some traditional PhD-degree-focused faculty remain skeptical. After all, Lee S. Shulman (2010), president emeritus of the Carnegie Foundation for the Advancement of Teaching and professor of education emeritus at Stanford University, recently stated, "Doctoral education shouldn't be a marathon" (p. 1).

The great advances of this degree in the profession include: (a) giving nurses a doctoral degree option other than the PhD; (b) more degree parity for highly educated nurse clinicians, nurse executives, and others; (c) enhanced credibility and prestige of DNP graduates in the corridors of the health practice environment and at the tables of health policy; and (d) more refined skills in knowledge management and in the translation and dissemination of evidence for health care utilization. However, unresolved issues remain: (a) how much scholarship (even the word "research" in nursing becomes a loaded word) belongs in the practice doctorate?; (b) should DNP graduates become leaders in practice knowledge development derived by generating practice-based evidence (versus evidence-based practice)?; (c) is 1,000 total clinical hours for the post-master's DNP degree reasonable and sound?; (d) should there be any crossover coursework between DNP and PhD students?; and (e) should the PhD and DNP degrees ultimately be the only nursing doctorates offered? Finally, after examining trends in the educational preparation of nursing faculty discussed in Chapter 11, we often now wonder if the resurgent EdD in nursing education ought to become the degree of choice especially for academics who do not teach in research-intensive universities, and who predominate in the teaching ranks across the country. As these issues are debated and hopefully resolved, it is still likely that the DNP degree may ultimately look different at research-intensive universities than at colleges where teaching is more of an emphasis. We, and the multiple contributors to this text, write with great optimism, but also with circumspect and critical analyses of the DNP degree. We view this approach to this text, retained from the first edition, as a strength.

This text is divided into three sections. The first section is titled "Historical and Theoretical Foundations for Role Delineation in Doctoral Advanced Nursing Practice." In this section, the historical and political evolution of the DNP degree is traced and an analytical view of the "state of the degree" is presented. This section continues with a historical orientation of professional roles in nursing as the discipline slowly emerged from simply "work" to a "field" and then ultimately to a "discipline." Role theory and a perspective on the meaning of nursing roles, from professional to advanced, to doctoral advanced practice, are offered. The concluding chapters in this section trace the historical evolution of advanced practice nursing roles (including nurse practitioner [NP], nurse-midwife, nurse anesthetist, and clinical nurse specialist), and ends with an opening discussion by two DNP graduates, who discuss how their doctoral advanced practice roles differ from their previous master's roles.

The second section is titled "Primary and Secondary Contemporary Roles for Doctoral Advanced Nursing Practice." Here the contributing authors first discuss the two primary roles of the DNP degree that the AACN has endorsed—practitioner and clinical executive. It would, however, be neglectful not to address the roles that other DNP graduates have assumed, and so the secondary roles of the educator, the DNP graduate's role in quality improvement and safety, and the important discussion on the roles of DNP graduates as clinical scholars to the profession are explored. One of the assumptions of this text is that there is a domain of practice beyond the master of science in nursing (MSN) degree and that with the doctoral credential the graduate is empowered and obliged to be a greater steward to the discipline. Part of this enhanced stewardship is a commitment to both the conduct and dissemination of clinical scholarship in its multiple forms.

The final section is titled "Operationalizing Role Functions of Doctoral Advanced Nursing Practice." This critical section of the text addresses the multifaceted aspects of the role of doctoral APRNs (DAPRNs) and doctoral advanced practice nurses (DAPNs) as they claim their new roles and enact them in the workplace. Smith Glasgow, Zoucha, and Johnson replicate the study, "Role Strain in the Doctorally Prepared Advanced Practice Nurse: The Experience of Doctor of Nursing Practice Graduates in their Current Professional Positions," published in the first edition of this book in 2010. It is this kind of empirical data that the discipline will need in increasing volume to best understand the competencies and outcomes of this critical mass of nurses who possess a practice doctorate. Career development is particularly important for DNPs, and because there are few role models (but certainly more than 5 years ago), the first graduate cohorts are now becoming the mentors of today and the future. Chapter 12 discusses the emerging roles of DNPs in academic partnerships. DNP graduates are educated to assume higher levels of leadership with enhanced skills, and therefore with doctoral preparation much more is expected from them. Chapter 14 specifically addresses how technology skills and competencies are critical for leadership preparation for the DNP-educated graduates in all types of roles. Chapters 13 and 15 outline the benefits of coaching for DNP students and the art of negotiation, two important aspects of any diverse DNP role. Chapter 16 explores the roles of mentors and the mentee in both the educational and trajectory professional career of the DNP graduate's professional career.

Chapter 17 examines the necessity for more interprofessional collaboration between DNPs and their peer health profession colleagues. Having a critical mass of new nurse clinicians with doctoral preparation may be new for some disciplines who will be working with and alongside these new graduates. Chapter 18 calls attention to what is expected of this new graduate—a higher level of involvement in health policy, especially at the activist grass roots of health advocacy. Chapters 21 and 23 address two controversial issues with the nursing practice doctorate—the still very controversial DNP examination and what challenges does the DNP-educated department chair face? As the AACN and CCNE do not recognize the DNP degree for the advanced role of the nursing educator, there are often institutional issues the DNP-educated department chair will likely face. This text is thought to be the first to discuss the issue of DNP-educated department or program chairs. Finally, this text focuses on why doctorally educated clinicians and practitioners in particular need to enhance their emphasis on reflective practice (Chapter 19), why DNP clinical scholars ought to have more real educational experiences in global health, and why a mandatory study-abroad program is one way to achieve this (Chapter 20). The final chapters are designed to leave the DNP student with thoughts of the present and future. Bloch (Chapter 22), with her some 35 years' experience as a veteran NP, has wise counsel and advice, particularly for MSN-prepared NPs who are heading back to graduate school and perhaps wondering how their doctoral degree might really improve their already fine-tuned practice. The text concludes with a critique (perhaps more a reflection) on the AACN's (2006) *Essentials of Doctoral Education for Advanced Nursing Practice* 10 years after its publication (Chapter 24) and some futuristic thoughts about the DNP degree by the text's two primary authors (Chapter 25). We end this text with some projections of how we see DNP roles and the degree evolving in the future.

After each of these chapters, Reflective Responses are provided by leading academics, administrators, and practitioners, including graduates from different DNP programs. These contributions by leading nursing scholars are one great innovation of this text. Sometimes, these additional viewpoints complement and sometimes contradict, but mostly add additional insight and perspective. The concluding Reflective Responses are written by Dr. Suzanne Prevost, former president of Sigma Theta Tau International and now professor and dean at the University of Alabama, Capstone College of Nursing, and by Dr. Margaret C. Slota, director of the DNP program at Georgetown University. In the end, we are certain that these reflective responses will markedly enhance the discussion that will likely take place in the classroom or online as these multiple positions are evaluated. Each chapter also has 10 critical thinking questions, which we highly recommend as discussion points, paper topics, debates, or even as weekly written assignments. We mostly hope they will be fodder for "tussling in the doctoral classroom," which is what late Dr. Susan K. Leddy (Dr. Dreher's dissertation chair and former dean at Widener University) said should occur in doctoral study. She had little affinity for polite or convenient agreement. Having completed a postdoctoral research fellowship late in her career, Dr. Leddy told us that she did not feel that conformist thinking advanced science much. She embraced vigorous debate, but she always required doctoral nursing students to provide principled rationales for their arguments.

We are both indebted to the many contributors to this text who are all paving the way for an improved DNP degree that will ultimately gain its proper place and foothold in the discipline. In many ways, the first edition of this text in 2010 could *not* have been written earlier. Only now, in the second edition, after a decade of experience with the DNP, have the substantive issues with the degree begun to surface in a constructive and perhaps less political way. The DNP degree is alive and thriving and it is up to you, your faculty, and all the other stakeholders (and there are many) to move forward, advance the nursing discipline, and improve the health of this nation and the globe.

■ NOTE

1. Many revisionists considered the nursing doctorate (ND) degree the first "practice nursing doctorate," when in reality, the title "practice doctorate" was not yet in the common vernacular nor a recognized term when the degree was first offered at Case Western Reserve University in 1979 (Schlotfeldt, 1978).

■ REFERENCES

Affordable Care Act. (2010). Retrieved from https://www.gpo.gov/fdsys/pkg/BILLS-111hr3590enr/pdf/BILLS-111hr3590enr.pdf

American Association of Colleges of Nursing. (2006). *The essentials of doctoral education for advanced nursing practice.* Retrieved from http://www.aacn.nche.edu/DNP/pdf/Essentials.pdf

American Association of Colleges of Nursing. (2009). Institutions offering doctoral programs in nursing and degrees conferred. Retrieved from http://www.aacn.nche.edu/IDS/pdf/DOC.pdf

American Association of Colleges of Nursing. (2010). Doctor of nursing practice (DNP) programs. Retrieved from http://www.aacn.nche.edu/DNP/DNPProgramList.htm

American Association of Colleges of Nursing. (2015a). DNP fact sheet. Retrieved from http://www.aacn.nche.edu/media-relations/fact-sheets/dnp

American Association of Colleges of Nursing. (2015b). The doctor of nursing practice: Current issues and clarifying recommendations. Retrieved from http://www.aacn.nche.edu/aacn-publications/white-papers/DNP-Implementation-TF-Report-8-15.pdf

Carnegie Project on the Education Doctorate. (n.d.). Resource library. Retrieved from http://www.nursingworld.org/MainMenuCategories/ANAMarketplace/ANAPeriodicals/OJIN/TableofContents/Vol-16-2011/No3-Sept-2011/Articles-Previous-Topics/DNP-as-the-Single-Entry-Degree-for-Advanced-Practice-Nursing.html

Christensen, C. (1997). *The innovator's dilemma: When new technologies cause great firms to fail.* Cambridge, MA: Harvard Business Press.

Collinge, C., Burfitt, A., & MacNeill, S. (2006). *The impossibility of innovation: Towards a knowledge-based approach to Eurodite.* Paper presented at the EURODITE, Regional Trajectories to the Knowledge Economy Meeting, DG Research, European Commission, Brussels, Belgium, March 30–31.

Fulton, J., & Lyon, B. (2005). The need for some sense making: Doctor of nursing practice. *The Online Journal of Issues in Nursing, 10*(3), Manuscript 3. Retrieved from www.nursingworld.org/MainMenuCategories/ANAMarketplace/ANAPeriodicals/OJIN/TableofContents/Volume102005/No3Sept05/tpc28_316027.aspx

Horn, M. (2014). Disruptive innovation and education. *Forbes.com.* Retrieved from http://www.forbes.com/sites/michaelhorn/2014/07/02/disruptive-innovation-and-education/#ec4a2f65cc87

Krugman, P. (2009). The Great Recession versus the Great Depression. *New York Times.* Retrieved from http://krugman.blogs.nytimes.com/2009/03/20/the-great-recession-versus-the-great-depression

Maxwell, T. (2003). From first to second generation professional doctorate. *Studies in Higher Education, 28*(3), 279–291.

Rhodes, M. (2011). Using effects-based reasoning to examine the DNP as the single entry degree for advanced practice nursing. *The Online Journal of Issues in Nursing, 16*(3). Retrieved from http://www.dcmsonline.org/jax-medicine/1999journals/december99/index.htm

Roy, C. (2007). Advances in nursing knowledge and the challenge for transforming nursing practice. In C. Roy & D. A. Jones (Eds.), *Nursing knowledge development and clinical practice* (pp. 3–38). New York, NY: Springer Publishing.

Schlotfeldt, R. M. (1978). The professional doctorate: Rationale and characteristics. *Nursing Outlook, 26,* 302–311.

Shulman, L. S. (2010). Doctoral education shouldn't be a marathon. *The Chronicle Review of Higher Education,* April 4. Retrieved from http://chronicle.com/article/Doctoral-Education-Isnt-a/64883

Townsend, B. K. (2002). *Rethinking the Ed.D., or what's in a name.* Paper presented at the Annual Meeting of the Association for the Study of Higher Education, Sacramento, CA, November 21–24, 2002.

Tucker, N. H., III. (1999, December). President's message—Medicine: Art versus science. *Jacksonville Medicine, 15*(12), 1–2.

The Historical and Political Path of Doctoral Nursing Education to the Doctor of Nursing Practice Degree

H. Michael Dreher

This opening chapter examines the history of the Doctor of Nursing Practice (DNP) degree in the United States. It is the historical and sociological evolution of the degree and its reception in our health system labor market that will ultimately shape the role of this new doctoral advanced practice nurse or the nurse who engages in doctoral advanced nursing practice (ANP; Dreher & Montgomery, 2009). The chapter draws on contexts, both historical and political, that illustrate the progress of the degree—from the earliest attempts, the failures, and successes in our discipline—to first create a professional doctorate (EdD), then a research doctorate (PhD), a clinical doctorate (doctor of nursing science [DNSc]), another professional doctorate (doctor of nursing [ND]), and finally a DNP, including other various degree iterations splattered along the way—doctor of science in nursing (DSN), doctor of nursing science (DNS), and DrNP.[1] Some of the important benefits and unresolved issues with this still relatively new DNP degree are also summarized. Finally, this chapter concludes with final points on how the American iteration of the DNP degree interfaces with the prevalent international professional doctorate degree model, highlighting how today's global health issues can impact anyone anywhere, and the need for the health professions' education that advances health best for all.

A new doctorate in any discipline is rarely created without some controversy. The DNP degree is no different. However, the largely subsided controversy today is more "Where do we go from here?" Some of the earliest programs are now about 10 years old, and curriculum evaluation and revision have been completed by many of the early programs. Different from most historical analyses in nursing education, this chapter attempts to provide an honest and objective (as much as possible) narrative critique of both the problems and progress of this new nursing doctorate as it has emerged over this past decade. This author was not at the table of the American Association of Colleges of Nursing (AACN) when members (restricted to college, schools of nursing deans, and/or the chief nursing administrator in any given AACN-affiliated program) cast a very narrow vote in 2004 to require the DNP degree instead of the MSN degree for advanced practice registered nurses[2] (APRNs) by 2015 (which ultimately did not happen in 2015). However, this author has nonetheless been a keen observer of the practice doctorate movement from the beginning and even prior to 2004 (AACN, 2004a; Dreher, 2005; Dreher, Donnelly, & Naremore, 2005; Smith Glasgow & Dreher, 2010). And now as a dean starting its college's first doctorate, a DNP in advanced clinical care, the contemporary realities of DNP education are even more apparent, especially the cost models to launch a degree that looks different than in 2005.

In a previous academic appointment, my own university sponsored what was the very first national conference on the practice nursing doctorate in Annapolis, Maryland, in 2007 titled Practice Doctorate: Where Is It Headed? The First National Conference on the Doctor of Nursing Practice: Meanings and Models and the third held in Hilton Head Island, South Carolina, in 2009 titled Doctor of Nursing Practice: The Dialogue Continues... Later the conference morphed into something to attract a different audience, including PhD programs. At each of these venues, many of the contemporary discussion points were highly visible in the podium papers, poster sessions, and in the conversations and networking that took place among faculty, some of the first graduates with the degree in the country, and current students. Actually, as the conference chair for each of those conferences, one of the primary objectives of the organizing committee was to attempt to provide a safe platform for nursing scholars with diverse points of view. We thought that the profession was in need of more critical discourse about the DNP degree, especially from a broader subset of doctoral nursing faculty who were not necessarily academic administrators or not tied more publicly to the mission or position statements of various nursing organizations. We even invited a very prominent anesthesiologist (herself a former certified registered nurse anesthesiologist [CRNA]) who had been publicly criticizing the CRNA-to-doctorate movement, to share her professional perspective.

Internal debate, nonetheless, is nothing new to nursing. We only have to look at our profession's failure, now about 45 years and counting, to require the bachelor of science in nursing (BSN) degree for entry into professional nursing for example (Donley & Flaherty, 2008). Labor historian Barbara Melosh (1982), in her outstanding sociological analysis of nursing in *The Physician's Hand: Work, Culture and Conflict in American Nursing*, calls the history of nursing a battle between the "professionalizers" and the "traditionalists." The battle lines again appear to be drawn (perhaps less visibly these days) between those perceived to be the most in favor of replacing the master's degree with the practice doctorate—the professionalizers (nursing academics), and those who prefer the post-master's DNP (against phasing out the master's)—the traditionalists (the masses of currently practicing advanced practice nurses and many nursing academics, too). This divide exists because APRNs, despite being only master's prepared (and without a DNP degree), astutely know the literature, which touts their outstanding outcomes as widely acknowledged (American College of Nurse-Midwives [ACNM], 2012a; Horrocks, Anderson, & Salisbury, 2002; Malina & Izlar, 2014; Mundinger et al., 2000). Of course, this description is partly an oversimplification, as these lines are not so black and white. There are nursing faculty who oppose the DNP degree (increasingly fewer it seems) and APRNs who support it (increasingly more it seems). And of course, if you are a DNP student reading this book, you are likely matriculating in a DNP program of your own volition, and therefore absolutely not a traditionalist! Nonetheless, discourse, debate, and critique are very healthy for our discipline. Absolute division is not. Maybe with the surge of the DNP degree (and make no mistake, nursing education has never seen a degree captivating the profession so quickly), professionalizers and traditionalists can learn from each other. It would be helpful in the spirit of egalitarianism (not elitism) and continuous improvement, however, if the nursing profession's members could work more cohesively toward the broader benefit of increased access to health services and ultimately to the improvement of health in our nation.

Hopefully, as we reflect on from where we have come, we can emphasize graduate nursing education policy that is both evidence based and does not do what Melosh says happened in our earlier history when "Nurses on the job were sometimes threatened by the strategies leaders adopted, for the rising standards of professionalization often meant downgrading or even eliminating current practitioners" (1982, p. 5). Dracup and Bryan-Brown (2005) also express these concerns, stating "We also worry that the current advanced practice nurses who hold MS degrees will feel disenfranchised" (p. 280). And in very frank language, Dracup and Bryan-Brown echo much of Melosh's (1982) early analysis:

> When nursing education moved from the hospital to the university or college setting, diploma nurses found themselves with an education that provided little or no college credit. We had an entire generation of embittered nurses who saw nursing academics as out of touch with clinical practice. (p. 280)

We implore the nursing profession not to forget its history and, this time, to learn from some of these very painful growing pains in our discipline, and respond differently in the future. As Dracup and Bryan-Brown beseech, we must avoid disenfranchising a large number of nurse practitioners (NPs), nurse-midwives, nurse anesthetists, and clinical nurse specialists (CNSs) who believed they were properly prepared for their roles when they entered advanced practice with a master's degree.

■ BACKGROUND

This book may be the first to have ever declared that the first doctorate in nursing, the EdD in nursing education at Teachers College, Columbia University, in 1933, was actually a professional (or practice) doctorate.[3] Globally, the EdD degree is viewed as the professional doctorate in education, whereas the PhD in education is viewed as the research degree (Maxwell, 2003; Townsend, 2002). Herein lies one of the issues that still plague the nursing academy with the DNP degree. The EdD graduate also completes a dissertation (like the PhD graduate), but the EdD dissertation is more practice oriented and work based. Some even view the EdD as a research degree, too, but it is worth noting that the Harvard School of Education does not offer the PhD in Education (only in collaboration with the School of Arts and Sciences); it offers only the EdD (Baez, 2002; Courtenay, 1988; President and Fellows of Harvard University, 2016). And like Harvard's doctor of business administration (DBA) degree, both are viewed as professional doctorates, but include practice-oriented, rigorous research (Fink, 2006). The DNP degree, however, is very similar to other professional doctorates that do not normally include an original research project—the doctor of medicine (MD), the doctor of pharmacy (PharmD), and the doctor of physical therapy (DPT), for example. Nonetheless, in 2016, this question remains one of the most contentious discussion points among doctoral nursing educators (both DNP and PhD): What is the role of research in the DNP degree, and should DNP students and graduates generate new nursing knowledge or be restricted to expertly translating and disseminating what is currently known? As the AACN (2015a) has recently published a white paper that clarifies this knowledge production role some, we will revisit this issue later in this chapter as we discuss the central unresolved issues with the degree. Nevertheless, maybe what we are attempting now with the largely DNP degree is simply a return to nursing's orientation as a practice discipline in the way the EdD was first created to advance nursing education practice. Some would applaud this return to our disciplinary roots, whereas others would see this as a diversion.

As there was very sluggish growth of doctoral programs in nursing after the Teachers College experiment in 1933, it is noteworthy that three of the next four doctoral nursing programs were aimed at clinical specialization in the discipline rather than a doctorate awarded in the general discipline of nursing itself. The first doctor of philosophy (PhD) program in nursing was started at New York University in 1934. There is not a lot written about this very early PhD and this author has wondered "Who taught in this program?" Furthermore, because nursing was often not allowed to offer a PhD degree by many university faculties beginning in the 1960s and into the 21st century,[4] with other disciplines arguing "is nursing a real science?" it is remarkable that the New York University faculty was progressive enough to position itself at the literal forefront of nursing as a recognized academic discipline (Meleis & Dracup, 2005). It would take until the mid-1980s, at least 50 years, before nursing science would clearly evolve into a scientific discipline (Dreher, 2010a); and as stated in an issue of *The Academic Nurse* (2010),

> In late 1985...In nursing schools where faculty were active in moving the profession forward, research was now becoming a significant part of the academic role, while at the same time faculty clinical practice was falling out of favor. (p. 21)

The third and fourth doctorates in nursing were developed with a clinical focus too. The PhD in nursing at the University of Pittsburgh was started in 1954 with a clinical nursing and clinical research emphasis and the DNSc at Boston University in 1960 with a psychiatric–mental health focus (Grace, 1989; Nichols & Chitty, 2005). Two important distinctions should be made about these two programs, as they both created two distinctive pathways to nursing science knowledge development and shaped doctoral nursing education differently.

First, it is the historic inability of the profession to truly develop a widely viewed "clinical doctorate" for the profession as an alternative to the research-intensive PhD that has led to the surge of the DNP degree. Fitzpatrick (2003) made a very strong case for the clinical doctorate in nursing in 2003 (prior to the 2004 AACN vote), even advocating a clinical doctorate for teachers of nursing. Over the years, much has been written about the DNSc, DSN, and DNS degrees. Although all three were initially designed to be clinically oriented doctorates, the profession has come to view them all as de facto PhD degrees (AACN, 2006; Carlson, 2003). To that measure, in 2016, almost all of them have now converted to a PhD mostly in the last decade (except for one DNSc degree at the University of Tennessee Health Sciences Center, which oddly converted to a DNP program perhaps because they already had a PhD degree). Table 1.1 lists most of the schools that attempted the clinical doctorate and also traces one school's history from its earliest nursing education, to the conversion of its clinical doctorate (DNS) to a PhD, and finally to the approval of the DNP degree (Exhibit 1.1).

The unanswered question is: Why did the profession ultimately abandon the idea of a clinical doctorate? The discipline of psychology faced this very issue in the 1960s when many felt the PhD in psychology had become too research oriented, too experimental, and not client focused. As a result, the doctor of psychology degree (PsyD) was first started in 1968 as a clinical doctorate (Murray, 2000). The PsyD degree, however, did not eliminate the research enterprise in the new degree, only de-emphasized it, and its founders developed a clinical dissertation model in lieu of the traditional PhD dissertation, which is still integral to the degree (Sayette, Mayne, & Norcross, 2010). Peterson (1997), in referring to the PsyD degree versus the PhD, succinctly said that it is not that science and practice do

TABLE 1.1   **The First Quest for an Alternative Nursing Doctorate to the PhD**

Iteration #1: The "Doctor of Nursing Science" degree: DNSc	First at Boston University 1960, later at University of California San Francisco (UCSF), Penn, Columbia, Yale, Catholic, Rush, Widener, etc...all phased out now
Iteration #2: The "Doctor of Science of Nursing" degree: DSN	First at the University of Alabama-Birmingham 1975, later at East Tennessee State, U Texas Health Sciences-Houston, West Virginia, etc...all phased out now
Iteration #3: The "Doctor of Nursing Science" degree: DNS	First at Indiana University 1976, later at Arizona State, LSU Health Sciences Center (LSUHSC), University of Buffalo, etc... all of these are phased out except LSUHSC, Kennesaw State University, and the Sage Colleges

LSU, Louisiana State University.

EXHIBIT 1.1   **The Indiana University Nursing Story**

University-based nursing education began in 1914

Sigma Theta Tau founded in 1922 by six educators from Indiana University Training School for Nurses

BSN curricula first established 1932

MS first offered 1945

MSN first offered 1966

DNS approved 1976

First DNS degree awarded 1981

Planning for PhD began 1990

DNS converts to PhD 1996

DNP degree approved 2009

BSN, bachelor of science in nursing; DNP, Doctor of Nursing Practice; DNS, doctor of nursing science; MS, master of science; MSN, master of science in nursing; PhD, doctor of philosophy.

not belong in the same program, but that it is a matter of emphasis. The AACN, however, is quite precise in stating that the DNP degree should not be described as a clinical doctorate, but a "practice doctorate" stating: "The Task Force recommended that the terminology, practice doctorate be used instead of clinical doctorate" (2004a, p. 4). Is the reason for this distinction (i.e., calling the DNP a "practice" doctorate and not a "clinical" doctorate) the realization that our earlier clinical doctorate nursing models did include both a clinical and research emphasis (and the desire, at least by the AACN leadership at the time, was to move away from this type of degree model)? We will later revisit two universities that tried to resurrect different models of the "clinical doctorate" in 2005, but their curricular innovations were not adopted by others (Dreher et al., 2005; Mundinger, 2009).

Second, the arrival of the PhD at the University of Pittsburgh in 1954 was perhaps better timed than the PhD at New York University in 1934 for the slow maturation of the field of nursing to a discipline. The profession's first research journal, *Nursing Research*, was founded in 1952, and this author discusses at length the early struggles of the journal to attract enough high-level, true research-oriented submissions in Chapter 15 in *Philosophy of Science for Nursing Practice: Concepts and Applications* (Dreher, 2010a, 2016a). The profession also benefited, especially the specialty of psychiatric–mental health nursing, with the publication and work of Dr. Hildegard Peplau's *Interpersonal Relations in Nursing* in 1952. Her work spurred interest in this specialty, and the editor of *Nursing Research* at one early point emphasized (or complained about?) the overrepresentation of articles specific to psychiatric–mental health nursing (Bunge, 1962). Nevertheless, the momentum was slowly growing toward nursing as a scientific discipline. With the first federal research grants in nursing established in 1955 through a new research and fellowship branch within the federal Division of Nursing Resources (founded in 1948) and the first grants awarded that fall, and following later implementation of the Nurse–Scientist Training Program in 1961, the growing need for nurses with a doctorate was emerging (Gortner, 1986, 2000). Interestingly, with so few doctoral programs in nursing in 1961 (there were only three), this innovative research training program prepared nurses for PhDs in other fields besides nursing. The idea was that hopefully these early nurse scientists from the fields of sociology, anthropology, and psychology, for example, would graduate and then pursue nursing scientific inquiry and establish new doctoral programs in nursing. Table 1.2 lists the first 10 doctoral programs in nursing, and the prevalence of the PhD degree or the clinical doctorate (the DNSc in particular) should be noted. What is perhaps fascinating is why the Teachers College degree model EdD in nursing education was never replicated until the last several years where we have seen several EdD in nursing education programs started. There have recently been new PhDs in nursing education (the University of Northern Colorado established in 2004), but they appear to be less common than the EdD in Nursing Education.[5]

It is obvious, especially with the further establishment of the First Division of Nursing Field Research Center founded in San Francisco in 1962, that nursing was aiming toward a scientific orientation (Vreeland, 1964).[6] Whether that would evolve at the expense of the discipline's original practice orientation is another question. This author would add that it is the failure of the discipline to bridge its two disciplinary orientations, what Peplau

TABLE 1.2 **First Doctoral Nursing Programs in the United States**

Rank	Institution	Degree	Year
1	Teachers College, Columbia University	EdD	1933
2	New York University	PhD	1934
3	University of Pittsburgh	PhD	1954
4	Boston University	DNSc	1960
5	University of California San Francisco	DNSc	1964
6	Catholic University	DNSc	1967
7	Texas Woman's University	PhD	1971
8	Case Western Reserve University	PhD	1972
9	University of Pennsylvania	DNSc	1974
	University of Texas-Austin	PhD	1974
10	University of Alabama-Birmingham	DSN	1975
	University of Illinois—Chicago	PhD	1975
	University of Michigan	PhD	1975
	Wayne State University	PhD	1975
	University of Arizona	PhD	1975

aptly called the "art and science [or art versus science] of nursing" (1988, p. 8), that has led many practicing nurses (both professional and advanced) to view the "nursing ivory tower" as too removed from practice (and its realities) and, in some eyes, even irrelevant.

■ THE EVOLUTION OF THE NEED FOR THE NURSE WITH A DOCTORATE

With the first step in the movement of nursing into the university setting—which included various landmark events such as: (a) the first constituted nursing school in a university (albeit under Medicine) at the University of Minnesota in 1909; (b) the first individual (Professor Adelaide Nutting) appointed as a nursing professor at Teachers College in 1910; and (c) the first independent nursing school at Yale University in 1924—nursing began its slow path to perceiving the need for the profession to produce nurses with doctorates (Donohue, 1996). If nurses were indeed going to be full members of the academy (a rather oblique term that includes the members of the formal academic community) with other disciplines, this would be essential. The Flexner Report on the state of medical education in 1910 also had implications for nursing education. Although this report was in many ways very critical of institutionalized medicine,[7] medicine's dominance over nursing was under way (Hiatt, 1999). Further, and perhaps most importantly, the derision of medicine did not elevate nursing or the status of nurses. This widely publicized report on medicine also made it obvious to nursing leaders that they would likewise need to evaluate the state of nursing education even as the profession was in its early formative years. A subsequent 1912 report titled *The Educational Status of Nursing* (Nutting, 1912), which became the first comprehensive survey of schools of nursing, was likewise critical of the about 1,100 schools of nursing that responded. Of this report Melosh (1982) writes, "315 schools, or nearly 45%, reported that they did not have a single paid instructor, and 299 did not maintain a library. Instead the nursing 'curriculum' in many hospitals consisted of two or three years of ward work" (p. 41).

■ THEN: THE DOCTORAL-PREPARED NURSE EMERGES FROM A MINISCULE POOL

The ultimate movement of nursing into the college and university from the hospital-based diploma settings has taken place ever so slowly in the past 100 years or so (diploma programs are still in operation in Pennsylvania and Ohio and sparingly elsewhere). And while, according to Edward Salsberg (2015) in the prestigious blog Health Affairs, the average nurse is first educated in a community college, 4-year college or university (more than 98% of all new nurse graduates in 2014), it is certain that the early nursing leaders who sought the increasing professionalism of nursing did not intend that nursing education should be from a community college rather than from a university or other 4-year degree granting institution (National League for Nursing [NLN], 2007). Among the 1.4 million nurses who entered the profession between 1970 and 1994 with either an associate degree (AD) or BSN, 59% entered with an AD and 41% a BSN (Aiken, Cheung, & Olds, 2009). NLN (2007) data from 2006 to 2007 indicated that 60% of new graduates were AD prepared and 31% BSN prepared. Only in 2011 did BSN-prepared nurses become predominant over associate degree in nursing (ADN)/diploma-prepared nurses and more recent data from 2013 indicate that the BSN degree is proliferating with between 55% and 61% of nurses now having a BSN degree or higher (Budden, Zhong, Moulton, & Cimiotti, 2013; Health Resources & Services Association [HRSA], 2013; Robert Wood Johnson Foundation, 2015). Furthermore, in California (our largest state), and sometimes called the most progressive state, a decade ago, some 70% of all RNs had an ADN degree; 2014 data indicate that 61.5% now have a BSN degree, a remarkable shift (California Board of Registered Nursing, 2014; Dreher, 2008a).

Because data from Aiken, Cheung, and Olds in 2009 indicated that only 6% of nurses who first get an ADN go on to advanced practice (the master's degree or higher), this trend away from an initial community college nursing education may have an important impact on the profession. Moreover, even as we enter a period of uncertain supply and demand of RNs with the Great Recession blunting the retirement of many older nurses, a continuing shortage of nursing faculty (with doctorates), and a shortage of nurse scientists (with the projected retirements of so many senior faculty), the prospects for an adequate supply of nurses in different sectors remains predictably uneven. Furthermore, the movement to end advanced practice at the master's degree, or at least the transition away from the MSN to the DNP, has caused some to warn that this move may cause a drop in the number of new NPs each year (Bloch, 2007; Dreher & Gardner, 2009; Ford, 2008). As the expense and time commitment to skip the MSN can be burdensome and can take longer than obtaining the MSN, the Great Recession that began in the Bush administration and ended during the Obama administration, negatively impacted the employer-based tuition reimbursement system that so many RNs who seek higher education have always relied on (Azam, 2010; Babcock, 2009; Krugman, 2009). Bloch warns that NPs, particularly those who work with vulnerable professions, may see declining numbers, and this would be tragic, especially now that about 30 million or more individuals are transitioning into the health care system and all need primary care (National Association of Community Health Centers, 2009). No data have been reported whether the move to the entry-level DNP has specifically curtailed the NP supply, but 2012 data report a slowing of growth of individuals who identify themselves as a "nurse practitioner" (Auerbach, 2012). According to the Society for Human Resource Management (2013), some 61% of employers offer undergraduate tuition assistance in greatly varying amounts. But while graduate tuition assistance is slightly less prevalent (59%), this author has had doctoral students whose employers specifically did not support doctoral tuition reimbursement. We mention this in particular because the 2004 AACN vote must be placed in this context—the vote occurred before this substantial economic downturn and this author wonders whether it would still pass today?

Likely, and partly due to economic factors that have impacted the United States since the 2004 AACN vote (2004a), we are seeing that while more schools are offering the post-master's DNP degree, they are increasingly reticent about closing their MSN advanced practice tracks out of fear of potential declining enrollments and loss of tuition revenue. We now hear of schools indicating that they plan to offer both options (MSN and DNP entry) permanently. The slow rate of actual conversions of master's advanced practice programs to the DNP actually caused the AACN to commission the RAND Corporation to study this problem (Auerbach et al., 2015). We discern the four most important conclusions from this report as:

- The DNP continues to expand steadily.
- The MSN remains the dominant pathway for APRN entry-into-practice education, though there is some limited movement toward replacement with the BSN to DNP.
- There will likely be two tracks toward the DNP for the near future (defined by schools' planning horizons): a single-step process (BSN to DNP) and a two-step process (BSN to MSN followed by an MSN to DNP at a later date).
- The value of the added content of the DNP education is almost universally agreed upon (p. x).

In reflecting back, it is interesting to note that at the 2010 National Organization of Nurse Practitioner Faculties (NONPF) meeting, the sense was that both degrees would continue and be supported at least for the time being (*Academic Nurse*, 2010). That characterization does not appear to be prescient, but it is concerning that with these continual trends of support for both master's and DNP preparation for the entry-level NP (in particular), the focus on master's APRN practice at the AACN master's education annual conference has been largely absent for many years. This disconnect is recognized by the RAND Corporation, but attention to quality master's advanced practice nursing (APN) programs needs to continue with a higher level of visibility and support, despite the politics of the profession. My previous employer has robust enrollments in all their online master's NP programs and it is unlikely they are planning any conversion to DNP only entry level for NPs. At my current institution, enrollment in our master's Family Nurse Practitioner (FNP) program is at capacity and we are challenged like many institutions to secure a steady supply of master's-prepared FNP preceptors. We hypothesize that perhaps prospective NP applicants were anxious to enroll in master's NP programs ahead of the "feared 2015 mandate for DNP entry" (which was never a mandate and which would have grandfathered everyone imaginable), and that perhaps our enrollments will flatten out. Further, the greater Philadelphia region is saturated with nursing schools, and yet in fall 2010, only one nursing program was offering a BSN-to-DNP program for NPs. In 2016, that number has grown to three and only one school has phased out the master's for the DNP. In a 2009 article in *The American Nurse*, then Dean and Professor Linda Cronenwett of the School of Nursing at the University of North Carolina Chapel Hill was quoted stating, "I support the DNP *Essentials* outlined by the AACN and the important emphasis on quality and safety competencies, but I think society would be better served by a postmaster's DNP" (Trossman, 2009, p. 8). This issue will obviously continue to be debated over the next decade at least.

So the question remains: Does the profession really need nurses with doctorates? The answer is unequivocally "yes." In our history, the burden of a burgeoning discipline has always necessitated that nurses possess doctorates to achieve parity with other faculty in other disciplines in colleges and universities (the academy). Superimposed on this need for nurses with doctorates with research skills was the realization that if the scientific basis of nursing was going to grow, the profession would need them in larger numbers, and thus we saw mostly new PhD and DNSc programs opening in the 1970s. Certainly, this supply would have to grow in order for more rigorous nursing science to be conducted and for our science to be perceived more as a "real science" by others. We should mention that as the science of nursing slowly evolved, there was initially a focus on nursing administration and nursing education research and an absence of focus on clinical research. Indeed, with the founding of the Association of Collegiate Schools of Nursing in 1935, with its mission to promote nursing education in the collegiate/university environment and away from the hospital-based programs, one of the aims of the new organization was "to promote study and experimentation in nursing service and nursing education" (Goodrich, 1936, p. 767). This may very well have been one of the earliest visible policy statements to encourage nursing research. Yet, over time, although nursing administration research has been aligned with health services research, the predominance of clinical research over all other types (with the devaluation of nursing education research), the debate has largely waned, and clinical research, favoring quantitative methods, now predominates as it has more and more extensive funding sources (Hutchinson, 2001; Werley & Westlake, 1985).

Despite significant advances in nursing education, however, education-focused research in the discipline has unfortunately suffered, and this author believes that this did not need to happen. For example, nursing health systems research (oriented toward the administrative indirect care role in nursing) has grown in sophistication over the decades. One only has to look at the extensive work of Dr. Linda Aiken and Claire M. Fagin, leadership professor in nursing, professor of sociology, and director of the Center for Health Outcomes and Policy Research at the University of Pennsylvania School of Nursing, to see the kind of high impact that nursing health system research can make. Nursing education research, however, has suffered from a lack of innovation and too many education-oriented dissertations that have focused on minor issues of importance inside and outside the profession. Maybe this will change as the NLN ramps up its nursing education funding, and if DNP faculty scholars and graduates seriously conduct and publish outcome data.

Severely complicating this early drive to the doctorate were data in 1965 indicating that only approximately 22% of all nurses had been prepared in academic programs (this included associate degree graduates; Nelson, 2002). As mentioned earlier, the American Nurses Association (ANA) in 1965 first tried to change this percentage by mandating that nursing education should take place in a college or university setting, and that the BSN be required for entry into professional nursing (Donley & Flaherty, 2008). Today, this percentage exceeds 50%; hence, although the mandate was never realized, perhaps we can recognize there has been success at upgrading the overall preparation of RNs. Next, the emergence of the NP role at the University of Colorado, Denver, in 1965 and the rise of NP programs offering MSN degrees in the 1970s increased the need for the doctoral credential for faculty NPs, as nurses without common university credentials (typically the PhD) were marginalized in academia (Dunphy, Smith, & Youngkin, 2009; Silver, Ford, & Day, 1968). What is not known, however, is how broadly current faculty NPs (or other APN faculty) are indeed prepared at the doctoral level. This author's cursory review of many nursing school websites across the country indicates that there are still a plethora of NP track coordinators, particularly nurse anesthesia program coordinators, who do not possess the doctorate. Perhaps the DNP degree will help alleviate this.

■ NOW: THE DWINDLING SUPPLY OF NURSING FACULTY WITH THE PhD

In 2008, the AACN published a white paper *The Preferred Vision of the Professoriate in Baccalaureate and Graduate Nursing Programs* indicating that nurses who teach in university settings (not the community college) should have a doctorate degree at minimum (AACN, 2008). Unfortunately, in challenging economic times, the profession faces two issues on this front to accomplish this: (a) how to attract more nurses to doctoral study and to the educator role and (b) how can we help the masses of MSN-prepared faculty across the country complete a doctorate? These two issues are critically important because it is the nursing faculty role that most drives the need for nurses with doctorates. For instance, DNP programs would not be offered, nor would you be sitting in your classroom (or behind your computer), if there were not a faculty member in front of you or online.[8] Similarly, it will likely take time for the consumer health care market to expect the nurse clinician (certified registered nurse practitioner [CRNP], CRNA, certified nurse-midwive [CNM], or CNS) to have a doctorate in the same way that it is expected in academia.

The complete answer to the first question previously mentioned—how to attract more nurses to doctoral study and to the educator role—is beyond the scope of this chapter. There is, however, a protracted nursing faculty shortage that has now existed for more than a decade and is predicted to persist (AACN, 1999, 2005a, 2015a; Aiken et al., 2009). The reasons why the shortage is likely to continue include the following:

- A predicted surge in faculty retirements that will exceed predicted replacements (AACN, 2015a; Smith Glasgow & Dreher, 2010)
- Lack of competitive salaries for nursing professors versus what they can earn in industry (Ingeno, 2013; Smith & Dreher, 2003)
- Lack of adequate role modeling in undergraduate nursing education to foster pursuing the doctorate and a teaching career (Potempa, Redman, & Anderson, 2008)
- Perhaps even gender bias in the academy that disenfranchises nursing schools, largely composed of women, from their full exercise of power, influence, and benefit in many colleges and universities (Curtis, 2010; Smith & Dreher, 2003)

One example of the previously mentioned gender bias,[9] is the low comparative research start-up packages reported for tenure-track nursing faculty versus start-up packages for business, law, medicine, and engineering faculty (Valian, 2005). Although Rudy and Grady (2005) reported that among 31 biological nurse scientists engaged mostly in animal-model research (48% had formal postdoctoral training and all had received previous National Institute of Nursing Research funding), their mean research start-up package was for $50,000 (in the range from $2,000 to $105,000); this author has heard numerous doctoral faculty at the annual AACN Doctoral Nursing Education meeting complain about their comparative research start-up packages in their own universities.[10] Furthermore, administrative stipends for nursing administrators pale in comparison to stipends for faculty administrators from the disciplines mentioned previously and perhaps others (Kirkpatrick, 1994). Although Kirkpatrick in 1994 reported stipends as low as $1,000 for the nursing department chair, this type of data admittedly is hard to substantiate, because the university power structure that favors one discipline (for whatever reason) over another has reason to keep these data hidden. Nevertheless, this author (and others) has had multiple confirmations of this practice, and there is no reason to believe that this inequity has been rectified in the past 15 years. It is also not unusual for colleges or universities to internally cap permanent administrative promotions to 10% of the base salary, thus exposing an internally imposed salary compression that can generally be circumvented by an external candidate who may have more salary negotiation opportunities on the front end of the hire (University of South Florida, 2015). This critique of the "status of the nurse in the academy" is not meant to discourage readers from the professoriate or to academic nursing administrators, but to identify some of the challenges that the current generation and next generation of nursing professors will face. A critical mass of DNP faculty educators in particular, whose own entrance into the academy is going to spark a multitude of additional issues, may be particularly vulnerable.

The second item, encouraging MSN-prepared faculty to pursue the doctorate, is equally problematic. I am reminded of Melosh's (1982) and Dracup and Bryan-Brown's (2005) critiques of the disenfranchisement of nurses in an earlier generation (and the risk to current MSN-prepared APRNs), and of the current lack of flexible transitioning to the next degree as the profession suddenly mandates a doctorate for all university nursing professors (AACN, 2008). On the surface, this is a realistic expectation—that nurses who teach in a university setting should possess a doctorate. But again, as a practice profession, is this realistic? Foremost, what is needed most in undergraduate and APN education is to have faculty who are current and competent in the nursing practice they are teaching. I recall very vividly in my own master's education in the late 1980s how a very talented pathophysiology instructor (with an MSN) was removed from the teaching roster in favor of a faculty member with a doctorate who had very little background or currency in the topic. We literally taught ourselves each week with class presentations. Most current MSN-prepared nursing faculty have no aim to be nurse scientists, and thus the PhD option (which takes an average of 8.3 years to complete post a master's degree!) for many reasons is not attractive (Valiga, 2004). Since Valiga's report, some PhD programs tried to decrease the total time to complete the degree. We suspect there may have been marginal improvements, but this is another area where reliable, contemporary data are elusive. Further, many nursing schools prohibit their own master's-prepared faculty from matriculating internally in their own doctoral nursing programs due to potential conflicts of interest. Instead, they must go to another university for the nursing doctorate or attend a non-nursing, internally offered doctorate where they might get tuition support as an employee benefit. And even in those universities that do permit internal matriculation, "faculty-as-students" face conflicts of interest when nursing faculty attend classes taught (and graded) by their peers and colleagues (Anselmi, Dreher, Smith Glasgow, & Donnelly, 2010). If the PhD is not an option, then what other nursing degree can faculty attend?

The DNP degree is being increasingly suggested as a solution to the nursing faculty shortage. But despite internal disagreements within the profession on this issue, the nursing educator role is not a role supported by the AACN within the confines of the normal DNP curriculum (AACN, 2006; Fitzpatrick, 2008). Authors in this text argue for this to change, especially because Zungolo (2009) indicates that more than 30% of all DNP graduates are going into academia. This more than supports earlier data from Loomis, Willard, and Cohen (2006) indicating that 55% of a sample of current DNP students ($N = 69$) had intentions of pursuing a career in nursing education postgraduation. A 2013 Texas study found that 58% of nursing college/university faculty or staff who were pursuing a doctorate, were pursuing the DNP degree. The fear is that these graduates may be unprepared for the faculty role and may experience even more inequities in the academy. McKenna (2005) has similarly suggested that "However, a word of warning; without an adequate background in the knowledge and skills necessary for teaching and scholarship, these people [graduates from practice doctorate programs] may be set up for failure in the University setting" (p. 246). The AACN (2006) has suggested that DNP graduates may take extra courses to add the educator role to the DNP degree. Again, this seems reminiscent of Melosh's (1982) earlier critique of nursing leadership's professionalizers. The NLN (2007), however, has indicated some displeasure with the DNP degree being promoted as a solution to the nursing faculty shortage, especially as the NLN (2007) has a central mission to conduct nursing education research and most DNP graduates are not educated to do this. In their Reflection and Dialogue web series, they write:

> However, foundational essentials for DNP curriculum design do not include courses related to pedagogy, evaluation, academic role issues and elements, and educational theory, and the NLN fears that graduates of such programs will lack the complex and specialized knowledge intrinsic to the advanced practice role of nurse educator. (p. 1)

In 2010, the NLN clearly pronounced that "Advanced practice nurses must have in-depth clinical knowledge of nursing practice; similarly, both part- and full-time faculty must have an in-depth knowledge of nursing education and nursing practice" (p. 1). This indicates that the proper preparation for the nursing faculty role is to have coursework and practica in the teaching role to ensure the effectiveness of the graduate. Our continued concern is whether the move to properly and expertly prepare the DNP graduate for the academic role will nonetheless result in the burden of extra coursework at an additional cost.

What, then, is the solution? Certainly, the answer is not to create easy or quick doctorates that MSN-prepared nurse educators can complete. In my own 2014 survey for external feedback on the development of the DNP, one respondent wrote that the best program would take less than a year to complete and be totally online. Nor should work experience be credited to the awarding of the doctorate. The new AACN (2015a) white paper on the DNP has suggested that DNP students who are nationally certified should be considered for automatic credit toward their 1,000 total practice hours post the awarding of the BSN:

> One commonly used process adopted by programs is to award credit to students who hold national certification in an area of advanced nursing practice, most commonly for national certification in one of the four APRN roles. Some programs also currently waive practice hours for other national advanced nursing practice certifications e.g. ANCC's [American Nurses Credentialing Center] Advanced Public Health Nursing certification and ANCC's Advanced Nurse Executive certification. (pp. 8–9)

This is going to result in a Pandora's box for DNP programs as one program may waive a certain percentage of practice hours and the next program will attempt to attract more students by waiving even more practice hours. This is a new descriptive element of the DNP, not previously expanded upon, and it has the potential to be detrimental to the rigor of the DNP degree to many stakeholders.

To enhance the transition of MSN-prepared faculty to achieve the doctorate and establish common credentials as the majority of members of the academy, Anselmi et al. (2010) suggest nursing faculty exchange programs (e.g., "you take two of our MSN faculty for free and we will take two of yours for free") and mention that internal matriculation of nursing faculty in their own doctoral nursing program could be allowed reputably if the potential conflicts of interest can be minimized. Such a "doctoral nursing program exchange" is now in operation between Duquesne University School of nursing and Saint Louis University School of Nursing to assist their own internal MSN-prepared faculty to complete a nursing doctorate without having to experience internal conflicts of interest by enrolling in their own PhD programs, which was prohibited. Large numbers of the current nursing professoriate are pursuing the DNP and many schools of nursing have more applicants for vacant teaching positions with the DNP instead of the PhD or EdD. What is one to do? This is where nursing innovation is needed and where accreditors too often become the barriers to innovation (Dreher, 2008a; Melnyk & Davidson, 2009; Neal, 2008; Stewart, 2009).

Finally, large numbers of MSN faculty are not going to return for the doctorate with the likelihood of only marginal increases in compensation. It is disturbing that in the aforementioned recent study and white paper from the Texas Higher Education Coordinating Board reported limited upward mobility of graduates with only 37% achieving higher levels of compensation after the DNP. Certainly, Texas is just one market and every individual DNP graduate has the ability to negotiate new employment terms, including compensation. This author has seen incredible upward career mobility with his own DrNP graduates and in other DNP graduates as well. But both nursing accreditor agencies, the Commission on Collegiate Nursing Education (CCNE) and Accrediting Commission for Education in Nursing (ACEN), and now a new third nursing accrediting agency—the NLN Commission for Nursing Education Accreditation (CNEA)—which began nursing accreditation services in Spring 2016, need to be more proactive (like the Association to Advance Collegiate Schools of Business) and include adequate faculty compensation to their review criteria. The AACN does publish extensive salary data each year and it is an excellent resource when academic nursing administrators need to negotiate internal salary adjustments and external competitive offers to new faculty.

■ THE SECOND PROFESSIONAL DOCTORATE IN NURSING: THE ND DEGREE

To be completely true to history, Case Western Reserve University's (CWRU) initiation of the extraordinarily innovative ND degree in 1979 was never called nor classified as a "practice" doctorate. Indeed, it was called a "professional doctorate" (p. 308) by its founder Dean Rozella Schlotfeldt (1978) of the Frances Payne Bolton School of Nursing at CWRU. Only now do revisionists call it the "first practice doctorate" (AACN, 2006; Case Western Reserve University, 2016; Hathaway, Jacob, Stegbauer, Thompson, & Graff, 2006; Lenz, 2005). Again, the 1970s was a time of rapid growth in nursing education. The DSN and DNS clinical doctorates were initiated, more PhD and DNSc programs were founded, MSN NP programs began to flourish, and the ANA was still battling to require the BSN for professional nursing (Nelson, 2002). Then Schlotfeldt (1978), followed by Dean Luther Christman (1980) of the Rush University School of Nursing in Chicago, affirmed this vision that the doctorate should be the entry-level degree for nursing (Nelson, 2002). If there were ever a larger gap in the nursing profession between the professionalizers and the masses of practitioners or traditionalists, it was at this time. The ND degree at CWRU was designed after the MD degree. Students entered the doctoral nursing program with any basic college degree (just like medicine) and then completed a 3-year full-time curriculum including the completion of an ND thesis (somewhat differentiated from the university's PhD dissertation). Without a doubt, this was a professional doctorate model, and graduates initially were not prepared for advanced practice roles. This changed in 1990 when alternate pathways to the ND were created, including a post-master's option for nurses with an MSN, and indeed graduates at this time were prepared for advanced practice roles (Dr. Joyce Fitzpatrick, personal communication, April 13, 2010). Technically, this degree modification could be termed "a practice doctorate" (entry level vs. advanced practice), but again the term practice doctorate was not yet part of the nursing vernacular. In the end, the ND was a failure of innovation and only three other schools ever adopted the degree model (Rush University in 1987, the University of Colorado in 1990, and the University of South Carolina in 1999). All four of these programs subsequently closed and transitioned to DNP programs in 2004 and 2005.

One day someone will write the history of the ND degree and why it failed. Was it the unrealistic initial concept that any nurse needed a doctorate for entry into practice? In hindsight, and with apologies to Christman, a true pioneer in nursing, retrospectively this idea seems absurd or, more kindly, extremely idealistic. For whatever reason, the first working group on the clinical doctorate established by the AACN in 2002 did not see much of a future for the degree. Were the initials "ND" perhaps too foreign? Was the degree confusing to some outside the discipline who thought it was a doctor of naturopathy—also an ND degree as the AACN has noted (AACN, 2004a)? Certainly, the post-master's ND model was an alternative doctorate model to the PhD. But this author thinks it was more properly a "second generation clinical doctorate" (the DNSc,

DSN, and DNS degrees were the first generation), in that its graduates did complete an ND thesis and were generating evidence for the discipline.[11] In other words, this post-master's model emphasized practice and practice-based research. And in the transition from the ND to the DNP, it is perplexing why the practice mission of the degree was retained but the practice–evidence-generating mission eliminated (at least until the current DNP white paper; AACN, 2015b).

■ THE CONTEMPORARY PRACTICE DOCTORATE MOVEMENT: DNP (MOSTLY) AND DRNP

The contemporary practice doctorate movement can be largely attributed to the innovators at Columbia University School of Nursing and its dean, Mary Mundinger (who retired in 2010). In the late 1990s, a team of investigators conducted a randomized clinical trial to determine whether, under comparable primary care protocols, MSN-prepared NPs and doctorally prepared physicians would have similar or different patient outcomes? In 2000, Mundinger et al. published their findings in the prestigious *Journal of the American Medical Association (JAMA)* and indeed reported that the outcomes were equivalent. This was certainly a landmark study for the nursing profession and caused quite a controversy in medicine. This author, if possible, would give a special courage award to the physician investigators and participants who even agreed to participate in the study (at seemingly some risk to the prestige of their discipline and the superiority of physician practice). The first outcome of this study set the stage for an innovative comprehensive care practice by Columbia University faculty NPs (Rubenstein, 2009). With this evidence, they gained admitting privileges (albeit with great passionate, political maneuvering by Dean Mundinger) to hospitals, and participated in the first model of comprehensive care where the NP sees and follows patients throughout their hospital stays, and not just seen by the APRN in the confines of a primary care clinic (Mundinger, 2005).

The second outcome of this study was the initiation of the Doctor of Nursing Practice (DrNP) degree model. Although the inventors first described this as a "clinical doctorate" and a "Doctor of Nursing Practice in Primary Care," they later dropped the primary care emphasis, largely out of the realization that many of their APRNs were not practicing just primary care and they embraced their comprehensive care model more explicitly (Dreher et al., 2005; Mundinger, 2005). They have since retained the idea that their degree is a clinical doctorate, as the overwhelming emphasis in their curriculum is on direct clinical practice and focuses on Essential VII: Advanced Practice from the AACN's *Essentials of Doctoral Education for Advanced Nursing Practice* (2006; Dr. Janice Smolowitz, personal communication, June 25, 2010). This author is in a quandary whether this iteration is really a clinical doctorate. It does not have the thesis or dissertation knowledge generation model that the earlier clinical doctorates all had. Instead, they have implemented a DNP portfolio that is innovative, but does not have an emphasis on generating new practice knowledge; rather, it emphasizes translation of evidence to practice (which is technically more in line with the AACN conception of the DNP degree as a nonresearch degree; Honig & Smolowitz, 2009). Nonetheless, there is no DNP program in the United States that has more emphasis on clinical practice, and it even includes a 1-year full-time practicum in the second year of study. For whatever reason, the Columbia DrNP degree model has never been replicated. Indeed they changed their initials to "DNP" in 2009, probably in order to be accredited by the CCNE, which elected to only accredit DNP programs that subscribe to the "DNP" initials (AACN,

2005b). Consequently, is this degree model a clinical doctorate as the profession has traditionally defined this term? As this author is aware that some Columbia graduates are actually assuming primary investigator roles and obviously going to be at the forefront of creating new evidence for the profession, the conclusion is yes, the Columbia DNP model with its intensive emphasis on clinical practice is a new type of third-generation clinical doctorate (despite the use of the DNP degree initials).

Historically, credit for the first DNP degree in 2001 belongs to the faculty of the University of Kentucky. However, this DNP focused on the clinical/executive management role and not advanced practice. As Montgomery and Byrne detail in Chapter 4, it is perplexing why the AACN membership chose to endorse the Kentucky DNP model that *did not* emphasize advanced clinical practice, instead of the Columbia DrNP degree model *that did*. It is also unfortunate that the inventors of the Kentucky DNP model did not publish the reasoning behind their new degree in the peer-reviewed literature. Thus, we are left only with the dean's deliberations at the AACN membership to ascertain why the DNP degree model was preferred and why it was altered (from the Kentucky degree model) to include the traditional advanced practice role in the organization's first endorsement of the degree (AACN, 2004a). Interestingly, the addition of the clinical executive role[12] (termed aggregate/systems/organizational focus) was only done after minor language in the AACN draft document was changed from the January 2004 *AACN Draft Position Statement on the Practice Doctorate in Nursing* (AACN, 2004b). From the January 2004 draft, it is stated in Recommendation 8 that:

> The practice doctorate should eventually be identified as the preferred graduate degree for APN preparation in the four current roles: clinical nurse specialist, nurse anesthetist, nurse midwife, and nurse practitioner. (2004b, p. 10)

Two months later, in March 2004, *AACN Draft Position Statement on the Practice Doctorate in Nursing* in Recommendation 10 (originally Recommendation 8), the language changed to:

> The practice doctorate should eventually be identified as the preferred graduate degree for *advanced nursing practice preparation, but not limited to* [italics my emphasis] the four current roles: clinical nurse specialist, nurse anesthetist, nurse midwife, and nurse practitioner. (AACN, 2004c, p. 12)

The change in language from APN to ANP is important, because the administrative role could never technically be equated with the advanced practice roles of the four traditional APRN roles. But if it were under the umbrella of ANP, it could. This inclusion of the clinical executive role, however, was not widely realized or perhaps promoted (again we reaffirm the clinical executive has been granted an advanced role by this definition, but not the advanced role of the educator). Even in the October 27, 2004 press release by the AACN titled *AACN Adopts a New Vision for the Future of Nursing Education and Practice*, the AACN states:

> In a historic move to help shape the future of nursing education and practice, the American Association of Colleges of Nursing (AACN) has adopted a new position which recognizes the Doctor of Nursing Practice degree as the highest level of preparation *for clinical practice*" [italics my emphasis]. (AACN, 2004d, p. 1)

Further in the press release, the AACN states:

> Currently, advanced practice nurses (APNs), including Nurse Practitioners, Clinical Nurse Specialists, Nurse Mid-wives, and Nurse Anesthetists, are

prepared in master's degree programs that often carry a credit load equivalent to doctoral degrees in the other health professions. AACNs newly adopted *Position Statement on the Practice Doctorate in Nursing* calls for educating APNs and *other nurses seeking top clinical roles* [italics my emphasis] in Doctor of Nursing Practice (DNP programs). (AACN, 2004d, p. 1)

Certainly, this is just a press release and not the official policy of the AACN, but the reader is left to believe that APRNs are the target and who are the "other nurses seeking top clinical roles?" That is indeed a very odd way to describe the job description of a chief nursing officer or vice president for nursing. These are not clinical roles. All the indirect functions in nursing (e.g., administration, teaching, clinical trials management) are classified differently from direct care roles, and the point made here is that the nursing professor who oversees students in the clinical area is as close to clinical as the administrator in charge of clinical services. Ultimately, the clinical executive role was made explicit in the AACN's (2006) *Essentials of Doctoral Education for Advanced Nursing Practice* and became an official ANP specialty.

A further examination of the final 2004 AACN position statement document does indicate that there was no consensus over endorsing only the DNP degree initials, but the argument that multiple degree initials would create confusion and perhaps lead to the DNSc, DNS, and DSN conundrum again apparently won (AACN, 2004a). It is largely unknown, however, how the practice of the nurse executive was deemed "advanced practice" by the AACN in 2006, but the practice of the nurse educator was excluded. The authors of Chapter 7 also raise this issue. This author has covered this unfolding history in detail, mostly because it is unrealistic to assume that PhD enrollment is going to alleviate the nursing faculty shortage, especially with there being a 3.1% decline in PhD enrollment (and a 19.1% increase in DNP enrollments) in 2015 to 2016 (Fang, Li, Stauffer, & Trautman, 2016). Throughout this book, and especially in the last chapter, the very erratic enrollments and graduations from PhD programs noted do not look promising. For instance, in 2008, there were only three net new PhD graduates in the United States with an overall increase of 0.1%, while there was an increase of 5.1% in 2009 with 201 net new graduates (AACN, 2009a; Fang, Tracy, & Bednash, 2010). Eight years later in 2016, enrollment in doctoral, research-focused programs decreased by 3.2% (minus 168 students) and graduations decreased by 3.5% (net loss of 26 graduates; Fang, Li, Stauffer, & Trautman). Nevertheless, what is worrisome is that these stagnant enrollments and graduation from largely PhD programs declines do not represent a trend that will adequately resupply the number of PhD-prepared, senior faculty teaching in the academy. Already, according to recent data from the Tri-Council of Nursing[13] (April 2, 2014):

> The U.S. Bureau of Labor Statistics expects that by year 2022, the number of practicing RNs will grow by 19% and that employment of NPs, CRNAs, and CNMs will grow by 31%. Moreover, a 2013 HRSA report anticipates that waves of retirements in the nursing workforce will leave a significant burden on the pipeline. Over the next 10 to 15 years, the nearly one million RNs over age 50 (comprising approximately one-third of the current workforce), will reach retirement age. (p. 1)

Because the DNP degree is still the "sizzling hot nursing degree" it was when we published the first edition of this book (simply based on numbers and new programs), a reengineered curriculum that allows at least some inclusion of the educator role without penalizing students with extra coursework seems to be one realistic option because the trends are very clear—DNP graduates are going into academia in significant numbers and the nursing faculty shortage continues.

■ THE AACN'S EARLY DEVELOPMENTAL WORK ON THE DNP DEGREE

While Columbia started down one track toward what it called a new clinical doctorate (DrNP), which would ultimately become a practice doctorate, and with Kentucky boldly introducing a practice doctorate (DNP) that did not actually emphasize clinical practice, we should trace the third track by the AACN that in the end had the most influence. In March 2002, the AACN Board of Directors charged a task force to examine the current status of clinical or practice doctoral programs and other related charges (AACN, 2004b). What is interesting about this 2004 document is that the task force reported that it had established a collaborative relationship with the NONPF, and therefore there was a strong faculty–NP connection in these early deliberations. Yet, there was also no liaison to the major practicing APRN organizations including the ACNM, the American Association of Nurse Anesthetists (AANA), the National Association of Clinical Nurse Specialists (NACNS), the American Academy of Nurse Practitioners (AANP), or the American College of Nurse Practitioners (ACNP). Further, none of the 10 external reaction panel members invited by the AACN to comment on deliberations represented these organizations, and the formal exclusion of the ANA is noteworthy (AACN, 2004c). This lack of diversity of decision makers and formal consultants to the exclusion of organizations representing members (and future members) who would be the most impacted by any proposed change in educational requirements led to early criticism of the AACN for not fully vetting its proposal with audiences not inclined to agree with them. As Fulton and Lyon wrote back in 2005, "In proposing the practice doctorate AACN has engaged only a limited number of stakeholders in meaningful dialogue" (Fulton & Lyon, 2005, p. 3).

As of the writing of the chapter in 2016, only national groups representing nurse anesthesia and CNSs (two of the four traditional APRN specialties) have endorsed mandatory doctoral entry. The Council on Accreditation's (2007; which accredits nurse anesthesia programs) requirement that doctoral entry be required by 2015 (the DNP was not specified as the only option) was actually announced in 2007. In 2015, the NACNS called for the DNP requirement for entry-level practice by 2030. The NACNS had remained neutral on the DNP degree, neither endorsing it nor discouraging it for future CNSs (NACNS, 2009). Part of the NACNS argument was a study presented at the 2007 DNP Conference in Annapolis, Maryland, indicating significant duplication of curriculum outcomes between MSN and DNP degrees, and thus the need for another degree was questioned (Jacobson et al., 2007). Furthermore, because many CNS positions have a strong research role component (and many have a PhD), a degree that de-emphasizes the conduct of research was seen as problematic (Fulton, 2010; McNett, 2006). Even today, this author questions why master's preparation for the CNS with additional education at the PhD level in nursing is not offered as an option.

The ACNM Accreditation Commission for Midwifery Education has gone on record of endorsing the DNP but not to the exclusion of its other educational entry-level degree options for nurse-midwives (ACNM, 2009). In 2012b, they updated their 2009 statement with:

> There is inadequate evidence to support the DNP as the entry-level requirement for midwifery education. While it is true that additional time spent in an educational environment would likely benefit graduates, no data are available addressing the need for additional education to practice safely as a midwife. (p. 1)

Finally, with regard to the preparation of NPs, in 2016, the NONPF called for the preparation of future NPs at the DNP level *without a first exit point* for the awarding of the master's degree, but they did not identify or recommend any specific date by which would be mandated (or recommended; 2016). The decision to not suggest a date by which to accomplish this was prudent because the elusive 2015 date previously suggested by the AACN for broad adoption of the DNP by APRNs came and went, practically without comment. Moreover, because conversion to the entry-level DNP (BSN to DNP) had been so sluggish (with programs overwhelmingly maintaining their master's APRN degree programs while adding post-master's DNP degree options), as previously mentioned in this chapter, the AACN commissioned the prestigious RAND Corporation to study the barriers to the entry-level DNP (Auerbach et al., 2015). Many of the major NP specialty organizations have endorsed the NP DNP *Education, Certification and Titling: A Unified Statement* (Nurse Practitioner Roundtable, 2008), which states:

> Current master's and higher degree nurse practitioner programs prepare fully accountable clinicians to provide care to well individuals, patients with undifferentiated symptoms, and those with acute, complex chronic and/or critical illnesses. The DNP degree more accurately reflects current clinical competencies and includes preparation for the changing health care system. It is congruent with the intense rigorous education for nurse practitioners. This evolution is comparable to the clinical doctoral preparation for other health care professions. (p. 1)

This unified statement is actually quite progressive. It does not appear to disenfranchise current MSN-prepared NPs (I note the emphasis on "current" however), while acknowledging that they endorse the evolution of clinical doctoral preparation for NPs. More recently, the American Association of Nurse Practitioners (2013), a member of the Roundtable and the largest organization representing NPs, essentially reaffirmed this statement.

After the constitution of the AACN Task Force on the clinical doctorate in 2002, the NONPF and the AACN cohosted the National Forum on the Practice Doctorate in December 2003. What is interesting about the executive summary of this document is the following: (a) The constituent attendees identified that "practice" might encompass the clinical role, administrator, educator, or informaticist; (b) "Also clinically expert, doctorally prepared faculty will have to be recognized and have parity with other doctorally prepared faculty" (p. 3); and (c) "If the scope of practice remains unchanged, certification could accommodate an evolution from master's to doctoral preparation" (National Forum on the Practice Doctorate, p. 4). Although this forum had much more representation than the AACN Task Force, it still had only 51 attendees plus the invited speakers, and it appears that concerns expressed about moving forward with an acute nursing shortage and aging population, as reported by Hawkins-Walsh (2004), went unheeded. Along with Hawkins-Walsh, this author and colleagues Donnelly and Naremore in 2005 also questioned why the AACN undertook a new doctorate for advanced practice and a new generalist master's degree role (i.e., clinical nurse leader) when there were already two more critical nursing issues facing the nation: (a) a protracted nursing shortage and (b) a nation that was woefully preparing for an aging population with a meager production of geriatricians and gerontological NPs (Dreher, 2008b; Dreher et al., 2005). Both physician and nursing leadership can be faulted for this poor health policy planning. What is also interesting about this meeting was that the seeds were already planted that this degree would not be for practitioners only. On the conference's second point, the disenfranchisement of DNP faculty nevertheless took place, as many research-intensive and research-oriented universities have denied them tenure-track positions, but smaller, largely liberal arts colleges have been more accommodating. In a small, but recent study by Agger, Oermann, and Lynn (2014) titled Hiring and Incorporating Doctor of Nursing Practice–Prepared Nurse Faculty Into Academic Nursing Programs, they write, "we found that in many baccalaureate schools, DNP-prepared faculty are still held to similar tenure expectations as PhD-prepared faculty, which is why many are not or will not be considered for tenure" (p. 443).

Finally, with regard to scope of practice, the AACN in 2004(a) stated, "master's prepared advanced practice nurses identify additional knowledge that is needed for a higher level of advanced practice" (p. 7) and "a new and higher level of preparation for APN is justified if and only if it results in sufficient knowledge and skill above that already included at the master's level" (p. 12). Even the National Panel for Nurse Practitioner Practice Doctorate Competencies (2006) states: "The practice doctorate for the NP includes additional competencies that are to be combined with the existing Domains and Core Competencies of Nurse Practitioner Practice" (p. 1). It is for this reason that the term *doctoral advanced practice* is used to refer to practice by nurses with the DNP or DrNP to differentiate their practice from master's-prepared advanced practice nurses (Dreher & Montgomery, 2009). Extending this definition, we now suggest that the term "DAPRN" be used for "doctoral advanced practice registered nurse" instead of simply "APRN." For nonclinicians, the term suggested is "DANP" for "doctoral advanced nursing practice" instead of "ANP." This issue of the doctoral ANP role is actually the focus of this text. Much has been written about the effectiveness of master's-level APN, but with a paucity of outcome data on the DNP degree, a solid decade after it was launched, these authors and contributors agree it is time to focus more deliberatively on this new level of practice, with an emphasis on the role. Other books conflate DNP role development with DNP-related issues. We continue to think that a particular emphasis on role remains essential, especially because the success of this degree will depend on how the role of the DNP graduate evolves and is embraced or rejected by other health professions and the health care market. Despite the degree's surge in popularity, there is no guarantee that the degree will enact all that it was intended to do. Dr. David G. Campbell-O'Dell's comments as a DNP practitioner in Chapter 24 illuminate this. Only with conscientious attentiveness and concern by stakeholders for the degree, professional development of graduates in their new roles, and the elevated stewardship of its graduates to the discipline beyond what master's degree preparation has historically provided, will the degree's future success be ensured. If the degree becomes watered down and "quick to get," it will simply become a replacement for the master's, and not perceived by employers as having additional skills they need (or should pay for). If the degree, however, helps improve the health care delivery system (and with opportunities for us to prove its worth with millions of more getting new primary care under the Affordable Care Act), and simultaneously advance the profession, then the degree's creation will have been a triumph. As enthusiastic as this author has been toward DNP education, the story of this degree is still a new one and will continue to evolve, and not necessarily along predictable lines. Remember, just the explosiveness of this degree was not foreseen by its founders.

These two groups, the AACN and the NONPF, therefore, became the drivers of the DNP degree. And as reported to this author by attendees at various subsequent AACN meetings (remember that only deans could vote and only recently have nonvoting associate deans been invited to attend one of the two annual meetings if the dean is in attendance), it was evident that the PharmD and DPT degree models were being promoted over the research-oriented hybrid professional doctorates like the PsyD. This decision was likely made by conference conveners to perhaps better differentiate a new practice doctorate from the PhD. But in retrospect, the decision to exclude empirical research or some form of "dissertation or doctoral thesis" was for some nursing academics a reactionary overreach. This decision, left unchallenged for many years, ultimately harmed the notion of "what is nursing knowledge development?" In recent years, this issue was revisited as it has been acknowledged that DNP graduates are actually involved in the development of new knowledge, explicitly "clinical knowledge" or "practice knowledge" derived from practice evidence or internal evidence (AACN, 2015a; Dreher, 2013; Melnyk & Fineout-Overholt, 2011) practice. But even with the AACN white paper on the DNP, this is not a settled issue and good nursing scholars can disagree on this point. Some feel the degree should be made more accommodating to practice scholars who have every right to conduct research, others feel just as strongly that this is precisely what the PhD is for. Thus, with the early train headed toward a nonresearch DNP, the dialogue at open meetings leading up to the 2004 vote and the post-vote "team building" nevertheless, for some, seemed unstoppable.

■ THE AACN'S 2015 POSITION AND THE RUSH BEGINS

As we reflect on the history that both Columbia University and the University of Kentucky have provided to the contemporary practice doctorate, it is also important to examine the first critical mass of schools that began DNP programs in 2005. At the time, despite the October 25, 2004, vote[14] by the AACN to require the DNP degree for all advanced practice nurses—NPs, CRNAs, CNMs, and CNSs—by 2015, the landscape and the curricula of the DNP degree had not yet evolved. Table 1.3 lists the DNP programs (both DNP and DrNP) that existed in August 1, 2005, the first critical mass of DNP programs.

Right after Columbia University introduced their DrNP model in early 2005, Drexel University developed its own DNP degree model in March 2005 and labeled it a "clinical research doctor of nursing practice degree." It combined both advanced practice and the conduct of practical clinical research, concluding with a clinical dissertation. The degree was modeled after the PsyD and DrPH degrees (both professional doctorates that include a research emphasis), and the authors detailed their new degree model in *The Journal of Online Issues in Nursing* in 2005 (Dreher et al., 2005). As the former chair of that doctoral nursing program development committee, I can say that the faculty-working group began contemplating this particular degree model in 2000 in an innovative quest to find a practice-oriented degree as an alternative to the PhD. However, the Drexel nursing faculty felt very strongly that the research mission of the degree should only de-emphasize the PhD degree's focus on conducting research and creating new knowledge, not eliminate it. Certainly, since 2005 the Drexel program was an obvious outlier, but other programs using the DNP initials quietly let its students engage in clinical research as this was probably what the faculty felt more comfortable mentoring its students to perform. The DrNP was actually modeled on the PsyD clinical dissertation; so in many ways, the professional psychology doctorate was the "hybrid professional doctorate," which the AACN in 2004 was not actively considering, despite the open-review process it was publicly claiming it was conducting (Murray, 2000). All hybrid doctorates in the health professions complete a research project, usually in the form of a dissertation (Dreher, Fasolka, & Clark, 2008; Hawkins & Nezat, 2009; Smith Glasgow & Dreher, 2010). Figure 1.1 indicates that the DrNP degree was theoretically designed to fall in between the PhD and the DNP degrees, and Figure 1.2 indicates how this is similarly approached (from a practice doctorate with the smallest emphasis on research to the most, the PhD) in occupational therapy. Finally, as the DrNP degree model at the time included four roles (practitioner, clinical executive, educator, and clinical scientist), it is interesting to note that 50% of first 16 current graduates who entered the doctoral program in a role other than that as an educator (most were full-time practicing certified NPs) went into academia postgraduation, and 56% of these

TABLE 1.3   Inaugural Doctor of Nursing Practice Programs in the United States (as of August 1, 2005)

University	Year Founded	Type of Program	Notes
Case Western Reserve University	2005	DNP	Founded as ND and converted to DNP
Columbia University	2005	DrNP	Founded as DrNP and converted to DNP in 2008. Founders still refer to the degree as a "clinical doctorate"
Drexel University	2005	DrNP	A hybrid professional doctorate combining the practice doctorate and the academic research doctorate. Founders refer to degree as a "clinical research Doctor of Nursing Practice degree"; it converted to a DNP in 2014
Rush University	2005	DNP	Founded as ND and converted to DNP in Leadership and the Business of Health Care (only)
Tri-College University Nursing Consortium[a]	2005	DNP	NDSU left consortium in 2007; consortium disbanded in 2008
University of Colorado, Denver	2005	DNP	Founded as ND and converted to DNP
University of Kentucky	2001	DNP	First DNP—Clinical Leadership (only)
University of South Carolina	2005	DNP	Founded as ND and converted to DNP. First school to offer the BSN-to-DNP option to prepare entry level NPs
University of Tennessee, Memphis	2005	DNP	Founded as DNSc and converted to DNP

[a] Concordia College; Minnesota State University, Moorhead; North Dakota State University.
Modified from Dahnke and Dreher (2010).
BSN, bachelor of science in nursing; DNP, Doctor of Nursing Practice; DrNP, doctor of nursing practice; DNSc, doctor of nursing science; ND, doctor of nursing; NDSU, North Dakota State University; NPs, nurse practitioners.

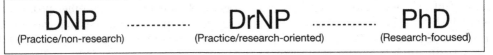

FIGURE 1.1   Practice/non-research, practice/research-oriented, and research-focused nursing doctorates.

DNP, Doctor of Nursing Practice; DrNP, doctor of nursing practice.

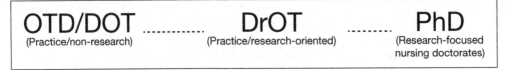

FIGURE 1.2   Practice/non-research, practice/research-oriented, and research-focused occupational therapy doctorates.

DOT, doctor of occupational therapy; DrOT, doctor of occupational therapy; OTD, occupational therapy doctorate.

graduates were in full-time academic appointments.[15] We suggest that at that time this degree model had a high rate of producing new full-time nursing faculty (three of whom have even procured tenure-track positions) and the average time from matriculation to graduation was approximately 3.29 years.

The hybrid degree is particularly facile in academia, because all students complete a clinical dissertation and therefore have common research skills. And although their research skills are not typically as extensive as that of the PhD graduate, they are nonetheless comparable. Other health professions have also dealt with the realities of professional doctorates and the difficult transition of their graduates into academic roles, particularly when the degree emphasis was on practice, not scholarly productivity. For this reason, physical therapy and occupational therapy both developed a hybrid professional degree after their introduction of their doctor of physical therapy and occupational therapy doctorate or doctor of occupational therapy (DPT and OTD or DOT) degrees, respectively, with the doctor of science in physical therapy and doctor of science (DScPT and DSc degrees), and in occupational therapy, the doctor of occupational therapy (DrOT degree). Table 1.4 identifies other health professions that have hybrid doctorates and indicates the differences among the research, hybrid professional, and professional doctorates.

What is interesting is that the National Institutes of Health (NIH) has opened up research funding (at least in the Parent K23 mechanism) to both graduates of "doctoral nursing research and nursing practice" programs (NIH, 2009a, section 1.B) and a few schools are revisiting the role of research in the DNP; in one case, the University of Connecticut has added courses in research methods that they previously did not

TABLE 1.4   **Types of Doctorates for Health Professions Disciplines in the United States**

Academic Research Doctorate (Research-Intensive Emphasis)	Hybrid Professional Doctorates (Practice/Research-Oriented Emphasis)	Professional Doctorates (Practice/Nonresearch Emphasis)
PhD—doctor of philosophy	DrPH—doctor of public health	MD/DO—doctor of medicine, doctor of osteopathy
ScD—doctor of science	DSc—doctor of science	DPT—doctor of physical therapy
DNS—doctor of nursing science	PsyD—doctor of psychology	PharmD—doctor of pharmacy
DSN—doctor of science in nursing	DSW—doctor of social work	DNP—Doctor of Nursing Practice
DNSc—doctor of nursing science	DScPT—doctor of science in physical therapy	DDS/DMD—doctor of dental surgery, Dentariae Medicinae Doctoris
	DrNP—doctor of nursing practice	DVM/VMD—doctor of veterinary medicine, Veterinariae Medicinae Doctoris
	DCN—doctor of clinical nutrition	DOT—doctor of occupational therapy

Modified from Smith Glasgow and Dreher (2010).

have and now require a clinical practice dissertation that was previously only a project (Dr. Regina Cusson, personal communication, June 25, 2010). In some ways, it seems un-egalitarian to say that one doctoral nursing graduate will create the evidence and the other will then translate and disseminate it. Good science, especially science grounded in practice, is not really conducted that way. That is part of the critique that Florczak (2010) had made querying "just how and where one could [could one] arbitrarily uncouple the practice of nursing from nursing research" (p. 16)?

The University of Washington School of Nursing faculty's initially promoted the concept of "practice inquiry" (which some schools adopted; Magyary, Whitney, & Brown, 2006). Although this scholarly approach did not prohibit the conduct of nursing research, it was designed to frame their DNP scholarly end product with a practice orientation and called it a clinical investigative project.[16] The call to revisit the particular "scholarly/research mission" of the DNP was heard over the last decade (Bellini & Cusson, 2010; Reel, 2009; Smith Glasgow & Dreher, 2010; Terry, 2014; Vincent, Johnson, Velasquez, & Rigney, 2014; Webber, 2008) and again with the new white paper on the DNP (AACN, 2015), what lies ahead is hopefully a maturing of scholarship from DNP graduates and a more precise mentoring and supervision from their DNP faculty. This author has studied DNP curricula intensely for years. Having chaired two national conferences on the practice doctorate and presented at the first International Conference on Professional Doctorates in London in 2009, this author has come to hypothesize that the DNP graduate may be best positioned to create "Practice Knowledge" for the profession (Dreher, 2010b, 2016b). In my view, it is in the focus on creating practice-based evidence where DNP graduates may excel, even beyond the PhD graduate. Moreover, although this author does support BSN-to-PhD options for some exceptionally talented students, at matriculation into their post-baccalaureate PhD program, they will have less a frame of reference to know what questions should be asked.

In my own proposed model of scientific inquiry in nursing (see Figure 1.3), I suggest that it is practice knowledge or mode 2 knowledge (represented by the right circle of the Venn diagram) that the DNP graduate is most prepared to conduct (Dreher,

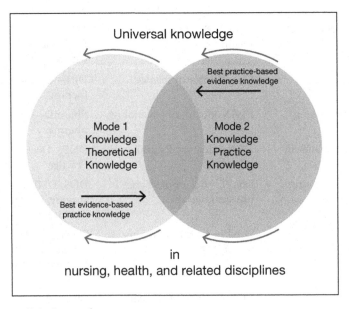

FIGURE 1.3 A model of scientific inquiry in nursing.
Source: Dahnke and Dreher (2016).

2010b, 2016b). This knowledge is created through practice-based research and inquiry that leads to practice-based evidence (Barkham & Mellor-Clark, 2003; Hellerstein, 2008; San Francisco AIDS Foundation, 2008). The left circle represents theoretical knowledge or mode 1 knowledge, and it is here where the PhD student is more prepared to conduct theoretical knowledge and generate evidence-based practice knowledge using larger data sets. The knowledge emanating from the best DNP programs, however, would be more practice oriented, closely connected to the work or clinical environment, and likely conducted in real time. Then, after rigorous but efficient analysis, the findings are translated into practice on a smaller scale until larger, more empirical work (evidence-based practice) can be conducted. Indeed, this drive for practice-based evidence should not be construed as a lesser research function. Some new or novel phenomena are just not ready for multisite, clinical trial investigation, or even multivariate analysis. The practitioner or clinical executive scholar closest to practice is in the best position to identify new clinical problems that need clinical investigation. The intersection of the two circles in the Venn diagram represents research that is highly contextualized to both practice-based evidence and evidence-based practice domains. Here the final research project (whatever it is called), whether PhD or DNP, is simply *indistinguishable*. Herein lies the rigor of the best DNP programs and the PhD programs where clinical practice problem solving is the overwhelming emphasis. This author believes that this is where the knowledge development is the most highly developed and relevant to the discipline. These DNP or PhD student-led studies include both large and small data sets (again, depending contextually on the clinical or practice question), with some DNP projects/clinical dissertations/DNP theses (you name it!) more focused on practice-based evidence and others on creating knowledge for evidence-based practice. A more complete description of this model (Figure 1.3) can be found in Chapter 16, "Next Steps Toward Practice Knowledge Development: An Emerging Epistemology in Nursing," in Dahnke and Dreher's (2016) recently published second edition *Philosophy of Science for Nursing Practice: Concepts and Applications.*

■ WHERE WE STAND NOW: A RELATIVELY NEW DEGREE, PROGRESS, AND UNRESOLVED ISSUES

PROGRESS

This chapter concludes with a short overview of some of the progress and central challenges or unresolved issues that the DNP degree now faces after a decade of implementation. Resolving these is essential as this still relatively new doctoral degree tries to gain a foothold in academic nursing circles and into the consciousness of the health care market. This market is extensive and very competitive and includes peer health professionals, the consumer public, and individuals from all walks of life who have substantive policy input and authority that impacts nursing. Certainly, three Institute of Medicine (IOM) reports, *To Err Is Human: Building a Safer Health System* (1999), *Crossing the Quality Chasm, A New Health System for the 21st Century* (2001), and *Health Professions Education: A Bridge to Quality* (2003), influenced the AACN leadership in their deliberations about moving forward with the DNP degree. Florczak (2010), however, writes creatively and extensively about the influence of the IOM reports and concludes "she remained somewhat confused about the link between the IOM reports and the push toward the DNP" (p. 15). Perhaps a more influential report was by the National Academy of Sciences (NAS, 2005), which then called for nursing to consider developing a nonresearch clinical doctorate to prepare expert practitioners who could also serve as faculty.

However, even the NAS recognized that "the concept of a nonresearch clinical doctorate in nursing is controversial" (NAS, 2005, p. 7). Today, in 2016, we are still wrangling with this question and we now ask instead: What kind of research (or scholarship) should the DNP graduate produce?

The first of the chief positive outcomes of the DNP degree is the realization that with the complexity of health care today, there is indeed curricular content and specialized knowledge beyond the MSN to give DNP graduates additional, enhanced skills. This has been detailed earlier both by the AACN (2004a) and the National Panel for Nurse Practitioner Practice Doctorate Competencies (2006). And even with the NONPF (2012) now abandoning specific DNP only competencies, this text implores the profession to seek the next domain of doctoral ANP. How can there not be skills, competencies, and expectations of doctorally educated clinicians over master's-prepared clinicians? Obviously, there will be continuous resistance, however, to claiming that there is a domain of practice and a skill set above and beyond basic advanced practice. Whether the DNP degree ultimately changes the scope and practice of the advanced practice nurse is another question. Although the AACN (2009b) says, "No, transitioning to the DNP will not alter the current scope of practice for APRNs" (p. 1), it is somewhat illogical to require additional skills and competencies for more ANP and then assume that the scope of practice will not change. Maybe that is actually what the American Medical Association (AMA) fears the most: not nurses using the title "Dr." but real fears about the possibility that the scope and boundaries of their practice will expand (AMA, 2009). Nevertheless, if there was ever an argument against the DNP, it would be a situation in which MSN programs simply added a few credits and called the degree a "doctorate" without any forthright attention to educating a more highly prepared practitioner.

A second positive outcome is that there is now a widely established nursing doctorate that gives nurses an alternative to the PhD (Buchholz, Yingling, Jones, & Tenfelde, 2015; Sperhac & Clinton, 2008). For decades, nurses only had a research-intensive degree, clinical doctorates that were de facto research-intensive degrees, and four NDs and one lone EdD—degree models that never gained a foothold within the profession. Whether it really is in the interest of nursing for there to be only one alternative to the PhD, the DNP, with the CCNE's refusal to recognize any form of the practice doctorate except the initials "DNP," is still debatable (AACN, 2005b). However, because of the power and influence of the AACN and CCNE, they are not likely to endorse a third doctorate at this time. The National League for Nursing Accrediting Commission (NLNAC, 2005) indicated a more progressive stance on titling, however, stating in their *NLNAC Statement on Clinical Practice Doctorates*:

> Other health care professionals such as dentists (DDS and DMD), psychologists (PhD and PsyD), and physicians (MD and DO) are able to define their roles, qualifications, and expertise to their patients and the public with more than one type of degree. We have confidence that doctorally prepared advanced practice nurses will be able to do so as well. (p. 1)

Nevertheless, in graduate nursing education circles, the AACN and CCNE seem to be more influential in some ways, but we must recognize that the former NLNAC, now ACEN since 2013, and now the NLN CNEA began accrediting nursing programs in Spring 2016. It should be noted that both ACEN and CNEA will accredit DNP programs with a focus on nursing education, whereas the CCNE will not (CNEA, 2016). In the end, often the determining factor of influence is whether it is the CCNE, ACEN, or CNEA that is accrediting the individual nursing school and sometimes different programs can be accredited by different agencies as nurse anesthesia, for example, must be accredited by the Council on Accreditation and sometime additionally by the CCNE or the newer options.

A third positive outcome of this doctoral option gives doctoral advanced practice nurses more parity with other health professionals (O'Sullivan, 2005). Although this was one of the goals for the creation of this degree, it really should not be a leading reason for individuals to seek it. The incentive to be called "Dr." ought to be driven more by what the doctorate adds to the master's-prepared practitioner to warrant the higher degree. Furthermore, the doctorate ought to be credible, have rigor, and must be seen by others as legitimate. This happens with every new doctorate: Public critical analyses by degree supporters, detractors, and skeptics, and not just toward the DNP. Furthermore, with a new degree, some DAPRNs are going to experience some difficulty in the workplace while working alongside master's-prepared APRNs who may feel resentment or deny that there is any difference in practice. Doctoral-prepared physical therapists, working alongside master's-prepared physical therapists, have already experienced this, and it is likely to happen in nursing, too (Salzman, 2010). But parity is important. It allows us to sit at the table as an equal contributor. Noted health care and nursing journalist Suzanne Gordon (2006) has written about the "invisibility of nursing" (p. 184). Maybe the DNP degree can help increase our visibility and permit our practitioners and clinicians (and others) to be seen as full partners in both practice and policy.

A final positive outcome (and surely there are others) is that this degree was designed to emphasize the translation and dissemination of research findings (AACN, 2006). Although this author and others believe that generating practice knowledge through practice inquiry (Dreher, 2010b; Magyary et al., 2006) should be incorporated into the degree, the opportunity this degree presents the profession is nonetheless unique. Magyary et al. (2006) write of the DNP student's role in practice inquiry:

> How to frame researchable questions generated from clinical observations and discourse is an essential practice inquiry competency. Clinical observations discrepant with habitual ways of knowing and doing may reveal new insights into clinical phenomena that have received limited or no empirical inquiry. These types of revelations may generate questions that beg to be answered through rigorous scientific investigation. (p. 144)

Furthermore, if properly and rigorously educated, the DNP degree graduate should be a skilled professional who should be able to data-mine (even skillfully scour) the endless databases that warehouse the enormous amount of research conducted every year in nursing and the health sciences. These graduates should be experts in knowledge management, poised to extract information and apply it in a novel or utilitarian way, and then efficiently translate and disseminate this new conceptualization of the evidence (Dreher, 2009). However, this theoretical rubric for what this graduate can be trained and educated to do can only be accomplished if the DNP student is exposed to coursework that indeed enables the student to truly participate credibly in this kind of practice inquiry. Philosophy of science courses are unusual in DNP programs, although this content is sometimes dispersed or integrated into other courses. But how else will these doctoral students understand the concepts of evidence, causation, empirical data, deduction, induction, probability, bias, scientific truth, and other important concepts all necessary to practice inquiry and the evaluation of evidence, if this content is absent in curricula? How can a student perform a meta-analysis or secondary analysis of existing data, conduct outcomes research, or engage in basic interpretive inquiry if the student does not have the advanced research methods courses (beyond the master's degree) to prepare one for this level of inquiry? The DNP student will likely be at the forefront of making the impractical practical and Fink (2006) suggests that the professional doctorate graduate should be well prepared for the knowledge economy simply based on the very practice orientation of the degree.

DNP graduates should also help broaden the definition of evidence through their work-based problem solving. Very traditional definition of "what is evidence in the health professions" was challenged by Pearson, Wiechula, Court, and Lockwood (2007) at the Joanna Briggs Institute at the University of Adelaide in Adelaide, Australia, and American DNP (and PhD) nursing faculty would benefit from exploring this literature. Initially, Pearson and colleagues describe four different types of clinical evidence that are posited based on a clinical question: (a) evidence of feasibility; (b) evidence of appropriateness; (c) evidence of meaningfulness; and (d) evidence of effectiveness. More recently, the Joanne Briggs Institute has expanded their taxonomy of evidence and offered a more detailed, descriptive reorganization of levels of evidence based on: (a) levels of evidence for effectiveness, (b) levels of evidence for diagnosis, (c) levels of evidence for prognosis, (d) levels of evidence for economic evaluations; and (e) levels of evidence for meaningfulness (Joanna Briggs Institute Levels of Evidence and Grades of Recommendation Working Party, 2013). It is highly recommended that both DNP faculty and students review this document as the clinical problem is identified and the methodology developed.

DNP-generated knowledge can also be described as mode 2 knowledge, which is work based, practice oriented, is derived differently and disseminated differently than mode 1 knowledge (Gibbons et al., 1994; Nowotny, Scott, & Gibbons, 2001; Reed, 2006; Smith Glasgow & Dreher, 2010). Mode 1 knowledge is mostly traditional, empirical, theoretical, and disseminated very typically according to academy norms. Mode 2 is where the professional/practice doctorate graduate should excel. This author has proposed that the DNP graduate generate practice knowledge (output) through the lens of practice inquiry (input) and by utilizing practice research methods (process; Dreher, 2010b, 2016b). This is illustrated in Figure 1.4.

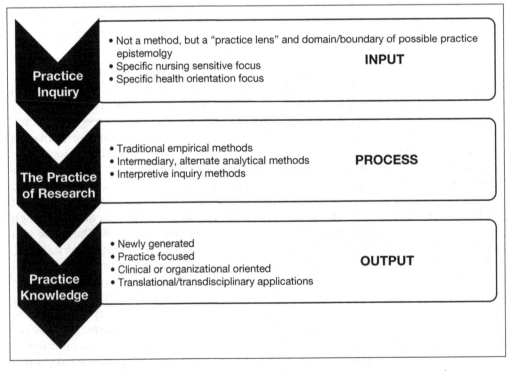

FIGURE 1.4 Path of practice knowledge generation in an emerging nursing epistemology.
Modified from Dahnke and Dreher (2010, 2016).

UNRESOLVED ISSUES

The chief unresolved issues surrounding the DNP degree can be summarized as follows:

1. Continuing controversy over the domain of knowledge development within the DNP degree and whether empirical research should be generally acceptable or not
2. Disagreement over the required number of clinical hours necessary for the degree, particularly for post-master's students
3. Controversy over the mandate, at least by the CCNE, that the "accredited" DNP degree may not formally prepare educators
4. An ongoing discussion over whether PhD and DNP students should share any common coursework.

Some of these issues, particularly the first and third, will be discussed at length in this text by various authors, and because this chapter has addressed these to some degree already, only a few summary points will be made here.

The issue over the role of research in the DNP degree is likely to continue despite the recent white paper that offered a little clarity (AACN, 2015). Our inclination is to predict that ultimately the DNP degree may look different at research-extensive and research-intensive universities where knowledge generation and scholarship are central to the mission. DNP programs that reside in colleges where the teaching mission and scholarship are emphasized, however, may be less inclined to design curricula that generate practice knowledge. However, these generalizations need not be used indiscriminately to prevent practice inquiry or even formal empirical inquiry by any DNP student anywhere. If we are honest, the same reality is present in PhD nursing/nursing science programs all across the country. Although some PhD programs emphasize the nurse scientist model (with a focus on generating nursing science), other PhD programs emphasize teaching and education research, and are less focused on producing graduates for research careers. The DNP degree should be no different. It will continue to evolve, and it will evolve best when both doctoral advanced nursing practitioners who simply want to practice and those who want to practice and generate practice knowledge (e.g., generate primary care, clinical, or organizational nursing knowledge) are both seated at the table and can respect the role each wants to play as stewards of the discipline. Medicine is actually no different as many practicing physicians are not involved in research or have no interest in it. They simply want to practice the art of medicine. Other physicians, however, see problems in their practice and are interested in initiating or participating in research related to these problems.

The other previously discussed issue—the role of the DNP degree in the preparation of nurse educator—will be discussed further by Wittman-Price, Waite, and Woda in Chapter 7. As mentioned earlier, there are unfortunately no aggressive strategic plans by nursing's current leadership to adequately replenish the supply of retiring nursing professors and nurse scientists. This is most unfortunate, because without nursing faculty, we cannot admit more nursing students and help alleviate the long-term nursing shortage. It seems highly unlikely, however, that we can increase the number of PhD students and graduates in the critical mass that is needed. The only solution that seems plausible is to reengineer the DNP graduate, especially those interested in teaching in MSN and DNP programs, for pathways that include a specific curriculum focus on teaching doctoral advanced practice. But as the leader of accrediting graduate nursing programs, the CCNE is unlikely to support this modification in the near future. This author has come to an alternate conclusion to address the nursing faculty shortage at least. I actually encourage my own master's-prepared faculty to seek EdD preparation in nursing education over DNP or PhD education if their goal is to remain in the academy and focus on teaching, not practice or clinical research. There are still many, many educational issues that need investigative inquiry and the small resurgence of EdD in nursing education programs is probably reflective of the disconnect between the original intent of the DNP and formal preparation for the teaching role. The results of our second doctoral nursing faculty survey, found in Chapter 11, reports the rising prominence of DNP preparation in the academy—an unintended consequence of the DNP the AACN in 2014 did not foresee. The last two unresolved issues (the second and fourth listed previously) are not discussed sufficiently in this text, so they will be addressed here. First, there continues to be debate over the required number of clinical hours necessary for the degree, particularly for post-master's students. Most programs have interpreted the statement from the AACN's *Essentials of Doctoral Education for Advanced Nursing Practice* (2006) "In order to achieve the DNP competencies, programs should provide a minimum of 1,000 hours of practice post-baccalaureate as part of a supervised academic program" (p. 19) very, very liberally. Even the usually supportive NONPF never fully endorsed the mandate that every post-master's clinical DNP student needs 400 more hours of actual practice (if the original MSN degree in pediatrics, e.g., had 600 hours). According to the NONPF (2006), "The evidence for the AACN recommendation for 1,000 clinical hours for all practice doctorate students has not been presented" (p. 1). This issue was debated at length at the 2007 DNP Conference in Annapolis, Maryland. For some it seemed unrealistic that part-time students (who work full-time) would need a total of 1,000 clinical hours (including whatever was earned for the master's degree), plus coursework (and still remain fully employed, particularly if they were receiving employer-based tuition benefits), to complete the degree. At Drexel, almost all of the students work full time and attended doctoral study as part-time students, and they barely seemed able to complete the rigorous intense curriculum that was structured year round (four quarters) over 3 years (the third year was devoted exclusively to the completion of the clinical dissertation). The Drexel program did not require 1,000 hours, but it focused more on the quality of the two required doctoral practice practica and not the quantity of hours. According to the new DNP white paper (AACN, 2015), it is again reinforced that students are not allowed to count work (paid hours) toward the minimum number of required hours. But this white paper (even unintentionally), may have unnecessarily muddied the water on this clinical hour requirement with the aforementioned statement that programs may award doctoral practice hours "credit" to students in DNP tracks who have national certification. What if DNP Program A will award XX credits toward the 1,000 clinical hour requirement to the ANCC certified FNP doctoral student, but competitor DNP Program B decides to award "more" hours.

More over, this author wonders if this will ultimately be an available option where some programs may require little if any new doctoral practice clinical hours. I remain skeptical that the monitoring of practice hours is vigorously enforced in all programs and worry that this is an area of compliance (even for accreditation that again is not required for post-master's programs) that is open to abuse. Additionally, many of these students did not complete hundreds of hours of precepted time during their MSN degrees in nursing administration, and therefore it seems it would be exorbitant to require them to complete 1,000 total hours for the degree. This is not logical. One DNP track requires 1,000 hours and one perhaps does not, even if the requirement is there, but it is tacitly not enforced. There is an inequity here. This absolute requirement needs revisiting, given the NONPF's (2006, p. 1) lack of enthusiasm for this requirement, stating "The NONPF Board has significant concern in establishing a random standard" (of required number of clinical hours). The NONPF has recognized this since the inception of the DNP and more recently published further comment on this issue, stating in 2016 "For post-baccalaureate DNP programs, a minimum of 1,000 practice hours must be acquired in the DNP program" (p. 3), but there is no specificity on post-master's programs, leaving this issue at least operationally unresolved.

The last issue—shared coursework between the two degree programs—was debated extensively by attendees in one session focusing on the future of the PhD at the January 2009 AACN Doctoral Nursing Education Conference in Coronado Island, California. From this author's point of view, there seem to be two camps of nursing faculty perspectives. One camp firmly believes that students from both degrees can learn from each other and therefore support some joint coursework between the two programs. The other camp is firmly against crossover between the two curricula fearing dilution of the PhD degree and the slow trajectory to one day "the DNP becoming the same as the PhD." Interestingly, I have not heard DNP faculty similarly state they do not want their DNP students taking courses with PhD students. It appears, however, that across the country there is some minimal coursework that students in the two degrees share. For administrators, it is also more cost-effective to offer some courses to both groups, especially if the class size (usually the PhD class these days) is small. Some of the comments I have heard, however, come from post-master's DNP graduates who took some common coursework with BSN-to-DNP students and who complained of the level of the content and its appropriateness for experienced master's-prepared APRNs. This is very similar to complaints sometimes from RNs who share coursework with generic BSN students. It is good to see in the white paper (AACN, 2015) that more collaboration between DNP and PhD students is being encouraged stating "DNP and PhD graduates will [should] have the opportunity to collaborate and work synergistically to improve health outcomes" (p. 3). Absolute separatism, which I am aware exists in some schools where there is a PhD and a DNP program might foster elitism among PhD students and in PhD programs (or even among faculty), and indeed we fear this. Deans and chairs need to actively promote collegiality among students (and faculty) in both cohorts, and if these students are going to be involved in PhD/DNP translational research teams, as some are now suggesting, then what better time to begin to work together than during doctoral study (Cacchione, 2007; Hastings, Mitchell, & Loud, 2010)?

One important point, however, needs to be emphasized. "Translation of research" and "translational research" are not the same thing. The NIH (2009b) has very clear definitions of what constitutes translational research, indicating:

> Translational research includes two areas of translation. One is the process of applying discoveries generated during research in the laboratory, and in preclinical studies, to the development of trials and studies in humans. The second area of translation *concerns research* [italics mine] aimed at enhancing the adoption of best practices in the community. Cost-effectiveness of prevention and treatment strategies is also an important part of translational science. (Section 1.1)

The AACN *Essentials of Doctoral Education for Advanced Nursing Practice* (2006) document makes it clear that "translational research" is not what it is referring to when it states:

> The scholar applies knowledge to solve a problem via the scholarship of application (referred to as the scholarship of practice in nursing). This application involves the *translation of research* [italics mine] into practice and the dissemination and integration of new knowledge, which are key activities of DNP graduates. (p. 11)

The nuance is nevertheless very clear. Translational research involves very formal traditional methods of scientific inquiry (Rubio et al., 2010). Supporting this in their description of practice inquiry, Magyary and colleagues (2006) indicate, "Practice inquiry entails a wide spectrum of designs, methods and statistical approaches. Emerging conceptual and technological advances in clinical epidemiology and informatics provide APNs the instruments to identify and monitor clinical patterns over time" (p. 145). To this author at least, the skill set of the DNP graduate described here is different from the more narrow focus of the scholarship of application. Therefore, until there is more clarity about the direction of the scholarship focus of the DNP degree, we are likely to see individual DNP programs undertaking very different forms of scientific and practice inquiry.

■ INTERNATIONAL IMPLICATIONS FOR THE DNP DEGREE

Finally, this chapter concludes with some thoughts about the DNP degree in the larger professional doctorate and larger universal doctoral nursing community.[17] With the exception of medicine, dentistry, and veterinary medicine, there are no doctoral programs outside of the United States that do not include the conduct of research. Indeed, the European Union (EU) in their Bologna Third Doctoral Cycle deliberations are trying to establish some uniformity among EU nations to better standardize both the PhD and the professional doctorate so that the transferability of scholars' credentials across borders is not an issue (Bologna Process, 2010; Davies, 2008). First, it may not be common knowledge, but professional nursing doctorates have existed globally, particularly in Australia, Northern Ireland, and Great Britain, since the 1990s (Ellis & Lee, 2005; McKenna & Cutcliffe, 2001). What is common among them (and professional doctorates in all other disciplines aside from those disciplines identified previously) is that the conduct of research is an integral part of their core competencies. Stew (2009), author of Chapter 19, and his colleagues from the University of Brighton indicate the difference between the PhD and the professional doctorate is that the PhD prepares the "professional researcher" and the professional doctorate prepares the "researching professional." But does the DNP degree fit into this international professional nursing doctorate degree model? The answer is that some do, but that most do not. However, what the DNP and other U.S.-based professional doctorates do that the international professional doctorates largely do not[18] is to emphasize and actually require additional practice hours beyond the MSN or other health professions master's degree. Even as I attended the first Professional and Practice-Focused Doctoral Research Special Interest Group meeting in London in July 2010 as the only U.S. attendee, I queried a fellow colleague who indicated that their professional doctorate graduates do gain advanced practice hours at their work site, although absolute hours are not required. I argued that it would be controversial (even open the university to liability, which I understand is less prevalent in the British legal system) to award credit in the United States for actual work the student completed as the agent of the employer (hospital) and not primarily as the agent of the university. Further, I am skeptical that one can prepare a more advanced practitioner just by gaining more clinical research skills that can be applied in the practice environment. Nevertheless, especially with the emerging codified language from the Bologna Third Cycle, it is very unlikely that a nursing doctorate without a research project would be accepted outside the United States. Therefore, any American DNP nurse who might seek a teaching position outside the United States should be aware of this expectation. On the other hand, the proximity of Canada to the United States has already got Canadian nursing scholars wondering how the DNP might impact the Canadian nursing educational system (Brar, Boschma, & McCuaig, 2010; Joachim, 2008), but the DNP degree is still absent outside the United States. I conclude by writing humorously that I did warn my mostly British colleagues in London once that they should not ignore what is happening in the United States with the professional doctorate or with the DNP degree. Our ideas, both good and bad, can easily make a transatlantic voyage or flight.

■ SUMMARY

As the DNP degree continues to evolve, more than 15 years since the first DNP degree and over 10 years since the first large cohort of programs were first established, it is now time to take a deep breath and evaluate how far we have come and what direction this degree should now take. Only recently, in the spring of 2010, did the ANA undertake its first analysis of the DNP degree and take public comment. As far as this author can tell, the ANA has never offered a final public document on the DNP degree. In the first edition of this text, I predicted it would likely be a 2-year process before the ANA House of Delegates voted on this degree and that it would either: (a) endorse it; (b) offer cautionary approval or suggest a slower period of transition (rather than 2015 which has now passed); or (c) possibly reject the idea that all advanced practice nurses one day must have an entry-level doctorate. But more realistically, I suggested the ANA's ultimate position may not be determinative and I still agree with that point. This degree has arrived and graduates are going out into the professional work force and starting to make their mark. New DNPs are working in roles that the health care system has never seen before. Some PhD nursing graduates have unfairly, but sometimes fairly, had their relevance to the clinical practice environment questioned (Wilkes & Mohan, 2008). The clinical practice environment, however, is fertile ground for the DNP graduate, and it is here where they are educated to excel.

This author has tried to provide a descriptive analysis of the trajectory of this degree, particularly in the context of doctoral nursing education. Sometimes history and its analysis and commentary are not pretty, especially as an author may suggest or affirm views a reader may disagree with. But mostly history and its politics are complex. In the end, the history of the DNP degree can be summarized as follows: Initially there was great opposition to the DNP degree, but the opposition was largely quelled quickly. Now what we have left is the fine tuning of the degree and a need to generate outcome data that will help enable our graduates to better define and "live" this new role so that nursing's mission to improve health and alleviate suffering can advance.

■ CRITICAL THINKING QUESTIONS

1. *How do you view the state of critical discourse in nursing? Do we debate enough? Do we need more agreement and more consensus? Or should we embrace difference more and be less concerned with conformity?*

2. *The nursing profession appears to have abandoned the idea of clinical doctorate as an alternative to the PhD and has embraced the title "practice doctorate" to describe the DNP. Discuss whether you think the profession needs a research doctorate (PhD), a practice doctorate (DNP), and a clinical doctorate?*

3. *Why do you think the EdD in nursing education degree model at Teachers College is suddenly being replicated after decades (since its founding) passed by in which it was never replicated?*

4. *What can be done to combat the aging nursing workforce, which faces imminent retirements that will not be replaced by the current pool of those entering the profession at all levels?*

5. *Debate the following: "Resolved, nursing is a profession."*

6. *The ND degree and now the DNP were partly modeled after the MD degree. What are your thoughts about this?*

7. *Discuss whether you think 1,000 total clinical hours should be required for the DNP degree, including practice and clinical executive tracks.*

8. *Discuss whether original research ought to be part of the formal DNP curriculum.*

9. *Do you agree that the DNP degree might offer something the PhD degree cannot? Provide your rationale.*

10. *Discuss why you have chosen the particular DNP program you are currently matriculating in.*

■ NOTES

1. To be completely historically accurate, we can add two nurse anesthesia-oriented doctorates developed: the increasingly popular Doctor of Nurse Anesthesia Practice (DNAP degree) and the Doctor of Management Practice of Nurse Anesthesia (DMPNA degree) at Marshall University. Furthermore, because degree initials "DNP" and "DrNP" are both Doctor of Nursing Practice degrees, for simplification (and because the only two DrNP programs at Columbia University and Drexel University ultimately changed to the "DNP" initials), the initials "DNP" will be used in most cases in this chapter and text except when the difference between the two is noted.

2. CRNPs, CNMs, CRNAs, and CNSs.

3. Because "professional doctorate" and "practice doctorate" are nearly synonymous, for simplicity, we use the term "practice doctorate" to include both. Where the nuance between each is indeed important, we will use the terms separately and indicate why.

4. Why did some university faculties not allow the PhD in nursing? Certainly, for many the issue was prejudice against nursing as a discipline as Meleis and Dracup (2005) affirm. Senior faculty (who often predominate in conservative university faculty senates), were often the elected members who viewed nursing despairingly as a scientific discipline. In other cases, like Widener University, the university charter did not permit the awarding of any PhD, so an alternate doctorate was offered. Many of those charter restrictions have been modified over the years, and almost all programs that awarded the DNSc, DNS, or DSN, retroactively converting those degrees to the PhD (as Widener and University of Alabama–Birmingham did for instance).

5. This author has always thought that PhD programs that emphasize the nurse scientist model should be titled PhD in nursing science, and other PhD programs that emphasize the teaching or other mission in nursing should be titled PhD in nursing. The PhD in nursing education seems redundant and unnecessary, with the EdD in nursing education historically more consistent with the discipline.

6. Two examples of the kinds of research projects that were funded by this new field research division was a study that examined pre–post knowledge of diabetic patients after teaching and another that looked at classifying patients and distributing nursing staff according to patients' nursing needs (*American Journal of Nursing*, 1965).

7. Examples of his critique of institutionalized medicine among the 155 graduate and 12 postgraduate medical schools in the United States and Canada, he claimed to have visited included findings of equipment at one school "dirty and disorderly beyond description" (Flexner, 1910, p. 190) and another institution had "in place of laboratories, laboratory signs" (p. 165). Additionally, Flexner was actually criticized for being too critical and his methods of his data collection came under heavy fire (Hiatt, 1999).

8. Moreover, scholarship such as this text needs to be better recognized by nursing deans and traditional tenure and promotion committees because, again, if there are no nursing texts, then there is no nursing curricula period, and ultimately no tuition revenue.

9. A 2010 report found that female law partners at elite law firms made on average $66,000 less than their male counterparts, and this disparity was largely attributed to stereotyping, gender bias, and even bullying and intimidation (Williams & Richardson, 2010). More recently, *The Guardian* has reported that global economic disparity between men and women is rising, with levels now similar to those during the 2008 financial crisis. At this pace of sustained gender pay inequity, it will take 170 years according to data from the World Economic Forum (Treanor, 2016).

10. I cannot help but also mention that when these discussions of "research start-up packages" takes place, there are always gaps among other nursing faculty who received zero research support on hire. What is more typical is nursing faculty have no idea how equitable their packages are respective to other faculty in other departments in their universities.

11. Similarly, with the EdD at Teachers College a first-generation professional doctorate, the initial ND degree at CWRU could also be termed a second-generation professional nursing doctorate.

12. The original Kentucky DNP degree model.

13. Tri-Council for Nursing represents leaders from the AACN, the National League for Nursing, the ANA, and the American Organization of Nurse Executives.

14. The actual vote was 162 yes, 101 no, 13 abstain, and no proxy or in absentia votes were permitted. Indeed, the power and influence of 162 individuals are substantial (Dreher et al., 2005).

15. The Drexel DrNP degree was fully approved by the Pennsylvania Department of Education (PDOE) on April 29, 2010. As it included a clinical dissertation, it was classified as a research degree by the PDOE.

16. They, however, initially called it a clinical investigative project, even though the faculty workload of supervising one of these projects can be near that of a dissertation (Dr. Marie-Annette Brown, personal communication, July 24, 2010). Will this become a trend in nursing academia (especially at research universities) where faculty are assigned or expected to chair more DNP Final Projects because they are not "dissertations?" At present, the DNP curriculum on their website terms this a "Practice Doctorate Project/Capstone," which addresses a clinical or systems problem using an evidence-based, practice relevant approach (May 22, 2016).

17. This issue is discussed thoroughly in Dreher and Smith Glasgow (2011).

18. The DCPsych degree is one exception. This professional doctorate in counseling psychology uniformly requires additional practicum hours to complete the degree. But this degree is an exception among professional doctorates globally outside the United States.

■ REFERENCES

Academic Nurse. (2010). Ten years of progress: The Council for the Advancement of Care: The academic nurse. *The Journal of Columbia University School of Nursing and its Alumni, Spring*, 21–27.

Accrediting Commission for Education in Nursing. (2013). Accreditation manual. Retrieved from http://www.acenursing.net/manuals/GeneralInformation.pdf

Agger, C., Oermann, M. H., & Lynn, M. R. (2014). Hiring and incorporating doctor of nursing practice-prepared nurse faculty into academic nursing programs. *Journal of Nursing Education, 53*(8), 439–446.

Aiken, L. H., Cheung, R. B., & Olds, D. M. (2009). Education policy initiatives to address the nurse shortage in the United States. *Health Affairs, 28*(4), 646–656.

American Association of Colleges of Nursing. (1999). Faculty shortages intensify nation's nursing deficit. Retrieved from http://www.aacn.nche.edu/publications/issues/IB499WB.htm

American Association of Colleges of Nursing. (2004a). AACN position statement on the practice doctorate in nursing October 2004. Retrieved from http://www.aacn.nche.edu/DNP/pdf/DNP.pdf

American Association of Colleges of Nursing. (2004b). *AACN draft position statement on the practice doctorate in nursing January 2004*. Washington, DC: Author.

American Association of Colleges of Nursing. (2004c). *AACN position statement on the practice doctorate in nursing March 2004*. Washington, DC: Author.

American Association of Colleges of Nursing. (2004d). AACN adopts a new vision for the future of nursing education and practice. Retrieved from http://www.aacn.nche.edu/Media/NewsReleases/DNPRelease.htm

American Association of Colleges of Nursing. (2005a). Faculty shortages in baccalaureate and graduate nursing programs: Scope of the problem and strategies for expanding the supply. Retrieved from http://www.aacn.nche.edu/publications/pdf/05FacShortage.pdf

American Association of Colleges of Nursing. (2005b). Commission on Collegiate Nursing Education moves to consider for accreditation only practice doctorates with the DNP degree title. Retrieved from http://www.aacn.nche.edu/Media/NewsReleases/Archives/2005/CCNEDNP.htm

American Association of Colleges of Nursing. (2006). *The essentials of doctoral education for advanced nursing practice.* Retrieved from http://www.aacn.nche.edu/DNP/pdf/Essentials.pdf

American Association of Colleges of Nursing. (2008). The preferred vision of the professoriate in baccalaureate and graduate nursing programs. Retrieved from http://www.aacn.nche.edu/Publications/pdf/PreferredVision.pdf

American Association of Colleges of Nursing. (2009a). *2008–2009 Enrollment and graduations in baccalaureate and graduate programs in nursing.* Washington, DC: Author.

American Association of Colleges of Nursing. (2009b). Frequently asked questions, position statement on the practice doctorate in nursing. Retrieved from http://www.aacn.nche.edu/DNP/dnpfaq.htm

American Association of Colleges of Nursing. (2015a). Nursing faculty shortage. Retrieved from http://www.aacn.nche.edu/media-relations/fact-sheets/nursing-faculty-shortage

American Association of Colleges of Nursing. (2015b). The doctor of nursing practice: Current issues and clarifying recommendations, report from the task force on the implementation of the DNP. Retrieved from http://www.aacn.nche.edu/aacn-publications/white-papers/DNP-Implementation-TF-Report-8-15.pdf

American Association of Nurse Practitioners. (2013). Discussion paper: The doctor of nursing practice. Retrieved from https://www.aanp.org/images/documents/publications/doctorofnursingpractice.pdf

American College of Nurse-Midwives. (2009). ACNM Division of Accreditation (now the Accreditation Commission for Midwifery Education) statement on midwifery education. Retrieved from http://www.midwife.org/siteFiles/DNPstatementedited.doc

American College of Nurse-Midwives. (2012a). Midwifery: Evidence-based practice: A summary of research on midwifery practice in the United States. Retrieved from http://www.midwife.org/acnm/files/cclibraryfiles/filename/000000002128/midwifery%20evidence-based%20practice%20issue%20brief%20finalmay%202012.pdf

American College of Nurse-Midwives. (2012b). Position statement: Midwifery education and the doctor of nursing practice. Retrieved from http://www.midwife.org/ACNM/files/ACNMLibraryData/UPLOADFILENAME/000000000079/Midwifery%20Ed%20and%20DNP%20Position%20Statement%20June%202012.pdf

American Journal of Nursing. (1965). The Division of Nursing USPHS. *American Journal of Nursing, 65*(7), 82–85.

American Medical Association. (2009). *AMA scope of practice data sets: Nurse practitioners.* Chicago, IL: Author.

Anselmi, K. K., Dreher, H. M., Smith Glasgow, M. E., & Donnelly, G. F. (2010). Faculty colleagues in your classroom as doctoral students: Does a conflict of interest exist? *Nurse Educator, 35*(5), 213–219.

Auerbach, D. I. (2012). Will the NP workforce grow in the future? New forecasts and implications for healthcare delivery. *Medical Care, 50*(7), 606–610.

Auerbach, D. I., Martsolf, G. R., Pearson, M. L., Taylor, E. A., Zaydman, M., Muchow, A. N., . . . Lee, Y. (2015). *The DNP by 2015: A study of the institutional, political, and professional issues that facilitate or impede establishing a post-baccalaureate doctor of nursing practice program.* Santa Monica, CA: RAND. Retrieved from http://www.rand.org/pubs/research_reports/RR730.html

Azam, M. S. (2010). Fewer employers paying for tuition, corporate training. *Orlando Business Journal.* Retrieved from http://orlando.bizjournals.com/orlando/stories/2010/04/19/focus1.html

Babcock, P. (2009). Always more to learn. Society for Human Resource Management. Retrieved from http://www.shrm.org/Publications/hrmagazine/EditorialContent/Pages/0909babcock.aspx

Baez, B. (2002). *Degree of distinction: The EdD or the PhD in education.* Paper presented at the Annual Meeting of the Association for the Study of Higher Education, Sacramento, CA, November 21–24, 2002.

Barkham, M., & Mellor-Clark, J. (2003). Bridging evidence-based practice and practice-based evidence: Developing a rigorous and relevant knowledge for the psychological therapies. *Clinical Psychology and Psychotherapy, 10*(6), 319–327.

Bellini, S., & Cusson, R. (2010). The role of the practitioner. In H. M. Dreher & M. E. Smith Glasgow (Eds.), *Role development for doctoral advanced nursing practice* (pp. 123–135). New York, NY: Springer Publishing.

Bloch, J. R. (2007). *The DNP/DrNP degree as entry into NP practice: Is this nursing's answer to eliminate disparities in health care access for vulnerable populations?* Paper presented at the First National Conference on The Doctor of Nursing Practice: Meanings and Models, Annapolis, MD, March 28–30, 2007.

Bologna Process. (2010). Third cycle: Doctoral education. Retrieved from http://www.ond.vlaanderen .be/hogeronderwijs/bologna/actionlines/third_cycle.htm

Brar, K., Boschma, G., & McCuaig, F. (2010). The development of nurse practitioner preparation beyond the master's level: What is the debate about? *International Journal of Nursing Education Scholarship, 7*(1), Article 9, 1–15.

Buchholz, S. W., Yingling, C., Jones, K., & Tenfelde, S. (2015). DNP and PhD collaboration: Bringing together practice and research expertise as predegree and postdegree scholars. *Nursing Educator, 40*(4), 203–206.

Budden, J. S., Zhong, E. H., Moulton, P., & Cimiotti. J. P. (2013). The National Council of State Boards of Nursing and The Forum of State Nursing Workforce Centers 2013 National Workforce Survey of Registered Nurses. *Journal of Nursing Regulation, 4*(2), S1–S72.

Bunge, H. (1962). The first decade of "nursing research." *Nursing Research, 11*(3), 132–138.

Cacchione, P. Z. (2007). What is clinical nursing research? *Clinical Nursing Research, 16*(3), 167–169.

California Board of Registered Nursing. (2014). 2014 survey of registered nurses. Retrieved from http:// www.rn.ca.gov/pdfs/forms/survey2014.pdf

Carlson, L. H. (2003). The clinical doctorate—Asset or albatross? *Journal of Pediatric Health Care, 17*(4), 216–218.

Case Western Reserve University. (2016). The next level in nursing. Retrieved from https://nursing .case.edu/dnp

Christman, L. (1980). Leadership in practice: Image. *Journal of Nursing Scholarship, 12*, 31–33.

Commission on Nursing Education Accreditation. (2016). FAQs: National League for Nursing Commission for Nursing Education Accreditation (CNEA)—General questions. Retrieved from http://www.nln.org/accreditation-services/faqs

Council on Accreditation. (2007). AANA announces support of doctorate for entry into nurse anesthesia practice by 2025. Retrieved from http://www.aana.com/newsandjournal/News/Pages/092007 -AANA-Announces-Support-of-Doctorate-for-Entry-into-Nurse-Anesthesia-Practice-by-2025.aspx

Courtenay, B. C. (1988). Eliminating the confusion over the EdD and PhD in colleges and schools of education. *Innovative Higher Education, 13*(1), 11–20.

Curtis, J. (2010). Faculty salary equity: Still a gender gap? *On Campus With Women, 39*(1). Retrieved from https://archive.aacu.org/ocww/volume39_1/feature.cfm?section=2

Dahnke, M. D., & Dreher, H. M. (2016). *Philosophy of science for nursing practice: Concepts and applications.* (2nd ed.). New York, NY: Springer Publishing.

Davies, R. (2008). The Bologna process: The quiet revolution in nursing higher education. *Nurse Education Today, 28*, 935–942.

Donley, R., & Flaherty, M. J. (2008). Revisiting the American Nurses Association's first position on education for nurses: A comparative analysis of the first and second position statements on the education of nurses. *The Online Journal of Issues in Nursing, 13*(2). Retrieved from http:// www.nursingworld.org/MainMenuCategories/ANAMarketplace/ANAPeriodicals/OJIN/ TableofContents/vol132008/No2May08/ArticlePreviousTopic/EntryIntoPracticeUpdate.aspx

Donohue, P. (1996). *Nursing the finest art: An illustrated history* (2nd ed.). St. Louis, MO: Mosby.

Dracup, K., & Bryan-Brown, C. (2005). Doctor of nursing practice—MRI or total body scan? *American Journal of Critical Care, 14*(4), 278–281.

Dreher, H. M. (2005). The doctor of nursing practice: Has this train left the station? If so, just where is it going? *The Pennsylvania Nurse, 60*, 17–19.

Dreher, H. M. (2008a). Innovation in nursing education: Preparing for the future of nursing practice. *Holistic Nursing Practice, 22*(2), 77–80.

Dreher, H. M. (2008b). A dearth of geriatric specialists: Will invention and gerotechnology save us? *Holistic Nursing Practice, 22*(5), 255–260.

Dreher, H. M. (2009). How do RNs today best stay informed? Do we need "knowledge management?" *Holistic Nursing Practice, 23*(5), 263–266.

Dreher, H. M. (2010a). The path to nursing science today, 1910–2010. In M. D. Dahnke & H. M. Dreher (Eds.), *Philosophy of science for nursing practice: Concepts and applications* (pp. 269–300). New York, NY: Springer Publishing.

Dreher, H. M. (2010b). Next steps toward practice knowledge development: An emerging epistemology in nursing. In M. D. Dahnke & H. M. Dreher (Eds.), *Philosophy of science for nursing practice* (pp. 355–391). New York, NY: Springer Publishing.

Dreher, H. M. (2013). Differentiating "clinical evidence" and "clinical knowledge." *Clinical Scholars Review: The Journal of Doctoral Nursing Practice, 6*(1), 9–12.

Dreher, H. M. (2016a). The path to nursing science today, 1910–2010, with epilogue 2010-2015. In M. D. Dahnke & H. M. Dreher (Eds.), *Philosophy of science for nursing practice: Concepts and applications* (2nd ed., pp. 315–354). New York, NY: Springer Publishing.

Dreher, H. M. (2016b). Next steps toward practice knowledge development. In M. D. Dahnke & H. M. Dreher (Eds.), *Philosophy of science for nursing practice: Concepts and applications* (2nd ed., pp. 353–391). New York, NY: Springer Publishing.

Dreher, H. M., Donnelly, G., & Naremore, R. (2005). Reflections on the DNP and an alternate practice doctorate model: The Drexel DrNP. *The Online Journal of Issues in Nursing, 11*(1). Retrieved from www.nursingworld.org/ojin/topic28/tpc28_7.htm

Dreher, H. M., Fasolka, B., & Clark, M. (2008). Navigating the decision to pursue an advanced degree. *Journal of Men in Nursing, 3*(1), 51–55.

Dreher, H. M., & Gardner, M. (2009). *With the rise of the DNP, who will conduct primary care research?* Paper presented at the Second National Conference on the Doctor of Nursing Practice: The Dialogue Continues…, Hilton Head Island, SC, March 24–27, 2009.

Dreher, H. M., & Montgomery, K. E. (2009). Let's call it "doctoral" advanced practice nursing. *The Journal of Continuing Nursing Education, 40*(12), 530–531.

Dreher, H. M., & Smith Glasgow, M. E. (2011). Global perspectives on the professional doctorate. *International Journal of Nursing Studies, 48*, 403–408.

Dunphy, L. M., Smith, N. K., & Youngkin, E. Q. (2009). Advanced practice nursing: Doing what has to be done—Radicals, renegades, and rebels. In L. Joel (Ed.), *Advanced practice nursing: Essentials for role development* (2nd ed., pp. 2–22). Philadelphia, PA: F. A. Davis.

Ellis, L. B., & Lee, N. (2005). The changing landscape of doctoral education: Introducing the professional doctorate for nurses. *Nurse Education Today, 25*(3), 222–229.

Fang, D., Li, Y., Stauffer, D. C., & Trautman, D. E. (2016). *2015–2016 enrollment and graduations in baccalaureate and graduate programs in nursing.* Washington, DC: American Association of Colleges of Nursing.

Fang, D., Tracy, C., & Bednash, G. D. (2010). *2009–2010 enrollment and graduations in baccalaureate and graduate programs in nursing.* Washington, DC: American Association of Colleges of Nursing.

Fink, D. (2006). The professional doctorate: Its relativity to the PhD and relevance for the economy. *International Journal of Doctoral Studies, 3*, 35–44.

Fitzpatrick, J. (2003). The case for the clinical doctorate in nursing. *Reflections on Nursing Leadership, First Quarter, 8–9, 37*, 52.

Fitzpatrick, J. (2008). Doctor of nursing practice programs: History and current status. In J. Fitzpatrick & M. Wallace (Eds.), *The doctor of nursing practice and clinical nurse leader: Essentials of program development and implementation for clinical practice* (pp. 13–30). New York, NY: Springer Publishing.

Flexner, A. (1910). *Medical education in the United States and Canada: A report to the Carnegie Foundation for the Advancement of Teaching. Bulletin No. 4.* New York, NY: Carnegie Foundation for the Advancement of Teaching.

Florczak, K. L. (2010). Research and the doctor of nursing practice: A cause for consternation. *Nursing Science Quarterly, 23*(1), 13–17.

Ford, J. (2008). Editorial: DNP a bad idea. Retrieved from http://community.advanceweb.com/blogs/np_1/archive/2008/07/23/editorial-on-dnp.aspx

Fulton, J. S. (2010). Evolution of clinical nurse specialist role and practice in the United States. In J. S. Fulton, B. L. Lyon, & K. A. Goudreau (Eds.), *Foundations of clinical nurse specialist practice* (pp. 3–14). New York, NY: Springer Publishing.

Fulton, J., & Lyon, B. (2005). The need for some sense making: Doctor of nursing practice. *The Online Journal of Issues in Nursing, 10*(3), Manuscript 3. Retrieved from www.nursingworld .org/MainMenuCategories/ANAMarketplace/ANAPeriodicals/OJIN/TableofContents/ Volume102005/No3Sept05/tpc28_316027.aspx

Gibbons, M., Lomoges, C., Nowotny, H., Schwartzman, S., Scott, P., & Trow, M. (1994). *The new production of knowledge*. London, UK: Sage.

Goodrich, A. A. (1936). Modern trends in nursing education. *American Journal of Public Health, 26,* 764–770.

Gordon, S. (2006). *Nursing against the odds: How health care cost cutting, media stereotypes, and medical hubris undermine nurses and patient care*. Ithaca, NY: Cornell University Press.

Gortner, S. R. (1986). Impact of the division of nursing on nursing research development in the U.S.A. In S. M. Stinson & J. Kerr (Eds.), *International issues in nursing research* (pp. 113–130). Philadelphia, PA: Charles Press.

Gortner, S. R. (2000). Knowledge development in nursing: Our historical roots and future opportunities. *Nursing Outlook, 48*(2), 60–67.

Grace, H. (1989). Issues in doctoral education in nursing. *Journal of Professional Nursing, 5*(5), 266–270.

Hastings, C. E., Mitchell, S. A., & Loud, J. T. (2010). *Advancing nursing roles in clinical and translational science*. Paper presented at the 2010 Clinical and Translational Research and Education Meeting, ACRT/SCTS Joint Annual Meeting, April 5–7, 2010, Washington, DC.

Hathaway, D., Jacob, S., Stegbauer, C., Thompson, C., & Graff, C. (2006). The practice doctorate: Perspectives of early adopters. *Journal of Nursing Education, 45*(12), 487–496.

Hawkins, R., & Nezat, G. (2009). Doctoral education: Which degree to pursue? *American Association of Nurse Anesthetists Journal, 77*(2), 92–96.

Hawkins-Walsh, E. (2004, July–August). The "practice doctorate"—What's it all about? *The Pediatric Nurse Practitioner, 31*(4), 18.

Health Resources and Services Administration, National Center for Health Workforce Analysis. (2013). The U.S. nursing workforce: Trends in supply and education. Retrieved from http://bhpr.hrsa .gov/healthworkforce

Hellerstein, D. (2008). Practice-based evidence rather than evidence-based practice in psychiatry. *Medscape Journal of Medicine, 10*(6), 141.

Hiatt, M. D. (1999). Around the continent in 180 days: The controversial journey of Abraham Flexner. *The Pharos, 62*(1), 18–24.

Honig, J., & Smolowitz, J. (2009). Clinical doctorate at Columbia University School of Nursing: Lessons learned. *Clinical Scholars Review, 2*(2), 51–59.

Horrocks, S., Anderson, E., & Salisbury, C. (2002). Systematic review of whether nurse practitioners working in primary care can provide equivalent care to doctors. *British Medical Journal, 324,* 819–823.

Hutchinson, S. A. (2001). The development of qualitative health research: Taking stock. *Qualitative Health Research, 11,* 505–521.

Ingeno, L. (2013). Who will teach nursing? Retrieved from https://www.insidehighered.com/ news/2013/07/22/nursing-schools-face-faculty-shortages

Institute of Medicine. (1999). *To err is human: Building a safer health system*. Washington, DC: National Academies Press.

Institute of Medicine. (2001). *Crossing the quality chasm: A new health system for the 21st century*. Washington, DC: National Academies Press.

Institute of Medicine. (2003). *Health professions education: A bridge to quality*. Washington, DC: National Academies Press.

Jacobson, A., Stern, C., Gaspar, P., Spross, J., Heye, M., France, N., . . . Sedhorn, L. (2007). *Comparison of National Association of Clinical Nurse Specialist Statement Competencies with DNP Essentials: What is the fit?* Paper presented at the First National Conference on The Doctor of Nursing Practice: Meanings and Models, Annapolis, MD, March 28–30, 2007.

Joachim, G. (2008). The practice doctorate: Where do Canadian nursing leaders stand? *Nursing Leadership, 21*(4), 42–51.

Joanna Briggs Institute Levels of Evidence and Grades of Recommendation Working Party. (2013). New JBI levels of evidence. Retrieved from http://joannabriggs.org/assets/docs/approach/JBI -Levels-of-evidence_2014.pdf

Kirkpatrick, M. (1994). The department chair position in academic nursing. *Journal of Professional Nursing, 10*(2), 77–83.

Krugman, P. (2009). The Great Recession versus the Great Depression. *New York Times.* Retrieved from http://krugman.blogs.nytimes.com/2009/03/20/the-great-recession-versus-the -great-depression

Lenz, E. R. (2005). The practice doctorate in nursing: An idea whose time has come. *The Online Journal of Issues in Nursing, 10*(3), Manuscript 1. Retrieved from www.nursingworld.org/ MainMenuCategories/ANAMarketplace/ANAPeriodicals/OJIN/TableofContents/Volume 102005/No3sept05/tpc28_116025.aspx

Loomis, J. A., Willard, B., & Cohen, J. (2006). Difficult professional choices: Deciding between the PhD and the DNP in nursing. *The Online Journal of Issues in Nursing, 12*(1), 6.

Magyary, D., Whitney, J. D., & Brown, M. A. (2006). Advancing practice inquiry: Research foundations of the practice doctorate in nursing. *Nursing Outlook, 54*(3), 139–151.

Malina, D. P., & Izlar, J. J. (2014). Education and practice barriers for CRNAs. *The Online Journal of Issues in Nursing, 19*(2), Manuscript 3. Retrieved from http://www.nursingworld.org/ MainMenuCategories/ANAMarketplace/ANAPeriodicals/OJIN/TableofContents/Vol-19-2014/ No2-May-2014/Barriers-for-Certified-Registered-Nurse-Anesthetists.html

Maxwell, T. (2003). From first to second generation professional doctorate. *Studies in Higher Education, 28*(3), 279–291.

McKenna, H. (2005). Doctoral education: Some treasonable thoughts. *International Journal of Nursing Studies, 42*, 245–246.

McKenna, H., & Cutcliffe, J. (2001). Nursing doctoral education in the United Kingdom and Ireland. *The Online Journal of Issues in Nursing, 6*(2). Retrieved from www.nursingworld .org/MainMenuCategories/ANAMarketplace/ANAPeriodicals/OJIN/TableofContents/ Volume62001/No2May01/ArticlePreviousTopic/UKandIrelandDoctoralEducation.aspx

McNett, M. (2006). The PhD-prepared nurse in the clinical setting. *Clinical Nurse Specialist, 20*(3), 134–138.

Meleis, A., & Dracup, K. (2005). The case against the DNP: History, timing, substance, and marginal-ization. *The Online Journal of Issues in Nursing, 10*(3), Manuscript 2. Retrieved from www.nursing world.org/MainMenuCategories/ANAMarketplace/ANAPeriodicals/OJIN/TableofContents/ Volume102005/No3Sept05/tpc28_216026.aspx

Melnyk, B., & Davidson, S. (2009). Creating a culture of innovation in nursing education through shared vision, leadership, interdisciplinary partnerships, and positive deviance. *Nursing Administration Quarterly, 33*(4), 288–295.

Melnyk, B. M., & Fineout-Overholt, E. (2011). *Evidence-based practice in nursing & healthcare: A guide to best practice* (2nd ed.). Philadelphia, PA: Wolters Kluwer/Lippincott Williams & Wilkins.

Melosh, B. (1982). *The physician's hand: Work culture and conflict in American nursing.* Philadelphia, PA: Temple University Press.

Mundinger, M. O. (2005). Who's who in nursing: Bringing clarity to the doctor of nursing practice. *Nursing Outlook, 53*, 173–176.

Mundinger, M. O. (2009). The clinical doctorate 15 years hence. *Clinical Scholars Review, 2*(2), 35–36.

Mundinger, M. O., Kane, R., Lenz, E., Totten, A., Tsai, W., Cleary, P., . . . Shelanski, M. L. (2000). Primary care outcomes in patients treated by nurse practitioners or physicians: A randomized trial. *Journal of the American Medical Association, 283*, 59–68.

Murray, B. (2000). The degree that almost wasn't: The PsyD comes of age. *The Monitor, 31*(1), 52.

National Academy of Sciences. (2005). *Advancing the nation's health needs: Committee for monitoring the nation's changing needs for biomedical, behavioral, and clinical personnel.* Washington, DC: National Academies Press.

National Association of Clinical Nurse Specialists. (2009). Position statement on the nursing practice doctorate. Retrieved from http://www.nacns.org/LinkClick.aspx?fileticket=TOZlongI258%3D& tabid=116

National Association of Clinical Nurse Specialists. (2015). NACNS position statement on the doctor of nursing practice. Retrieved from http://www.nacns.org/docs/DNP-Statement1507.pdf

National Association of Community Health Centers. (2009). America needs more primary care. Community Health Forum. Retrieved from http://www.nachc.com/client/documents/200909_ Forum_Feature_Doctors.pdf

National Forum on the Practice Doctorate. (2003). *Executive summary.* Washington, DC: Author.

National Institutes of Health. (2009a). Mentored patient-oriented research career development award (Parent K23), program announcement (PA) Number: PA-10-060. Retrieved from http://grants2 .nih.gov/grants/guide/pa-files/PA-10-060.html

National Institutes of Health. (2009b). Part II full text of announcement. Section I. Funding opportunity description. 1. Research objectives. In: Institutional Clinical and Translational Science Award (U54), RFA-RM-07-007. Retrieved from http://grants.nih.gov.ezproxy2.library.drexel.edu/grants/ guide/rfa-files/RFA-RM-07-007.html

National League for Nursing. (2007). Master's education in nursing June 2010. Retrieved from http:// www.nln.org/about/position-statements/nln-reflections-dialogue/read/dialogue-reflection/ 2010/06/02/reflection-dialogue-6---master's-education-in-nursing-june-2010

National League for Nursing Accrediting Commission. (2005). NLNAC statement on clinical practice doctorates. Retrieved from http://www.nlnac.org/statementClinPrac.htm

National League for Nursing Commission for Nursing Education Accreditation. (2016). General questions. Retrieved from http://www.nln.org/accreditation-services/faqs

National Organization of Nurse Practitioner Faculties. (2006). Doctor of Nursing Practice (DNP) Related Statements: Response to recommendations on clinical hours & degree title. Retrieved from http:// www.nonpf.com/displaycommon.cfm?an=1&subarticlenbr=16 [Historical document, verified 11/29/2016, under Protected View]

National Organization of Nurse Practitioner Faculties. (2012). Nurse practitioner core competencies, amended 2012. Retrieved from http://c.ymcdn.com/sites/www.nonpf.org/resource/resmgr/ competencies/npcorecompetenciesfinal2012.pdf

National Organization of Nurse Practitioner Faculties. (2016). Background paper: Transitioning to a seamless, integrated DNP NP curriculum. Retrieved from http://c.ymcdn.com/sites/www.nonpf .org/resource/resmgr/Docs/DNPSeamlessTransitionNONPFFi.pdf

National Panel for Nurse Practitioner Practice Doctorate Competencies (2006). Practice doctorate nurse practitioner entry-level competencies. Retrieved from http://c.ymcdn.com/sites/www.nonpf .org/resource/resmgr/competencies/dnp%20np%20competenciesapril 2006.pdf

Neal, A. (2008). Seeking higher-ed accountability: Ending federal accreditation. *Change: The Magazine of Higher Education Regulation*, 25–29.

Nelson, M. (2002). Education for professional nursing practice: Looking backward into the future. *The Online Journal of Issues in Nursing, 7*(3), Manuscript 3. Retrieved from www.nursingworld .org/MainMenuCategories/ANAMarketplace/ANAPeriodicals/OJIN/TableofContents/ Volume72002/No2May2002/EducationforProfessionalNursingPractice.aspx

Nichols, E. F., & Chitty, K. K. (2005). Educational patterns in nursing. In K. K. Chitty & B. P. Black (Eds.), *Professional nursing: Concepts and challenges* (3rd ed., pp. 31–62). Philadelphia, PA: Saunders.

Nowotny, H., Scott, P., & Gibbons, M. (2001). *Re-thinking science: Knowledge and the public in an age of uncertainty.* Cambridge, UK: Polity Press.

Nurse Practitioner Roundtable. (2008). *Nurse practitioner DNP education, certification and titling: A unified statement.* Washington, DC: Author.

Nutting, M. A. (1912). *The educational status of nursing: U.S. Bureau of Education Bulletin. No. 7.* Washington, DC: U.S. Government: Printing Office.

O'Sullivan, A. L. (2005). The practice doctorate in nursing. *The Mentor: The NONPF Newsletter, 16*(1), 1–2, 12.

Pearson, A., Wiechula, R., Court, A., & Lockwood, C. (2007). A re-consideration of what constitutes "evidence" in the healthcare professions. *Nursing Science Quarterly, 20*(1), 85–88.

Peplau, H. E. (1952). *Interpersonal relations in nursing.* New York, NY: G. P. Putnam.

Peplau, H. E. (1988). The art and science of nursing: Similarities, differences, and relations. *Nursing Science Quarterly, 1*(1), 8–15.

Peterson, D. R. (1997). *Educating professional psychologists: History and guiding conception.* Washington, DC: American Psychological Association.

Potempa, K. M., Redman, R. W., & Anderson, C. A. (2008). Capacity for the advancement for nursing science: Issues and challenges. *Journal of Professional Nursing, 24,* 329–336.

President and Fellows of Harvard University. (2016). Doctor of philosophy in education. Retrieved from http://www.gse.harvard.edu/doctorate/doctor-philosophy-education

Reed, P. G. (2006). The practice turn in nursing epistemology. *Nursing Science Quarterly, 19*(1), 36–38.

Reel, S. (2009). *The role of research and rigor in DNP programs: The ongoing debate.* Paper presented at the Second National Conference on the Doctor of Nursing Practice: The Dialogue Continues..., Hilton Head Island, SC, March 24–27, 2009.

Robert Wood Johnson Foundation. (2015). In historic shift, more nurses graduate with bachelor's degrees. Retrieved from http://www.rwjf.org/en/library/articles-and-news/2015/09/more-nurses-with-bachelors-degrees.html

Rubenstein, D. (2009). The nurse-crusader goes to Washington. *New York Observe.* Retrieved from http://www.observer.com/2009/nurse-crusader-goes-washington

Rubio, D. M., Schoenbaum, E. E., Lee, L. S., Schteingart, D. E., Marantz, P. R., Anderson, K. E.,…Platt, L. D. (2010). Defining translational research: Implications for training. *Academic Medicine, 85*(3), 470–475.

Rudy, E., & Grady, P. (2005). Biological researchers: Building nursing science. *Nursing Outlook, 53,* 88–94.

Salsberg, E. (2015, April 9). Recent trends in the nursing pipeline: U.S. educated BSNs continue to increase. Health Affairs Blog. Retrieved from http://healthaffairs.org/blog/2015/04/09/recent-trends-in-the-nursing-pipeline-us-educated-bsns-continue-to-increase

Salzman, A. (2010). The DPT degree: Our destiny or a cosmetic change? *Advance for Physical Therapy & PT Assistants, 14*(4), 55.

San Francisco AIDS Foundation. (2008). Confronting the "evidence" in evidence-based HIV prevention: Summary report. *HIV Evidence-Based Prevention,* 1–5.

Sayette, M. A., Mayne, T. J., & Norcross, J. C. (2010). *Insider's guide to graduate programs in clinical and counseling psychology.* New York: NY: Guilford.

Schlotfeldt, R. M. (1978). The professional doctorate: Rationale and characteristics. *Nursing Outlook, 26,* 302–311.

Silver, H. K., Ford, L. R., & Day, L. R. (1968). The pediatric nurse–practitioner program: Expanding the role of the nurse to provide increased health care for children. *Journal of the American Medical Association, 204*(4), 298–302.

Smith Glasgow, M. E., & Dreher, H. M. (2010). The future of oncology nursing science: Who will generate the knowledge? *Oncology Nursing Forum, 37*(4), 393–396.

Smith, M. E., & Dreher, H. M. (2003). Wanted, nursing faculty! If you think the nursing shortage is bad, the nursing faculty shortage is worse. *Advance for Nursing, 5,* 31–32.

Society for Human Resource Management. (2013). 2013 Employee benefits: An overview of employee benefits offerings in the U.S. Retrieved from https://www.shrm.org/research/surveyfindings/articles/documents/13-0245%202013_empbenefits_fnl.pdf

Sperhac, A. M., & Clinton, P. (2008). Doctorate of nursing practice: Blueprint for excellence. *Journal of Pediatric Health Care, 22*(3), 146–151.

Stew, G. (2009). *The professional/practice nursing doctorate in the United Kingdom.* Paper presented at the Second National Conference on the Doctor of Nursing Practice: The Dialogue Continues…, Hilton Head Island, SC, March 24–27, 2009.

Stewart, D. (2009). *Challenges and opportunities for the professional doctorate: A North American perspective.* Paper presented at the European Conference on the Professional Doctorate, London, England, November 5–6, 2009.

Terry, A. J. (2014). *Clinical research for the doctor of nursing practice degree* (2nd ed.). Burlington, MA: Jones & Bartlett.

Texas Higher Education Coordinating Board. (2013). *White paper: The doctor of nursing practice degree.* Retrieved from http://www.thecb.state.tx.us/reports/PDF/2963.PDF?CFID=41003217&CFTOKEN=99921138

Townsend, B. K. (2002). *Rethinking the EdD, or what's in a name.* Paper presented at the Annual Meeting of the Association for the Study of Higher Education, Sacramento, CA, November 21–24, 2002.

Trainor, J. (2016, October 25). Gender pay gap could take 170 years to close, says World Economic Forum. *theguardian.* Retrieved from https://www.theguardian.com/business/2016/oct/25/gender-pay-gap-170-years-to-close-world-economic-forum-equality

Tri-Council for Nursing. (2014). Tri-Council for nursing senate letter. Retrieved from http://www.aacn.nche.edu/government-affairs/FY15-TC-Senate-Request.pdf

Trossman, S. (2009). Nurses discuss economy, DNP degree, care in the ED. *The American Nurse,* 1, 8.

University of South Florida. (2015). Faculty salary adjustment. Retrieved from http://health.usf.edu/facultyaffairs/facultysalary

Valian, V. (2005). Beyond gender schemas: Improving the advancement of women in academia. *Hypatia, 20*(3), 198–213.

Valiga, T. (2004). *The nursing faculty shortage: A national perspective.* Congressional briefing presented by the A. N. S. R. Alliance, Hart Senate Office Building, Washington, DC.

Vincent, D., Johnson, C., Velasquez, D., & Rigney, T. (2014). DNP-prepared nurses as practitioner-researchers: Closing the gap between research and practice. *Web NP Online*. Retrieved from http://www.doctorsofnursingpractice.org/wp-content/uploads/2014/08/Vincet_et_al.pdf

Vreeland, E. M. (1964). Nursing research programs of the public health service: Highlights and trends. *Nursing Research, 13*(2), 148–158.

Webber, P. (2008). The doctor of nursing practice degree and research: Are we making an epistemological mistake. *Journal of Nursing Education, 47*(10), 466–472.

Werley, H. H., & Westlake, S. K. (1985). Impact of nursing research on public policy: An examination of ANA research priority statements. *Journal of Professional Nursing, 1*(3), 148–151, 154–156.

Williams, J. C., & Richardson, V. T. (2010). New millennium, same glass ceiling? The impact on law firm compensation systems on women. A joint report of the Project for Attorney Retention, Minority Corporate Counsel Association. Retrieved from http://www.pardc.org/Publications/SameGlassCeiling.pdf

Wilkes, L. M., & Mohan, S. (2008). Nurses in the clinical area: Relevance of a PhD. *Collegian, 15,* 135–141.

Zungolo, E. (2009). *The DNP and the faculty role: Issues and challenges.* Paper presented at the Second National Conference on the Doctor of Nursing Practice: The Dialogue Continues..., Hilton Head Island, SC, March 24–27, 2010.

Reflective Response

Lynne M. Dunphy

This first chapter of the second edition of this book provides a vigorous, excellently argued overview of the rich discourse that follows throughout the textbook, as references are cited throughout the chapter to later content. Dreher has made a strong choice on the use of the term *political path* in the title, as the convoluted story of the evolution of this role is fraught with political (and social) implications that are difficult to summarize, synthesize, and explain. Here, Dreher succeeds admirably. He also does not attempt to bring premature closure to some of these complex and deep (in the sense of knowledge development and philosophy of science) issues. These issues have only intensified and multiplied. He challenges the reader to think through the many potential implications of the previous courses of action in *nursing* that have influenced the evolution of doctoral education in nursing in general and the development of the doctorate of nursing practice in particular. I would suggest, this chapter could use additional work—and I would direct the readers of the text to this task—in the further description of nursing in the context of broader historical trends and sociopolitical disciplinary environments in general. Dreher cites the work of labor historian Barbara Melosh, as well as provides the context to ideas about knowledge development by comparing and contrasting the doctorate of nursing practice programs with the evolution of the PysD, for example, in psychology, and similar disciplinary endeavors in pharmacology (the PharmD), physical therapy, and public health, and even occasionally medicine.

However admirable the work of Melosh (which this author by and large endorses), it is only one viewpoint on nursing's rich history. Also, it begs the question of larger issues in the evolution of science, technology, and therapeutics in general across the 20th century, as well as the rise (and fall) of other health professions in the same time frame (medicine comes to mind), and the even broader cultural, political, and social changes that framed the times and these issues. So, I would see the readers of this text being guided to a broader variety of other historical and sociological readings with which to frame the nursing-specific *debates, power plays, and dissension.*

I would also direct the reader to the work of David Allen, critical social theorist in nursing, who was one of the first in nursing to raise the issue (along with Melosh, to be fair) of the limits of advanced education as a "professionalizing strategy" for nursing (Allen, 1986). Historians and sociologists have also pointed out the use of "education" as a pseudonym for class, pointing out that in medicine, requiring the prerequisite of a baccalaureate degree prior to admission to medical school, assured a steady stream of well-educated (read: "well-bred" as in "invariably well-off enough" to be able to AFFORD education) young gentlemen, of a certain class. Has anything *really* changed here? If anything, this situation has exacerbated. How many bright young individuals, male or female, interested in a career in health care, are able to sustain the arduous path of admission to medical school without major support, be it economic, social, or psychological? Equally, any historical and political analysis cannot afford to ignore the gender issue in nursing, as tedious as this discussion may be to some. How many nurses in their 40s and 50s that return for the PhD have spent years raising children, supporting family, putting their own educational aspirations aside? When it is time for "them" they choose *pursuit of knowledge* rather than mere pleasure, perhaps having been frustrated in their early youth by economic demands, or perhaps as part of an ongoing quest toward social status and respect. Ethel Manson Fenwick, organizer of the British Nurses Association and the editor of the first British journal of nursing (*Nursing Record*), aptly summed up the situation in 1887 when she said, "The Nurse question is the Women question, pure and simple. We have to run the gauntlet of those historic rotten eggs" (Fenwick, quoted in Baer, 1997, pp. 256–257). Has anything *really* changed?

When one examines the evolution of the nurse practitioner (NP) role broadly speaking, within its social context, one gets a sense of the "grass-roots" nature of its development—a response to a social need for primary care (Dunphy, 2012). NP programs sprung up willy-nilly; certifications and continuing education programs abounded for practicing diploma-prepared nurses to become "nurse practitioners." In contrast, as broadly observed and described in this chapter, the DNP evolved as a much more "top-down" movement, springing from ideas of influential nurse leaders and educators (nurse *professionalizers*) as actualized in various nursing organizations like the American Association of Colleges of Nursing (AACN) and the National Organization of Nurse Practitioner Faculties (NONPF). Against the broader backdrop of history, and societal need for health care, debates over titling, splitting hairs over the differentiation of the PhD, DNS, DNSc, and DNP (so well outlined in this chapter!) will in all likelihood continue. Critical issues face us in terms of the need for numbers of future nursing faculty and nurse educators. Is nursing knowledge advancing and contributing to positive change? The unresolved issues of education and research in DNP education continue to be "clear as mud." And the speed of change is only accelerating. How can we best position ourselves as a discipline and a profession to meet current challenges and anticipate future demands? Medicine provides a pathway for MD/PhD education. With a large pool of DNP graduates, many of who *want* to teach—or ideally have a mix of practice and teaching and in some cases research—why not develop DNP–PhD pathways that may enhance both? Most programs have students who have switched from one to the other once on the "path" to doctoral education.

Although as an academic I applaud the need for "tight" definition and appreciate fully the implications in this endeavor in defining knowledge development, curriculum, and the like, some of these issues emerge as "small"—and possibly petty—when confronted with the magnitude of human need for health care and the subsequent need for nursing *action*. Thus, I posit a broader frame for examining these continually important and compelling issues in nursing.

Role Theory and the Evolution of Professional Roles in Nursing

H. Michael Dreher and Jeannine Uribe

In the most explicit sense, the "role" of the RN *defines* the work of the RN. In other words: What are the job functions of the RN? What are the role boundaries of the RN? How did the evolution of the work of the RN advance to be a professional role? (Fritter & Shimp, 2016; Haase, 1990; Zerwekh & Claborn, 2009). As one reflects on the history of nursing, one can appreciate the struggles of the profession today. The very first formal program for nursing in the United States was a 6-month training curriculum established at the Women's Hospital in Philadelphia in 1863 by physician Emmeline Horton Clevelend, MD, an 1855 alumna of the Women's Medical College of Pennsylvania, the world's first medical college for women (Robinson, 1946).[1] The historical and operational creation of the job description of an RN is discussed in this chapter, because one can make assumptions about the role of the advanced practice nurse only after having some clarity about the role of the RN. Furthermore, with the advent of the still relatively new Doctor of Nursing Practice (DNP) degree, the role of the *doctoral advanced practice nurse* (DAPN) then needs to be reflected on and addressed (Dreher & Montgomery, 2009).[2] Moreover, some serious questions need to be asked and answered: What should the *role* of the DAPN be? How is it or how should it be different from the roles of the master's-prepared advanced practice nurse? If the roles are not different now and will not differ substantively in the future, then the nursing profession has a problem. Finally, if a more highly educated advanced practice nurse with a doctorate degree does not improve health, then why bother with the expense and effort of another degree? This chapter lays some of the groundwork with which to answer these questions in this text. Moreover, after more than a decade with nurses in critical impact numbers attaining the DNP degree, is it not time for a new acronym to describe this—*DAPN* for the doctoral advanced practice nurse and *DAPRN*—for a description of the practice-doctorate-educated traditional advanced practice registered nurse (APRN) who is a nurse practitioner, nurse-midwife, nurse anesthetist, or clinical nurse specialist?

This chapter is not meant to be a history of American nursing, which has been excellently provided by Donohue (1996) in *Nursing, the Finest Art: An Illustrated History* (1996); Reverby's (1987) *Ordered to Care: The Dilemma of American Nursing, 1850–1945*; and by Judd, Sitzman, and Davis (2009) in *A History of American Nursing: Trends and Eras*.

Robinson (1946) has also written an outstanding text that focuses on the history of nursing globally, but it ends with nurses still active in World War II. This chapter, however, is historical in its approach. What we wish to do differently is to trace the role of nurses (their work) from its early American origins to the emergence of professional nursing roles. Dreher reviews the meaning of *role* or *work roles* and discusses how the theoretical aspects of role theory have influenced nursing as a profession. Uribe, a nurse historian, will then trace the evolution of these roles (or work roles) in nursing from Nightingale to just after the turn of the 20th century in the United States, and then through the evolution of the "professional registered nurse" educated at the baccalaureate level in the mid-1960s. As we all know, the American Nurses Association's (ANA's) historic 1965 position statement, which called for all RNs to be educated at the baccalaureate level, tragically was never realized (Donley & Flaherty, 2002). Despite the ANA's reaffirmation of that position in 1985, the majority of nurses in the United States is still not first educated at the bachelor of science in nursing (BSN) level, with associate degree (AD)-level nurses (and to lesser, but additive effect) predominating (Aiken, Cheung, & Olds, 2009; Dreher, 2008a; Health Resources and Services Administration, National Center for Health Workforce Analysis, 2013; Kraus, 1980).[3] Linda Aiken et al., have long reported better health-related outcomes for hospitals that deliver care by BSN-prepared nurses over the care delivered by non-BSN-prepared nurses (Aiken et al., 2011, 2014; Aiken, Clarke, Cheung, Sloane, & Silber, 2003). More recently, she and her new European colleagues indicated a 10% increase in the proportion of nurses with BSNs was associated with a 7% decrease in patient deaths. Although trends point to increasing percentages of all RNs attaining the baccalaureate degree, the question is whether there are forces that can still undermine BSN education and thwart the new goals of the Institute of Medicine report from 2010 *The Future of Nursing: Leading Change, Advancing Health,* which calls for 80% BSN-prepared nurses by 2020. What is still driving AD nursing education? Is it an issue of economics: A 2-year degree obviously costs less than a 4- or 5-year baccalaureate degree?[4] The Magnet® movement that encourages (some think they require 80% of the staff to have the BSN, but this cannot be verified) hospital-based RNs to pursue higher education, probably is helpful. But does the public not view nursing as a profession and, as a result, a significant number of potential nurses are steered toward AD programs, which still predominate (approximately 1,100+ associate degree in nursing [ADN] programs versus 700+ BSN programs; American Association of Colleges of Nursing [AACN], 2015)?

Whether this decades old issue over the entry level for basic professional nursing practice will ever be fully resolved is unknown. The politics behind the support of AD (and thus Community College education) is enormous. Furthermore, a very antiquated federal formula that funnels Medicare's "pass-through" funds still favors hospital-based (or hospital-connected) RN diploma, CRNA nurse anesthesia, and medical education, over BSN and graduate nursing education (AACN, 2015; Aiken et al., 2009). It is therefore not surprising that there is continuing controversy over whether the doctorate will ever fully replace the master's degree for entry-level advanced nursing practice. Do you envision all 50 various state legislatures changing their respective nurse practice acts to eliminate the master's degree requirement in favor of the doctorate? This is an interesting question.

Having defined what the roles of the professional nurse were through the mid-1960s, Chapter 3 focuses on the evolution of what came to be known as "advanced practice nursing" roles. The first iteration of advanced practice nursing began with the certificate pediatric nurse practitioner movement at the University of Colorado in 1965 and culminated in the 1990s with the master's of nursing science as the requirement for all advanced practice nurses (Dreher, 2009; Ford & Silver, 1967). Finally, Chapter 4 builds on these chapters and provides both a contemporary and futuristic analysis of what roles the DAPN possesses or should possess. The central thesis of Chapter 4 is: "How do doctoral advanced practice nursing roles differ, or how should they differ, from master's advanced practice nursing roles?" In a real sense, the specific role of DAPNs, the sphere of influence they will cast, the boundaries of their work, and what they will do with a DNP degree that is explicitly different, are still evolving. In other words, the history of the role of the DNP graduate is being written as you live it.

■ ROLE AND ROLE THEORY IN THE PROFESSION OF NURSING

Perhaps the seminal book on role theory in the health professions is *Role Theory: Perspectives for Health Professionals*, first published by Hardy and Conway in 1979 followed by a second edition in 1988. Unfortunately, the book did not have a third edition. This chapter extends only some of the work of their contributors and analyzes the content that would specifically pertain to role theory for present-day DAPNs. The term *role* is largely a sociological one (Biddle, 1986). However, its sociological application has universal meaning for society at both the individual and the group level and for disciplines that are accorded the status of a profession where roles and role functions are important.

ROLES IN THE PROFESSION

Although the early classical professions were divinity, law, and medicine (Klass, 1961), more contemporary definitions of a *profession* include nursing, dentistry, engineering, architecture, social work, accountancy, and others. Professions such as nursing are different from other types of work, as the work of the professional nurse is characterized by the following: professional autonomy; a clearly defined, highly developed, specialized, and theoretical knowledge base; control of training, certification, and licensing of those newly entering the profession; self-governing and self-policing authority; an explicit ethical code especially pertaining to professional ethics; and a commitment to public service (Burbules & Densmore, 1991). A very recent analysis of the word *profession* emphasizes that what makes the work of the professional nurse different from, for example, the work of an engineer is that there is a distinctive reliance on interpersonal skills and on ethical codes of work behavior (Dreher & Dahnke, 2016).

A separate discussion, and not the focus of this chapter, is whether nurses with associate degrees in nursing are also professionals. Although the Carnegie Foundation and the Institute of Medicine (2010) have both come out strongly in support of a more highly educated nursing workforce (Benner, Sutphen, Leonard, & Day, 2009), many take the position that, while nursing *is* a profession, some practitioners (without a baccalaureate degree) are technically *not professionals* (AACN, 2000; Barter & McFarland, 2001). Liaschenko and Peter (2004) even declare that nursing is not a profession, but simply "work." Melosh (1982) also flatly writes: "nursing is not and cannot be a profession" (p. 15). Certainly, Melosh was historically correct in her critique in 1982 when she wrote: "Clearly, nurses never gained the large measure of control over their work that defines a profession" (p. 19). She further indicated that, by classical definitions of a profession, "Professionals are their own bosses" (p. 15) and "If professions maintain their authority through controlling the division of labor related to their work...then doctors' own professionalization organizes and requires nurses' subordination" (p. 19). Perhaps this was true in 1982 (except where military nurses could outrank their physician colleagues then and now), but in 2016, 23 states (including the District of Columbia) allow completely independent nurse practitioner practices (American Association of Nurse Practitioners, 2016; Ferris, 2001; Pearson, 2010).[5] There is even a very reputable blog (its authors have previously won *American Journal of Nursing* [*AJN*] Book-of-the-Year awards) that presents a very modern case for why nursing is a profession (truthaboutnursing.org, 2015). By contemporary standards, at least by Melosh's definition, some nurses are indeed autonomous and classically "professional." Furthermore, that would mean that the profession of nursing is legitimately partly professional, too. This chapter, however, focuses on the roles of doctoral-educated advanced practice nursing professionals that have evolved from the emergence of professional nursing roles, but the ongoing debate about the nature of the professionalism of nursing continues. Because the health of our citizenry is so important, the roles of nursing professionals are particularly critical to both the development of the profession itself and their impact on society because of the highly skilled work they perform.

Role and Its Meaning for New DNP Graduates

At its most basic level, *role* can be defined as "a socially expected behavior pattern usually determined by an individual's status in a particular society" (Role, 2010). A more precise sociological view would characterize *role* as occurring within systems (or organizations, or relationships), and therefore a *role* can be considered a "set of systems states and actions of a subsystem, of an organization, including its interactions with other systems of nonsystem elements" (Kuhn, 1974, p. 298). These definitional frameworks lead us to conceptualize an operational definition of the word *role* for nursing. It is suggested that nursing roles are professional, socially constructed, operationalized behaviors that form the boundaries of what a professional nurse does. It is only through a thorough analysis of the work of RNs and the roles they play, enact, or fulfill in the course of their professional work can one ascertain what are *advanced (practice) nursing roles*.

Finally, what differs or extends the boundaries of advanced practice to doctoral advanced (practice) nursing roles? In theory, it sounds very simple. In actuality, we believe that it is more complex. Multiple discussions have ensued in our DNP seminars in the past 5 years about nursing roles and the nature of advanced practice nursing. For example, in the scenario of an overweight or obese patient with accompanying negative health conditions that need intervention, how does the 20-minute primary care interaction of an adult nurse practitioner and patient differ operationally from the physician–patient interaction (Dreher, 2008b)? This kind of discussion is particularly germane to DAPNs, who must now identify how their roles and role functions will be different and *more advanced* than when they had a master's degree. Again, the authors contend that if the skill set is the same, then nursing has a weakened debate calling for a practice nursing doctorate. Meleis's work (1975; Meleis & Trangenstein, 1994) on role transitions is still very well applicable to today's doctoral advanced practice graduate, especially one who practiced previously with the master's degree. In her 2011 book, Meleis suggests, "Role insufficiency may be manifested in assuming any new roles..." (p. 2), and further indicates that there are "some losses and gains in their different roles and support systems" (p. 3). Smith Glasgow et al. addressed some of the role strain among DNP students in this text's first edition and in a replication study in Chapter 10. But we suspect there is more role strain among DNP graduates than has penetrated the nursing literature. Cusson (Cusson & Strange, 2008; Cusson & Viggiano, 2002) has written extensively about nurse practitioner role transitions, especially among neonatal nurse practitioners. The authors are aware that Dr. Cusson is currently extending her work to role transitions among doctoral advanced practice graduates and it is precisely this kind of outcome data that the profession needs.

Sociological Schools of Thought on Roles

There are two very prominent sociological schools of thought on roles and social inter-actions that serve as frameworks or even paradigms in which individuals, institutions, and systems operate. In Table 2.1, the *functionalist* view, as mostly attributed to the emi-nent sociologist Emile Durkeim (1964), and the competing *symbolic interaction* perspec-tive best articulated by Mead (1934), Cooley (1964), and Blumer (1969) are summarized.

In a functionalist view, or in structural–functional theory, the roles that individu-als play in society evolve out of very organic systems that constantly interact and are somewhat predictable. For example, in the case of the professional nurse, there is a need in society for nurses to perform certain roles (e.g., health educator, caregiver, advocate), and thus most nurses employ those roles in their daily work. DAPNs, however, are in a

TABLE 2.1 **Two Perspectives on Roles in Social Interactions**

Functionalist View (Macro-Sociological Analysis)	Symbolic Interactionist View (Micro-Sociological Analysis)
Focus of perspective is on the group and its demarcation into smaller subgroups, units, and systems.	Focus of perspective is on the individual interacting and the symbolic interpretation of both verbal and nonverbal behavior and cures.
Objects and persons are stimuli that act on an individual.	An individual constructs objects on the basis of his ongoing activity. He gives meaning to objects and makes decisions on the basis of his judgments.
Action is a release or response to what the situational norms demand.	The individual decides what he wishes to do and how he will do it. He takes account of external and internal cues, interpreting their significance for his action.
Environmental forces act to "produce" behavior.	By a process of self-indication, an individual accepts, rejects, or transforms the meaning (impact) of such forces.
Prescriptions for action, or norms, dictate appropriate behaviors. They are social facts.	Others' attitudes are the basis for individual lines of action.
An act is a unitary, bounded phenomenon; that is, it starts and stops.	An act is disclosed over time and what the end of the act will be cannot be foretold at the start.
The act (of an actor) will be followed by the response of another with or without any interpretation taking place on the part of the other.	An act is validated by the response of another.
Persons act on the basis of a generally objective reality; that is, learned responses.	Reality is defined by each actor; one defines a situation as he "sees it" and acts on this perception.
People are socially molded, not forced, to perform societal functions.	Social order is maintained when people share their understanding of everyday behavior.
Group action is the expression of societal demands and shared social values.	Group action is the expression of individuals confronting their life situations.

Adapted from Conway (1988, p. 65).

very different place functionally. Society does not yet know exactly what roles they will play (or be required to fill), and the new domain of this *doctoral advanced practice* is being created in real time, even as this text is published.

We, therefore, propose that the functionalist view of the roles of the professional nurse, where a common socialization of RNs creates stability in the social system, may not theoretically or properly explain the unfolding role of a new type of advanced practice nurse. In a discussion of the roles of professionals, a symbolic interactionist view of DAPNs would indicate that their emerging roles would evolve from an ongoing examination of their meaning, to a vigorous self-analysis of how satisfying, effective, or well received the exhibition of the role is. In other words, the critical feedback this new practitioner receives, processes, interprets, and reinterprets will ultimately reinforce the role being integrated and assimilated in a new domain of practice. In the study "What Do People Need Psychiatric and Mental Health Nurses For?," Jackson and Stevenson (2000) describe the utility of using this critical feedback from patients (which may not be explicit) to answer this question. Similarly, Erving Goffman's (1955) original theory of "face work," which is described by Shattell (2004) as the face of the nurse interacting with the face of the patient in the simplicity or ordinariness of any basic nurse–patient interaction, is an example of how symbolic interaction theory may be highly useful in explaining how two different dyadic DAPN roles may evolve.

First, what is the new DAPN/patient role? Second, what is the new DAPN role in relation to professional clinicians in other health care disciplinary colleagues? On an operational level, these questions are: (a) How will the individual patient perceive Dr. Jane Smith's role as a nursing primary care provider now using the title "Dr."? (b) How will fellow health profession colleagues perceive the new role of the DAPN as *doctoral prepared*, not master's prepared? Will patients have different expectations? Will colleagues have different expectations? Indeed, Goffman in his classic sociological text *A Presentation of Self in Everyday Life* (1959) writes, "When an individual enters the presence of others, they commonly seek to acquire information about him or to bring into play information about him already possessed" (p. 1). Will this new type of advanced practice nurse use the face-to-face feedback to create solutions to any new role conflict or role strain that may occur? Although role conflict and role strain in the DAPN are addressed in Chapter 10 by Smith Glasgow, Zoucha, and Johnson, both sociological concepts are not new to nursing. However, there are likely particular nuances that are different from the role conflict and role strain of the newly educated, master's-prepared advanced practice nurse.

Another important concept in symbolic interaction is that of *role-taking*. Role-taking is a key mechanism of interaction that permits us to take another person's perspective and to see what our actions might mean to the other actors with whom we interact (Schell & Kayser-Jones, 1999). One scholar suggests that the outcome of role-taking is not just the *processing of the influence of the interaction* on behavior, but requires overt behavioral change based on the processing of those interactions (Cast, 2004). In other words, in the DAPN role, the new practitioner is likely to not just think differently, but also to act differently as new face–work interactions with patient and colleagues are experienced. We contend that this change in perspective and change in thinking is more likely to occur as the new practitioner engages in more reflective practice. Johns and Freshwater (2005) are leading scholars supporting the practice of reflection in advanced nursing practice and they build and extend the classical work of Schön (1983) who coined the concepts of "reflection in action" and "reflection on action." In Chapter 19, Stew writes about how reflective practice ought to be even more mature and developed in the DNP/ professional doctorate nursing graduate. With deep reflection about this new role and consideration of what it is or should be (and conversely what it is no longer), the new practitioner is thus likely to experience ambiguity as he or she tries to "figure this new role out." Our view is that the experience of ambiguity is not detrimental, but a sign of progress. As the new practitioner engages in activities that lead to more secure role delineation, we think the ambiguity will lessen. Hopefully, patients will respond differently and positively to the confidence and enhanced skill set of the DNP graduate. Over time, we predict that health profession colleagues will respond similarly.

A vigorous curricular focus on the concept of role is particularly important for the student pursuing a DNP degree. However, it is not likely that the expansion and ultimate role delineation of the DNP graduate will be entirely noncontroversial or always well received. There will be resistance from current master's-prepared nurse practitioners, nurse-midwives, nurse anesthetists, and clinical nurse specialists who will claim your practice is not different (or better?) than theirs. If their argument prevails, then a given institution, perhaps, may not compensate the doctoral graduate more highly. Thus, in supporting doctoral advanced nursing practice, we are unyielding in our plea that the necessary outcome data must be conducted and disseminated. Nevertheless, there is a bountiful amount of optimism in the profession about your future and this new degree, and as one recent graduate has recently written:

> Since attaining my doctorate, I find myself better equipped to build upon my master's level training. I'm no longer satisfied with doing the "how to," but indeed now relish and crave the "why?" and the "why not?" As a doctoral advanced practice nurse, I am different! (Dreher and Montgomery, 2009, p. 530)

We anticipate that in your new role you will also be different.

■ EMERGENCE OF PROFESSIONAL ROLES IN NURSING: RISING FROM THE TOIL OF PUBLIC HEALTH NURSES

It is with some incredulity that public health nurses are not more duly recognized for their role in the evolution of our discipline. Furthermore, while Nightingale's preeminence still reigns over nursing, her vision for nursing was enacted very differently in the United States. In many ways, the rise of modern nursing has been accomplished despite tension from two equally dogmatic nursing subcultures—the *conservative traditionalists* and the *elite professionalizers* (Melosh, 1982; Reverby, 1987). And as quarrelsome as these two camps have been, progress has indeed been made, and nursing is probably more advanced here than in any other place on the globe.

THE IMPACT OF NIGHTINGALE

The Nightingale Influence

Florence Nightingale wrote about patients and nursing, beginning a revolution of the roles of nurses, represented up to that point by religious sisters or inmates living in the almshouses where they served. Her ideas on nursing included a reformed vision of employment for women, a profession removing the societal attachment to the idea of womanly work and feminine intuition, and replacing the characterization of a nurse with an educated, highly moral, and stable woman to run the wards. Her nurses required both theoretical and practical training. In Deloughery's (1977) book on the nursing profession, Nightingale changed nursing to "a career and not a last resort" (p. 61) for women in need of employment. Nightingale's ideal plan separated ward service from nursing education by making student nurses' practical experiences on the hospital wards opportunities for learning with nurse instructors and physicians, rather than just providing service to the hospital.

Scientific progress in medicine, combined with the growing promotion of social reforms in many areas, helped formulate the idea that for better outcomes physicians needed assistants to carry out their complex medical treatments. Recognizing that they were following the physician's orders, Nightingale wanted her nurses to understand the reasons for their actions, and thus promoted the idea of education. She wanted public support for nursing education, which included some medical education—a shift in thinking that was not readily accepted.

In opposition to Nightingale's educational plan for nurses were widely supported societal ideas characterizing what constituted the natural traditional work of women, and views that too much education would take away the feminine instinct that was related to delivering care. The transfer of the Nightingale tenets to hospitals in the United States altered important educational objectives, which were different from just using student nurses to fulfill the service needs of the hospital.

The Nightingale Nursing Model Becomes "Americanized"

Hospital administrators, physicians, and women in the United States studied Nightingale's ideas and brought them to hospitals that had been established since the late 18th century, staffed with employees providing care without formalized training (Rosenberg, 1987). The first nursing schools were formed by separate nursing school boards charged with planning and financing the institution. Unfortunately, poor funding removed Nightingale's ideal of student nurses in the hospitals to learn. Instead, students became the sole hospital care providers, in effect paying for their training, which lacked public support (Rosenberg, 1987). Their education became ward service, as theoretical classroom time decreased and practical experience became the teacher. The proliferation of hospitals in the 1870s increased the need for student nurses and the growth of schools of nursing, which led to a diffusion of nursing education and the graduation of a variety of levels of nurses. The reputation of nurses, as well as the quality of the care they provided both in the hospitals and in private duty positions in the home after completing training, varied.

In the late 19th and early 20th centuries, nursing leaders, including a group of women nursing superintendents, shaped nursing education and work and attempted to require prescriptively a level of consistency to nursing care, thus protecting the reputation of the schools and the work done by their graduate nurses. Although the superintendent title was mostly associated with the directors of training schools in the profession's infancy, the "nurse superintendent" was later clarified by Davis (1929) as:

> The administrator or executive head of the hospital, *not* the director of the training school. In some of the smaller hospitals (unfortunately) the two positions are combined. The nurse superintendent has her chief field in the nongovernmental charitable hospital of less than 100 beds. (Davis, 1929, p. 386)

This early cohort of leaders worked together to form committees to evaluate school curricula and the education of specialized tasks performed by nurses. They actively promoted the formation of alumni groups (and their obvious financial philanthropy) and became a formidable and interested group of active nurses. The American Society of Superintendents of Training Schools, founded in 1894, promoted leadership, higher entrance requirements for potential students, and better training schools in an effort to increase the professionalization of nursing and protect trained nurses' legitimate role in society. Renamed as the National League of Nursing Education in 1912, members aimed to encourage more women to enter nursing by pushing for progressive reforms, including shorter days, a university education, and a standard curriculum (Dock & Stewart, 1938).

The reputation of hospitals during the 1800s kept many ill people at home to be cared for by their families. With the growth of nursing training schools, those who could afford supplementary care hired a private duty nurse to come to the home to carry out physician treatments and provide skilled nursing care to the sick individual. Demand for private duty nurses increased as female family members increasingly joined the workforce. After the turn of the 20th century, hospitals also arranged for private duty nurses to provide care within the institution, which created employment opportunities for the majority of graduate nurses (Whelan, 2005). These nurse-owned and operated registries were formed to assist nurses with finding work while granting them the freedom to choose the job, although this type of autonomy did not add to the professional image of nurses. When caring for patients in their homes, nurses fought against the image of subservience, especially African American nurses, who had been kept in inferior positions by a White majority of nurses and society alike (Young, 2005). Following Nightingale's promotion of highly moral and educated women, nursing leaders from the first half of the 20th century promoted the ideal nurse to have "the exercise of superior intelligence, a large body of knowledge and skills, sensitiveness, and imagination" (Harmer & Henderson, 1939, p. 4). However, middle- and upper-class women did not join nursing in large numbers, leaving women of the lower socioeconomic class with a high school diploma to enter training (Dock & Stewart, 1938; Rosenberg, 1987).

THE TOIL AND CONTRIBUTION OF PUBLIC HEALTH NURSES TO NURSING

Nursing's Role in the Public's Health

Public health nurses had specialized knowledge and skills obtained by furthering their education after hospital training and required to be effective in the communities where they worked. Advances in medicine and science during the late 1800s, specifically the wide acceptance of the germ theory, helped change the thinking about infections and debunked the previously held moral aspects of the causes of disease (Rosen, 1993). Identifying controllable germs as the root cause for illness and disability a global initiative sprang up asking governments to take responsibility to respond to the public welfare and to subsidize improvements in community sanitation, water supplies, and other alterable situations that, if left unattended, could lead to higher morbidity and mortality rates from infectious disease. The federally funded U.S. Public Health Service (USPHS) is one example of the U.S. government's attention to the need for community services to protect the health of citizens. Although the USPHS can trace its early history back to 1798 with an act designed for the relief of sick and disabled seamen, its history was more formally established by legislation in 1889 forming the USPHS Commissioned Officer program (Williams, 1951). At first, only physicians were admitted to the Commissioned Officer Association, with the first nurses not commissioned as officers until July 1945 (Parascandola, 2007; U.S. Public Health Service Nursing, 2009). Nevertheless, nurses in the 20th century would serve a fundamental role in this agency.

At the turn of the 20th century, the continuing influx of immigrants from around the world and overcrowding in urban areas led to a renewal of social reforms in which nurses participated and started a new role for nurses: short term caring for and educating families in their homes. The settlement house movement, which flourished in many cities beginning in the late 1800s, interested many individuals from all walks of life who subscribed to a belief in social welfare, and who sought to help raise the lives of the poor immigrants (Wade, 1967). Their social activism was intentional and aimed at the social determinants of health by assisting immigrant families to acculturate to urban life in America by improving their employment, the sanitation of their living arrangements, and their health. Lillian Wald, Mary Brewster, and other nurses formed the world famous Henry Street Settlement House in New York in 1893, financed by wealthy patrons who saw the value of improving the health and welfare of the urban working poor (Buhler-Wilkerson, 1991). Living in the neighborhoods they served, nurses visited tenement homes providing nursing care and health education to all members of the family, and providing information to educate them about their capacity to care for themselves and to enhance their health. In the new role of the public health nurse another opportunity was provided to increase the professionalism of nurses due to its requirements of higher education, specialized knowledge, and a more autonomous practice (Brainard, 1985).

During the early 1900s, public health initiatives aimed to decrease disease, but the social issues connected with disease remained. Despite great efforts by public health nurses, poverty often limited individual choices and the ability to live a healthy life. Public awareness of growing health problems created the perfect link between public health and social reforms, forging a place for nurses to address health policies caused by urbanization, poverty, and disease (Porter, 1994). In recognition of this need for more specialized training for this role, Simmons College in Boston in 1904 began an 8-month course for public health nurses (Nutting, 1904). These public health nurses, referred to as *visiting nurses*, worked for two types of agencies, voluntary and official. The privately funded voluntary organizations were funded by communities and philanthropies were run by board members who hired public health nurses. Official agencies of the federal and state governments funded public health nurse positions supported by tax dollars.

The National Organization of Public Health Nurses (NOPHN), started in 1912, played a role in shaping public health nursing and attempted to bring this branch of nursing to a higher professional level. The NOPHN promoted standards of education, leadership, supervision, and employment and gave advice to groups looking to employ a public health nurse. Their journal *Public Health Nurse*, founded in 1912, was a resource for nurses and committees looking for legislation, statistics, health information, and programs. Physicians contributed to the journal, writing about communicable diseases and treatments carried out by the nurses in the home. Although NOPHN recommendations were available, there was a very limited number of employable, educated public health nurses who met them. As a result, many organizations overlooked the NOPHN's minimum standards and hired unprepared nurses to public health positions, which in many cases did not have supervisors or other nurses to assist the newly hired nurses to fulfill their job requirements (Buhler-Wilkerson, 1987). Although the hiring of public health nurses continued to rise, it was due to the increasing number of agencies hiring a single public health nurse, ultimately limiting the number of citizens who came into contact with this service (Giacomo, 1953).

With the continued rise of organized nursing and a growing diverse population, philanthropic organizations pushed for national policy reforms and programs that included positions for public health nurses and helped promote an increase in government support for employing nurses (Magat, 1989). These official agencies were funded at a variety of government levels, and employed public health nurses to address health issues in the hope of decreasing the incidence and prevalence of disease. As public funding increased with the increased incidence of communicable diseases, public health nurses had a choice of employment in official agencies sponsored by the government at the state and federal levels or in voluntary agencies, usually run by a board of community women and men (Beckemeier, 2008).

Public health nurses working in privately-funded voluntary agencies specialized in caring for the entire family in their home. They routinely visited many families each day to provide nursing care and to improve public health education practices in the home. These nurses determined the needs of the families and worked in cooperation with local boards and agencies to get services delivered. There were distinct skills required by public health nurses that were not gained from private duty or hospital experience (Dock, 1906). Hospital training did not provide the education to prepare the public health nurse to work with the acute and chronic health care needs seen in the community. In the early 1900s, public health nurses worked autonomously, caring for patients who could not afford to seek treatment from a physician (Craig, 2003). Their role thus changed with the growing organization of public health and the interest by the federal government in providing services.

Physicians Emerged Dominant Over Nurses in Public Health Role

C.-E. A. Winslow, a Yale professor, physician, and leader in public health, ranked the physician as the head of the team, but he strongly promoted nurses as integral to public health campaigns. Indeed, early on, Winslow (1911) wrote very supportively of visiting nurses, stating:

> Yet it is, I think, more and more clear that the real strategic point is by the bedside of the patient and at the elbow of the convalescent or the carrier. Here the chain of infection can be broken far more surely and more economically than at any point. (Winslow, 1911, p. 909)

In his view, however, physicians would still make the diagnosis or program decisions that public health nurses then carried out in the homes, schools, and workplaces in the community. Winslow pushed health education as the change factor for successful public health campaigns, giving the task to nurses to interpret and translate health information to groups, families, and individuals. Attempting to decrease the individual's exposure to communicable diseases, public health nurses broke down scientific health information into doable tasks to be carried out by mothers, workers, children, and teachers. Yet, although he respected their work and realized the necessity of their work in conjunction with public health education, his writings show the continued ambivalent thoughts about the professional role of the nurse. He described a public health nurse as "a community mother but armed with expert knowledge which few mothers can possess" (Winslow, 1923, p. 56).

Supported by administrators in the powerful, pro-medicine Rockefeller Foundation in the 1920s, physicians were formally designated as the public health team leaders in the governmental agencies. Universities, medical schools, and schools of public health joined to educate physicians in bacteriology, statistics, and public health principles and administration (Winslow, 1925). Graduates took positions in health departments and were given the official title of health officer. Public health nurses in official agencies were once again viewed in the position of assisting physicians to carry out public health principles and programs. Under this model, public health nurses thus lost some of the autonomy of practice in the homes of their clients and responded by shifting their focus to prevention instead of treatment.

The Public Health Nurse: More Specialized and More Professional?

The public health nurse of the first half of the 20th century had several unique roles described in the textbooks as translator, educator, advocate, and conservator of the public's health (Gardner, 1936). Debate heightened in the 1930s over whether their role should be further specialized into the different services provided, such as child health, maternal health, orthopedics, tuberculosis care, and others (Footner, 1998; Melosh, 1982). With significant medical advances (the first antimicrobial drugs were introduced and new surgical procedures invented), the profession of medicine was becoming more specialized, leading to the idea that physicians needed more specialized nurses *to assist them* (Schulz & Johnson, 2003). However, a generalist role still worked best for most agencies to deliver community nursing care efficiently, although nurses debated this issue. Families usually had several problems among various members of the household, and in order to avoid the duplication of services, a public health nurse generalist was able to enter the home and tackle whatever problem the family presented to her. The special tasks of public health nurses, the requirement for additional education, as well as their autonomy in the field outside of the agency, boosted the view of professionalization in nursing.

Indeed, even before the severance of the generalist nurse into the specialist, public health nursing became the first specialty in nursing (Allen, 1991; Alpi & Adams, 2007; Gardner, 1936). Various postgraduate courses educated graduate nurses in public health, sanitation, sociology, ethics, and other subjects to give them a better understanding of the problems as well as approaches to assist different immigrant and impoverished families. Seeing the need for specialized knowledge, nursing leaders promoted the idea of a university education for public health nurses that culminated in 1949 with the Russell Sage Foundation–sponsored Brown Report, calling for nurses to be educated in colleges and universities (Gebbie, 2009; Maraldo, Fagin, & Keenan, 1988). However, nursing continued to be burdened with a label and reputation of "women's work," rather than work that was valued as a "profession." Furthermore, physician control over nursing continued. Group and Roberts (2001) wrote "By the 1930's the American Medical Association (AMA) had established a set of committees on nursing that tightened its control" (p. 148), and the tensions between nursing and medicine would continue for decades.

THE FEDERAL RECLASSIFICATION OF NURSING CHANGES THE PROFESSION

The Emergence of the Recognized Professionalism of Nursing

Professionalism for nurses gained momentum just after the turn of the 20th century with endorsements from state and federal legislation. Lusk (1997) points out in her historical study that nursing leaders pushed and promoted the professional classification for nurses based on criteria established in the literature. However, nurses' link to service sometimes placed them in the laborer category, especially students in training whose work hours were limited to 8-hour days similar to unionized factory workers. Some nursing leaders fought against these limits to autonomous practice and gained the right for graduate nurses to set their own work hours (Lusk, 1997). Government institutions denied professional status to nurses, which left army nurses during World War I without rank or authority in battlefield hospitals (Donahue, 1985). Now with women holding the right to vote, nurses fought the federal government classification of nurses as "subprofessionals" in the 1923 legislation (Minnigerode, 1923). However, they did not have enough influence to change the category until 1935, when Harry L. Hopkins of the federal Work Progress Administration (WPA) reclassified nurses from "skilled non-manual workers" to "Class 4 professional and technical workers" in a simple federal memo (*AJN*, 1935). Nevertheless, this historic subclassification of nurses' work negatively affected their social standing, and more importantly affected the salaries they earned. Even after this important 1935 regulatory memo, the status of nurses and their work did not substantively change as the ravages of the Great Depression (1929–1940) continued and left nurses with stagnant opportunities for educational advancement (D'Antonio, 2004). However, Byers (1999) views this period as a time of an emerging liberation for all women writing:

> Women's roles began to change with World War II as many were forced to find employment and to assume more family responsibilities as a result of the financial devastation of the Great Depression and men being forced to *serve* with the Armed Forces. (Byers, 1999, p. 12)

In reality, nurses used expert knowledge, indeed some of the same knowledge used by physicians and often taught to nurses by physicians, but they were not seen as colleagues of the physicians. The public health hierarchy maintained the role of the physician as the head, responsible for making the assessments and the program decisions that directed the care and education to be delivered by the nurse. Therefore, while public health nurses developed a role in a new venue outside of the hospital and changed their work from bedside treatment of illness to health promotion and education requiring specialized knowledge, their work was still viewed within the maternal role of women and not considered by society to be "professional level work." The contemporary nursing leadership held a different view and developed education programs to promote the use of scientific knowledge when addressing issues affecting the public. Two pioneers of nursing, Lavinia Lloyd Dock and Isabel M. Stewart, both wrote very provocatively (in an almost unheard language of the day by nurses) in 1938 that nursing is not:

> A subordinate or "satellite" vocation…nursing is as old if not older than medicine and has had an independent existence for hundreds of years. The Nightingale concept of nursing was not that of a sub-caste of medicine or a "handmaid of medicine." (pp. 365–366)

They both further stated that:

> The experience of years in many countries tends to show that nursing flourishes best when it is directed and controlled by skilled and experienced nurses and given the largest possible measure of freedom for the exercise of its particular functions. (p. 367)

Earlier, the Rockefeller Foundation, a leader in public health research and education, wanted to evaluate the effectiveness of public health nursing education in order to have workers adequately trained in public health. Nurses effectively bridged the gap between science and home, bringing health teaching to families in terms they understood in incremental steps that they could take to improve their health within their surroundings. The Committee for the Study of Nursing Education, funded by the Rockefeller Foundation in 1919, studied the education requirements for public health nurses. However, due to the requirement of nurses' training, the committee decided to study hospital training also (Winslow, 1922). Josephine Goldmark subsequently wrote the influential Goldmark Report, published in 1923 (Gebbie, 2009), which found that the long and difficult hospital training using nursing students as cheap labor for the hospitals did not attract the interest of middle-class women who were thought to be able to grasp the higher level of knowledge needed to be a public health nurse. The recommendations that came out of the report called for higher entrance standards to nursing school, as well as 3 years of hospital training plus postgraduate training, which included classroom education as well as public health field work. The committee felt that these steps would encourage more middle-class women to enter nursing, thus bringing more respect to the profession. Ultimately, public health nursing became an expensive funding endeavor, because their service remained limited to the poor rather than expanding health education to all levels of society (Buhler-Wilkerson, 1985). Public health nurses' numbers decreased with the draw of nurses to meet war needs; furthermore, changes in the financial arrangements to pay nurses' salaries at the public health agencies did not garner public support (Buhler-Wilkerson, 1993).

Nursing's Status Post–World War II—The 1960s

After World War II, the specialized knowledge of the public health nurse became a basic part of nursing education, and the NOPHN blended into the ANA. In pursuing the agenda of professionalization, public health nurses attempted to bring status to all of nursing and to control their nursing work, job qualifications, and education globally. However, a shortage of educated public health nurses hampered the tremendous need to develop health programs in countries recovering from war. Many countries were building their nursing education programs and did not have established public health nursing agencies so the leaders of the World Health Organization (WHO) endorsed the usage of lesser trained workers in public health work (Cueto, 2007).

Post–World War II advancements in medicine and pharmaceuticals, and federal funding of the Hill-Burton Act (which increased the number of hospitals) changed the U.S. health care system. Nurses experienced innovative programs, such as military flight nurses caring for wounded soldiers on cargo planes and in mobile surgical units close to the battles in the Korean War (Kalisch & Kalisch, 2003). The Truman administration's promotion of the community college system in conjunction with a nursing shortage ultimately made acceptable the idea of a 2-year AD producing a college-educated nurse. However, community colleges lacked hospital affiliations and raised educational costs by the needed employment of additional clinical staff (Halloran, 1995). Public health nursing changed from a post-diploma specialty to a standard part of the baccalaureate nursing program. The Nurse Training Act (NTA) of 1964 helped fund nursing education; however, a smaller percentage funded baccalaureate nursing education, although the apprentice system of diploma training schools (still very prevalent, but decreasing in number) and community college ADN programs received a larger share of the money. Incredulously, this inequity still persists some 40-plus years later with the famed researcher, Dr. Linda Aiken, co-chair of the Council on Physician and Nurse Supply (2007), reporting:

> However, nurse education is currently balanced toward associate degree nursing (ADN) programs, which receive the bulk of federal funding for nurse education, yet few ADN graduates progress to advanced practice and faculty roles, both of which are needed. The Council urged a national effort to substantially expand BSN training. (Aiken, 2007, p. 1)

The ANA's leaders published their stance on nursing education in 1965 promoting the baccalaureate degree as the entry level for professional nurses, but with support for the associate degree for technical nursing practice (ANA, 1965). The intention was to limit the scope of practice of the technical nurse, and develop the leadership aspect of the baccalaureate nurse (Freund, 1990). Ultimately, an increased demand for nurses related to increased health care funding from the Medicare and Medicaid programs added to the persistent nursing shortage in hospitals (Lynaugh, 2007). Despite their best intentions, the nursing leadership had difficulty quantifying the intended levels of care and the lack of differentiation between roles that seemed to blend nurses together. Today, the nursing profession is well aware of its failed efforts to ensure that all nurses have a BSN. However, Donley and Flaherty (2008) write, "If you view the 1965 statement as a call to close hospital schools of nursing and to move all nursing education inside the walls of colleges or universities, then the ANA was successful in implementing its vision" (p. 1). Notwithstanding, they further state, "If, however, you view the 1965 Position Paper as a mandate for a more educated nurse force to enhance patient care, the goal has not been achieved" (Donley & Flaherty, 2008, p. 1).

The sustained progress in medical technology and nursing's emergence as a discipline in the mid- to late 1960s, again offered nurses specialized knowledge and skill in hospital settings in the newly established cardiac care units (Dreher, 2010). Small groups of specially trained nurses in these intensive observation units used the skills usually completed by physicians, which gave nurses a larger scope of practice and perhaps a boost to their professionalism (Keeling, 2004). Through skilled observation, these nurses made independent decisions to administer the needed medications based on standing orders and used the technology to save patients' lives. Keeling referred to it as "the blurry line" between medicine and nursing, because these nurses gave medications to stop arrhythmias and *then* wrote the verbal orders for physicians to sign at a later time. Increasingly in the 1960s, many nursing tasks involved using new machines and taking new measurements from them, although previously these functions had been limited to the realm of physicians. Physicians, however, embraced the capacity of the RNs to manage this ever increasing technology, as they ultimately could not manage and monitor all of this technology themselves.

Was this real progress toward more nursing professional autonomy? Or was it simply acquiescence by physicians that their work depended on the good functioning of nurses and nursing?

■ SUMMARY

From the origins of American nursing in the 1800s through the 1960s, nursing leaders gradually sought and established higher standards for nurses largely with changes in society. Woods (1996) has also recognized that the rise of professional nursing has been led primarily by nurse educators and public health nurses. Ultimately, however, those "traditionalists" and "professionalizers" (again despite their disagreement on change) did succeed in raising nursing from being simply everyday women's work to a professional career choice for women (and men to a lesser extent), giving women an economic position in the market, albeit undercompensated and still unnecessarily stereotyped. The struggle of nurses to gain true professional status continues today, as their scope of practice and their role in health care expand into the realm of a new doctoral degree, one day possibly to be required for entry into advanced practice nursing. We can only imagine how long that will take! But first, the authors of Chapter 3 will characterize the rise of the role of the first advanced practice nurses in the mid-1960s.

■ CRITICAL THINKING QUESTIONS

1. *How do you think the controversy over whether nursing is truly a profession might impact the perception of the DNP graduate by other, more common doctoral-prepared health care professionals?*
2. *As you read, there are many times in history when nursing roles changed but continued to be limited by internal and external forces. Can you identify any particular forces that might support or work against the proliferation of this new degree?*
3. *Do you agree that the role of the professional nurse is best described using a functionalist perspective, and the role of the DAPN is best described using a symbolic interactionist perspective? What about the role of the master's-prepared advanced practice nurse—is their role more structural–functional or symbolic interactionist?*
4. *Your new role will interact with two different populations: patients and colleagues. How do you envision your new role evolving with each one?*
5. *As you are most likely very early in your DNP curriculum, do you already have ideas about how you want your doctoral role to be different from your master's role?*
6. *As a future nursing leader, how can you use historical research for problem solving? In other words, can knowledge of the past prepare one for the future?*
7. *The information in this chapter points out some of the external influences that affected the nursing profession, leaving nursing leaders with their hands tied. Do you think nursing leaders are ably ascertaining the external influences that are affecting nursing today? Discuss.*
8. *Do you think this chapter points to nurses actively promoting their professionalism or passively accepting the judgment of others? Discuss. How will you advance your role as a DNP graduate: active promotion or passive acceptance or maybe somewhere in between?*
9. *Discuss whether nurses were handed their place in the health care system or did they endeavor to develop roles for nurses in the health care system, placing nurses where they were most effective.*
10. *Discuss why you are either a conservative traditionalist or an elite professionalizer.*

■ NOTES

1. Robinson (1946), who has written a meticulous and gripping history of nursing in *White Caps: The Story of Nursing*, indicates that five separate entities lay claim to the status of the "first nursing school or first training program for nurses," including New York Hospital (1798), Nurse Society of Philadelphia (1828), and the New York Infirmary (1857). However, Robinson favors the authenticity of the more substantial programs established first at the Women's Hospital of Philadelphia in 1863, which was the first 6-month curriculum, and then next a 12-month curriculum founded at New England Hospital in 1872.
2. Is it time for a new acronym to describe this—*DAPN* for the doctoral advanced practice nurse and *DAPRN* for a description of the practice-doctorate-educated traditional APRN who is a nurse practitioner, nurse-midwife, nurse anesthetist, or clinical nurse specialist?
3. As diploma nurses only accounted for 5% of all new RNs, they were not analyzed in this calculation (Aiken et al., 2009).
4. Northeastern University founded the first 5-year BSN co-operative education degree in 1971 and Drexel University followed in 2000.
5. We should note this number *has not changed* since 2010, the year of publication of the first edition of this book.

■ REFERENCES

Aiken, L. H., Cheung, R. B., & Olds, D. M. (2009). Education policy initiatives to address the nurse shortage in the United States. *Health Affairs (Project Hope)*, 28(4), w646–w656.

Aiken, L. H., Cimiotti, J. P., Sloane, D. M., Smith, H. L., Flynn, L., & Neff, D. F. (2011). Effects of nurse staffing and nurse education on patient deaths in hospitals with different nurse work environments. *Medical Care, 49*(12), 1047–1053.

Aiken, L. H., Clarke, S. P., Cheung, R. B., Sloane, D. M., & Silber, J. H. (2003). Educational levels of hospital nurses and surgical patient mortality. *Journal of the American Medical Association, 290*(12), 1617–1623.

Aiken, L. H., Sloane, D. M., Bruyneel, L., Van den Heede, K., Griffiths, P., Busse, R.,... RN4CAST Consortium. (2014). Nurse staffing and education and hospital mortality in nine European countries: A retrospective observational study. *The Lancet, 383*(9931), 1824–1830.

Allen, C. E. (1991). Holistic concepts and the professionalization of public health nursing. *Public Health Nursing, 8*(2), 74–80.

Alpi, K. M., & Adams, M. G. (2007). Mapping the literature of public health and community nursing. *Journal of the Medical Library Association, 95*(1), e6–e9.

American Association of Colleges of Nursing. (2000). The baccalaureate degree in nursing as minimal preparation for professional practice. Retrieved from http://www.aacn.nche.edu/Publications/positions/baccmin.htm

American Association of Colleges of Nursing. (2015). MEDICARE at 50: A look at nursing education. Retrieved from http://www.aacn.nche.edu/government-affairs/ian/2015/September-2015.pdf

American Association of Nurse Practitioners. (2016). Safe practice environment. Retrieved from https://www.aanp.org/legislation-regulation/state-legislation/state-practice-environment

American Journal of Nursing. (1935). The WPA and nursing: The nurse's status; projects; state committees [Unsigned Editorial]. *The American Journal of Nursing, 35*(12), 1154–1156.

American Nurses' Association. (1965). American Nurses' Association's first position on education for nursing. *The American Journal of Nursing, 65*(12), 106–111.

Barter, M., & McFarland, P. L. (2001). BSN by 2010. A California initiative. *The Journal of Nursing Administration, 31*(3), 141–144.

Beckemeier, B. (2008). History of public health and public health nursing. In L. L. Ivanovov & C. L. Blue (Eds.), *Public health nursing: Leadership, policy, & practice* (pp. 2–26). Clifton Park, NY: Delmar Cengage Learning.

Benner, P., Sutphen, M., Leonard, V., & Day, L. (2009). *Educating nurses: A call for radical transformation.* Hoboken, NJ: Jossey-Bass.

Biddle, B. J. (1986). Recent developments in role theory. *Annual Review of Sociology, 12*, 67–92.

Blumer, H. (1969). *Symbolic interactionism: Perspective and method.* Berkeley: University of California Press.

Brainard, A. M. (1985). *The evolution of public health nursing.* Philadelphia, PA: W. B. Saunders.

Buhler-Wilkerson, K. (1985). Public health nursing: In sickness or in health? *American Journal of Public Health, 75*(10), 1155–1161.

Buhler-Wilkerson, K. (1987). Left carrying the bag: Experiments in visiting nursing, 1877–1909. *Nursing Research, 36*(1), 42–47.

Buhler-Wilkerson, K. (1991). Lillian Wald: Public health pioneer. *Nursing Research, 40*(5), 316–317.

Buhler-Wilkerson, K. (1993). Guarded by standards and directed by strangers. Charleston, South Carolina's response to a national health care agenda, 1920-1930. *Nursing History Review: Official Journal of the American Association for the History of Nursing, 1*, 139–154.

Burbules, N., & Densmore, K., (1991). The limits of making teaching a profession. *Educational Policy, 5*(1), 44–63.

Byers, B. K. (1999). *The lived experience of registered nurses, 1930–1950: A phenomenological study.* A Dissertation in Higher Education submitted to the Graduate Faculty of Texas Tech University. Retrieved from https://ttu-ir.tdl.org/ttu-ir/handle/2346/9563 [Restricted access for full source.]

Cast, A. (2004). Role-taking and interaction. *Social Psychology Quarterly, 67*(3), 296–309.

Conway, M. E. (1988). Theoretical approaches to the study of roles. In M. E. Hardy & M. E. Conway (Eds.), *Role theory: Perspectives for health professionals* (2nd ed., pp. 63–110). Norwalk, CT: Appleton and Lange.

Cooley, C. (1964). *Human nature and social order.* New York, NY: Schocken Books.

Council on Physician and Nurse Supply. (n.d.). New council calls for immediate increase in physician and nurse education. Retrieved from http://www.physiciannursesupply.com/news-press-releases.aspx

Craig, P. (2003). The development of public health nursing. In S. Cowley (Ed.), *Public health in policy and practice: A sourcebook for health visitors and community nurses* (pp. 25–43). London, UK: Elsevier Science.

Cueto, M. (2007). *The value of health: A history of the Pan American Health Organization.* Washington, DC: Pan American Health Organization.

Cusson, R. M., & Strange, S. N. (2008). Neonatal nurse practitioner role transition: The process of reattaining expert status. *The Journal of Perinatal & Neonatal Nursing, 22*(4), 329–337.

Cusson, R. M., & Viggiano, N. M. (2002). Transition to the neonatal nurse practitioner role: Making the change from the side to the head of the bed. *Neonatal Network, 21*(2), 21–28.

D'Antonio, P. (2004). Women, nursing, and baccalaureate education in 20th century America. *Journal of Nursing Scholarship, 36*(4), 379–384.

Davis, M. (1929). The nurse as hospital superintendent. *The American Journal of Nursing, 29*(4), 385–387.

Deloughery, G. (1977). *History and trends of professional nursing.* St. Louis, MO: Mosby.

Dock, L. L. (1906). Training for visiting nursing. *The American Journal of Nursing, 7*(2), 109–111.

Dock, L. L., & Stewart, I. M. (1938). *A short history of nursing from the earliest times to the present day.* New York, NY: G. P. Putnam's Sons, The Knickerbocker Press.

Donahue, P. (1985). *Nursing, the finest art.* St. Louis, MO: Mosby.

Donohue, P. (1996). *Nursing, the finest art: An illustrated history* (2nd ed.). St. Louis, MO: Mosby.

Donley, R., & Flaherty, R. (2002). Revisiting the American Nurses Association's first position on education for nurses. *Online Journal of Issues in Nursing, 7*(2). Retrieved from http://www.nursingworld .org/MainMenuCategories/ANAMarketplace/ANAPeriodicals/OJIN/TableofContents/ Volume72002/No2May2002/RevisingPostiononEducation.aspx

Donley, R., & Flaherty, M. J. (2008). Revisiting the American Nurses Association's first position on education for nurses: A comparative analysis of the first and second position statements on the education of nurses. *The Online Journal of Issues in Nursing, 13*(2). Retrieved from http://www.nursingworld .org/MainMenuCategories/ANAMarketplace/ANAPeriodicals/OJIN/TableofContents/ Volume72002/No2May2002/RevisingPostiononEducation.aspx

Dreher, H. M. (2008a). Innovation in nursing education: Preparing for the future of nursing practice. *Holistic Nursing Practice, 22*(2), 77–80.

Dreher, H. M. (2008b). Is poor weight management a failure of primary care? *Holistic Nursing Practice, 22*(6), 312–316.

Dreher, H. M. (2009). Education for advanced practice: The question: Is the PhD or the DNP the right degree model for future advanced practice nurses? In L. Joel (Ed.), *Advanced practice nursing: Essentials for role development* (2nd ed., pp. 58–71). Philadelphia, PA: F. A. Davis.

Dreher, H. M. (2010). The path to nursing science today, 1910–2010. In M. D. Dahnke & H. M. Dreher (Eds.), *Philosophy of science for nursing practice: Concepts and application* (pp. 269–300). New York, NY: Springer Publishing.

Dreher, H. M., & Dahnke, M. D. (2016). Philosophy of science in a practice discipline. In M. D. Dahnke & H. M. Dreher (Eds.), *Philosophy of science for nursing practice: Concepts and application* (2nd ed., pp. 71–96). New York, NY: Springer Publishing.

Dreher, H. M., & Montgomery, K. A. (2009). Let's call it "doctoral" advanced practice nursing. *Journal of Continuing Education in Nursing, 40*(12), 530–531.

Durkeim, E. (1964). *The division of labor in society.* New York, NY: Free Press.

Ferris, D. (2001). Military intelligence. Retrieved from http://www.nurseweek.com/news/features/ 01-06/military.html

Footner, A. (1998). Nursing specialism or nursing specialization? *Nursing Outlook, 2*(4), 219–223.

Ford, L. C., & Silver, H. K. (1967). Expanded role of the nurse in child care. *Nursing Outlook, 15,* 43–45.

Freund, C. M. (1990). *The unity of education, research, and practice.* Kansas City, MO: American Nurses Association.

Fritter, E., & Shimp, K. (2016). What does certification in professional nursing practice mean? *Med-Surg Matters, Academy of Medical-Surgical Nurses, 25*(2), 8–10.

Gardner, M. S. (1936). *Public health nursing.* New York, NY: Macmillian.

Gebbie, K. M. (2009). 20th-century reports on nursing and nursing education: What difference did they make? *Nursing Outlook, 57*(2), 84–92.

Giacomo, R. (1953). The 1953 census of nurses in public health work. *Nursing Outlook, 1*(11), 645–646.

Goffman, E. (1955). On face-work; an analysis of ritual elements in social interaction. *Psychiatry, 18*(3), 213–231.

Goffman, E. (1959). *The presentation of self in everyday life.* Edinburgh, Scotland: University of Edinburgh, Social Sciences Research Centre.

Group, T. M., & Roberts, J. I. (2001). *Nursing, physician control, and the medical monopoly: Historical perspectives on gendered inequality in roles, rights, and range of practice.* Bloomington: Indiana University Press.

Haase, P. T. (1990). *The origins and rise of associate degree nursing education.* Durham, NC: Duke University Press.

Halloran, E. (1995). *A Virginia Henderson reader: Excellence in nursing*. New York, NY: Springer Publishing.

Hardy, M., & Conway, M. (1979). *Role theory: Perspectives for health professionals*. East Norwalk, CT: Appleton & Lange.

Hardy, M., & Conway, M. (1988). *Role theory: Perspectives for health professionals* (2nd ed.). East Norwalk, CT: Appleton & Lange.

Harmer, B., & Henderson, V. (1939). *Textbook of the principles and practice of nursing*. New York, NY: Macmillan.

Health Resources and Services Administration, National Center for Health Workforce Analysis. (2013). The U.S. nursing workforce: Trends in supply and education. Retrieved from http://bhpr.hrsa.gov/healthworkforce

Institute of Medicine. (2010). The future of nursing: Leading change, advancing health. Retrieved from http://www.nationalacademies.org/hmd/Reports/2010/The-Future-of-Nursing-Leading -Change-Advancing-Health.aspx#sthash.ECAsL6ya.dpuf

Jackson, S., & Stevenson, C. (2000). What do people need psychiatric and mental health nurses for? *Journal of Advanced Nursing, 31*(2), 378–388.

Johns, C., & Freshwater, D. (2005). *Transforming nursing through reflective practice* (2nd ed.). Hoboken, NJ: Wiley-Blackwell.

Judd, D., Sitzman, K., & Davis, G. M. (2009). *A history of American nursing: Trends and eras*. Boston, MA: Jones & Bartlett.

Kalisch, P. A., & Kalisch, B. J. (2003). *American nursing: A history* (4th ed.). Philadelphia, PA: Lippincott Williams & Wilkins.

Keeling, A. W. (2004). Blurring the boundaries between medicine and nursing: Coronary care nursing, circa the 1960s. *Nursing History Review: Official Journal of the American Association for the History of Nursing, 12*, 139–164.

Klass, A. A. (1961). What is a profession? *Canadian Medical Association journal, 85*, 698–701.

Kraus, N. (1980). "The 1985 proposal" for entry into nursing practice: How should the ACNM respond? *Journal of Nurse-Midwifery, 25*(1), 1–3.

Kuhn, A. (1974). *The logic of social systems*. San Francisco, CA: Jossey-Bass.

Liaschenko, J., & Peter, E. (2004). Nursing ethics and conceptualizations of nursing: Profession, practice and work. *Journal of Advanced Nursing, 46*(5), 488–495.

Lusk, B. (1997). Professional classifications of American nurses, 1910 to 1935. *Western Journal of Nursing Research, 19*(2), 227–242.

Lynaugh, J. (2007). Hospitals, nurses, and education—Eternal triangle. In J. Lynaugh, H. Grace, G. Smith, R. Sena, M., & de Villabos (Eds.), *The W. K. Kellogg Foundation and the nursing profession: Shared values, shared legacy*. Indianapolis, IN: Sigma Theta Tau International.

Magat, R. (Ed.). (1989). *Philanthropic giving: Studies in varieties and goals*. New York, NY: Oxford University Press.

Maraldo, P. J., Fagin, C., & Keenan, T. (1988). Nursing and private philanthropy. *Health Affairs (Project Hope), 7*(1), 130–136.

Mead, G. (1934). *Mind, self, and society*. Chicago, IL: University of Chicago Press.

Meleis, A. I. (1975). Role insufficiency and role supplementation: A conceptual framework. *Nursing Research, 24*(4), 264–271.

Meleis, A. I. (2011). Transitions from practice to evidence-based. In A. Meleis (Ed.), *Transitions theory: Middle range and situation specific theories in nursing research and practice* (pp. 1–10). New York, NY: Springer Publishing.

Meleis, A. I., & Trangenstein, P. A. (1994). Facilitating transitions: Redefinition of the nursing mission. *Nursing Outlook, 42*(6), 255–259.

Melosh, B. (1982). *The physician's hand: Work culture and conflict in American nursing*. Philadelphia, PA: Temple University Press.

Minnigerode, L. (1923). Report of committee on federal legislation. *American Journal of Nursing, 24*(3), 223.

Nutting, A. (1904). A school for social workers. *The American Journal of Nursing, 4*(9), 679–681.

Parascandola, J. (2007). Public health history. *Commissioned Officer Association for the USPHS*. Retrieved from http://www.coausphs.org/phhistory.cfm

Pearson, L. (2010). The Pearson Report 2010: The annual state-by-state national overview of nurse practitioner legislation and healthcare issues. *The American Journal for Nurse Practitioners, 14*(3).

Porter, D. (1994). The history of public health and the modern state: Introduction. *Clio Medica, 26*, 1–44.

Reverby, S. (1987). *Ordered to care: The dilemma of American nursing, 1850–1945.* Cambridge, MA: Cambridge University Press.

Robinson, V. (1946). *White caps: The story of nursing.* Philadelphia, PA: J. B. Lippincott.

Role. (n.d.). *Merriam-Webster's online dictionary.* Retrieved from http://www.merriam-webster.com/dictionary/role

Rosen, J. (1993). *A history of public health.* Baltimore, MD: Johns Hopkins University Press.

Rosenberg, C. (1987). *The care of strangers: The rise of America's hospital system.* New York, NY: Basic Books.

Schell, E. S., & Kayser-Jones, J. (1999). The effect of role-taking ability on caregiver-resident mealtime interaction. *Applied Nursing Research, 12*(1), 38–44.

Schön, D. (1983). *The reflective practitioner: How professionals think In action.* New York, NY: Basic Books.

Schulz, R., & Johnson, A. C. (2003). *Management of hospitals and health services: Strategic issues and performance.* Washington, DC: Beard Books.

Shattell, M. (2004). Nurse-patient interaction: A review of the literature. *Journal of Clinical Nursing, 13*(6), 714–722.

Truthaboutnursing.org. (2015). Q: Are you sure nurses are autonomous? Based on what I've seen, it sure looks like physicians are calling the shots. Retrieved from http://www.truthaboutnursing.org/faq/autonomy.html

U.S. Public Health Service Nursing. (2009). Nurse resource manual: USPHS nursing—Mission, responsibilities, and challenge. Retrieved from http://phs-nurse.org/nurse-resource-manual/usphs-mission

Wade, L. C. (1967). The heritage from Chicago's early settlement houses. *Journal of the Illinois State Historical Society (1908–1984), 60*(4), 411–441.

Whelan, J. C. (2005). "A necessity in the nursing world": The Chicago Nurses Professional Registry, 1913-1950. *Nursing History Review: Official Journal of the American Association for the History of Nursing, 13*, 49–75.

Williams, R. C. (1951). *The United States Public Health Service, 1798–1950.* Washington, DC: Commissioned Officers Association of the United States Public Health Service.

Winslow, C.-E. A. (1911). The role of the visiting nurse in the campaign for public health. *American Journal of Nursing, 11*(11), 909–929.

Winslow, C.-E. A. (1922). From the report of the committee on nursing education. *American Journal of Nursing, 22*(11), 882–884.

Winslow, C.-E. A. (1923). *The evolution and significance of the modern public health campaign.* New Haven, CT: Yale University Press.

Winslow, C. E. (1925). The place of public health in a university. *Science, 62*(1607), 335–338.

Woods, C. Q. (1996). Evolution of the American Nurses Association's position on health insurance for the aged: 1933-1965. *Nursing Research, 45*(5), 304–310.

Young, J. (2005). Revisiting the 1925 Johns Report on African-American nurses. *Nursing History Review: Official Journal of the American Association for the History of Nursing, 13*, 77–99.

Zerwekh, J., & Claborn, J. (2009). *Nursing today: Transitions and trends* (6th ed.). Philadelphia, PA: Elsevier Health Sciences.

CHAPTER TWO

Reflective Response

Sheila P. Davis

Does the role of a more highly educated advance practice nurse result in improved patient outcomes as compared to the traditional master's-prepared advanced practice nurse? These and other questions are posed by Dreher and Uribe in an attempt to describe evolution of the advanced practice role. Does the public more clearly understand and embrace us now that we have introduced the doctoral role? How are the 20 minutes of care provided by the doctoral advanced practice nurse (DAPN) significantly different from the care provided by the physician, master's-level advanced practice nurse, and the physician assistant? What is the value added by the DAPN? We are reminded that since 1965, the American Nurses Association (ANA) position statement called for all RNs to be educated at the baccalaureate level. Fifty years have passed and in the United States, the majority of RNs are still educated at the associate degree nursing (and) level. Since that time, the ANA reaffirmed its position and, recently, the Institute of Medicine report, *The Future of Nursing: Leading Change, Advancing Health*, recommended 80% BSN-prepared nurses by 2020. Given the progression of our past compelling mandates, one has to wonder if current recommendations will translate into practice policies. Perhaps, it is time to study the politics that feed the ADN movement. Although we may recommend, the reality is that we fall short in legislating. Consequently, DAPN are tasked with carving out a place in the practice community where, in many instances, there is not only confusion, but resentment to the title of doctor. How can one be the "thing" that they are educationally prepared to be without acknowledgment of the title? The title is the first step in acknowledgment of the role, in my opinion. To give a personal example, I became a family nurse practitioner after having had the doctorate of philosophy for more than 20 years. Hence, I am very accustomed to the title doctor. Well, one day while attending a staff meeting in the clinical setting, before long, I realized that the meeting was about me. The physician's assistant expressed his extreme discomfort with me being called doctor. I explained that I always introduced myself as a nurse practitioner with a doctorate. In most instances, patients referred to me as "their doctor" even if I did not refer to myself as doctor. What's in a name? I submit that as we seek to advance the role of the doctorate advanced practice nurse, the discussion and ownership of the name has to be paramount.

Small wonder, as alluded in the chapter, more role strain is being experienced by the DNP graduates. For this and other reasons, I agree with Dreher and Urbide that "A vigorous curricular focus on the concept of role is particularly important for the student pursing a doctorate of nursing practice degree." An old adage in many oppressed ethnic communities is: *it does not matter what they call you. It's what you answer to.* In other words, unless you know who you are, you will be defined by others. And, in most instances, their definition of you is less favorable.

In a previous reflective response to the doctorate of nursing practice degree role (Davis, 2011), I advocated that now is the time for radical change for the DANP. Have we made the change? Are we mimicking other practice professionals or, are we adding something that will distinguish us in practice? Nightingale would never have won the recognition as the Mother of Modern Nursing had she duplicated the work of other health care practitioners. Rather, she forged a new identity for nurses. I know that we are trained differently, but how is that training understood, demonstrated, and embraced in practice? Although I do not have the answers, I would like to pose an area of practice for consideration. This is a somewhat overlooked past role of the nurse, which is creeping back into modern practice. It was once the requirement of all nurses to render massage therapy to patients as part of the nightly duties. Now, massage, hydrotherapy, and countless other complementary and alternative methods (CAMs) for health and healing are making a remarkable comeback. The National Institute of Health reports that approximately 38% of adults (4 out of 10) use some form of CAMs (nccih.nih .gov). Not only that, a growing body of practitioners are questioning traditional medical approaches to treatment (Barnard, 2007; Esselstyn, 2007; Fuhrman, 2012; Marcum, 2013; Ornish, 2010; Youngberg, 2012). Could it be that this is an opportunity for DAPNs to participate in bringing the scientific evidence to the practice community for select CAMs? In our curriculum, how much attention are we giving to the prevailing trends of the population? By all popular estimates, CAMs are here to stay and will continue to explode. My kind suggestion is that we seize the opportunity to embrace this emergent practice opportunity while providing the clinical, scientific evidence for its use. To me, curing is much better than treating. I wish you every success.

■ REFERENCES

Barnard, N. (2007). *Dr. Neal Barnard's program for reversing diabetes: The scientifically proven system for reversing diabetes without drugs.* New York, NY: Rodale.

Davis, S. (2011). Reflective response to role theory and the evolution roles in nursing. In H. Dreher & M. Smith-Glasgow (Eds.), *Role development for advanced doctoral nursing practice* (Chapter 2). New York, NY: Springer Publishing.

Esselstyn, C. (2007). *Prevent and reverse heart disease: The revolutionary, scientifically proven nutrition-based cure.* New York, NY: Avery.

Fuhrman, J. (2014). *The eat to live plan to prevent and reverse diabetes: The end of diabetes.* New York, NY: Harper Collins.

Marcum, J. (2011). *The ultimate prescription: What the medical profession is not telling you.* Carol Stream, IL: Tyndale.

Marcum, J. (2013). *Medicines that kill: The truth about the hidden epidemic.* Carol Stream, IL: Tyndale.

Ornish, D. (2010). *Dean Ornish program for reversing heart disease: The only system scientifically proven to reverse heart disease without drugs or surgery.* New York, NY: Random House.

Youngberg, W. (2012). *Goodbye diabetes: Preventing and reversing diabetes the natural way.* Fallbrook, CA: Hart Books.

CHAPTER THREE

The Evolution of Advanced Practice Nursing Roles

Marcia R. Gardner, Bobbie Posmontier, Michael E. Conti, and Mary Ellen Roberts

Nursing, as a discipline, has struggled since the Florence Nightingale era to articulate the unique contribution of its practitioners to health and illness care. This tension comes in part from its own history and in part from its link with, and historical dependence on, other disciplines including medicine for certain types of scientific knowledge, practice skills, and to a large degree access to patients. Functional skills (e.g., physical examination) and functional knowledge (e.g., pharmacology, pathophysiology of disease, or psychology of illness) are shared with (some might say "borrowed" from) other health disciplines. Mastery of higher level biomedical and pharmacological knowledge, clinical reasoning, and clinical and/or diagnostic skills has emerged as a hallmark of advanced practice nursing as enacted by nurse practitioners (NPs), nurse anesthetists, nurse-midwives, and clinical nurse specialists (CNSs). Yet, at the same time, nursing has also labored to establish a distinctive knowledge and practice structure separate from these shared domains.

Nursing's scope in the United States has expanded, contracted, and re-expanded in concert with, and in response to, a variety of social, political, technological, and theoretical forces such as:

- The influx of poor immigrants into overcrowded tenements at the turn of the century, culminating in Lillian Wald's creation of the Henry Street Settlement (Keeling, 2009)
- Congress's establishment of the Army and Navy Nursing Corps in the early 1900s (Keeling, 2009)
- The advent of World War I and the 1918 influenza epidemic (Buhler-Wilkerson, 2001; Wald, 1922)
- The Great Depression of the 1930s, resultant closing of hospital nursing programs, and movement of graduate nurses into hospitals (Keeling, 2009)
- Nursing's shortage during World War II resulting in the Bolton Act that established funding for basic nursing education and postgraduate education for the preparation of certified nurse anesthetists, educators, and administrators (Spalding, 1943)

- Post–World War II development of the acute care hospital system (Fairman & Lynaugh, 1998)
- The Brown Report of 1948, funded by the Carnegie foundation, advocating the transition of nursing education from hospital-based diploma programs into colleges and universities, and recruitment of men and minorities (Donahue, 1996)
- Explosions in scientific, biomedical, and pharmaceutical knowledge, as well as related technologies (Keeling, 2009)
- President Johnson's "Great Society" legislation in 1964 enacting Medicare and Medicaid (Keeling, 2009)
- The growth of the third-party payment system in 1965 (Keeling, 2009)
- Economic pressures and expanding costs of health care and health care coverage (Keeling, 2009)
- The need to fill the "provider gap" in rural and underserved geographic areas (Keeling, 2009)
- Title VIII funding for advanced practice nursing education through the Health Resources and Services Administration (HRSA; American Nurses Association [ANA], n.d.)
- Creation of the National Center for Nursing Research in 1985 and the National Institute of Nursing Research (NINR) in 1993 (National Institute of Health [NIH], n.d.), providing greater opportunities for funded research helping to document outcomes associated with advanced nursing practice, among other issues
- Publication of the Institute of Medicine (IOM)'s "Future of Nursing" Report in 2010 (IOM, 2010)
- Approval and implementation of the federal Affordable Care Act (ACA), beginning in 2010

In the midst of these social and scientific changes (and possibly in response to them), nursing leaders and innovators in the mid-20th century embraced a growing theoretical and practice focus on individuals and their experiences, rather than on medical diagnoses and treatment (Fairman, 1999). This disciplinary, cognitive shift offered a means to recognize and consolidate nursing's distinctive knowledge and practice methods, to break away from a purely medicalized approach to patient care, and to situate nursing as an independent, collaborative health care discipline with a differentiated knowledge base, focus, skill set, and language—particularly differentiated from medicine. Such efforts led to the development, articulation, and scientific testing of conceptual models and related descriptive grand theories for the understanding of human responses to health and illness, such as Orem's Self-Care Framework, the Roy Adaptation Model, or Rogers's Science of Unitary Human Beings. Other crucial developments included elucidation of the generally accepted meta-paradigm for nursing practice, research, and theory construction: *human/person, environment, health, nursing*, and synthesis and testing of midrange and other theories to guide practice (Baer, 1987; Fawcett & Alligood, 2005; Phillips, 1996). These efforts were integral to and important in the examination and expansion of nursing's knowledge and practice structures, including its taxonomy, processes, strategies for knowledge generation, scope of practice, and practice strategies (Blegen & Tripp-Reimer, 1997; Fawcett & Alligood, 2005; Moorhead, Head, Johnson, & Maas, 1998; Roy, 2007). Knowledge and clinical practice set the stage for the more recent evolution of, and revolution in, nursing advanced practice roles and scope of practice. The four advanced practice nursing roles, addressed subsequently, include the nurse-midwife, nurse anesthetist, NP, and CNS, all of whom contributed via their own unique history to shaping advanced practice nursing in the 21st century. We have provided a lengthier analysis of nurse-midwifery, as its emergence as an advanced practice role is often minimized in the broader nursing literature.

■ DEVELOPMENT OF THE NURSE-MIDWIFE ROLE

Although records of midwifery practice date back to the 370 to 460 BCE at the time of Hippocrates, it was the midwives of the 18th and 19th centuries who shaped the evolution of nurse-midwives in the 21st century in the United States (McCool & Simeone, 2002). Midwifery skills among colonial midwives ranged from those formally trained in Europe to illiterate women who became midwives in response to community need. In addition to assisting with childbirth, bathing women after childbirth, and cooking, most midwives also provided primary care to their communities. When the first boat of African slaves arrived from West Africa, the first granny midwives began to practice midwifery on plantations in the rural south for both White and Black women, which was based on West African tribal folklore (Graninger, 1996; Morrison & Fee, 2010). The safety and skill of midwives varied widely during the first 250 years in America because there were no educational standards. Although some were well educated, others relied on herbs and poultices (Manocchio, 2008). Most midwives were either self-taught or learned by apprenticeship from others.

Dr. William Shippen, a protégé of Dr. William Smellie in England, established the first formal educational program for midwives in Philadelphia in 1765 (Rooks, 1997). Because illiterate women could not qualify for or afford the private education, and midwifery was considered beneath the stature of educated women, Dr. Shippen limited the education to men. By the end of the 18th century, colonial men traveled to England for medical training, and returned to provide obstetric care to upper class women. Morally outraged by men providing care for women, Dr. Samuel Gregory, a graduate of Yale University, established the first formal midwifery education program for women at the Boston Female Medical College in 1848 (Rooks, 1997). The 3-month midwifery program graduated 12 midwives between 1848 and 1851, but was forced to close in 1874 due to strong opposition from the Boston Medical Society (Rooks, 1997). By the late 19th century, there was massive immigration into the United States from southern and eastern Europe (Dawley, 2003). New immigrants were densely packed into urban areas and suffered poor working conditions, long hours in factories, and overcrowding in tenements (Keeling, 2009). High maternal–infant mortality was blamed on granny and immigrant midwives, who managed 50% of all U.S. births. Public health nursing leaders, including Carolyn Conant van Blarcom, who wrote the first obstetric nursing textbook; Lillian Wald, the founder of the Henry Street Settlement in New York City; Mary Beard, who developed prenatal care; and Mary Breckinridge, who founded the first midwifery service in America, joined with obstetricians to eliminate lay midwives in the United States (Dawley, 2005; Stone, 2000). These nursing leaders sought to combine public health nursing and midwifery to create the nurse-midwife. Dr. Fred Taussig, a Missouri physician, is credited with coining the term *nurse-midwife* in 1925 (Stone, 2000).

The 1920s were framed by several pivotal events including:

- Middle- and upper-class women embracing "twilight sleep" (a combination of morphine and scopolamine for childbirth analgesia and amnesia to decrease and forget labor pain)
- Physicians gaining higher esteem (because upper- and middle-class women chose them for labor and pain management)

- Physicians becoming more politically organized
- The increased use of intervention methods (forceps, episiotomies, scopolamine, and morphine) recommended for all women by obstetrician Joseph Delee (McCool & Simeone, 2002)

Despite the findings in several New York– and New Jersey–based studies, and the 1925 White House Conference on Child Health and Protection, that midwives had much better maternal–infant outcomes than obstetricians, middle and upper class women felt that the use of midwives should be reserved only for poor women who could not afford the prestigious care of an obstetrician (Keeling, 2009; Rooks, 1997).

The Bellevue School of Midwifery opened in 1911 to train lay midwives, but was forced to close in 1935 by the New York City Commissioner of Hospitals because he considered midwifery superfluous in the current social climate as well as below current medical standards (Varney, Kriebs, & Gegor, 2004). In 1923, the Maternity Center Association's (MCA) Hazel Corbin, RN, and obstetrician Ralph Lobenstine, MD, sought to open a nurse-midwifery educational program in conjunction with Bellevue Hospital in New York City, but they were thwarted by the New York City commissioner who worried that well-educated nurse-midwives would be harder to eliminate than the lay midwives (Dawley, 2003; Dawley & Burst, 2005).

In 1921, Mary Breckinridge conducted a maternal–child needs assessment and lay midwifery survey in Leslie County Kentucky while she was studying public health nursing at Columbia University Teachers College (Dawley, 2005; Dawley & Burst, 2005). When Corbin and Lobenstin's nurse-midwifery education program failed to open in New York, Mary Breckinridge's friend and colleague Carolyn Conant van Blarcom assisted her with enrolling in an English midwifery school. On her graduation in 1925, Breckinridge returned to Hyden, Kentucky, to establish the Frontier Nursing Service (FNS). With the help of Louis Dublin, statistician from Metropolitan Life Insurance, Breckinridge compiled statistics that showed positive outcomes among the first 10,000 births assisted by midwives and public health nurses from the FNS (Dawley, 2003; Raisler & Kennedy, 2005).

In 1923, the Preston Retreat Hospital added a midwifery course, which continued to operate despite dwindling enrollment until 1960 (Varney et al., 2004). In 1927, the FNS and MCA joined forces to draft plans for developing a nurse-midwifery educational program and to examine state laws governing midwifery practice. By 1931, the MCA opened its own home-birth service (Lobenstin Midwifery Clinic) and by 1932 it opened an educational program, the Lobenstine Midwifery School (Burst & Thompson, 2003; Dawley & Burst 2005; Stone, 2000).

By the late 1930s, after the introduction of penicillin and sulfonamides, improved nutrition, improved sanitation, and improved housing, the maternal death rate dropped dramatically for all women in the United States (Rooks, 1997). Changes in the U.S. health care system then influenced midwifery education after World War II (Dawley, 2003). In 1943, the federal government established the Emergency Maternity and Infant Care Program for the wives and children of returning servicemen who could not otherwise afford a hospital birth. In addition, the Hill–Burton Act of 1946 provided funding for the construction of hospitals. Although 9% of all U.S. citizens had health insurance in 1940, by 1950, the percentage had increased to 50%. However, despite more widespread health insurance coverage, there was a shortage of obstetricians providing hospital maternity services. In response to the shortage, there was an accelerated increase in midwifery programs from 1940 to 1950. The Medical Mission Sisters of Philadelphia designed and developed a midwifery service and educational program (Catholic Maternity Institute) in New Mexico (Barger, 2005; Dawley, 2005). Once established, the New Mexico program provided partial funding for the education of black nurse-midwives in Tuskegee, Alabama (1941), as well as in the Flint Goodrich Hospital Nurse Midwifery program (1942) in New Orleans. Racial tensions, however, eventually resulted in closing the programs in 1946 (Burst & Thompson, 2003). By 1947, the Medical Mission Sisters of Philadelphia established the first master's in nursing program for nurse-midwives at the Catholic University of America to respond to the needs of underserved families in Washington, DC.

Despite the innovations in natural childbirth methods based on Dr. Grantly Dick Read's work developed after World War II, and with increasing public dislike of "twilight sleep," 88% of women chose to deliver in hospitals (Rooks, 1997). During the 1950s, 25 university affiliated hospitals offered graduate nursing programs for maternal–child nursing to provide leaders in teaching, education, and public health. Their socialization was different from that of the nurse-midwife, because they were taught to follow physician standing orders, recognize abnormal labor, and call the physician to the labor room when delivery was imminent. Midwifery was never part of these nursing programs.

In the meantime, MCA recommended moving midwifery education into recognized universities and formulating standard admission requirements and curriculums (Burst & Thompson, 2003; Rooks, 1997). In 1955, Columbia University opened the first graduate nurse-midwifery education program with clinical training in an academic medical center. Yale University opened its own program in 1956. By 1958, three of six national midwifery education programs offered a master's degree for nurse-midwives.

In 1954, 20 nurse-midwives attended the ANA convention and formed the Committee on Organization because the National League for Nursing (NLN) and ANA would not create a special niche for nurse-midwives (Rooks, 1997). In May 1955, the Committee on Organization voted to form the American College of Nurse-Midwives (ACNM) as a separate accrediting body to develop and evaluate nurse-midwifery standards, improve nurse-midwifery education, sponsor nurse-midwifery research, and participate with the International Confederation of Midwives (Burst & Thompson, 2003).

The social changes of the 1960s were marked by the counterculture activities, rejection of authority, and the enactment of Medicare and Medicaid by President Lyndon Johnson (Keeling, 2009). After Senator Robert Kennedy visited the Mississippi Delta in 1965, federal funding was established for the County Health Improvement Program for Holmes County Mississippi starting in 1969. In addition, the Federal Division of Nursing provided funding for nurse-midwifery education in the Department of Obstetrics and Gynecology at the University of Mississippi School of Medicine. As the requirements for admission initially included a bachelor's degree in nursing, most nurses in Mississippi could not participate. In response, the requirements were revised to allow non-degreed nurses to obtain a certificate in midwifery (Keeling, 2009).

During the 1970s, the number of infants delivered by nurse-midwives doubled, there was a shortage of physicians providing obstetric care to the poor, and the concept of using a nurse-midwife for birth moved into the middle class (McCool & Simeone, 2002). Nurse-midwifery educational programs increased from seven in 1960 to 19 in 1979, and nurse-midwifery became legal in most states. The National Health Service Corps began to offer scholarships to nurse-midwife students willing to work in underserved areas after graduation. In 1973, in response to the increased births and the shortage of physicians, the University of Mississippi began a modular curriculum for nurse-midwifery students, based on self-mastery learning that could be completed in less time than traditional education. The modular program included a list of objectives for the entry-level nurse-midwife, learning materials in self-contained packages, independent and self-paced learning, and self-assessment measures by which students could decide if they were ready for testing. By 1979, the ACNM established core competencies in nurse-midwifery, which specified the body of knowledge, skills, and behaviors expected of nurse-midwife graduates (Avery, 2005). The core competencies served as a guide for formulating curricula, accrediting nurse-midwifery programs, and setting the standards for the national certification exam.

As the three branches of military service in the United States had difficulty recruiting and retaining obstetricians, the Air Force started its own nurse-midwifery program at Andrews Air Force Base in Maryland in 1973 (Rooks, 1997). The ACNM, however, would not accredit its program. The Air Force affiliated with Georgetown University in 1975 and offered its base as a clinical site. The Army formed its own graduate nurse-midwife program in 1974 in affiliation with the University of Kentucky and offered Fort Knox as the clinical site. The Navy chose to send its personnel to already-established nurse-midwifery programs (Rooks, 1997).

By the 1980s there were 21 accredited nurse-midwife educational programs ranging from 9- to 18-month certificate programs to two to three master's-level programs (Burst & Thompson, 2003). In 1980, the Education Program Association opened the first distance learning program for family NPs and physician assistants desiring to practice midwifery in publicly funded clinics in California. This innovation allowed students to continue to live in their own communities, while rapidly completing the requirements for graduation. By 1989, the FNS had established its own distance learning by establishing the Community-Based Nurse Midwifery Program (CNEP) in order to increase rural access to nurse-midwifery education. CNEP affiliated with Francis Payne Bolton School of Nursing at Case Western Reserve University in order to offer a master's degree in nursing (Burst & Thompson, 2003).

Although the number of midwifery programs increased to 28 by 1984, enrollment dropped between 1984 and 1986, largely as a result of the malpractice crisis (Burst & Thompson, 2003; Rooks, 1997). By 1988, however, the Robert Wood Johnson Foundation provided a grant for scholarships to educate and recruit nurse-midwifery students to work in West Virginia after graduation (Burst & Thompson, 2003). The program increased the number of nurse-midwives in West Virginia from four in 1989 to 20 in 1992. Between 1991 and 1993, federal financial support provided nurse-midwifery education in exchange for working in underserved areas. In 1991, the ACNM task force also identified barriers for nurse-midwives and established the goal of 10,000 practicing nurse-midwives by 2001. In response to a 50% decrease in practicing obstetricians and 20% increase in births, the Florida Midwifery Resource Center established a call to action in 1993 to educate 600 additional nurse-midwives by the year 2000. By 1993, 67% to 70% of nurse-midwives were master's prepared and 4% to 5% were doctorally prepared (Burst & Thompson, 2003; Rooks,1997).

Between 1982 and 1997, ACNM Division of Accreditation (now the Accreditation Commission for Midwifery Education [ACME]) only provided accreditation for nurse-midwifery programs (2010). In 1997, however, the ACNM Division of Accreditation recognized the certified (direct entry) midwife credential. There are only two direct-entry midwifery programs recognized by the ACNM, including the Midwifery Institute at Philadelphia University in Philadelphia, Pennsylvania, and State University of New York (SUNY) Downstate Medical Center Midwifery Education Program in Brooklyn, New York. Graduates of this program must meet the core competencies and may sit for the national certification exam. The ACNM issued a position statement (Mandatory Degree Requirements for Entry Into Midwifery Practice) in 2010 that a graduate degree (minimum master's degree) is required for entry into clinical practice for both nurse-midwife and direct-entry midwifery students. The Doctor of Nursing Practice (DNP) degree, however, is not a requirement for entry into clinical practice. Nurse-midwives and cer-tified midwives educated before 2010 without a graduate degree are permitted to retain licensure to practice. As of February 2015, there are currently 11,018 nurse-midwives and 88 certified midwives, and 39 accredited graduate nurse-midwifery programs in the United States (ACNM). In 2013, nurse-midwives and certified midwives attended 320,983 births in the United States.

■ DEVELOPMENT OF THE NURSE ANESTHETIST ROLE

The roots of the certified registered nurse anesthetist (CRNA) emerged during the American Civil War (1861–1865) when surgeons needed the assistance of the Catholic sis-ters and Lutheran deaconesses trained as nurses to administer chloroform to wounded soldiers during surgery (Wall, 2005). Ten years after the Civil War, Dr. William Mayo of St. Mary's Hospital in Rochester, Minnesota, recognized the value of training nurse anesthetists, because unlike medical students who watched the surgery while admin-istering anesthesia, nurses observed the patient, which resulted in reduced mortality rates (Keeling, 2007). In 1889, Dr. Mayo trained and hired nurses Edith Granham and Alice Magaw to serve as his anesthetists. By 1913, his 6-month program included theo-retical education and clinical practice.

Despite the success of the Mayo training program for nurse anesthetists, other phy-sicians began to question the authority of nurses to administer anesthesia (Keeling, 2009). Both the New York State Medical Society and the Ohio State Medical Board tried unsuc-cessfully to bar nurse anesthetists from practicing medicine without a license. In *Frank vs. South* (1917), a landmark case, the Kentucky appellate court ruled in favor of nurse anesthetist Margaret Hatfield, stating that she was not practicing medicine because she was under the supervision of and subordinate to licensed physician Dr. Louis Frank. During World War I, Mayo physicians and Dr. George W. Crile of the Lakeside Hospital anesthesia program in Cleveland, Ohio, advocated for nurse anesthetists to provide pain relief to wounded soldiers (Keeling, 2009). In addition, nurse anesthetist Agatha Hodgins and Dr. George Crile developed novel anesthetic techniques, including the use of nitrous oxide–oxygen combinations, and scopolamine and morphine as anesthetic adjuncts.

As medicine was laying claim to the specialty of anesthesiology during World War II due to scientific advances, shortages of anesthesiologists on the battlefield necessitated the training of nurse anesthetists (Keeling, 2009). In 1945, certifica-tion became a practice requirement for CRNAs (National Board of Certification and Recertification of Nurse Anesthetists, 2010). The Korean War provided yet another opportunity for the expansion of the profession. By the early 1960s, the army estab-lished nurse anesthesia programs at Walter Reed Hospital and Letterman General Hospital. Although the number of nurse anesthesia programs decreased during the 1970s due to decreased funding, lack of affiliation with universities, and physician opposition, by 1998, nurse anesthesia educational programs were offered at the mas-ter's level (Diers, 1991; Keeling, 2009).

Anesthesia delivery is currently accomplished by three main methods: anesthesi-ologists working as the sole provider, an anesthesia care team (ACT), or by independ-ent CRNAs. The ACT, where a physician anesthesiologist may supervise one to four CRNAs, is the most common form of delivery. CRNAs work independently, mostly in rural areas, where they deliver approximately 70% of anesthetics in rural hospitals (Fallacaro, Obst, Funn, & Chu, 1996).

Nationally, 18 states have enacted the "opt out," where physician anesthesiologist supervision is no longer required for Medicare and Medicaid patients. This was intended to increase access to care for those patients who resided in primarily rural areas (Agres, 2010). According to 2004 data by the AANA, approximately 39% of CRNAs were employed by hospitals; 36% were employed by physician anesthesia groups; 15% were employed by nurse anesthesia groups; and 10% were employed by a physician office (dentist, podiatrist), were self-employed, or were employed by a university (AANA, 2013). Military CRNAs have had a distinguished history of autonomous practice. On Navy ships, smaller military and Veterans Administration (VA) hospitals, and on the battlefield they have provided and continue to practice without anesthesiologist supervision as the sole provider to the U.S. military (Jenkins, Elliott, & Harris, 2006).

The current scope of practice according to the practice guidelines, published by the AANA, includes:

- Preoperative assessment
- Development and implementation of an anesthetic plan
- Anesthesia delivery (sedation, general anesthesia, regional and neuraxial anesthesia)
- Selection and implementation of noninvasive and invasive monitoring (arterial lines, pulmonary artery [PA] catheters, and central lines)
- Airway management (natural airway, endotracheal intubations, laryngeal mask airway [LMA] placement and implementation of alternative airway techniques, fiber-optic intubations [FOI], needle cricothytotomy)
- Facilitation of emergence from anesthesia; transfer to the post-anesthesia care unit (PACU) and PACU management
- Chronic and acute pain management
- The ability to function as a member of emergency response teams (providing cardiopulmonary support) (AANA, 2010)

It is important to note that the scope of practice for CRNAs is determined by individual state nursing boards and by each facility where the CRNA practices, as determined by their bylaws.

Nurse anesthesia has, from its nascence, had to continuously and diligently prove its important contribution to the delivery of anesthetic care within the matrix of the U.S. health care system. Two important, recent studies examined the effect of the anesthesia provider on mortality rates (Canadian Coordinating Office for Health Technology Assessment, 2004). First, Pine, Holt, and Lou (2003) examined risk-adjusted mortality rates for the following provider models: anesthesiologist as sole provider, CRNAs as sole provider, and the ACT model. Medicare patients undergoing eight surgical procedures were the focus of the study. Results indicate that there was no statistically significant difference between provider types. Similar results were found among the sole CRNA provider, anesthesiologists, and ACT personnel (Pine et al., 2003), meaning anesthesia care outcomes were equivalent regardless of provider type. Second, Jordan, Kremer, Crawforth, and Shott (2001) found no statistical difference in adverse outcomes between type of provider and preoperative physical status, patient age, surgical procedure, or method of anesthesia in a study that reviewed 223 closed claims studies from 1989 to 1997. In 2010, Dulisse and Cromwell's retrospective study of Medicare data from 1999 to 2005 reported no adverse outcomes when CRNAs are not supervised by a physician. This study, published in *Health Affairs*, was important in that it was not biased and the authors recommended that the Centers for Medicare & Medicaid allow CRNAs to practice without physician supervision in every state. Although only two studies have been cited, it is important to note that CRNAs, who now almost universally have a master's degree and by 2025 a practice doctorate, DNP, or a doctor of nurse anesthesia practice (DNAP), have a long history of providing quality, cost-effective patient care with positive patient outcomes

■ DEVELOPMENT OF THE NP ROLE

The NP's role has been prominent in terms of controversies, visibility in public and social policy, and scope of practice considerations, particularly in the role's uniqueness and overlap with medical practice. The history of the NP movement can be seen as another exemplar for advanced practice nursing's developmental journey. The NPs step beyond the range of extended health care services, including education, direct care, chronic illness management, and community services that public health nurses had been providing since the 1920s. Formal NP practice was "birthed" in 1965 through the joining of primary care pediatrics and public health/family-community nursing. This was the vision of Dr. Henry Silver, a pediatrician associated with the University of Colorado, School of Medicine, and Dr. Loretta Ford from the University of Colorado School of Nursing. The NP role emerged at a time when pediatric medicine was struggling to extend care to underserved populations during a shortage of health care professionals. At the same time, nursing was also struggling to expand its scope beyond hospital care to develop autonomous practice, to fully embed nursing education in higher education, and to professionalize as a workforce (Bullough, 1976; Ford, 1975; Richmond, 1965).

The new breed of pediatric care providers in the original University of Colorado program were baccalaureate-prepared clinicians with: (a) advanced clinical and diagnostic skills and knowledge; (b) the ability to monitor child health, growth, and development; and (c) the ability to provide guidance to families, manage minor acute health problems in pediatric primary care, and function within health care teams—particularly for medically underserved populations. The program involved 4 months of university-based education, followed by clinical training in underserved rural community/primary care pediatric settings. Dr. Ford subsequently argued strongly for embedding NP education fully within a graduate nursing education framework; both Ford and Silver were instrumental in communicating the effectiveness of this pediatric NP model and in ensuring its replication (Ford, 1975; Mason, Vaccaro, & Fessler, 2000; Silver, Ford, & Day, 1968).

A comparable brief pediatric NP program for the care of children from underserved urban families developed soon after at the Massachusetts General Hospital in Boston. In addition, other academic medical care settings also developed NP programs that would similarly extend the skills of public health nurses, address access to care for urban underserved children, as well as serve the needs of children in underserved rural areas (Murphy, 1990).

In the following decade, NP certificate training programs began to proliferate across the country. Most of these had a particular emphasis on pediatrics and/or family health, and on extending primary care to underserved urban and rural children, and families in a time of expanding health care needs, and growing recognition of disparities in access to care (Davidson et al., 1975; Mason et al., 2000). Most required a short-time commitment (less than 1 year), and not all required a bachelor's degree for entry (Mason et al., 2000). The scope of NP practice expanded to include family planning and women's health within 10 years after Ford and Silver's innovation (Lewis,

2000) and continues to expand in response to current health care needs nationally and globally.

Federal funding through Title VIII of the Nurse Training Act (American Association of Colleges of Nursing, 2009) provided opportunities for the expansion of NP use in family-focused primary care, in women's health, and then in other populations. In addition, regional programs funded by the federal Title X family planning initiative prepared NPs, therefore significantly expanding the NP workforce in women's health (Bednash, Worthington, & Wysocki, 2009; Manisoff, 1981). By 1978, the IOM had taken the stand that state regulations should be revised to accommodate an increased scope of practice and prescription authority for NPs, albeit under physician supervision (Mason et al., 2000). As the advanced nursing role began to fully take hold, university-based schools of nursing began to integrate NP education and training at the graduate level. Title VIII funding was essential in supporting nurses' completion of these programs (AACN, 2009), and thus, expanded the advanced practice nursing workforce. Scope of practice expanded beyond family and pediatric foci, and beyond primary care to include adult health, as well as highly specialized and/or system-focused practice (e.g., oncology, cardiology, and psychiatric specialties).

Coincidentally, a variety of forces created opportunities for expansion of the NP role. There were regulatory changes for medical education, including pass-through funding adjustments and state-level regulatory restrictions for physician residency training of physicians (hours permitted on duty). There was also a growing body of evidence supporting cost and treatment outcome effectiveness of NPs, as well as a growing and better educated NP workforce. Along with other forces, these recognized improvements created opportunities for greater inclusion of NP scope and practice into high acuity patient care. As fewer physician residents were able/available to provide acute patient care coverage, additional opportunities for NP employment developed (American Academy of Pediatrics Committee on Hospital Care, 1999; American Academy of Pediatrics Committee on Pediatric Workforce, 2003). Adult, pediatric, and neonatal acute care NP education was introduced and solidified, as nurse clinicians were poised to fill gaps in the acute care system (Hinch, Murphy, & Lauer, 2005). In the 1990s, the National Council of State Boards of Nursing (NCSBN); American Academy of Nurse Practitioners Certification Board; American Nurses Credentialing Center; National Certification Board for Pediatric Nurse Practitioners and Nurses, now the Pediatric Nursing Certification Board (PNCB); and National Certification Corporation (NCC) began to jointly consider a cohesive approach to regulation of NP practice (NCSBN, 1998).

The NP movement, particularly in its overlap with medicine's functions, created and continues to create controversies both within and outside of its own discipline. The IOM's landmark report *The Future of Nursing: Leading Change, Advancing Health* (IOM, 2010) calls for nurses to practice to the full scope of their skills and full extent of their education, as equal partners in both designing and providing health care services. Great strides have been made toward this goal. According to Stanley (2012), the consensus model for advance practice registered nurse (APRN) regulation (described later in this chapter) demonstrates the evolving leadership roles that advanced practice nurses (APNs) are taking on in the redesign of the U.S. health care system. In 2015, 21 states allowed NPs to have full, independent practice authority by statute and/or regulation. The VA now advocates for all advanced practice nurses in all specialties to have full practice authority across all VA facilities in the United States. NPs continue to press legislative initiatives promoting full practice authority on the federal and local levels. Educational preparation, and qualifications for practice, role functions, and differentiation from other providers (e.g., physicians, physician assistants, and CNSs) are among the areas continuing to need clarification for legislation, regulation, and reimbursement. NP practice has expanded beyond health professions, shortage areas into the mainstream of primary and acute care. Furthermore, NP clinicians, through their lobbying efforts, have made inroads in reimbursement for the provision of health care services, such as the formal ability to order durable medical equipment for their patients, the inclusion of NPs in the first year of the Merit-Based Incentive Payment System (MIPS), and ensuring that NP-led patient-centered medical homes are eligible to receive incentive payments for the management of patients with chronic disease, all part of the sustainable growth rate repeal for Medicare Part B. The American Medical Association (AMA), American College of Physicians, and the American Academy of Pediatrics (AAP), among others, have periodically attempted to limit NP scope of practice, particularly related to autonomous practice, through the creation of policies and standards for physician supervision of nonphysician providers (Buppert, 2005; Hedger, 2009). The Federal Trade Commission (FTC), in a landmark report, *Policy Perspectives: Competition and Regulation of Advanced Practice Nurses* (2014), encourages state legislatures to look closely at state regulations for NP practice and notes that

> Mandatory physician supervision and collaborative practice agreement requirements are likely to impede competition among health care providers and restrict APRNs' ability to practice independently, leading to decreased access to health care services, higher health care costs, reduced quality of care, and less innovation in health care delivery. (FTC, 2014, p. 38)

The FTC policy paper cites research documenting that APRNs provide safe and effective care within the scope of their training, certification, and licensure, noting that, in addition, significant shortages of primary care practitioners can be alleviated by reduction of undue regulatory burdens. NPs are still facing some challenges on the federal and state levels, including current inability to certify their patients' eligibility for home health care services and permitting assignment of NP's patients to Medicare Shared Savings accountable care organizations (ACOs). In 2015, there is at minimum, universal master's preparation for NPs, and increasingly, NPs prepared at the doctoral level, despite the fact that the DNP is not a requirement for entry into practice. In addition to post-master's DNP program development, there has been a proliferation of BSN to DNP programs across the United States.

■ DEVELOPMENT OF THE CNS ROLE

Concurrent with expansion of NP practice, programs preparing CNSs were proliferating. For example, the first CNS program in psychiatric nursing was established in the 1954 at Rutgers University in New Jersey. Subsequently, CNS programs expanded throughout the United States in the 1950s, 1960s, and later (MacDonald, Herbert, & Thibeault, 2006). The CNS role was conceived and then further evolved to an advanced, specialized, nursing clinician focused on expert practice, improvement of care at the bedside, and intertwining roles as "clinician, consultant, researcher, educator and manager" (Page & Arena, 1994, p. 316). More recent conceptualization of the "research" function of the master's-prepared nurse in an advanced role, regardless of specific role, is translation and integration of evidence into clinical practice (AACN, 1996). In its evolution, the CNS scope of practice would expand to include direct patient care services, as well as staff education and macrosystem management of a specialized population, embedded within a nursing or a systems model, rather than the medical model of care.

While the focus of NP practice was conceived as the individual at the direct care level, the focus of CNS practice was to be both individual and macro levels, in a specialized population (versus the generalist focus of the clinical nurse leader role), incorporating nursing diagnosis and management, as well as systems assessment and synthesis of improved approaches to nursing care. Psychiatric–mental health CNS practice was a forerunner in extending the focus beyond acute care. In 2000, only about one third of psychiatric–mental health clinical specialists were practicing in hospital-based settings, while a majority were practicing in other types of settings, providing a variety of mental health therapies (e.g., in clinics; private or collaborative practices offering counseling and/or psychotherapies; and forensic settings) (Delaney, 2009).

During the 1980s and 1990s, CNS and NP education were similar in some domains—coursework, caseload, practice strategies—although education and scope of practice for both were rapidly evolving (Lindeke, Canady, & Kay, 1997). Some suggested that both CNS and NP clinicians had similar competencies and could overlap in roles and functions. For example, in acute care or psychiatric–mental health care, some graduate programs established joint curricular pathways for both CNS and NP education (Elder & Bullough, 1990; MacDonald et al., 2006; Page & Arena, 1994). However, regulatory authority over CNS titling practice is a relatively recent innovation. Clinicians working as CNSs typically were not required by hiring organizations to have specific preparation in the role until late in the 20th century. Many nurses functioned as CNSs based on their clinical experience and expertise, without formal education preparation or certification in the role. In the 1990s, only about half of state nursing boards had statutes or regulations governing CNS scope of practice (Hudspeth, 2009). There remains wide variation at the state level in title protection, regulation, and scope of practice for the CNS. The consensus model for APRN practice, discussed subsequently, clarifies current and future vision for overlap and differences in education, licensure, regulation, and scope of practice for the CNS and other APRN clinicians, and, importantly, provides for uniform treatment and regulation of CNS scope of practice at the state level.

■ UNIFICATION OF APRN EDUCATION, REGULATION, AND PRACTICE

Professional and regulatory organizations continued to move toward a cohesive approach relative to the preparation of advanced practice nurses for entry into practice, and toward a unified vision of the scope of advanced practice nursing in general. Lewis (2000) notes that, in 1992, both the ANA and the NCSBN took similar positions regarding the need for advanced practice nursing education (with advanced practice nursing defined as NP, nurse anesthetist, nurse-midwife, and CNS) to be situated only at the graduate level, and made an initial effort to create a regulatory model (NCSBN, 1998). As nursing professional organizations began to take similar positions regarding advanced nursing practice and advanced nursing education, the transition of certificate programs preparing advanced practice nurse clinicians to formal graduate-level programs accelerated.

In the 1990s, the AACN convened a national group representing multiple organizations and specialty stakeholders for the development of consensus guidelines for advanced practice nursing education at the graduate (master's) level: *The Essentials of Master's Education for Advanced Practice Nursing* (AACN, 1996). This document recognized only four types of clinicians providing direct, advanced patient care as advanced practice nurses: nurse-midwives, nurse anesthetists, NPs, and CNSs. It specified clearly that education for advanced nursing roles should occur at the master's level. The National Task Force for Quality Nurse Practitioner Education, comprised of representatives from a variety of organizations, including the AACN, National Organization of Nurse Practitioner Faculties (NONPF), NP certifying bodies, and a variety of other stakeholder organizations, promulgated targeted educational guidelines for NP preparation. NONPF established a set of specialty-specific educational guidelines outlining competencies for NP education in both general and specialty areas of practice (NONPF, 2002, 2003, 2004). In 2008, the National Task Force produced the consensus document—*Criteria for Evaluation of Nurse Practitioner Programs.* Nurse anesthetist, nurse-midwife, and CNS education are, in addition, more specifically guided by the respective specialty accrediting organizations. Educational "landmarks" are critical, because they demonstrate the evolution of a cohesive view of advanced nursing practice on the part of those involved in preparing advanced clinicians for practice.

■ CONSENSUS MODEL AND *LACE*

Advanced practice nursing has continued to grow toward a unified licensure and practice model through the collaboration of a variety of advanced practice nursing stakeholder organizations, including the NCSBN, the APRN Consensus Workgroup, and representatives from multiple professional nursing organizations, building on a framework established in the 1990s. The *Consensus Model for Advanced Practice Registered Nurses* (APRN Consensus Workgroup and NCBSN APRN Advisory Committee, 2008), developed through this collaboration, prescribed the regulatory strategy for APRNs, identified the same four direct care providers as APRNs, and specified that other nurses prepared at the graduate level, whose scope is not direct care, do not fall under the rubric of the APRN as defined by the model. A proposed timeline for implementation of the model has been developed; as it is implemented and state regulations are amended, the title "advanced practice registered nurse" will be restricted. The model specifies that APRNs are licensed and practice in one of the following clinical roles: certified nurse practitioner (CNP), certified nurse-midwife (CNM), certified nurse anesthetist, or certified CNS. Education for practice will occur within six population foci (adult–geriatric, pediatric, neonatal, women's/gender-related health, psychiatric–mental health, or family/individual life span), with certification and licensing within the respective population focus as well. Specialization will involve an additional layer of certification, via professional organizations, beyond the population focus (e.g., adult-gerontology population focus, specialty of oncology; APRN Consensus Workgroup and NCBSN APRN Advisory Committee, 2008; Partin, 2009; Stanley, Werner, & Apple, 2009). It is important to note the definition of the CNS as an APRN with relevant licensing and regulatory expectations, because the title CNS is not currently universally restricted, nor are there license/certification requirements across all states for the CNS role.

The model offers a discrete definition of advanced practice nursing and outlines recommendations for uniform regulation of APRN practice via LACE: "licensure, accreditation [of APRN educational programs], certification, education" (APRN Consensus Workgroup and NCSBN APRN Advisory Committee, 2008, p. 7). Characteristics of an APRN as outlined in the consensus statement are that he or she is a clinician:

1. Who has completed an accredited graduate-level education program preparing him or her for one of the four recognized APRN roles
2. Who has passed a national certification examination that measures APRN role and population-focused competencies and who maintains continued competence as evidenced by recertification in the role and population through the national certification program
3. Who has acquired advanced clinical knowledge and skills preparing him or her to provide direct care to patients, as well as a component of indirect care;

however, the defining factor for *all* [sic] APRNs is that a significant component of the education and practice focuses on direct care of individuals

4. Whose practice builds on the competencies of RNs by demonstrating a greater depth and breadth of knowledge, a greater synthesis of data, increased complexity of skills and interventions, and greater role autonomy

5. Who is educationally prepared to assume responsibility and accountability for health promotion and/or maintenance as well as the assessment, diagnosis, and management of patient problems, which includes the use and prescription of pharmacologic and nonpharmacologic interventions

6. Who has clinical experience of sufficient depth and breadth to reflect the intended license

7. Who has obtained a license to practice as an APRN in one of the four APRN roles: CRNA, CNM, CNS, or CNP (APRN Consensus Workgroup and NCSBN APRN Advisory Committee, 2008, pp. 7–8)

■ UNIQUENESS OF APRN "PRACTICE"

Contemporary views of advanced nursing practice are grounded in the intersection of medical knowledge and skills with nursing's meta-paradigm and knowledge base. The unique contribution that APRNs can make in the current health care system can be conceptualized to emerge from a distinctive blend of biomedical and nursing perspectives, skills, and knowledge sets. One crucial challenge for contemporary and future advanced nursing practice is to fully elucidate and articulate the mechanisms by which this fusion occurs (resulting in excellent, cost-effective nursing and excellent patient outcomes). Our discipline's appreciation of holism incorporates an understanding of persons as integrated, continually interacting with their environment, and engaged in the creation of meaning, and our disciplinary attention to the influences of life transitions and health conditions on individuals, families, and communities form a matrix of underpinnings for advanced nursing practice. Holism, patient/client centeredness, respect for individual autonomy, respectful communication with active listening, focused preventive care, health education, and integration of services, all of which are combined with clinical knowledge and expertise, are potentially some of the essential components of APRN effectiveness that grow from the nursing meta-paradigm (Donnelly, 2003; Erikson, 2007; Neill, 1999).

Despite an evolving, but still small, evidence base for the uniqueness of APRN practice, many of these disciplinary dimensions of practice need to be systematically examined. For example, Charlton, Dearing, Berry, and Johnson (2008) reported findings of their integrative review of NP communication styles. Their review suggested that NPs patient-centered communication styles, which they termed "biopsychosocial," compared with "biomedical" styles (2008, p. 383), influenced patient satisfaction, adherence, and health indicators, and was consistent with a specialized model of APRN effectiveness based on nursing's disciplinary perspective. Dunphy and Winland-Brown (2006) proposed a model of APRN practice: the *Circle of Caring*, which accounts for, and formalizes, the overlapping multidisciplinary perspectives integrated in APRN practice through the standpoint of contextualized understanding in a scientific caring framework. Dunphy and Winland-Brown state that "caring is suggested as one way to bridge the gulf between holistic nursing theories and biomedical nursing praxis" (2006, p. 288). Table 3.1 offers other perspectives by summarizing a variety of studies that examined the influence of a nursing-disciplinary perspective as the underpinning for effective patient care by NPs.

TABLE 3.1 **Sample of Studies Examining Influence of Disciplinary Underpinnings on NP Practice Outcomes**

Authors	Design	Related Findings
Benkert, Hollie, Nordstrom, Wickson, and Bins-Emerick (2009)	Descriptive-correlational	African American subjects with moderate cultural mistrust of European Americans; high satisfaction/moderate trust of NPs
Benkert, Barkauskas, Pohl, Corser, Tanner, Wells, and Nagelkirk (2002)	Descriptive	Low-income African American subjects with significantly higher trust scores for NPs vs. MDs; no significant difference in mistrust or satisfaction between providers; significant higher trust scores for clinicians in nurse-managed vs. jointly managed clinics
Castro (2009)	Descriptive-correlational	Latina (female) subjects seen at least once by an NP clinician; all NP clinicians had cultural proficiency, competence, or awareness; no clinicians with cultural incompetence; higher NP cultural competence score correlated with higher patient satisfaction scores; higher time spent with provider correlated with higher satisfaction
Donohue (2003)	Descriptive, naturalistic	Middle-aged female subjects described resources expected and received from NP encounters; resources included services, information, support, time, respect, reassurance, affirmation, reinforcement, trust
Green and Davis (2005)	Predictive modeling	Predictors of patient satisfaction and relationships among NP demographic characteristics, components of Caring Behaviors Inventory, patient satisfaction measures; all NPs with high CBI scores; no differences between male and female; no significant relationships among CBI components and satisfaction
Hayes (2007)	Descriptive-mixed method	Patients aged 18–86 years receiving NP care; 86% female; high satisfaction with NP communication and style of interaction; high recall of instructions; intention to adhere to treatment plan very likely; themes connected with intention to follow treatment plan: trust, expertise, concern for own health
Kotzer (2005)	Descriptive survey	Advanced practice nurses in tertiary pediatric setting; 59% in NP role; 21% in combined CNS/NP role. Primary job functions: education/guidance/counseling, care coordination, direct care
Kozlowski, Lusk, and Melnyk (2015)	Pre-experimental single group pre/post	PNP's in primary care using evidence-based COPE model; decreased anxiety symptoms and improved anxiety measures in children aged 8–13 years

(*continued*)

TABLE 3.1 **Sample of Studies Examining Influence of Disciplinary Underpinnings on NP Practice Outcomes** (*continued*)

Authors	Design	Related Findings
Roots and McDonald (2014)	Descriptive, qualitative, case study	NPs added to rural Canadian fee for service practices; extended access and appointment times, emphasis on team approach, increased satisfaction, increased connection to community services for patients
Sawatsky, Christie, and Singal (2013)	Randomized trial	NP-directed care after cardiac surgery more likely to result in higher rating of functional status and fewer reported symptoms, higher satisfaction with amount and quality of services received
Van Leuven and Prion (2007)	Descriptive, naturalistic	Interview NPs for perspectives on health promotion activities in practice; health promotion viewed as implicit in nursing role; differentiates NP from MD; valued by NPs; obstacles: time, patient care needs, limitations of scope of practice, patient scheduling, practice model (HMO vs. other practice)

CBI , Caring Behaviors Inventory; CNS, clinical nurse specialist; COPE, creativity, optimism, planning, and expert information; HMO, health maintenance organization; NP, nurse practitioner; PNP, PhD in nursing program.

Sources: Benkert et al. (2002); Benkert, Hollie, Nordstrom, Wickson, and Bins-Emerick (2009); Castro and Ruiz (2009); Donohue (2003); Green and Davis (2005); Hayes (2007); Kotzer (2005); Kozlowski, Lusk, and Melnyk (2015); Roots and McDonald, 2014; Sawatsky, Christie, and Singal (2013); Van Leuven and Prion (2007).

■ APRN PRACTICE OUTCOMES

Compelling evidence of the effectiveness of APRN-managed care has been in the literature since the 1970s (Lenz, Mundinger, Kane, Hopkins, & Lin, 2004). A variety of patient outcomes of APRN-provided care have been studied, primarily in comparison to that provided by physicians. Patient satisfaction with, and quality outcomes of, APRN care have been studied extensively in the United States across the past three decades, and more recently in Canada, Britain and other European countries that have adopted advanced practice/NP roles. Satisfaction with the quality of NP-provided care in primary care, emergency departments, and specialty-care settings have consistently been found to be high, while researchers acknowledge that various methods, definitions, instruments, data sets, and time frames have been used in the measurement of these outcomes. However, across multiple studies and reviews, findings consistently documented quality of, and patient satisfaction with, APRN-provided care to be equivalent to or higher than physician-provided care (Carter & Chochinov, 2007; Cooper, Lindsay, Kinn, & Swann, 2002; Dierick-van Daele, Metsemakers, Derckx, Spreeuwenberg, & Vrijhoef, 2009; Horrocks, Anderson, & Salisbury, 2002; Jennings, Lee, Chao, & Keating, 2009; Kleinpell, Ely, & Grabenkort, 2008; Knudtson, 2000; Roblin, Becker, Adams, Howard, & Roberts, 2004). For example, Mundinger and associates' large randomized controlled trial of NP-provided primary care, compared with physician-provided care, with a 2-year follow-up, demonstrated no significant differences in patient satisfaction, utilization of services, self-reported health status and physiological measures related to diabetes, hypertension, and asthma outcomes (Lenz et al., 2004; Mundinger et al., 2000). Oliver, Pennington, Revelle, and Rantz (2014) found significantly improved health outcomes in Medicare and Medicaid patients in states where NPs have full, unrestricted practice authority.

In another large randomized controlled trial of 2,957 low-income, low-risk women, Jackson et al. (2003) found that birth outcomes of women receiving nurse-midwife collaborative care were equivalent to the group of women receiving traditional physician care, but had lower operative intervention, lower use of epidural anesthesia, more spontaneous vaginal deliveries, and less use of medical resources. Pine et al. (2003) and Jordan et al. (2001) studies of anesthesia morbidity and mortality, noted earlier, demonstrated in a similar fashion the effectiveness, safety, and quality of nurse anesthetist–delivered care. Both historical and recent literature continue to document the effectiveness of APN-provided care across multiple, diverse populations and in a diverse array of settings.

■ APRN CURRENT AND FUTURE OUTCOMES

Providers and researchers must, and are, extending the quality focus to a rigorous assessment of the influence of APRN-provided care across the health care system, including primary, acute, and specialty practice. There is evidence, evolving over several decades, that nurse anesthetist–provided care has resulted in high-quality patient outcomes that are at least equivalent to those achieved by physicians (AANA, n.d.). In addition, CNM-provided maternity care in the United States has resulted in excellent neonatal and maternal outcomes, including physical health of mothers and infants, and satisfaction with care, among others (Davidson, 2002; Oakley et al., 1996; Wilson, 1989). Overall, NP-directed care has achieved excellent outcomes, including care quality, cost-effectiveness, length of stay, and equivalence to physician-provided care (Lenz et al., 2004). However, all of these findings should be considered in the context of a changing health care system and rapidly changing population demographics.

Primary care needs of the population are expanding in an era of significant health reform, and many more primary care providers will be required to fill these needs. Management of chronic illness is a growing APRN focus, as the burden of chronic illness grows in our society. This is magnified by an increasingly aged population, by evolutionary technologies that extend life across the developmental continuum, and by health care reform that further pressures the economic bottom line, while additionally emphasizing chronic care management, medical homes, and primary care access (Blumenthal, Abrams, & Nuzum, 2015; Kocher, Emmanuel, & DeParle, 2010). APRNs are increasingly responsible for caseloads of chronically ill clients who have complex social, behavioral, mental health, and medical needs in primary, acute, and long-term care. Evidence of quality and effectiveness of APRN-provided care in past five decades is strong. The evidence foundation for outcomes of care as provided by NPs, CNMs, CRNAs, and CNSs, including their impact on client health in the short- and long-term, utilization of services, cost, access, quality, and other factors, should, and will, continue to grow in the now-transformed health care system of the 21st century.

■ SUMMARY: FROM SILOS TO COMMON VISION

On March 23, 2010, President Barack Obama signed into law the Patient Protection and ACA, the first overhaul of the American health care system since Lyndon Johnson signed Medicare and Medicaid into law on July 30, 1965. The ACA's planned focus on better access to and affordability of health insurance, health services integration and coordination, expanded use of electronic health records, expansion of primary care services, and redefinition of health care team member roles, especially those of NPs (Kocher et al., 2010) has helped solidify the importance of advance practice nurse providers in improving the health of American citizens. Despite controversies and state-level discrepancies related to its implementation, this historic legislation has indeed helped millions of Americans access health insurance and thus health care services, and has promoted expansion of primary care and chronic care management services (Blumenthal, Abrams, & Nuzum, 2015); APNs will continue to be needed to provide these crucial services (IOM, 2010). During the past two decades, significant changes that mesh with this historic health care reform have occurred. Advanced practice nursing has matured into a powerful force ready to determine its own future. Once separated by practice in separate professional silos, 100,000 APRNs (nurse-midwives, nurse anesthetists, NPs, and CNSs) stand ready to join forces under a uniform umbrella to push the profession forward through a common vision (Pearson, 2010).

During the past 15 years, APRNs have continued to fight for 100% insurance parity with physicians, universal coverage, and expansion of APRN practice to increase access to care, especially for the underinsured and underserved (Advance for Nurse Practitioners, 2010; Pearson, 2010). Utah and then Iowa adopted the APRN Compact, which allows APRNs in one compact state to practice in other compact states to further increase access to care (NCSBN, 2010). In several states, APRNs have decreased barriers to practice and have won the ability to receive Medicaid reimbursement for health care services. Progressive legislation has resulted in permitting APRNs to write prescriptions for the handicapped, placards for the disabled, order home health care, perform physical exams for drivers and students, sign death certificates, write "do not resuscitate" (DNR) orders, and become recognized as primary care providers. In many states, APRNs have won the ability to write for Schedule II through V controlled substances, and have their names printed on prescription labels.

Although there have been some losses, APRNs have held their ground in their struggles with Boards of Medicine across the United States to physicians' grip on regulation, supervision, and authority over their profession (Advance for Nurse Practitioners, 2010; Pearson, 2010). In several states, APRNs have managed to change legal language from "physician supervision" to "collaboration," or to "independent practice," and have removed mandatory APRN-to-physician ratios. Increasingly, state legislatures are removing barriers to independent NP practice; however, at this writing, fewer than half of the states allow fully independent practice. APRNs have continued to extend their scope with regard to referrals to other health care providers, prescribing rights, billing, and providing direction to RNs, school nurses, occupational therapists, and respiratory therapists.

APRNs have also increased their numbers in leadership positions on state boards of nursing. In several states, advanced practice nurses have won the protection of the title of APRN (Advance for Nurse Practitioners, 2010; Pearson, 2010). In addition, they have increased their involvement in the business of state legislatures and the federal government. Four NPs have been elected to powerful positions as state representatives. In several states, APRNs have become major players in malpractice reform, and have been integrally involved in state Medicaid legislation. As the profession has matured, APRNs have hired their own professional lobbyists and formed political action committees. In *Kentucky Association Health Plans, Inc. v. Miller, Kentucky Commissioner of Insurance* (2003) the United States Supreme Court upheld *any-willing provider* law where insurers must open their networks to any provider recognized by the state, including APRNs.

In addition to promoting external changes, APRNs have also focused inwardly to improve the quality of practice. APRNs are reexamining the essential degree for entry-level advanced nursing practice and moving toward unification through the *Consensus Model for Advanced Practice Registered Nurses* (Advance for Nurse Practitioners, 2010; Pearson, 2010). In addition, APRNs are moving toward uniform regulation of practice through licensing, accreditation, certification, and education. As the nation experiences dynamic changes in its health care system, APRNs—both master's and now including those doctorally prepared, stand ready to move the profession forward to provide the highest quality universally accessible health care.

■ CRITICAL THINKING QUESTIONS

1. *How have social, professional, and economic changes from the 1950s to the present influenced the APRN scope of practice?*
2. *How can historical factors in the evolution of the APRN shape the role and practice of future APRNs?*
3. *How is APRN practice different from generalist and medical practice? What accounts for its outcome in terms of patient satisfaction and health status?*
4. *APRN practice, particularly NP and CNM practice, may be conceptualized as built on a social justice foundation—to increase access to care for underserved and/or economically vulnerable populations. Current APRN practice has expanded beyond these boundaries, and many APRNs provide health services to clients who have access to adequate health care services, and who have adequate financial resources. How does this fit with nursing's values? How does this fit with the argument that APRNs should provide lower cost care than physicians and care that is more accessible?*
5. *What factors will influence full implementation of the consensus model for APRN practice? How? What are the barriers to fully autonomous APRN practice?*
6. *What strategies could be used to increase physician support of autonomous APRN practice?*
7. *What are the advantages and disadvantages of APRN movement toward the consensus model for APRNs and uniform regulation of practice through licensing, accreditation, certification, and education?*
8. *What are the factors of APRN practice that make it uniquely different from medical practice? How do they enhance or weaken the profession?*
9. *What are the theoretical factors that set APRNs apart from the discipline of medicine? How does this theory base influence research and practice?*

■ REFERENCES

Advance for Nurse Practitioners. (2010). Annual legislative updates 2000–2010. Retrieved from http://nurse-practitioners.advanceweb.com/Editorial/Search/SearchResult.aspx?KW=annual+legislative +update

Agres, T. (2010). California anesthesiologists buck governor over CRNA role. *Anesthesiology News*, 36(1). Retrieved from http://www.anesthesiologynews.com/index.asp?section_id=3&show= dept&issue_id=589&article_id=14427

American Academy of Pediatrics Committee on Hospital Care. (1999). Role of the nurse practitioner and physician assistant in the care of hospitalized children. *Pediatrics, 103*, 1050–1052. Retrieved from http://www.pediatrics.org/cgi/content/full/103/5/1050

American Academy of Pediatrics Committee on Pediatric Workforce. (2003). Scope of practice issues in the delivery of pediatric healthcare. *Pediatrics, 111*, 426–435. Retrieved from http://www.pediatrics .org/cgi/content/full/111/2/426

American Association of Colleges of Nursing. (1996). *The essentials of master's education for advanced practice nursing*. Retrieved from http://www.aacn.nche.edu/Education/pdf/MasEssentials96.pdf

American Association of Colleges of Nursing. (2009). Title VIII nursing workforce development programs achieving success: Student recipients report the benefits. Retrieved from http://www.aacn .nche.edu/government/pdf/FS_StudentSurvey.pdf

American Association of Nurse Anesthetists. (n.d.). Quality of care in anesthesia. Retrieved from http://www.aana.com/qualityofcare.aspx

American Association of Nurse Anesthetists. (2003). The cost effectiveness of nurse anesthesia practice. Retrieved from http://www.aana.com/crna/costeffect.asp

American Association of Nurse Anesthetists. (2010). Scope and standards for nurse anesthesia practice. Retrieved from http://www.aana.com/uploadedFiles/Resources/Practice_Documents/ scope_stds_nap07_2007.pdf

American Association of Nurse Anesthetists. (2013). Member survey data. Retrieved from http:// www.aana.com/myaana/AANABusiness/professionalresources/Documents/aana-membership -statistics0813.pdf

American College of Nurse-Midwives. (2010). Accreditation Commission for Midwifery Education. Retrieved from http://www.midwife.org/acme.cfm

American Nurses Association. (n.d.). Funding for nursing workforce development. Retrieved from http://nursingworld.org/DocumentVault/GOVA/Federal/Federal-Issues/Nursing WorkforceDevelopment.html

APRN Consensus Workgroup and NCBSN APRN Advisory Committee. (2008). Consensus model for advanced practice registered nurses. Retrieved from http://www.aacn.nche.edu/Education/pdf/ APRNReport.pdf

Avery, M. D. (2005). The history and evolution of the core competencies for basic midwifery practice. *Journal of Midwifery & Womens Health, 50*(2), 102–107.

Baer, E. D. (1987). "A cooperative venture" in pursuit of professional status: A research journal for nursing. *Nursing Research, 36*(1), 18–25.

Barger, M. K. (2005). Midwifery practice: Where have we been and where are we going? *Journal of Midwifery & Women's Health, 50*(2), 87–90.

Bednash, G., Worthington, S., & Wysocki, S. (2009). Nurse practitioner education: Keeping the academic pipeline open to meet family planning needs in the United States. *Contraception, 80*, 409–411.

Benkert, R., Barkauskas, V., Pohl, J., Corser, W., Tanner, C., & Wells, M. (2002). Patient satisfaction outcomes in nurse-managed centers. *Outcomes Management, 6*(4), 174–181.

Benkert, R., Hollie, B., Nordstrom, C. K., Wickson, B., & Bins-Emerick, L. (2009). Trust, mistrust, racial identity and patient satisfaction in urban African American primary care patients of nurse practitioners. *Journal of Nursing Scholarship, 41*(2), 211–219.

Blegen, M. A., & Tripp-Reimer, T. (1997). Implications of nursing taxonomies for middle range theory development. *Advances in Nursing Science, 19*(3), 37–49.

Blumenthal, D., Abrams, M., & Nuzum, R. (2015). The Affordable Care Act at 5 years. *New England Journal of Medicine, 372*, 2451–2458. Retrieved from http://www.nejm.org/doi/full/10.1056/NEJ Mhpr1503614?af=R&rss=currentIssue&

Buhler-Wilkerson, K. (2001). *No place like home: A history of nursing and home care in the United States*. Baltimore, MD: Johns Hopkins University Press.

Bullough, B. (1976). Influences on role expansion. *American Journal of Nursing, 76*(9), 1476–1481.

Buppert, C. (2005). Scope of practice. *Journal for Nurse Practitioners, 1*(1), 11–13.

Burst, H., & Thompson, J. (2003). Genealogic origins of nurse midwifery education programs in the United States, Brief report. *Journal of Midwifery & Women's Health, 48*(6), 464–472.

Canadian Coordinating Office for Health Technology Assessment. (2004). *Surgical anesthesia delivered by nonphysicians*, No. 37 [Report]. Retrieved from http://www.cadth.ca/media/pdf/273_No37_ surgicalanesthesia_preassess_e.pdf

Carter, A. J. E., & Chochinov, A. H. (2007). A systematic review of the impact of nurse practitioners on cost, quality of care, satisfaction and wait times in the emergency department. *Canadian Journal of Emergency Medical Care, 9*(4), 286–295.

Castro, A., & Ruiz, E. (2009). The effects of nurse practitioner cultural competence on Latina patient satisfaction. *Journal of the American Academy of Nurse Practitioners, 21*(5), 278–286.

Charlton, C. R., Dearing, K. S., Berry, J. A., & Johnson, M. J. (2008). Nurse practitioners' communication styles and their impact on patient outcomes: An integrated literature review. *Journal of the American Academy of Nurse Practitioners, 20*(7), 382–388.

Cooper, M. A., Lindsay, G. M., Kinn, S., & Swann, I. J. (2002). Evaluating emergency nurse practitioner services: A randomized controlled trial. *Journal of Advanced Nursing, 40*(6), 721–730.

Davidson, M. H., Burns, C. E., St. Geme, J. W., Cadman, S. G., Newman, C. G., & Bullough, B. (1975). A short term intensive training program for pediatric nurse practitioners. *Journal of Pediatrics, 87*(2), 315–320.

Davidson, M. R. (2002). Outcomes of high risk women cared for by certified nurse midwives. *Journal of Midwifery & Women's Health, 47*(1), 46–49.

Dawley, K. (2003). Origins of nurse-midwifery in the United States and its expansion in the 1940s. *Journal of Midwifery & Womens Health, 48*(2), 86–95.

Dawley, K. (2005). Doubling back over roads once traveled: Creating a national organization for nurse-midwifery. *Journal of Midwifery & Women's Health, 50*(2), 71–82.

Dawley, K., & Burst, H. V. (2005). The American College of Nurse-Midwives and its antecedents: A historic time line. *Journal of Midwifery & Women's Health, 50*(1), 16–22.

Delaney, K. R. (2009). Looking 10 years back and 5 years ahead: Framing the clinical nurse specialist debate for our students. *Archives of Psychiatric Nursing, 23*(6), 453–456.

Dierick-van Daele, A. T. M., Metsemakers, J. F. M., Derckx, E. W. C. C., Spreeuwenberg, C., & Vrijhoef, H. J. M. (2009). Nurse practitioners substituting for general practitioners: Randomized controlled trial. *Journal of Advanced Nursing, 65*(2), 391–401.

Diers, D. (1991). Nurse-midwives and nurse anesthetists: The cutting edge in specialist practice. In L. H. Aiken & C. M. Fagin (Eds.), *Charting nursing's future: Agenda for the '90s* (pp. 159–180). Philadelphia, PA: J. B. Lippincott.

Donahue, P. (1996). *Nursing, the finest art: An illustrated history* (2nd ed.). St. Louis, MO: Mosby.

Donnelly, G. (2003). Clinical expertise in advanced practice nursing: A Canadian perspective. *Nurse Education Today, 23*(3), 168–173.

Donohue, R. K. (2003). Nurse practitioner–client interaction as resource exchange in a women's health clinic: An exploratory study. *Journal of Clinical Nursing, 12*(5), 717–725.

Dulisse, B., & Cromwell, J. (2010). No harm found when nurse anesthetists work without supervision by physicians. *Health Affairs, 29*(8), 1469–1475.

Dunphy, L. M., & Winland-Brown, J. E. (2006). The circle of caring: A transformative model of advanced practice nursing. In W. K. Cody (Ed.), *Philosophical and theoretical perspectives for advanced nursing practice* (4th ed.). Sudbury, MA: Jones & Bartlett.

Elder, R., & Bullough, B. (1990). Nurse practitioner and clinical nurse specialist: Are the roles merging? *Clinical Nurse Specialist, 4*(2), 78–84.

Erikson, H. L. (2007). Philosophy and theory of holism. *Nursing Clinics of North America, 42,* 139–163.

Fairman, J. (1999). Thinking about patients: Nursing science in the 1950's. *Reflections, 23*(3), 30–32.

Fairman, J., & Lynaugh, J. (1998). *Critical care nursing: A history.* Philadelphia: University of Pennsylvania Press.

Fallacaro, M., Obst, T., Funn, I., & Chu, M. (1996). The national distribution of certified registered nurse anesthetists across metropolitan and nonmetropolitan settings. *Journal of the American Association of Nurse Anesthetists, 64*(3), 237–242.

Fawcett, J., & Alligood, M. R. (2005). Influences on advancement of nursing knowledge. *Nursing Science Quarterly, 18*(3), 227–232.

Federal Trade Commission. (2014). Policy perspectives: Competition and regulation of advanced practice nurses. Retrieved from http://www.ftc.gov/policy/reports/policy-reports/commission-and-staff-reports

Ford, L. (1975). An interview with Dr. Loretta Ford. *Nurse Practitioner, 1*(1), 9–12.

Frank vs. South. (1917). 175 Ky 416, 427–428; 194 SW 375, 380.

Graninger, E. (1996). Granny-midwives: Matriarchs of birth in the African-American community 1600–1940. *Birth Gazette, 13*(1), 9–13.

Green, A., & Davis, S. (2005). Toward a predictive model of patient satisfaction with nurse practitioner care. *Journal of the American Academy of Nurse Practitioners, 17*(4), 139–148.

Hayes, E. (2007). Nurse practitioners and managed care: Patient satisfaction and intention to adhere to nurse practitioner plan of care. *Journal of the American Academy of Nurse Practitioners, 19*(8), 418–426.

Hedger, B. (2009). ACP urges doctors and NPs to work together. *American Medical News.* Retrieved from http://www.ama-assn.org/amednews/2009/03/02/prsa0302.htm

Hinch, B., Murphy, M., & Lauer, M. K. (2005). Preparing students for evolving nurse practitioner roles in healthcare. *MEDSURG Nursing, 14*(4), 240–246.

Horrocks, S., Anderson, E., & Salisbury, C. (2002). Systematic review of whether nurse practitioners working in primary care can provide equivalent care to doctors. *British Medical Journal, 324*(7341), 819–823.

Hudspeth, R. (2009). Understanding clinical nurse specialist regulation by the boards of nursing. *Clinical Nurse Specialist, 23*(5), 270–275.

Jackson, D. J., Lang, J. M., Swartz, W. H., Ganiats, T. G., Fullerton, J., Ecker, J., & Nguyen, U. (2003). Outcomes, safety, and resource utilization in a collaborative care birth center program compared with traditional physician-based perinatal care. *American Journal of Public Health, 93*(6), 999–1006.

Jenkins, C. L., Elliott, A. R., & Harris, J. R. (2006). Identifying ethical issues of the department of the army civilian and army nurse corps certified nurse anesthetists. *Military Medicine, 171*(8), 762.

Jennings, N., Lee, G., Chao, K., & Keating, S. (2009). A survey of patient satisfaction in a metropolitan emergency department: Comparing nurse practitioners and emergency physicians. *International Journal of Nursing Practice, 15*(3), 213–218.

Jordan, L. M., Kremer, M., Crawforth, K., & Shott, S. (2001). Data driven practice improvement: The AANA foundation closed malpractice claims study. *AANA Journal, 69*(4), 304–311.

Keeling, A. (2007). *Nursing and the privilege of prescription, 1893–2000.* Columbus: The Ohio State University Press.

Keeling, A. (2009). A brief history of advanced practice nursing in the United States. In A. Hamric, J. Spross, & C. Hanson (Eds.), *Advanced practice nursing: An integrative approach* (4th ed.). St. Louis, MO: Elsevier.

Kentucky Association of Health Plans, Inc. vs. Miller. (2003). 538 U.S.329.

Kleinpell, R. M., Ely, E. W., & Grabenkort, R. (2008). Nurse practitioners and physician assistants in the intensive care unit: An evidence-based review. *Critical Care Medicine, 36*(10), 2888–2897.

Knudtson, N. (2000). Patient satisfaction with nurse practitioner service in a rural setting. *Journal of the American Academy of Nurse Practitioners, 12*(10), 405–412.

Kocher, R., Emmanuel, E. J., & DeParle, N. M. (2010). The Affordable Care Act and the future of clinical medicine. *Annals of Internal Medicine, 153*(8), 536–540.

Kotzer, A. M. (2005). Characteristics and role functions of advanced practice nurses in a tertiary pediatric setting. *Journal for Specialists in Pediatric Nursing, 10*(1), 20–28.

Kozlowski, J. L., Lusk, P., & Melnyk, B. M. (2015). Pediatric nurse practitioner management of child anxiety in a rural primary care clinic with the evidence-based cope program. *Journal of Pediatric Health Care, 29*(3), 274–282.

Lenz, E. R., Mundinger, M. O. N., Kane, R. L., Hopkins, S. C., & Lin, S. X. (2004). Primary care outcomes in patients treated by nurse practitioners or physicians: Two-year follow-up. *Medical Care Research & Review, 61*(3), 332–351.

Lewis, J. A. (2000). Advanced practice in maternal/child nursing: History, current status, and thoughts about the future. *The American Journal of Maternal/Child Nursing, 25*(6), 327–330.

Lindeke, L., Canedy, B., & Kay, M. (1997). A comparison of practice domains of clinical nurse specialists and nurse practitioners. *Journal of Professional Nursing, 13*(5), 281–287.

MacDonald, J., Herbert, R., & Thibeault, C. (2006). Advanced practice nursing: Unification through a common identity. *Journal of Professional Nursing, 22*(3), 172–179.

Manisoff, M. (1981). The nurse practitioner in family planning clinics. *Family Planning Perspectives, 13*(1), 19–22.

Manocchio, R. T. (2008). Tending communities, crossing cultures: Midwives in 19th-century California. *Journal of Midwifery & Women's Health, 53*(1), 75–81.

Mason, D. J., Vaccaro, K., & Fessler, M. B. (2000). Early views of nurse practitioners: A Medline search. *Clinical Excellence for Nurse Practitioners, 4*(3), 175–183.

McCool, W. F., & Simeone, S. A. (2002). Birth in the United States: An overview of trends past and present. *Nursing Clinics of North America, 37*(4), 735–746.

Moorhead, S., Head, B., Johnson, M., & Maas, M. (1998). The nursing outcomes taxonomy: Development and coding. *Journal of Nursing Care Quality, 12*(6), 56–63.

Morrison, S. M., & Fee, E. (2010). Nothing to work with but cleanliness: The training of African American traditional midwives in the South. *American Journal of Public Health, 100*(2), 238–239.

Mundinger, M. O., Kane, R. L., Lenz, E. R., Totten, A. M., Tsai, W. Y., Cleary, P. D., . . . Shelanski, M. L. (2000). Primary care outcomes in patients treated by nurse practitioners or physicians: A randomized trial. *Journal of the American Medical Association, 283*(1), 59–68.

Murphy, M. A. (1990). A brief history of pediatric nurse practitioners and NAPNAP 1964–1990. *Journal of Pediatric Health Care, 4*(6), 332–337.

National Board of Certification and Recertification of Nurse Anesthetists. (2010). Certification. Retrieved from http://www.nbcrna.com/certification.html

National Council of State Boards of Nursing. (1998). Using nurse practitioner certification for state nursing regulation: A historical perspective. Retrieved from https://www.ncsbn.org/428.htm

National Council of State Boards of Nursing. (2010). APRN compact. Retrieved from https://www.ncsbn.org/917.htm

National Institutes of Health. (n.d.). Important events in the National Institute of Nursing Research history. Retrieved from https://www.ninr.nih.gov/aboutninr/history#.VwJ82-a9-t4

National Organization of Nurse Practitioner Faculties. (2002). Nurse practitioner primary care competencies in specialty care areas: Adult, family, gerontological, pediatric, and women's health. Retrieved from http://www.aacn.nche.edu/education/pdf/npcompetencies.pdf

National Organization of Nurse Practitioner Faculties. (2003). *Psychiatric-mental health nurse practitioner competencies: National panel for psychiatric mental health NP competencies.* Washington, DC: Author.

National Organization of Nurse Practitioner Faculties. (2004). *Acute care nurse practitioner competencies: Faculties national panel for acute care nurse practitioner competencies.* Washington, DC: Author.

National Task Force on Quality Nurse Practitioner Education. (2008). Criteria for evaluation of nurse practitioner programs. Washington, DC: AACN. Retrieved from http://www.aacn.nche.edu/education/pdf/evalcriteria2008.pdf

Neill, K. M. (1999). A holistic interdisciplinary health care research model. *Holistic Nursing Practice, 13*(2), 54–60.

Oakley, D., Murray, M. E., Murtland, T., Hayashi, R., Anderson, H. F., & Mays, F. (1996). Comparison of outcomes of maternity care by obstetricians and certified nurse midwives. *Obstetrics & Gynecology, 88*(5), 832–829.

Oliver, G., Pennington, L. Revelle, S. & Rantz, M. (2014). Impact of nurse practitioners on health outcomes of Medicare and Medicaid patients. *Nursing Outlook, 62*(6), 440–447.

Page, N. E., & Arena, D. M. (1994). Rethinking the merger of the clinical nursing specialist and the nurse practitioner roles. *Image: Journal of Nursing Scholarship, 26*(4), 315–318.

Partin, B. (2009). Consensus model for APRN regulation. *The Nurse Practitioner, 34*(6), 8.

Pearson, L. (2010). *The Pearson report 2010.* Retrieved from http://www.pearsonreport.com

Phillips, J. R. (1996). What constitutes nursing science? *Nursing Science Quarterly, 9*(2), 48–49.

Pine, M., Holt, K. D., & Lou, Y. B. (2003). Surgical mortality and type of anesthesia provider. *AANA Journal, 71*(2), 109–116.

Raisler, J., & Kennedy, H. (2005). Midwifery care of poor and vulnerable women, 1925–2003. *Journal of Midwifery & Women's Health, 50*(2), 113–121.

Richmond, J. B. (1965). Gaps in the nation's services for children. *Bulletin of the New York Academy of Medicine, 41*(12), 1237–1247.

Roblin, D. W., Becker, E. R., Adams, E. K., Howard, D. H., & Roberts, M. H. (2004). Patient satisfaction with primary care: Does type of practitioner matter? *Medical Care, 42*(6), 579–590.

Rooks, J. (1997). *Midwifery and childbirth in America.* Philadelphia, PA: Temple University Press.

Roots, A., & McDonald, R. (2014). Outcomes associated with nurse practitioners in collaborative practice in rural settings in Canada: A mixed methods study. *Human Resources for Health, 12*(69). doi:10.1186/1478-4491-12-69

Roy, C. (2007). Advances in nursing knowledge and the challenge for transforming practice. In C. Roy & D. A. Jones (Eds.), *Nursing knowledge development and clinical practice* (pp. 3–37). New York, NY: Springer Publishing.

Sawatsky, J. A., Christie, S., & Singal, R. K. (2013). Exploring outcomes of a nurse practitioner managed cardiac surgery follow up intervention: A randomized trial. *Journal of Advanced Nursing, 69*(9), 2076–2087.

Silver, H. K., Ford, L. R., & Day, H. C. (1968). The pediatric nurse practitioner program: Expanding the role of the nurse to provide increased health care for children. *Journal of the American Medical Association, 204*, 298–302.

Spalding, E. (1943). The Bolton Act provides federal funding for postgraduate programs. *American Journal of Nursing, 43*, 833.

Stanley, J. M. (2012). Impact of new regulatory standards on advanced practice registered nursing: The APRN Consensus Model and LACE. *Nursing Clinics of North America, 27*(2), 241–250.

Stanley, J. M., Werner, K. E., & Apple, K. (2009). Positioning advanced practice registered nurses for healthcare reform: Consensus on APRN regulation. *Journal of Professional Nursing, 25*(6), 340–348.

Stone, S. E. (2000). The evolving scope of nurse-midwifery practice in the United States. *Journal of Midwifery & Women's Health, 45*(6), 522–531.

Van Leuven, K., & Prion, S. (2007). Health promotion in care directed by nurse practitioners. *Journal for Nurse Practitioners, 3*(7), 456–461.

Varney, H., Kriebs, J., & Gegor, C. (2004). *Varney's midwifery* (4th ed.). Sudbury, MA: Jones & Bartlett.

Wald, L. (1922). *The origin and development of the Henry Street Settlement Text for Broadcasting.* [Reel #25 Lillian Wald Papers]. In The Westinghouse Electric Manufacturing Co. (Producer). New York, NY: The New York Public Library.

Wall, B. M. (2005). *Unlikely entrepreneurs: Catholic sisters and the hospital marketplace, 1863–1925.* Columbus: The Ohio State University Press.

Wilson, B. (1989). Delivery outcomes of low risk births: Comparison of certified nurse midwives and obstetricians. *Journal of the American Academy of Nurse Practitioners, 1*(1), 9–13.

CHAPTER THREE

Reflective Response 1

Ann L. O'Sullivan

My first response after reading this succinct history of an advanced practice registered nurse's (APRN's) growth and development was to say, "It was the best of times, it was the worst of times" (p. 5) from Charles Dickens's (1859/2003) *A Tale of Two Cities*. He was speaking of London and Paris during the time of the French Revolution, just two decades after our own revolution, which certainly had influenced their French Revolution. So, each APRN has had revolutionary behavior to be able to serve people (and society) in the way they need and deserve. In order to have access to care by nurses in any of the four APRN roles, certified registered nurse anesthetists (CRNAs), certified nurse-midwives (CNMs), clinical nurse specialists (CNSs), and/or certified nurse practitioners (CNPs), scopes of practice often overlap with other health care professionals.

Another immediate response is to reflect on a picture from our Barbara Bates Center for the study of the *History of Nursing*,[1] of a young nurse carrying a velvet box, holding a thermometer for the physician to use to take a patient's temperature. Today, skill and knowledge, as depicted in this picture, which had traditionally been part of medicine, are part of everyday parenting, as we see a revolution in knowledge and skill acquisition by all. Sadly, when reading each profession's response to the American Medical Association's (AMA) 2005 *Scope of Practice Data Series*[2] that profiles 10 nonphysician professions'/professionals' (including audiologists, dentists, naturopaths, nurse anesthetists, nurse practitioners (NPs), optometrists, pharmacists, physical therapist, podiatrists, and psychologists) education, accreditation, certification, and licensure, I sense the revolution goes on into the 21st century. The AMA disputes that unwarranted scope of practice (SOP) expansions by nonphysician professionals will threaten the health and safety of patients (Devitt, 2006).

In fact, the Scope of Practice Partnership (SOPP) is a coalition of national medical specialty organizations and state medical societies established by the AMA in 2005 to study the qualifications, education, certification, and licensure of nonphysician providers. In addition to NPs, they are concerned about chiropractors, podiatrists, acupuncturists, naturopathic physicians, and psychologists. They will oppose inappropriate SOP expansion, or encroachments on physician practice. The AMA staffed the partnership and had allocated $170,000 to pay staff and fund studies that examined the education, accreditation, certification, and licensure of allied health professionals. The partnership had 12 founding members: six state medical associations and six medical specialty groups (Devitt, 2006).

Clearly, the authors of this chapter present data to dispute such claims of threatened patient safety, as do representatives from each profession in their letters of response to AMA's *Data Series*. On the other hand, if we keep in mind the 2006 collaborative document on *Changes in Healthcare Professions' Scope of Practice: Legislative Considerations* (revised in 2009)[3] developed by: the Federation of State Medical Board (FSMB), National Council of State Boards of Nursing, Inc. (NCSBN), Federation of State Board of Physical Therapy (FSBPT), National Board of Certification on Occupational Therapy (NBCOT), Association of Social Work Boards (ASWB), and National Association of Boards of Pharmacy (NABP), we can be hopeful with their statement, "overlapping scopes of practice are a reality in a rapidly changing healthcare environment. The criteria related to who is qualified to perform functions safely without risk of harm to the public are the only justifiable conditions for defining scopes of practice" (National Council of State Boards of Nursing, 2009, p. 15).

However, the AMA never gives up on an issue! In 2012, through their Advocacy Resource Center, they published a five-page white paper on the need for *Physician led health care teams—Advocacy on behalf of physicians and patients at the state level* (AMA 2012). They approached this topic with their values and opinions in seven areas, including:

1. Education and training makes physicians most qualified to lead the health care team—not advanced practice registered nurses.
2. Patients want physician leadership and one patient survey documented that patients care most about doctor's (of medicine) education, training and expertise not factors relating to convenience.
3. Top integrated health care institutions are physician lead.
4. Physician assistants (PAs) support the physician-led team model of care (because PAs cannot practice independently).
5. Increased utilization of APRNs does not lead to cost savings.
6. Increased use of APRNs is not the solution to access problems (because only 52% go into practicing primary care in the United States based on their geographic mapping).
7. Workforce shortages include both physicians and nurses.

In addition, in 2014, the AMA developed what it calls "Health Workforce Mapper," which is an interactive tool that illustrates the geographic locations of the health care workforce in each state, as well as other related trends including where to locate or expand your practice to reach patients without current access to care, and where not to locate due to an excess of providers for each patient currently (AMA, 2014).

Luckily, the ANA (2009) is an official observer at the AMA Annual Meeting, where the AMA proposes many resolutions and reports that could affect nursing practice.

The ANA publishes its observations in *Capital Update* after each annual meeting— so we are able to follow its assaults on our ability to practice to our full SOP.

We know the AMA tries constantly to stop any changes in SOP that it thinks will lessen its power and control of health care delivery in states. It continues to oppose the IOM's *The Future of Nursing* (2011) key message: "Nurses should practice to the full extent of their education and training" (p. 29).

In 2012, the AMA, feeling very threatened, worked with the Physicians Foundation-Empowering Physicians, Improving Healthcare on two documents regarding SOP: (a) *A Decision-Maker's Guide to Scope of Practice* (Issacs and Jellinek, October 2012) which covers nurse anesthetics, NPs, murse-midwives, and ten other professionals like audiologist, pharmacists, and psychologist; and (b) *Accept No Substitute: A report on Scope of Practice* (Issacs and Jellinek, November 2012) because in 2012 it had found through the

National Conference of State Legislation reports more than 350 SOP laws enacted in 48 states since January 2011.

As SOP is determined at the state level for professionals, they work at countering these intrusions state by state. NPs have full autonomy in 20 states and the District of Columbia; optometrists have gained simple surgical privileges in three or more states; and psychologists have won prescribing rights in two or more states. This paper also documents physicians' worries over the recent proliferation of doctorates in many of the 10 nonphysician professions. The worry is that a doctorate may strengthen the individuals in their advocacy for full practice authority, and they will engage consumer organizations and other nonmedical colleagues to increase their credibility and political clout with each state's legislators. In fact, they even worry about the additional fund-raising for advocacy that these non professionals are able to accomplish, and lack of funding of the professional medical organizations by salaried physicians.

In one case it was the Colorado Medical Society versus Hickenlooper 2015 CO 41 (Colo. 2015), where CRNAs had a win but it was a very unfavorable decision for physicians. This case had to go all the way to the Colorado Supreme Court because of the medical societies appeals but on June 1, 2015, the Colorado Supreme Court affirmed that the Colorado Nurse Practice Act allows CRNAs to provide health care services without physician supervision. In addition, the Colorado Supreme Court affirmed the finding that the governor of Colorado had acted within his discretion regarding the Medicare opt-out requirement!

Therefore, all Doctor of Nursing Practice (DNP) graduates will need to follow legislation that may influence their practice, positively as well as negatively, such as the new APRN Compact (NCSBN, 2015). The APRN Compact, approved on May 4, 2015, allows APRNs to practice in the other compact states with a single multistate license. Maintaining membership in one's professional nursing organization is essential in order to follow the dialogue on a particular issue, regardless of whether it will negatively or positively influence one's practice. The following are some examples of ongoing issues and organizations that can potentially affect DNP-APRN-CNP practice.

DNPs have every right to be called doctor and are very proud to be nurses and not physicians. They should have no problem being included in appropriate legislation, and like the dental hygienists, their education and training will not be confusing to patients.

Each year, state legislators are bombarded with bills related to SOP. The publication *Advance for Nurse Practitioners* (nurse-practitioners.advanceweb.com) is one source of such professional SOP information. For example, a July 29, 2009, posting shared the successful end to an NP Restraint-of-Trade Case from Butte, Montana. This case involved two NPs who owned and operated a clinic, whose referrals for imaging beyond routine x-rays were refused by a physician director of radiology and pathology at a nearby hospital, because they did not have physician supervision (which was not required in Montana). After an 8-month delay by the defendants (physician and hospital), the parties settled four days into the trial. Advice from these APRNs was, "Don't back down, don't allow it, stand up for our rights" (Ford, 2009, p. 1).

DNPs should also follow the calls for quick action from professional organizations regarding proposed federal legislation. The Nurse Practitioner Roundtable (NPR), a coalition of seven national NP organizations, works very hard to influence federal legislation (Nurse Practitioner Roundtable, 2008).

One hurdle in 2014 that the NPR took a stance on was documented in its paper *Nurse Practitioner Perspective on Education and Post-Graduate Training*. They made five evidence-based recommendations in their joint organizational paper. In addition, they clearly noted why "residency" is not a good description of NP postgraduate orientation into a new clinical practice.

An additional paper by Sheehan (2010) must not be forgotten because of the importance of the Roundtables message in "The Value of Health Care Advocacy for Nurse Practitioners." We must remember that NPs do win some legislative battles and lose some, but one success was getting language inserted into the Reconciliation Act, allowing Health and Human Services (HHS) secretary to include NP leaders in medical home demonstration projects.

The Coalition for Patients' Rights (CPR) was established in 2006 for the sake of giving patients a choice of providers and fighting barriers to quality care. As of 2016, CPR consisted of more than 35 organizations of a variety of licensed health care professionals who provide safe, effective, and affordable health care to millions of clients each year (CPR, 2010a). CPR was formed to prevent SOPP from implementing unnecessary actions against allied health professionals that "will impede, rather than enhance" (CPR, 2006, p. 1), patient access to evidence-based care by these nonphysician providers. CPR also advocates for "the practice rights of its members for the sake of their patients" (CPR, 2010b, p. 1). CPR seeks to have a balanced study of all health care providers' education, accreditation, certification, and licensure, and would like such a study to "assess whether state laws and regulations governing physicians practice contain outdated language that should be eliminated so that the unique skills of licensed healthcare professionals who do not hold a medical license are recognized" (CPR, 2006, p. 2).

In addition, such a study would "evaluate the implications of current state laws that allow physicians to practice in any specialty, regardless of the individual qualifications to do so" (CPR, 2006, p. 2). Support statements from more than 35 organizations can be found on CPR's website, as well as from media resources. In December 2008, the American Nurses Association (ANA, 2008) (a 2006 founding member of CPR) reaffirmed its support for patient access to licensed health care providers of their choice in a press release stated:

> Patients deserve to have access to the expert care that nurses can give them. Doctors do not have the right to impede nurses merely because we threaten their "territory." We can do more to improve patient care by working together rather than at odds with each other. (p. 1)

This statement by the ANA was made in concert with the aforementioned 35 other national health care organizations to rally toward the "common cause of ensuring that all patients have access to quality care" (CPR, 2010b, p. 1).

In 2015, CPR commended our colleagues at the American College of Cardiology (ACC) regarding its 2015 ACC Health Policy Statement on Cardiovascular Team- Based Care and the Role of Advanced Practice Providers. ACC stated, "team core leaders should be flexible, reflecting the specific needs of the patient at a particular time and setting. A nurse or pharmacist may lead a team that organizes a chronic anticoagulation clinic" (p. 1).

Each state's professional society tracks the number of providers that a state has and will need in the next 10 years. Sadly, the results of these studies document over and over again the shortage of physician providers to provide primary care to the clients of a particular state. In fact, the American College of Physicians (ACP) released a monograph in 2009, which stated, "NPs and physicians have common goals of providing high-quality, patient-centered care and improving the health status of those they serve" (p. 1). Furthermore, the ACP recommended that any demonstration project of the patient-centered medical home model should include one run by an NP (ACP, 2009). This is a perfect position for a DNP-APRN-CNP. AMA still states that DNPs must practice under physician supervision as part of a medical team, but this is much less apt to happen as the physician shortages increase. Clearly, the AMA and ACP have different views regarding a pilot of NPs as the leader of a medical home model—one that will, in the future, hopefully be called a "health home."

And in 2013 a paper for the National Institute of Health Care Reform by Yee, Boukus, Cross, and Samuel titled *Primary Care Workforce Shortages: Nurse Practitioner Scope of Practice Laws and Payment Policies* continued to discuss the influence of SOP and payer policies on effective care delivery. They outline how payer policies now have more impact than SOP laws on how and where NPs practice. In addition, the systematic review by Xue, Yee, Brewer, and Spetz (2016) of NP SOP shows promise that removing the remaining SOP restrictions could be one way to increase primary capacity in the United States.

One aspect of DNP education, accreditation, certification, and licensure about which the AMA and ACP do agree is that DNP certification should not be obtained through Step 3 of the medical licensing exam of the National Board of Medical Examiners. The discipline of nursing should certify and license the DNP, APRN, and CNP.

■ CONCLUSION

Our physician colleagues are alerted to four critical trends to keep in mind in 2016 by the Ray and Norbeck (2016). Perhaps we also should track them: (a) evidence-based policies regulating our practice; (b) health insurance market consolidation; (c) value-based care versus volume for Medicare payments; and (d) leadership challenges including administrative burdens (re-reporting requirement and prior authorization problems), financial pressures, and multiple health system changes influencing our practice.

Finally, the December 2015 Institute of Medicine Progress Report titled *The Future of Nursing* wants us to be sure to focus our attention on five important areas:

1. Removing APRN SOP restrictions and increasing interprofessional collaborations
2. Expanding educational opportunities for both baccalaureates and doctoral degrees as well as fostering lifelong learning
3. Collaborating and leading in the redesign of health care delivery and payment systems
4. Continuing to promote diversity
5. Improving workforce data collection by including all states and federal government in order to better measure and monitor the numbers of health professionals needed, where employed, and what roles

The challenges of APRN practitioners and their role in the delivery of client-care services to individuals in our society throughout their life span will go on for years; but clearly the time has come for better communications, collaboration, and commitment on the part of all health professionals in order to foster health care reforms in the 21st century.

■ NOTES

1. The center's website at the University of Pennsylvania School of Nursing: http://www.nursing.upenn.edu/history/Pages/default.aspx

2. The AMA Data Series on NPs can be found at: http://www.acnpweb.org/files/public/08-0424_SOP_Nurse_Revised_10_09.pdf
3. The revised 2009 version produced by the NCSBN can be found at: https://www.ncsbn.org/ScopeofPractice.pdf

■ REFERENCES

American Medical Association. (2014). Health workforce mapper. Retrieved from http://www.ama-assm.org/ama/pub/advoacy/state-ADVOCACY-ARC/health-workforce-mapper.page?

American Medical Association Litigation Center. (2015). Colorado Medical Society v. Hickenlopper, 2015 CO41 (Colo.2015) case summary. Retrieved from http://www.ama-assn.org/ama/pub/physician-resources/legal-topics/litigation-center/case-summaries-topics/scope-practice.page?

American College of Physicians. (2009). Nurse practitioners in primary care. Retrieved from http://www.acponline.org/advocacy/where_we_stand/policy/np_pc.pdf

American Medical Association. (2014) Geographic mapping initiative. Retrieved from http://www.medicalpracticeinsider.com/news/want-know-where-youre-most-needed-ama-has-tool

American Nurses Association. (2008). ANA supports patient access to licensed health care providers of their choice. Retrieved from http://www.patientsrightscoalition.org/About-Us/Statements-of-Support/ANA.aspx

American Nurses Association. (2009). ANA official observer at AMA annual meeting; AMA polices could affect nursing practice. Retrieved from http://www.rnaction.og/site/PageServer?pagename=CUP_07_09IntheAgencies_ANAOfficia/OberseratAMA&ct=1

Coalition for Patients' Rights. (2006). Healthcare professionals urge cooperative patient care; oppose SOPP & AMA Resolution 814. Retrieved from CPRJointStatement.doc

Coalition for Patients' Rights. (2010a). Homepage. Retrieved from http://www.patientsrightscoalition.org/default.aspx

Coalition for Patients' Rights. (2010b). Statements of support. Retrieved from http://www.patientsrightscoalition.org/About

Coalition for Patients' Rights. (2015). Letter to American College of Cardiology. Retrieved from www.patientsrightscoalition.org

Committee for Assessing Progress on Implementing the Recommendations of the Institute of Medicine Report The Future of Nursing: Leading Change Advancing Health. (2015). *Assessing progress on the institute of medicine report*. The future of nursing. Retrieved from www.ion.nationalacademies.org

Devitt, M. (2006). American Medical Association creates "partnership" to limit other providers' scope of practice: The next attempt to "contain and eliminate" chiropractic? *Dynamic Chiropractic, 24*(12), 1–7. Retrieved from http://www.dynamincchiropractic.com/mpacms/dc/article/php?id=51219

Dickens, C. (1859/2003). *A tale of two cities*. London, UK: Penguin Classics.

Ford, J. (2009). NP restraint-of-trade case settles. ADVANCE for nurse practitioners. Retrieved from http://nurse-practitioners.advanceweb.com/Article/Restraint-of-Trade-Case-Settles-2.aspx

Institute of Medicine. (2011). *The future of nursing: Leading change, advancing health*. Washington, DC: National Academies Press.

Isaacs, S., & Jellinek, P. (2012). *A decision-maker's guide to scope of practice*. Report prepared for the physicians' foundation. Retrieved from http://www.PhysiciansFoundation.org

Isaacs, S., & Jellinek, P. (2012, November). *Accept no substitute: A report on scope of practice*. Retrieved from www.PhysiciansFoundation.org

National Council of State Boards of Nursing. (2009). Changes in healthcare professions' scope of practice: Legislative considerations [revised from 2006]. Retrieved from https://www.ncsbn.org/ScopeofPractice.pdf

National Council of State Boards of Nursing. (2015). APRN compact. Retrieved from NCSBN.org

Nurse Practitioner Roundtable. (2008). Nurse practitioners: Medical home/coordinated primary care providers. Washington, DC: American Academy of Nurse Practitioners; American College of Nurse Practitioners; Association of Faculties of Pediatric Nurse Practitioners; National Association of Nurse Practitioners in Women's Health National Association of Pediatric Nurse Practitioners National Conference of Gerontological; Nurse Practitioners National Organization of Nurse

Practitioner Faculties. Retrieved from http://www.acnpweb.org/files/public/2009NPMedicalH omeCoordPrimaryCareProviders.pdf

Nurse Practitioner Roundtable. (2014). Nurse practitioner perspective on education and post-graduate training. Retrieved from https://www.aanp.org/education/82-legislation-regulation/state-policy -toolkit-accordion/445-aanp-and-the-np-roundtable-joint-statements

Ray, W., & Norbeck, T. (2016). Four critical trends physicians must keep top of mind in 2016. Retrieved from http://www.forbes.com/sites/physiciansfouation/2016/04/four-critical-trends -physicians-must-keep-top-of-mind-in-2016/#4a40d19ezdfa

Sheehan, A. (2010). The value of health care advocacy for nurse practitioners. *Journal of Pediatric Health Care, 24*(4), 280–282. doi:10.1016/j.pedhc.2010.04.001

Yee, T., Boukus, E. R., Cross, D., & Samuel, D. R. (2013). Primary care workforce shortages: Nurse practitioner scope of practice and payment policies (NIHCR Research Brief No. 13). Washington, DC: National Institute for Healthcare Reform. Retrieved from http://www.nihcr.org/ pcp-workforce-nps

Xue, Y., Ye, Z., Braver, C., & Spatz, J. (2016). Impact of state nurse practitioner scope of practice regulation on health care delivery: Systematic review. *Nursing Outlook, 64*(1),71–85. doi:10.1016/ j.outlook.2015.08.005

CHAPTER THREE

Reflective Response 2

Patti Rager Zuzelo

The authors correctly describe the historical "roots" of the clinical nurse specialist (CNS), nurse practitioner (NP), nurse-midwife, and nurse-anesthetist roles. However, it is critical to understand the important contrast between CNS role origins as compared to the genesis of other roles. Midwifery, anesthetist, and practitioner roles evolved from unmet public needs often in response to a lack of medical care and, many times, were birthed in practice models informed by medicine or by other non-nursing influences. These origins are in sharp contrast to those of the CNS role, a role *uniquely* grounded in professional nursing.

The term *clinical nurse specialist* was first used in 1938 (Peplau, 1965/2003), and the initial role description of CNS as an advanced practice nurse with expertise in nursing practice in the care of complex patients is credited to Dr. Hildegard Peplau (National Association of Clinical Nurse Specialists [NACNS], 2004). These underpinnings contribute to the significant differences found in the subsequent histories, practice barriers, regulatory challenges, and practice domains between advanced practice nursing roles.

Specialization is not unique to the CNS but is a hallmark of this role. The first edition of the *Nursing's Social Policy Statement* (American Nurses Association [ANA], 1980) described a CNS as a registered nurse holding a master's degree in nursing with a clinical focus. These clinical foci or areas of specialization often develop along lines of new knowledge, public needs and demands, nurse interests, and available opportunities (Peplau, 1965/2003). Nurse-midwife and nurse anesthetist roles are specialized fields but areas of expertise are confined to a particular demographic or a specific type of intervention. CNSs specialize in many practice areas with evidence-based competencies associated with a particular specialty (NACNS, 2004). CNS specialization taxonomy could be organized by population, problem type, setting, care requirement, or disease/pathology/medical specialty (NACNS, 2004). Regardless of the specialty area, *nursing* is the center of CNS practice. This observation reinforces the notion that the CNS is "first of all a generalist, so she [sic] can do what is expected of a staff nurse" (Peplau, 2003, p. 7).

The authors note that during the 1980s and 1990s, there was much discussion and published exchange about blending the CNS and NP roles. In part, this discussion was fueled by reduction in workforce decisions made by hospital administrators in response to reduced reimbursements and budget challenges (Barker, 2009). CNS positions were often threatened or lost. There were also educational programs touting blended role programs that typically provided minimal attention to developing the CNS skill set and specialized expertise. Because the CNS role was more vulnerable to workplace reductions and titling protections were often not provided at the state level, nurses interested in the CNS role often gravitated to this role after completing graduate education in a different area of study, including education, administration, or NP programs.

The authors point out threats related to CNS title protection, regulation, and scope of practice, and these issues are concerning. *The Consensus Model for Advanced Practice Registered Nurses* (APRN Consensus Workgroup and National Council of State Boards of Nursing [NCSBN] APRN Advisory Committee, 2008) offers both opportunities and challenges to CNS practitioners, particularly because specialization is a hallmark of the CNS role and this is an "optional" feature of the model. Limited access to and inadequate availability of necessary certification examinations are also priority CNS issues (Zuzelo, 2010). Many CNSs practice across the life span within a particular specialty. As an example, a CNS educated as an expert clinician in diabetes care management or a CNS with specialization in orthopedics or congestive heart failure care may work with people of varying ages. Their areas of expertise have been developed within a specialty, and their educational and employment experiences follow a trajectory reflective of this specialization.

The current "across the life span" population of the APRN Consensus Model poses challenges to this specialization model, and these challenges are associated with barriers and opportunities. The 2014 Clinical Nurse Specialists Census reports that 3,370 respondents practice in the population of family/across the life span (NACNS, 2015a). These particular CNSs ($n = 163$) capture only NACNS members who chose to respond. Data support the fact that the lack of a certification examination for CNSs practicing in this population is an important concern. NACNS is working to address this need.

A critical aspect of CNS history that is not noted by the authors relates to the conceptualization of the CNS role through efforts of the NACNS and the subsequent opportunities for a CNS "voice" at important national dialogues. This organization was formed in 1995 to represent CNSs, regardless of specialty. Its early work included explicating core competencies for CNS practice (Baldwin, Lyon, Clark, Fulton, & Dayhoff, 2007). Prior to this time, the CNS role was typically described in a functional, "laundry list" of sub-roles, including educator, clinician, consultant, researcher, and expert. Notably, other APRNs could reasonably claim to have similar expertise and responsibilities. This list did not provide an encompassing framework to inform CNS practice.

The essence of CNS practice is recognized as clinical expertise based on advanced nursing science knowledge (NACNS, 2004). Three interacting spheres of influence, guided by specialty knowledge and specialty standards, provide the conceptual framework for CNS practice (Figure 3.1). A process that included review of evidence, input and validation of experts, and public comment was used to develop CNS core practice competencies actualized in specialty practice (Baldwin et al., 2007). These core competencies were again validated in 2009 via a process that included input from practicing CNSs (Baldwin, Clark, Fulton, & Mayo, 2009). The conceptual framework provides a meaningful lens through which to explicate clear differences between CNS and NP practice (Zuzelo, 2003, 2010).

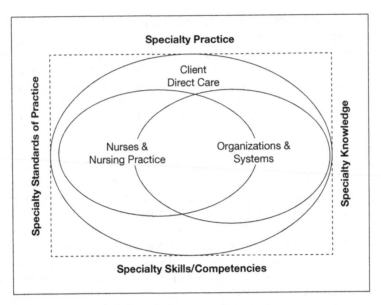

FIGURE 3.1 Conceptualization of clinical nurse specialist practice.

Source: Copyright Janet S. Fulton, PhD, RN, ACNS-BC, FAAN, professor of nursing, Indiana University, Indianapolis, IN. Reprinted with permission of the author. Contact author at jan_fulton@sbcglobal.net

■ RECENT WORK EFFORTS AND ONGOING ISSUES

Consistent with the experiences of other APRN groups, CNSs have needed to grapple with the implications of the Doctor of Nursing Practice (DNP) degree. The benefits of a CNS workforce that is prepared with doctoral education are obvious and understood. However, NACNS and its constituency have needed to carefully analyze the costs and benefits associated with taking an organizational position that calls for a DNP degree as a necessary requirement for entering CNS practice. This consideration process has been arduous and thoughtful. The NACNS Board of Directors recently endorsed the recommendations of the NACNS DNP Task Force (2015b) and its call for the DNP degree as required for entry into CNS practice by 2030 (NACNS, 2015b). Concurrently, NACNS endorsed a draft position statement on the PhD that is following NACNS process for member vetting prior to adoption (2016). This position statement asserts the importance of the terminal research degree as necessary to the development of nursing science.

Other ongoing issues have been revealed through the 2014 NACNS Census of CNSs (2015a). This first national consensus effort focused on CNSs provided data explicating barriers to CNS practice including state-regulated prescriptive authority and direct billing opportunities. One significant and persistent challenge is the U.S. Bureau of Labor Statistics (BLS) Standard Occupational Classification (SOC) system that federal agencies use to collect and manage data concerning 840 detailed occupations (BLS, 2010a). CNSs are currently grouped within the registered nurses classification. Other APRNs are specifically excluded and are categorized under health diagnosing and treating practitioners (BLS, 2010b). Various data collection efforts rely on SOC classifications and the failure of correctly classifying CNSs has potentially broad and negative public policy implications.

The authors have appropriately commented on wide state-level variation in regulation and scope of CNS practice, and have observed that there is a history of overlap in roles and functions between CNS and NP. The work of NACNS has provided a vehicle for making a clear case that CNS competencies are unique, built on clinical expertise and specialization, and directly connected to the science of nursing. Future opportunities for CNSs and their stakeholders will likely be positively energized by new possibilities provided in the Patient Protection and Affordable Care Act, and new curricular designs of both practice and research doctoral programs.

■ REFERENCES

American Nurses Association. (1980). *Nursing's social policy statement.* Kansas City, MO: Author.

Baldwin, K., Clark, A., Fulton, J., & Mayo, A. (2009). National validation of the NACNS clinical nurse specialist core competencies. *Journal of Nursing Scholarship, 2,* 193–201.

Baldwin, K., Lyon, B., Clark, A., Fulton, J., & Dayhoff, N. (2007). Developing clinical nurse specialist practice competencies. *Clinical Nurse Specialist, 6,* 297–303.

Barker, A. (2009). *Advanced practice nursing: Essential knowledge for the profession.* Sudbury, MA: Jones & Bartlett.

Bureau of Labor Statistics. (2010a). Standard occupational classification. Retrieved from http://www.bls.gov/soc

Bureau of Labor Statistics. (2010b). 29-0000 healthcare practitioners and technical occupations. Retrieved from http://www.bls.gov/soc/2010/soc290000.htm#29–1000

National Association of Clinical Nurse Specialists. (2015a). Key findings from the 2014 clinical nurse specialists census. Retrieved from http://www.nacns.org/docs/CensusInfographic.pdf

National Association of Clinical Nurse Specialists. (2015b). NACNS position statement on the doctor of nursing practice. Retrieved from http://www.nacns.org/docs/DNP-Statement1507.pdf

National Association of Clinical Nurse Specialists. (2016). Draft: PhD position statement. Retrieved from http://www.nacns.org/members/html/main.php

National Association of Clinical Nurse Specialists 2004 Statement Revision Task Force. (2004). *Statement on clinical nurse specialist practice and education* (2nd ed.). Harrisburg, PA: Author.

Peplau, H. (1965/2003). Specialization in professional nursing. *Clinical Nurse Specialist, 17*(1), 3–9.

Zuzelo, P. (2003). Clinical nurse specialist practice—Spheres of influence. *AORN Journal, 77*(2), 361–364, 366, 369–372.

Zuzelo, P. (2010). *The clinical nurse specialist handbook* (2nd ed.). Sudbury, MA: Jones & Bartlett.

How Doctoral-Level Advanced Practice Roles Differ From Master's-Level Advanced Practice Nursing Roles

Kym A. Montgomery and Sharon K. Byrne

Since the publication of the first edition of this book, two sentinel events have further transformed the landscape of nursing practice: the passage of the Patient Protection and Affordable Care Act (PPACA; U.S. Department of Labor, 2010) and the release of Institute of Medicine's (IOM) report *The Future of Nursing: Leading Change, Advancing Health* (IOM, 2010). The PPACA has challenged the U.S. health care delivery system to provide care to 30 million previously uninsured Americans, improve the health of our society, and to reduce the overall health care costs by providing the necessary health care services in a most efficient way. The IOM (2010) report is a prescription for the future of nursing's role in American health care through nursing leadership in decision making in a multidisciplinary arena, seamless academic advancement for all nurses, and the ability to achieve the maximum scope of nursing practice. The Doctor of Nursing Practice (DNP) graduate exemplifies the vision of the IOM report and is perfectly positioned to achieve the goals of the PPACA. In essence, the DNP is the answer to the future of nursing practice.

Globally, the ranks of advanced practice registered nurses (APRNs) have exploded over the past 50 years. Despite the number of APRNs in clinical practice, however, there has been a lack of consistency in education that is reflected in poor degree parity compared to other health care professions such as physical therapy, nutrition therapy, occupational therapy, and pharmacy that have successfully developed doctoral programs as entry into their fields of practice. Nursing's first foray into doctoral nursing education began in 1932 at Teachers College of Columbia University with the awarding of the first doctor of education (EdD) degree in nursing education (Nichols & Chitty, 2005). Since that time, the profession has been persistently and unsuccessfully seeking a true clinical doctorate degree that showcases the true intellectual triad of the nursing profession. In the past, the profession's support of the PhD, doctor of nursing science (DNSc), doctor of nursing science (DNS), and doctor of science in nursing (DSN), and lukewarm support of the EdD and doctor of nursing (ND) degrees, did not yield an appropriate pathway to the "clinical" doctorate. Is it possible that amid this chaos and ongoing scholarly debate about which is the right terminal degree for clinicians, opportunity knocks with the development of the Doctor of Nursing Practice (DNP)?[1] The authors of this chapter hopefully present a thought-provoking discussion regarding the roles of the long-standing and historically master of science in nursing (MSN)-prepared APRN, and contrast it with the newly heralded DNP-prepared APRN, as a new method of achieving a terminal degree that supports superior professional excellence.

■ THE EMERGENCE OF THE DNP DEGREE

The timeline leading up to the DNP degree for APRNs began with the call of the IOM (2001) for sweeping redesign of the entire health care system. The IOM outlined basic skills that all health care professionals should have and suggested that new educational options be developed to ensure the safety of patients and close the gap that impedes quality care. The IOM (2001) stated:

> Forced with rapid changes in the healthcare system, the nation's healthcare delivery system has fallen far short in its ability to translate knowledge into practice and to apply new technology safely and appropriately. And if the system cannot consistently deliver today's science and technology, it is less prepared to respond to the extraordinary advances that surely will emerge during the coming decades. There is a dearth of clinical programs with the multidisciplinary infrastructure required to provide the full complement of services needed by people with common chronic conditions. The healthcare system is poorly organized to meet the challenges at hand. (IOM, 2001, p. 1)

IOM's challenge ignited a series of responses by a myriad of organizations that called for better-prepared APRNs who could address the complexity of patient care requirements, improve the efficiency of health care environments, and provide for an increased knowledge base for practice and excellence in nursing leadership. Three years later in 2004, the American Association of Colleges of Nursing (AACN) adopted a position to move the level of preparation necessary for advanced practice roles from a master's degree to a doctoral degree. Initially, the AACN (2004) anticipated that the DNP would become the requisite credential for entry into advanced practice nursing by 2015. Although there has been significant movement toward this goal over the past decade, the lack of clarity regarding the definition of "nursing practice," the variety of curriculum existing among DNP programs, and the barriers inhibiting a school's implementation of a DNP program have prompted further reconsideration when to initiate this requirement (AACN, 2015a). Through a national survey of nursing schools offering APRN programs by the RAND Corporation, the AACN found great support and rising demand for DNP programs from nursing schools and nursing academic leaders (AACN, 2015a). The RAND study also identified obstacles inhibiting DNP programs such as lack of faculty, financial concerns, lack of clinical sites, resource issues regarding DNP scholarly projects, and confusion of potential employers surrounding the difference between master's-prepared and DNP-prepared APRNs. The Council on Accreditation of Nurse Anesthesia Educational Programs (American Association of Nurse Anesthetists [AANA], 2007) has mandated that all nurse anesthetists have doctoral education in order to practice by 2025. Could this possibly be the impetus for all APRN specialties to mandate the IOM's recommendation for nursing's seamless academic achievement (IOM, 2010)?

Similarly, the Commission on Collegiate Nursing Education (CCNE, 2005), the accrediting body of the AACN, decided that only practice doctorate degrees with the credential DNP would be considered for accreditation by the CCNE. At the time, this was a controversial stance since the initial 2004 vote was not unanimous (AACN, 2004).

Columbia University had proposed an older DNP degree model first, a DrNP, but there were concerns that multiple practice degrees might take the degree model down the path of the DNSc, DSN, DNS alphabet soup path again (AACN, 2004). As the first DNP degree founded at the University of Kentucky in 2001 did not prepare practitioners but only clinical executives, it is unclear why the Columbia degree model, which prepared advanced practitioners and clinicians, was not the preferred degree model.

Presently, CCNE continues to accredit master's in nursing programs leading to advanced practice (CCNE, 2010). In 2006, the National Organization of Nurse Practitioner Faculties (NONPF) also issued a position statement supporting the practice doctorate in nursing. The NONPF (2006) statement highlighted core competencies expected of entry-level nurse practitioners (NPs) with DNP preparation. This work, along with *The Essentials of Doctoral Education for Advanced Nursing Practice* (AACN, 2006), identified the competencies and outcomes necessary for quality DNP educational programs (Exhibit 4.1).

The DNP Roadmap Task Force stipulated steps to be taken to achieve the 2015 goal relative to educational programs. Having now identified that the DNP will be the terminal clinical practice doctorate supported by the previously mentioned organizations, the two major questions still remain: How will the DNP-educated APRN differ from the traditional master's-educated APRN? Can the health care system afford a workforce of exclusively doctoral-prepared APRNs, particularly in this economic climate?

■ THE MSN ADVANCED PRACTICE NURSE

The MSN-prepared APRN role as first outlined by the American Nurses Association (ANA) in 2004 has been historically restrictive and prescriptive. More recently, the ANA (2010) stated that an APRN is the regulatory title for one of the four advanced practice nursing direct care roles (e.g., certified nurse anesthetists, certified nurse-midwives, certified NPs, clinical nurse specialists).The requirements for licensure, accreditation, certification, and education for APRNs are outlined in the *Consensus Model for APRN Regulation: Licensure, Accreditation, Certification, and Education* (2008). The authors of this chapter acknowledge that well-educated master's-level APRNs provide safe, efficient, comprehensive, high-quality care to the population they serve. Mundinger and colleagues' (2000) classic article in the *Journal of the American Medical Association* reported equivalent master's APRN outcomes compared with physician primary care outcomes; these study findings were replicated 2 years later by Horrocks, Anderson, and Salisbury (2002) in the United Kingdom. These studies indicate the DNP degree was certainly not created because MSN APRN care was inferior. Unfortunately, the professional recognition of MSN-prepared APRNs outside of the nursing profession has been stunted because of numerous factors including "cookie cutter" educational training programs (e.g., overly restrictive, lacking innovation, or "designed for the past, not the future") and inaccurate and derogatory perceptions of these providers as being simply *physician extenders* or *mid-level providers*. These are terms that the nursing profession has fiercely tried to negate. As NPs, what we do is not midlevel anything: We certainly *do not* provide just mid-level care, and we certainly *do not* practice at a midlevel, nor is it mediocral! We suspect you, as well the authors of this chapter, provide high-quality care to the best of your ability all of the time. To us, that is not midlevel. We would prefer to be called by our title or be identified by the role that we hold within the health care domain with an emphasis on maintaining our nursing identity as APRNs, advanced practice nurses, doctoral APRNs, board certified nurses, or the designation provided by respective State Boards of Nursing.

EXHIBIT 4.1   AACN's *The Essentials of Doctoral Education for Advanced Nursing Practice*, With Commentary I

I. Scientific Underpinnings for Practice

The DNP program prepares the graduate to:

1. Integrate nursing science with knowledge from ethics, biophysical, psychosocial, analytical, and organizational sciences as the basis for the highest level of nursing practice
2. Use science-based theories and concepts to:
   - Determine the nature and significance of hearth and health care delivery phenomena; describe the actions and advanced strategies to enhance, alleviate, and ameliorate health and health care delivery phenomena as appropriate; and
   - Evaluate outcomes
3. Develop and evaluate new practice approaches based on nursing theories and theories from other disciplines

Our View: The MSN graduate should be aware of all current evidence and knowledge to provide quality patient care and remain current in practice.

In Addition: The DNP graduate should design, develop, implement, and publish scientific findings to improve patient care and health care systems; and utilize new scientific evidence to devise protocols and practice plans. Additionally, the DNP graduate should maintain an active professional development plan.

II. Organizational and Systems Leadership for Quality Improvement and Systems Thinking

The IDP program prepares the graduate to:

1. Develop and evaluate care delivery approaches that meet current and future needs of patient populations based on scientific findings in nursing and other clinical sciences, as well as organizational, political, and economic sciences
2. Ensure accountability for quality of health care and patient safety for populations with whom they work
   - Use advanced communication skills/processes to lead quality improvement and patient safety initiatives in health care systems
   - Employ principles of business, finance, economics, and health policy to develop and implement effective plans for practice-level and/or system-wide practice initiatives that will improve the quality of care delivery
   - Develop and/or monitor budgets for practice initiatives
   - Analyze the cost-effectiveness of practice initiatives accounting for risk and improvement of health care outcomes
   - Demonstrate sensitivity to diverse organizational cultures and populations including patients and providers
3. Develop and/or evaluate effective strategies for managing the ethical dilemmas inherent in patient care, the health care organization, and research

Our View: The MSN graduate should participate in professional organizations and lobby government officials for access to quality, cost-effective health care.

(continued)

EXHIBIT 4.1   AACN's *The Essentials of Doctoral Education for Advanced Nursing Practice*, With Commentary I   *(continued)*

In Addition: The DNP graduate should represent professional organizations at the table with government officials to ensure health care policy efficacy and quality. The DNP actively and prominently initiates and advances the health care agenda.

III. Clinical Scholarship and Analytical Methods for Evidence-Based Practice

The DNP program prepares the graduate to:

1. Use analytic methods to critically appraise existing literature and other evidence to determine and implement the best evidence for practice
2. Design and implement processes to evaluate outcomes of practice, practice patterns, and systems of care within a practice setting, health care organization, or community against national benchmarks to determine variances in practice outcomes and population trends
3. Design, direct, and evaluate quality improvement methodologies to promote safe, timely, effective, efficient, equitable, and patient-centered care.
4. Apply relevant findings to develop practice guidelines and improve practice and the practice environment
5. Use information technology and research methods appropriately to:
   - Collect appropriate and accurate data to generate evidence for nursing practice
   - Inform and guide the design of databases that generate meaningful evidence for nursing practice
   - Analyze data from practice
   - Design evidence-based interventions
   - Predict and analyze outcomes
   - Examine patterns of behavior and outcomes
   - Identify gaps in evidence for practice
6. Function as a practice specialist/consultant in collaborative knowledge-generating research
7. Disseminate findings from evidence-based practice and research to improve health care outcomes

Our View: The MSN graduate should understand the need for research to advance nursing science, actively participate in research agendas, and utilize current information to provide quality care.

In Addition: The DNP graduate should design, develop, implement, and evaluate clinical research to improve patient care and outcomes through the development of guidelines, protocols, and informed opinion. The DNP should ensure that organizational guidelines are congruent with current evidence-based practice, always with an open eye toward continuous improvement; and maintain a culture of excellence through continued scientific inquiry and personal and professional transformation.

(continued)

EXHIBIT 4.1   AACN's *The Essentials of Doctoral Education for Advanced Nursing Practice*, With Commentary I   *(continued)*

IV. Information Systems/Technology and Patient Care Technology for the Improvement and Transformation of Health Care

The DNP program prepares the graduate to:

1. Design, select, use, and evaluate programs that evaluate and monitor outcomes of care, care systems, and quality improvement including consumer use of health care information systems
2. Analyze and communicate critical elements necessary to the selection, use, and evaluation of health care information systems and patient care technology
3. Demonstrate the conceptual ability and technical skills to develop and execute an evaluation plan involving data extraction from practice information systems and databases
4. Provide leadership in the evaluation and resolution of ethical and legal issues within health care systems relating to the use of information, information technology, communication networks, and patient care technology
5. Evaluate consumer health information sources for accuracy, timeliness, and appropriateness

Our View: The MSN graduate should have a clear understanding of current technological advances to improve patient care and patient outcomes; and have the ability to evaluate new systems and suggest updates to fulfill the needs of rapidly changing clinical environment.

In Addition: The DNP graduate should participate in the design, development, implementation, and evaluation technology to meet the current and future needs of health care teams nationally and internationally; design, develop, implement, and evaluate databases to improve health care informatics and communications; and lead activist groups to lobby for global electronic medical records to ensure the quality and continuity of patient care.

V. Health Care Policy for Advocacy in Health Care

The DNP program prepares the graduate to:

1. Critically analyze health policy proposals, health policies, and related issues from the perspective of consumers, nursing, other health professions, and other stakeholders in policy and public forums
2. Demonstrate leadership in the development and implementation of institutional, local, state, federal, and/or international health policy
3. Influence policy makers through active participation on committees, boards, or task forces at the institutional, local, state, regional, national, and/or international levels to improve health care delivery and outcomes
4. Educate others, including policy makers at all levels, regarding nursing, health policy, and patient care outcomes
5. Advocate for the nursing profession within the policy and health care communities
6. Develop, evaluate, and provide leadership for health care policy that shapes health care financing, regulation, and delivery

(continued)

EXHIBIT 4.1   AACN's *The Essentials of Doctoral Education for Advanced Nursing Practice*, With Commentary I   *(continued)*

---

7. Advocate for social justice, equity, and ethical policies within all health care arenas

Our View: The MSN graduate should have a deep-rooted understanding of financial aspects of quality care, diverse ways to access care, and how to advocate for legislative changes to influence health care delivery systems.

In Addition: The DNP graduate should identify problems within the health care delivery system and actively spearhead legislation to improve and/or change health care policy utilizing advanced negotiating, consensus building, and partnering skills, particularly across other health care disciplines.

VI. Interprofessional Collaboration for Improving Patient and Population Health Outcomes

The DNP program prepares the graduate to:

1. Employ effective communication and collaborative skills in the development and implementation of practice models, peer review, practice guidelines, health policy, standards of care, and/or other scholarly products
2. Lead interprofessional teams in the analysis of complex practice and organizational issues
3. Employ consultative and leadership skills with intraprofessional and interprofessional teams to create change in health care and complex health care delivery systems.

Our View: The MSN graduate should collaborate and consult with health care providers as well as participate as a member of the health care team to advocate for both quality health care for patients and for the advanced practice role of the nurse.

In Addition: The DNP graduate should create and provide leadership in an interprofessional environment to advance health care agendas and improve patient care by utilizing critical and reflective thinking, scientific foundations, and research in all disciplines.

VII. Clinical Prevention and Population Health for Improving the Nation's Health

The DNP program prepares the graduate to:

1. Analyze epidemiological, bio-statistical, environmental, and other appropriate scientific data related to individual, aggregate, and population health
2. Synthesize concepts, including psychosocial dimensions and cultural diversity, related to clinical prevention and population health in developing, implementing, and evaluating interventions to address health promotion/disease prevention efforts, improve health status/access patterns, and/or address gaps in care of individuals, aggregates, or populations
3. Evaluate care delivery models and/or strategies using concepts related to community, environmental, and occupational health, and cultural and socio-economic dimensions of health

(continued)

EXHIBIT 4.1   AACN's *The Essentials of Doctoral Education for Advanced Nursing Practice*, With Commentary I   *(continued)*

Our View: The MSN graduate should provide comprehensive, culturally diverse, and competent care to patients in their scope of practice. The practitioner should investigate all resources to ensure quality care for their population.

In Addition: The DNP graduate should utilize problem-solving skills to generate new knowledge that affects patients within and outside their population. The DNP utilizes clinical experience, advanced analytic skills, and leadership abilities to target health care GLOBAL health care issues.

VIII. Advanced Nursing Practice

The DNP program prepares the graduate to:

1. Conduct a comprehensive and systematic assessment of health and illness parameters in situations, incorporating diverse and culturally sensitive approaches
2. Design, implement, and evaluate therapeutic interventions based on nursing science and other sciences
3. Develop and sustain therapeutic relationships and partnerships with patients (individual, family, or group) and other professionals to facilitate optimal care and patient outcomes
4. Demonstrate advanced levels of clinical judgment, systems thinking, and accountability in designing, delivering, and evaluating evidence-based care to improve patient outcomes
5. Guide, mentor, and support other nurses to achieve excellence in nursing practice
6. Educate and guide individuals and groups through complex health and situational transitions
7. Use conceptual and analytical skills in evaluating the links among practice, organizational, population, fiscal, and policy issues

Our View: The MSN graduate should practice in a collaborative environment.

However: The DNP graduate should "create" the environment he or she practices in utilizing principles of autonomy and independence, while fostering an interprofessional climate. *While some believe this is just a new degree with the same role, we disagree. We encourage more explicit development of doctoral advanced practice nursing competencies.*

AACN, American Association of Colleges of Nursing; DNP, Doctor of Nursing Practice; MSN, master of science in nursing.
Adapted from 2006 AACN *The Essentials of Doctoral Education for Advanced Nursing Practice*.

Conversely, the DNP degree is not prescriptive to the clinical specialty areas like master's education. The DNP degree builds on the MSN level of education, and the student learns to branch out of standard roles in order to assume greater responsibility and accountability for his or her patients, ensuring care continuity that will infiltrate through other disciplines (Mundinger, 2005). If the master's-prepared nurse wants to achieve a practice doctorate simply to earn the respect and the "doctor" title, we urge the matriculating student to stop now or proceed with extreme caution! Doctoral education differs dramatically from MSN education. It commands an overwhelming amount of dedication and an unwavering intellectual curiosity to "pry the lid off" of the road map point of care pathways and to understand the "why"; to think outside the box, to question practice, and to be the conduit to explore causation that might lead to new interventions (Dreher & Montgomery, 2009).

Since the first edition of this book in 2010, the 330-plus master's degree programs that have been accredited by the CCNE or by the National League for Nursing Commission for Nursing Education Accreditation (CNEA), which was established in 2013 and formerly known as the National League for Nursing Accrediting Commission (NLNAC), has grown to more than 450 master's or post-master's degree programs (CCNE, 2015; CNEA, 2013). Historically, master degree preparation for APRNs has existed with fairly standard and traditional curricula incorporating basic theoretical and conceptual aspects of nursing science, skills performance, research comprehension and application, and leadership proficiency to improve the health care system (AACN, 2006). The MSN graduate APRN is then molded within his or her practice environments to grow and mature in a specialty area. For many master's-prepared clinicians, contentment is found in providing high-quality care to the patients or systems they serve. For others, they may feel they have reached their full potential or the boundary of their practice ability. Their professional contentment slowly dissipates and results in the quest for "more." But just what exactly is *more*?

■ THE DNP-PREPARED APRN

The DNP is the answer to the prior resounding question! The emergence of this new title and its associated curricular structure may be just what the *doctor ordered* (no pun intended)[2] to lead APRNs with a progressive thirst for knowledge and armed with the assimilation and integration of new DNP NONPF competencies to merge into a different world of lifelong engagement and satisfaction in doctoral advanced practice nursing. In Exhibit 4.1, we have included a very specific commentary where we highlight what the DNP graduate is educated and trained to practice beyond the MSN. It is noted however that there is still variation in the academic preparation and transition within the health care system of the DNP student that appears outside of the eight substantive areas listed in the DNP *Essentials* (AACN, 2006). These variations in curriculum and the "real-life" roles of DNP graduates are discussed at length by Melnyk (2013). Both of us having now "lived" the *Essentials* (AACN, 2006) feel our perspective is very valuable as the profession tries to define what exactly is the domain of practice that exists beyond the MSN. As the number of DNP programs soar to more than 260 programs in 48 states and the District of Columbia with 125 programs accredited by the CCNE, the debate over academic preparation and role development is sure to continue (AACN, 2015b). The following two scenarios provide cases in-point for readers interested in sharing the journey and personal insight of two DrNP graduates from the start to completion of their terminal degree. We offer our two personal stories openly and hope they may be valuable to current DNP students.

■ CASE STUDY I: A Women's Health NP Who Continues to Want "More"

The first author of this chapter is a 50-year-old, well-seasoned practicing APRN. My 20-year practice, specializing in women's health in both clinical and academic arenas, centered on achieving success at providing empathetic, comprehensive care to my patients and was focused on health promotion and disease prevention. Each office day was packed with a full complement of patients with an array of issues ranging from the normal annual well visit to the extremely complex and potentially life-threatening disease situations. Booking an appointment with me typically necessitated a 6-month wait. My collaborating physicians' operating room schedules were also booked with referrals stemming from my robust practice. In addition, the number of my pregnant patients delivering with the collaborating physicians greatly contributed to the income of the practice. Needless to say, I successfully cultivated a large and loyal patient volume through dedication and hard work, and earned the respect of the medical community and my peers through my practice—my ideal clinical APRN professional career goal attainment.

However, as the years passed and as each professional milestone was attained, my office hours began to get longer and more mundane. Challenges were fewer and farther between. I did not feel as though I had to put much thought into providing high-quality, effective, and efficient care. I did, however, become more frequently frustrated by existing policies that were incongruent with high-quality health care options. Somehow, invisible to my patients and initially without my own complete self-awareness, I was intellectually stunted. But what grew out of this discomfiture was a gnawing desire to seek the unknown—to find "more," whatever that was. I thought about taking the Law School Admission Test (LSAT) for law school admission, but my unwavering self-identification and dedication as a nurse clinician halted that option. I also explored avenues in forensic nursing, defense law expert for nurses, and even medical school. However, my zest for my specialty and my profession continued to overpower my "wandering eye" into other career areas, until I found the practice doctorate, the DrNP.

In response to another IOM report (2003), *Health Professions Education: A Bridge to Quality*, the AACN interpreted the document's policy recommendations as supportive of more advanced nursing education, and thus the early planning and politicking toward a practice doctorate degree alternative to the PhD was underway. Many master's-level nursing programs had revamped their existing curricula by requiring an expansion of the already challenging and complex credit loads to deal with the IOM's requests. Some thought the MSN degree already conferred this advancement and was almost equal to similar entry-level health profession doctorates. Was nursing about to abandon its history of failed clinical doctorate models in favor of a new practice doctorate degree? The AACN ultimately indicated the new DNP degree was created to meet the demands of the present-day fragmentation of services and system failures in health care by preparing nurse clinicians (and later clinical executives) for practice with interdisciplinary, information systems, quality improvement,

(continued)

■ CASE STUDY I: A Women's Health NP
Who Continues to Want "More" *(continued)*

and patient safety expertise (AACN, 2006). Practically simultaneously, Mary O'Neil Mundinger, dean of the Columbia School of Nursing, pioneered the first DrNP program to revolutionize the nursing profession and prepare the nurse clinician for more sophisticated and complex advance nursing practices (Yox, 2005). At this juncture, a debate ensued that has really not abated. If the master's degree is still filled with rigor and produces capable and competent APRNs, why are some left asking for "more?" Why go for the DNP?

Before the DNP/DrNP degrees evolved, many passionate APRNs found themselves in PhD programs, not exactly certain what their role would be if they completed the PhD. Typically, APRNs who seek a doctoral nursing terminal academic degree still identify strongly with the clinician role (Bloch, 2005; Chism, 2009). The DNP program "requires competence in translating research in practice, evaluating evidence, applying research in decision-making, and implementing viable clinical innovations to change practice" (AACN, 2006, p. 6). In addition, a strong DNP curriculum should prepare the APRN clinician to become an integral part of a research team. In our program, and perhaps in some DNP programs, the graduate is also prepared to competently spearhead research initiatives, especially those deeply grounded in practice.

The expert APRN's journey into the DNP curricula is definitely not an easy one, Then again, is any doctoral program designed to be navigated effortlessly? For the clinician accustomed to being "on top of her game" in the clinical world, rejoining a very different academic world will often result in frustration. Being a doctoral student mentally means experiencing challenging workloads designed to reprogram the APRN's view of the world, the very same view that was accustomed to confidence and security in both judgment and performance (with a master's degree). In order for the APRN to attain the DNP, an extremely challenging metamorphosis needs to occur. These programs are designed to infuse a deep-rooted understanding of the multifaceted aspects of evidence-based practice, research skills, leadership, administration, and policy into the polished practitioner. The lens from which clinical practice was previously viewed is reinforced, but also changed so that a new broader landscape perspective is seen. The DNP clinician possesses newly acquired skills, which fortify critical thinking about the care provided and empower the nurse to authoritatively and credibly question the standard of care and to participate actively in the revision of current standards to improve patient care.

In my case, my quest to find something "more" and stay true to my clinical roots allowed me to build on my master's-level training. I was truly at the point in my professional career where I was no longer satisfied with doing the "how to," but I craved the "why" and the "why not" in order to *improve* "how to" learning. In this quest, my doctoral education encouraged and challenged me to find novel and creative ways to improve the care I deliver and enable me to make a greater impact on the lives of not only the patients I encounter but also the future generations of patients and providers through the dissemination of my clinical scholarship.

(continued)

■ **CASE STUDY I: A Women's Health NP
Who Continues to Want "More"** *(continued)*

Despite an economy in turmoil, the overall number of nursing students enrolled in doctoral programs continues to increase. There are currently 269 nursing schools in 48 states plus the District of Columbia accepting students into a DNP program with an additional 60 schools contemplating offering a DNP program (AACN, 2015b). Student enrollment in DNP programs has increased by 26.2% (14,688 in 2013 to 18,352 students nationwide) in 2014. Of particular interest, in research-focused doctoral programs, enrollments increased by only 3.2% from 2013 to 2014 with 5,290 students currently enrolled (AACN). As a critical mass of DNP clinicians accrues, their additional education, greater depth and breadth of knowledge, more refined leadership abilities, and enhanced skill set will propel graduates to exert more influence on patient care and demand equivalent input into joint decision making for their patients. At the same time, the DNP will "profoundly improve the nation's image of nursing" (Mundinger, 2005, p. 174). Mundinger also acknowledges that DNPs, based on their intense advanced education, coupled with their passion for patient care, are raising intriguing questions, offering resolutions, and stepping in with welcome wisdom to improve the care in the systems in which they work. The saga continues.

With the attainment of my DrNP, coupled with my scholarship productivity and expert clinical practice, I am no longer doing the same thing I was doing when I walked into my first doctoral seminar. I now have a joint appointment in both a prestigious nursing school and medical school, and published nine journal articles (three research related) in respected peer-reviewed journals in my first year of postgraduation. My clinical scholarship focuses on helping to raise public awareness concerning the issues of human papillomavirus (HPV) in women's health care, both nationally and internationally. I continue to be active in promoting optimal women's health care and I really believe my primary care has improved because of my enhanced abilities at formal clinical inquiry. My doctoral education (and the specific coursework I took) has given me (a clinician!) the tools to evaluate and strengthen women's health NP curricula and now educate future "foot soldiers" in women's health advanced practice nursing. I truly believe my doctoral education has enabled me to accept the challenge of the IOM (2001) to help close the gap that impedes the quality of care we give to patients. I also do not see practice on one side of the road and research on the other. Instead, my own degree has helped me professionally build a bridge between the two. I have been successful in writing and receiving funding for transdisciplinary education grants that combine diverse expert faculty instruction, multilevel simulation, and collaborative case study learning formats to educate OB/GYN medical students and resident physicians, women's health NP students, physician assistant students, and nurse anesthesia students *together* in a collaborative setting.

The focus of my work is to enhance knowledge of roles and responsibilities within the health care system, foster development of team-building skills, improve health care team communication, reduce medical errors, and improve the quality of patient care through simulation in a transdisciplinary environment.

(continued)

■ CASE STUDY I: A Women's Health NP
Who Continues to Want "More" *(continued)*

Coupled with my achievements of becoming a Fellow of Sigma Theta Tau's Nurse Faculty Leadership Academy (NFLA) and the American Association of Nurse Practitioners (FAANP), I am now the chair of a very large and successful NP program. My education and experience empowers me to mold the future of nursing practice! Had I kept my head to the grindstone in my clinical practice and never decided to continue on to get my DrNP, I do not believe I would have ever dreamed such issues existed in health care, or that I could be part of a solution. I feel as though the lenses of my clouded glasses were cleaned, and now I can see farther and more clearly than ever before. My DNP education has satisfied my desire for additional education, but my quest for "more" continues. I now see a new world of endless possibilities that will continue to assist me in my own personal and professional development, as well as help me be a better steward of my profession and discipline.

■ CASE STUDY II: Transitioning in Academia, Practice,
and Scholarship: One DrNP's (DNP) Story

The second author is an APRN who, after 30-plus years of practice evolving from a diploma-prepared registered nurse followed by a bachelor of science in nursing (BSN) degree and master's-level preparation as a clinical nurse specialist, sought and achieved post-master's certification as a family NP. After 3 years of competent practice in this role, at both a primary care setting and university medical center outpatient clinic setting, I had the personal drive to "do more." At first this urge was satisfied with supplemental adjunct faculty responsibilities in the clinical arena. This role, however, only fueled my desire to be both an expert practitioner and educator in my own realm. After exploring both PhD and DNP programs for more than a year, I knew that my future quest was doctoral education in nursing practice. As opposed to a PhD in nursing program, which emphasizes the philosophy of science, nursing science, and research, or the standard DNP, I chose a hybrid DrNP program as my educational pathway due to the ability to declare a dual track as a scholar in both nursing practice and nursing education. Coursework in the program appealed to the practitioner within me, as it included both a clinical and role practicum that could be tailored to expand my knowledge and translation of evidence-based practice. Specific to the ever growing discipline of oncology nursing advanced practice, this included such areas as genetics, multimodal treatment using a multidisciplinary team approach, and taking an active role in prevention and early detection of disease and cancer survivorship issues often overlooked by physician peers in their efforts to provide the latest technology based medical care. In addition to the chance to be an active participant in coordinating my education and securing

(continued)

■ CASE STUDY II: Transitioning in Academia, Practice, and Scholarship: One DNP's Story *(continued)*

expert mentorship, the program I choose included core courses in nursing science, leadership, legal issues in advanced practice, research methods, as well as cognates focused on nursing education. A major draw to this program was the ability to connect with international nursing scholars during a 2-week "DrNP-in-London" study abroad program.

The philosophy and tenets of the practice-oriented terminal degree program I chose coincided with my personal interests and ability to achieve subjective satisfaction and purposefulness in my professional role as a NP with dual national certification in both family practice and advanced oncology nursing. I felt strongly that on completion of the DrNP program, I would be prepared at the highest level, practice with the admiration of peers both inside and outside the discipline of nursing, and develop skills that were crucial to becoming a valued nursing faculty member and empowered nurse leader. The latter two skills have been found to be determinative in students' choosing a practice doctorate rather than a research-focused doctorate, and to support those who desire to focus their careers on clinical practice and nursing education (Loomis, Willard, & Cohen, 2007).[3] Likewise, Brar, Boschma, and McCuaig (2010) stated the DNP is the most recent credential and source of preparation of new nursing knowledge that has a strong emphasis on advanced leadership in clinical practice.

Following my coursework related to the terminal degree and successful defense of a clinical dissertation based on my practice and interest in breast cancer disparities in minority populations, I am pleased to say I was offered a full-time appointment as an assistant clinical professor in a College of Nursing and Health Professions within a large urban university. As noted in a discussion by Agger, Oermann, and Lynn (2014) related to the perceptions of deans' and directors' regarding hiring and utilization of new DNP prepared faculty, my main role was that of teaching across the curriculum at the baccalaureate and master's level. Within a short time frame, my clinical and leadership expertise were recognized by the department chair and I was offered and accepted the position of track coordinator for the MSN family NP program. It was in this position that I was able to apply many of the skills gained and mentorship given to me in the cognate educational courses within the terminal degree program to revamp the curriculum and transition the program from on-campus to on-line delivery.

Two years ago, I choose to move to a public collegiate institution that focused on the teacher–scholar model and offered the opportunity to join the tenure track. It is at this current setting that I have flourished beyond the initial intention of the DNP role and have realized my potential for shaping not only future nursing professionals but also have realized opportunities for shaping the health care system, a sentiment shared in the literature by Dunbar-Jacob, Nativio, and Khalil (2013). Within my current academic setting, I am up for promotion to associate professor as I am now 5 years out of my terminal degree and hold an appointment as cochair of the Department of Nursing. Over the past 2 years I have also had the distinct pleasure of giving back to the profession by serving as a mentor and/or preceptor to both master's-level advanced practice

(continued)

▪ CASE STUDY II: Transitioning in Academia, Practice, and Scholarship: One DNP's Story *(continued)*

nursing students as well as doctoral level DNP and PhD students. I have served on both capstone and dissertation committees, and am faculty for research and evidence-based practice coursework at the graduate level.

Dunbar-Jacob et al. (2013) feel that DNP prepared faculty foster scholarship in nursing. My own scholarship related to academia post DrNP continues on an active path with such activities as being a participant in one of the NLN's Scholarly Writing Retreat, being a primary author of manuscripts published in journals and certification review books, serving as a peer reviewer for specialty nursing practice, nursing education, and a nationally recognized public health journal, being principal investigator (PI) on a Health Resources and Services Administration (HRSA) grant submission focused on advanced nursing practice academic–practice partnerships, being awarded a 2-year Support of Scholarly Activities(SOSA) grant to engage in my program of research. I also fill the office of president of a chapter of Sigma Theta Tau.

Competency and engagement in clinical practice and providing high-quality care to underserved populations is what gives me the greatest satisfaction in my professional life. I feel strongly that my expertise as an advanced practice nurse (NP) was fostered by the application of evidence-based practice in my focused terminal degree program.

Currently, I am credentialed and practice within a university-based cancer center. In addition to serving as a provider, and as one of a half dozen APRNs (and the only one doctorally prepared) in an outpatient setting within the center, I have taken the lead in designing and developing educational outreach projects based on gaming strategies to increase participation of women in cancer screening and increase early access to services. These programs are the result of funding that was secured through grants from a nationally recognized cancer foundations and organization. This year I was chosen as coordinator-elect of the Prevention/Detection Special Interest Group within the Oncology Nursing Society and participated in 2015 Annual Congress by presenting a poster abstract at a session specifically focusing on research outcomes.

Dunbar-Jacob et al. (2013) described what they termed "the short-term impact in other areas" related to DNP education (p. 426). For me, the other area is one that I am growing ever more passionate about global health. I will soon embark on my fourth health outreach in Haiti where I serve as a primary care provider in the family NP role delivering care across the life span to individuals and families living in an extremely resource-poor environment. I also have had the opportunity to mentor nursing students at both the undergraduate and graduate level that have been involved in service learning within the area. Involvement with a nongovernmental organization (NGO) that provides sustainable health care and health education services in this country has strengthened my practice from one based on cultural competency to one of cultural humility. Although being involved in some type of international outreach effort was always in the back of my mind as a nurse or master's-prepared NP, the confidence and leadership skills related to capacity building gained throughout my doctoral education gave me the impetus to "jump in" and "round out" my role-development journey from a registered nurse to a doctoral advanced practice nurse.

APRN DNPs: SEE ONE, DO ONE, TEACH ONE?

As demonstrated in the case studies previously, both authors are expert clinicians, doctor nursing practice graduates, recognized leaders, and nurse educators. However, neither received formal training as a nurse educator (beyond one doctoral nursing education course each elected to take) during their doctoral program, necessitating independent study to attain the certified nurse educator (CNE) certificates. In contrast, other nursing terminal degree programs do include formal nurse educator curricula built into the program of study, but lack the advanced clinical component that provides the credibility for a clinical doctorate. Some nursing leaders postulate that one of the goals in the creation of the DNP was to help alleviate the nursing faculty shortage (Minnick, Norman, & Donaghey, 2013). In fact, more than 30% of DNP graduates do go into academia (Zungolo, 2009) and it makes perfect sense that APRN–DNP clinicians teach in all levels of nursing education, particularly in NP and DNP programs. Nursing accreditation bodies further require that the director of an NP program hold a doctoral degree (CCNE, 2013). The AACN as well as most state boards of nursing require directors of NP programs to be, at the minimum, master's-prepared. A survey of 220 nursing deans and directors identified the top five desired characteristics of novice faculty (Penn, Wilson, & Rosseter (2008):

- Teaching skills
- Knowledge, experience, and preparation for the faculty role
- Curriculum/course development skills
- Evaluation and testing skills
- Personal attributes

Ironically, formal education in the majority of these skills is specifically prohibited by the accreditation body to be included in DNP curriculum! Fortunately, many educational conferences, continuing nursing education programs, and faculty development agendas provide content to foster teaching excellence for clinician educators.

A quandary still exists. APRN DNP's are both needed in practice to further develop and improve the national health care agenda and needed in the educational settings to prepare the future nursing work force to provide the highest quality, safe, and efficient health care. As we envision the future of nursing as delineated in the IOM report (2010), is it time to reconsider a DNP clinical educator track as a solution to do more than "see one, do one, teach one?" The DNP graduate is being recruited to fill vacancies not only in practice and administrative roles within health care settings but also in academia particularly in programs that prepare master's-level advanced practice nurses, offer the DNP terminal degree, or are experiencing a shortage of PhD-prepared faculty.

The DNP prepared advanced practice nurse is also gaining more popularity in clinical practice. According to the *DNP Fact Sheet* (AACN, 2015b), employers are recognizing the contributions the DNP-prepared nurse bring to practice settings. It also appears that with this change many issues and questions arise, some of which have already been discussed previously. Questions that still linger include but are not limited to: What are the benefits of DNP versus MSN preparation of APRNs? Are practice settings recognizing the difference between doctoral-level advanced practice and master's-level advanced practice with respect to salary? When will the impetus for the DNP becoming the entry level for advanced practice actually occur?

For the most part, it appears the benefits of the DNP verses MSN are both personal and professional. Seeking and obtaining the DNP is both personally challenging and rewarding. It is the practitioner who does not accept the status quo that seems to be driven to obtain a terminal degree before it is actually formally mandated. In the ever-changing health care landscape, the DNP can assist advance practice nurses to increase their respective knowledge and skills in many areas already noted within this chapter. Having a DNP seems to "level the playing field" or create parity with other practice disciplines when working on multidisciplinary projects within health care settings. It is also a degree that is embraced by administrators as in many instances the DNP-prepared APRN has knowledge of organizational and systems thinking that can be applied to quality improvement projects or evidence-based practice initiatives that ultimately lead to improved patient care outcomes. Thus, in many instances the DNP-prepared APRN makes the institution, department, or program "look good" in the eyes of accreditors, patients, and other stakeholders. There has been concern raised about who will hire NPs with a practice doctorate and whether the pay they receive would be worth the additional education. A most recent 2014 salary survey conducted by Advance Healthcare Network (2015) estimated that NPs with a DNP are receiving an average salary of $113,618. This is approximately $13,000 more than the average salary of a master's-prepared NP. This is also close to a $4,500 gain since the same organization's 2011 salary survey. What will happen in the future across a larger geographic landscape, increased number of DNP-prepared graduates entering the profession and an influx health care system remain to be seen.

■ SUMMARY

The evolution of APRN education from the master's to the doctorate level appears to be here to stay. As Dreher (2005) stated: "Has this train left the station? If so, just where is it going?" (p. 17). The issues surrounding this transition will most likely continue to be debated for some time, and the ultimate direction of the DNP degree is still unfolding. We think that active, practicing DNP graduates can actually shape the future of this degree with our critical mass. We absolutely want more outcome data on what these graduates are accomplishing. We even welcome any constructive criticism, especially if there are DNP programs that proliferate that are not rigorous or that aim to create an easy path to the title "Dr." Weak DNP programs will harm us all and not advance the nation's health. We also call for the DNP graduate to advance "practice knowledge development" as has been advocated by Dreher (2010) who also contends the DNP graduate should be the leader in creating practice-based evidence for the discipline. DNP-prepared APRNs have quickly positioned themselves to become an integral part of our discipline's future. They not only carry with them a unique preparation for diverse health care roles, but a plethora of opportunities for advancement in the arenas of practice, leadership, education, and applied research awaits them.

So, exactly how is the MSN different from the DNP? Why take the leap into obtaining a practice doctorate in nursing? The answers to these questions will be different for every nurse practicing in the clinical arena. You will decide if you want *more*. However, one fact is clear: The MSN degree allows you to be part of the change to improve the quality of patient care you provide, while the DNP equips you to collaborate more inter-professionally (and with more confidence) to be the change and advance the discipline. This degree opens your professional world to a myriad of new lenses, new options, and new agendas with which to advance nursing and make a true impact on the patients you serve *and to the larger aggregate* through your disseminated clinical scholarship. To reiterate our warning at the beginning of the chapter, proceed with caution! When you obtain the DNP, you will be different. Your professional eyes will be open more widely to many more challenges. Your metamorphosis, we attest, will be profound.

■ CRITICAL THINKING QUESTIONS

1. *After review of the chapter, has your individual thoughts or views on the AACN's position to move the level of preparation necessary for advance practice roles from a master's degree to doctoral level as requisite credential for entry into advanced practice nursing changed? Why or why not?*
2. *If the DNP is mandated by regulatory bodies (licensure, accreditation, certification, and education), will it be held to the same prescriptive expectations as the master's-prepared ARPN?*
3. *Is there a need for a standardized, designated title to signify the educational preparation and national credentialing of DNPs? Explain.*
4. *Do you feel that the DNP degree will support the triad of academia, practice, and research related to the nursing profession? Discuss.*
5. *Will the DNP degree better prepare nurses to deal with the complexity of patient care environments, expand the knowledge base for practice, initiate and evaluate evidence-based practice through clinical research, and meet the need for nursing leadership in education and administration beyond that currently found within master's-level programs?*
6. *Can preparation at the DNP level contribute to and sustain the perfect balance between teaching and clinical practice competencies within the nursing profession? In other words, do you feel the DNP may lessen the "theory–practice gap" as discussed by Little and Milliken (2007)?*
7. *Based on the experience of these two DrNP graduates from the start to the completion of their terminal degree, can you see how the DNP supported a diverse perspective of roles and myriad of opportunities that may have not been otherwise fulfilled with traditional master's-level advanced practice nursing education?*
8. *Can the health care industry afford a workforce made up of exclusively doctoral-prepared ARPNs (DNPs)? Discuss.*
9. *The debate on how doctoral-level advanced practice nursing roles differ from master's-level advanced practice nursing roles is far from over. What areas of systematic evaluation related to the impact of the DNP on the advanced practice workforce do you see as most pressing?*
10. *The rationale for the shift in academic preparation of nurses in advanced practice has focused on several issues including how the transition to clinical doctoral preparation for APRNs can be conducted so that master's-prepared APRNs will not be disenfranchised in any way. Based on your knowledge and the information provided within this chapter, can this transition be handled smoothly? How should it proceed?*

■ NOTES

1. Both initials DNP and DrNP stand for *doctor of nursing practice*, although all programs now use DNP initials, except some doctoral programs in nurse anesthesia. Because the DrNP degree is termed a *hybrid professional doctorate* and emphasizes both advanced practice and the conduct of practical clinical research, it used different initials.
2. On a serious note, however, we *highly discourage* the use of the word *doctor* to describe one who is actually a physician. There are lots of *doctors* in health care, including DNPs who complete the doctorate. By using the proper title *physician*, we are describing their role and their profession. Even to a patient we recommend saying for example, "What did your physician prescribe for you?"
3. In nursing, a practice-focused doctorate is akin to the DNP while a research-focused doctorate is akin to the PhD.

■ REFERENCES

Advance Healthcare Network. (2015). NP results by degree. Retrieved from http://nurse-practitioners -and-physician-assistants.advanceweb.com/Web-Extras/Online-Extras/NP-Results-By-Degree .aspx

Agger, C. A., Oermann, M. H., & Lynn, M. R. (2014). Hiring and incorporating doctor of nursing practice-prepared nurse faculty into academic nursing programs. *Journal of Nursing Education, 53*(8), 439–446.

American Association of Colleges of Nursing. (2004). Position statement on the practice doctorate in nursing. Retrieved from www.aacn.nche.edu/DNP/DNPPositionStatement.htm

American Association of Colleges of Nursing. (2006). *The essentials of doctoral education for advanced nursing practice.* Retrieved from http://www.aacn.nche.edu/DNP/pdf/Essentials.pdf

American Association of Colleges of Nursing. (2015a). The DNP: A study of the institutional, political, and professional issues that facilitate or impede establishing a post-baccalaureate doctor of nursing practice program. Retrieved from http://www.aacn.nche.edu/dnp/DNP-Study.pdf

American Association of Colleges of Nursing. (2015b). The DNP fact sheet. Retrieved from http://www .aacn.nche.edu/media-relations/fact-sheets/dnp

American Association of Nurse Anesthetist. (2007). AANA announces support of doctorate for entry into nurse anesthesia practice by 2025. Retrieved from http://www.aana.com/newsandjournal/ News/Pages/092007-AANA-Announces-Support-of-Doctorate-for-Entry-into-Nurse-Anesthesia -Practice-by-2025.aspx

American Nurses Association. (2010). *Nursing: Scope and standards of practice* (2nd ed.). Nursesbooks .org. Retrieved from http://www.nursingworld.org/scopeandstandardsofpractice

APRN Joint Dialogue Group. (2008). Consensus model for APRN regulation: *Licensure, accreditation, certification and education.* Retrieved from http://www.nursingworld.org/ConsensusModelforAPRN

Bloch, J. (2005). Letter to the editor on "doctor of nursing practice." *Online Journal of Nursing Issues, 10*(3). Retrieved from http://www.nursingworld.org/MainMenuCategories/ANAMarketplace/ ANAPeriodicals/OJIN/LetterstotheEditor/JoanRosenBlochLetter.html

Brar, K., Boschma, G., & McCuaig, F. (2010). The development of nurse practitioner preparation beyond the masters' level: What is the debate about? *International Journal of Nursing Scholarship, 7*(1), 1–15.

Chism, L. A. (2009). *The doctor of nursing practice: A guidebook for role development and professional issues.* Sudbury, MA: Jones & Bartlett.

Commission for Nursing Education Accreditation. (2013). Retrieved from http://www.acenursing .org

Commission on Collegiate Nursing Education. (2005). Moves to consider for accreditation only practice doctorates with the DNP title. Retrieved from http://www.aacn.nche.edu/news/articles/2005/ commission-on-collegiate-nursing-education-moves-to-consider-for-accreditation-only-practice -doctorates-with-the-dnp-degree-title

Commission on Collegiate Nursing Education. (2010). CCNE reaffirms commitment to accrediting all types of master's degrees in nursing programs. Retrieved from http://www.aacn.nche.edu/ accreditation

Commission on Collegiate Nursing Education. (2013). Standards for the accreditation of baccalaureate and graduate nursing programs. Retrieved from http://www.aacn.nche.edu/ccne-accreditation/ Standards-Amended-2013.pdf

Commission on Collegiate Nursing Education. (2015). Amid calls for a more highly educated RN workforce, new AACN data confirm enrollment surge in schools of nursing. Retrieved from http:// www.aacn.nche.edu/news/articles/2015/enrollment

Dreher, H. (2005). The doctor of nursing practice: Has this train left the station? If so, just where is it going? *PA Nurse, 60*(5), 17, 19.

Dreher, H. M. (2010). Next steps toward practice knowledge development: An emerging epistemology in nursing. In M. D. Dahnke & H. M. Dreher (Eds.), *Philosophy of science for nursing practice: Concepts and application.* New York, NY: Springer Publishing.

Dreher, H. M., & Montgomery, K. (2009). Let's call it "doctoral" advanced practice nursing. *Journal of Continuing Education in Nursing, 40*(12), 530–531.

Dunbar-Jacob, J., Nativio, D. G., & Khalil, H. (2013). Impact of doctor of nursing practice education in shaping the healthcare systems for the future. *Journal of Nursing Education, 52*(8), 423–427.

Horrocks, S., Anderson, E., & Salisbury, C. (2002). Systematic review of whether nurse practitioners working in primary care can provide equivalent care to doctors. *British Medical Journal, 324*, 819–823.

Institute of Medicine of the Natural Academies. (2001). Crossing the quality chasm: A new health system for the 21st century. Retrieved from https://www.nationalacademies.org/hmd/~/media/Files/Report%20Files/2001/Crossing-the-Quality-Chasm/Quality%20Chasm%202001%20%20report%20brief.pdf

Institute of Medicine of the Natural Academies. (2003). *Health professions education: A bridge to quality.* Washington, DC: National Academies Press.

Institute of Medicine of the Natural Academies. (2010). The future of nursing: Leading change, advancing health. Retrieved from http://iom.nationalacademies.org/Reports/2010/The-Future-of-Nursing-Leading-Change-Advancing-Health.aspx

Loomis, J., Willard, B., & Cohen, J. (2007). Difficult professional choices: Deciding between the PhD and the DNP in nursing. *Online Journal Issues in Nursing, 12*(1), 1–16. Retrieved from http://proquest.umi.com.ezproxy2.library.drexel.edu/pqdweb?index=0&did=1737222291&SrchMode=1&sid=1&Fmt=6&VInst=PROD&VType=PQD&RQT=309&VName=PQD&TS= 1273105897&clientId=18133

Melnyk, B. M. (2013). Distinquishing the preparation and roles of doctor of philosophy and doctor of nursing practice graduates: National implications for academic curricula and health care systems. *Journal of Nursing Education, 52*(8), 442–448.

Minnick, A. F., Norman, L. D., & Donaghey, B. (2013). Defining and describing capacity issues in U.S. doctor of nursing practice programs. *Nursing Outlook, 61*(2), 93–101. doi:/10.1016/j.outlook.2012.07.011

Mundinger, M. (2005). Who's who in nursing: Bringing clarity to the doctor of nursing practice. *Nursing Outlook, 53*, 173–176.

Mundinger, M., Kane, R., Lenz, E., Totten, A., Tsai, W., & Cleary, P. (2000). Primary care outcomes in patients treated by nurse practitioners or physicians: A randomized trial. *Journal of the American Medical Association, 283*, 59–68.

National Organization of Nurse Practitioner Faculties. (2006). Competencies for nurse practitioners: Practice doctorate nurse practitioner entry level competencies. Retrieved from http://c.ymcdn.com/sites/www.nonpf.org/resource/resmgr/competencies/dnp%20np%20competenciesapril2006.pdf

Nichols, E. F., & Chitty, K. K. (2005). Educational patterns in nursing. In K. K. Chitty (Ed.), *Professional nursing: Concepts & challenges* (4th ed., pp. 31–63). St. Louis, MO: Elsevier Saunders.

Penn, B., Wilson, L., & Rosseter, R. (2008). Transitioning from nursing practice to a teaching role. *The Online Journal of Issues in Nursing, 13.* Retrieved from http://www.nursingworld.org/MainMenuCategories/ANAMarketplace/ANAPeriodicals/OJIN/TableofContents/vol132008/No3Sept08/NursingPracticetoNursingEducation.aspx. doi:10.3912/OJIN.Vol13No03Man0

U.S. Department of Labor. (2010). Patient Care and Affordable Care Act (PPACA) USC § 42 USC 18001.

Yox, S. (2005). Clinical doctorate in nursing: A newsmaker interview with Mary O'Neil Mundinger, DrPH. Retrieved from http://www.medscape.com/viewarticle/501769

Zungolo, E. (2009). *The DNP and the faculty role: Issues and challenges.* Paper presented at the 2nd National Conference on the Doctor of Nursing Practice: The Dialogue Continues . . . , Hilton Head Island, SC, March 24–27, 2009.

CHAPTER FOUR

Reflective Response 1

Connie L. Zak

The question of how doctoral-level education versus MS education impacts the role of advanced practice nurses (APNs) is asked by many nursing faculty and APNs nationally. The authors have eloquently presented their own experiences and impetus for pursuing the Doctor of Nursing Practice (DNP). The authors started their discourse with a historical recapitulation of doctoral education in nursing, leading up to the practice doctorate, and going on to give their personal journeys from seasoned practitioner to doctoral student and graduate.

It is important to understand that the inception of a practice doctorate in nursing is not a new concept, but one that has been around for 30 years. Nursing has been debating the need for a practice doctorate for a very long time. Unfortunately, the early practice doctorates, such as the doctor of nursing (ND) degree, were not generally accepted. Schools of nursing offering such degrees for nurse practitioners (NPs) lost students to MS programs and in the end had to phase out such programs.

Subsequently, with the position statement from American Association of Colleges of Nursing (AACN) in 2004 came the era of agreement (for the most part) within the nursing profession of the importance for APNs, and especially NPs, to have doctoral education as entry into advanced practice, as noted by the authors (AACN, 2004). This shift in nursing education is timely, given the changes in health care occurring in our nation today, which started with the Institute of Medicine's (IOM, 2001) report, outlining the skills needed for improving health care. It is important to highlight that translating research into practice, testing new models of care, and working in transdisciplinary teams, are the essentials of the role of DNP-prepared practitioners. Furthermore, the IOM emphasized the need for all health professions programs to educate students to be able to deliver patient-centered care as members of interdisciplinary teams that emphasize evidence-based practice, quality improvement, and informatics.

It is also important for the reader to understand that the DNP is a degree and not a role. The practice doctorate is not just role oriented, but it is advanced education that gives "added value" to the practitioner to better serve their patients and populations. One must keep in mind the AACN definition of *advanced nursing practice* as conceptualized in the DNP *Essentials* document refers to:

> any form of nursing intervention that influences health care outcomes for individuals or populations, including the direct care of individual patients,

management of care for individuals and populations, administration of nursing and health care organizations, and the development and implementation of health policy. (AACN, 2006, p. 4)

Although the authors point out that the DNP builds on MSN-level education, it should be understood that the DNP replaces MSN-level education for advanced practice with comprehensive and in-depth knowledge that is necessary to manage the complexities not only for individual patient care but also for populations and health care systems.

As outlined in Case Study I, A Women's Health NP Who Continues to Want "More," the DNP degree provides the education that practitioners need for responding to the health needs of the nation by being the bridge between research and practice. I would differ in opinion with this author who stated that this degree is for the NP who *wants more*, but I declare it is for the NP who *needs more* to continue to be effective in facing the challenges of taking care of patients in the ever-changing and expanding health care system. This is not to say that MS-prepared APNs are ineffective in their roles, but it is to say that continuing their education to the DNP will allow them to be even more effective, not only in their roles but also in improving the care they deliver. In doing so, it will be instrumental in changing practice to better serve their patients.

In Case Study II, Transitioning in Academia, Practice, and Scholarship: One DrNP's Story, the author highlights the importance of the DNP-prepared educator. Colleges of Nursing educate practitioners, and what better-prepared faculty is there than the "Practice Expert?" There is a national shortage of qualified nursing faculty that is further contributing to the nursing shortage nationally. The increasing number of DNP programs opening across the nation is one answer to the faculty shortage as it increases the number of faculty who can train nurses at both the entry and advanced levels. I agree with this author that it is very important to choose a DNP program that will fulfill the candidate's future career goals.

Finally, it is important to point out the importance of the DNP-prepared APN as a member of a research team, even as the leader of clinical research endeavors. This important point is still not appreciated in the AACN's revised White Paper on the DNP published August 2015, which attempts to clarify the scholarly role of the DNP student and graduate. When it comes to evidence-based practice, it is important to understand that there is not a linear pathway to improving patient care. Rather, it is a circular path that always feeds back into primary research. Without measuring outcomes of evidence-based changes in practice, there is no way to ascertain that such change has actually improved patient care and outcomes. It is imperative that DNP-prepared APNs are able to not only synthesize science, but also to apply it to practice and measure the impact of such change. The question here is, At what point is the generation of evidence-based practice knowledge considered 'research' and how do they differ? DNP-prepared practitioners are able to and should be prepared to measure the impact of their practice, whether by measuring the process of a program or practice change or by measuring individual patient outcomes. If this is considered "research," one can comfortably say that it is not primary knowledge generating research, but evidence-based practice that will actually benefit the health care system. Dreher (2016) has labeled this "practice knowledge" derived from practice evidence and Melynk and Fineout-Overholt (2014) label this "internal evidence" (p. 11) that is practice-generated. Webber (2008) raised an important question regarding the decision of DNP programs not to prepare graduates to be principal investigators of clinical research. She argues that such action "will limit the creation of a broader, more inclusive research environment and thus perpetuates marginalization of research for many faculty, students, and practicing nurses" (p. 466). Webber points out how NPs rely on medical research to support their practice. She urges the conduct of more practice-focused research based on phenomena unique to the nursing experience which will not happen if DNPs are marginalized from the research enterprise.

In conclusion, the authors have made a very important statement regarding the "added value" that DNP education gives to APNs. With the exciting changes going on in health care today, the road has been paved for DNPs to make their mark by advancing nursing practice, improving health care, and educating the future nursing workforce.

■ REFERENCES

American Association of Colleges of Nursing. (2004). AACN position statement on the practice doctorate in nursing October 2004. Retrieved from http://www.aacn.nche.edu/DNP/pdf/DNP.pdf

American Association of Colleges of Nursing. (2006). *The essentials of doctoral education for advanced nursing practice*. Washington, DC: Author.

American Association of Colleges of Nursing. (2015). New white paper on the DNP: Current issues and clarifying recommendations. Retrieved from http://www.aacn.nche.edu/news/articles/2015/dnp-white-paper

Dreher, H. M. (2016). Next steps toward practice knowledge development: An emerging epistemology in nursing. In M. D. Dahnke & H. M. Dreher (Eds.), *Philosophy of science for nursing practice: Concepts and application* (2nd ed., pp. 355–391, New York, NY: Springer Publishing.

Melnyk, B. M., & Fineout-Overholt, E. (2014). *Evidence-based practice in nursing & healthcare: A guide to best practice* (3rd ed.). Philadelphia, PA: Wolters Kluwer/Lippincott Williams & Wilkins.

Institute of Medicine. (2001). *Crossing the quality chasm: A new health system for the 21st century.* Washington, DC: National Academies Press.

Webber, P. B. (2008). The doctor of nursing practice degree and research: Are we making an epistemological mistake? *Journal of Nursing Education, 47,* 466–472.

Reflective Response 2

Karen Kaufman

Drs. Montgomery and Byrne provide a thought-provoking analysis of the differences between doctoral-level and master's-level practice roles. The personal stories and experiences they relate are powerful reminders that nurses with practice doctorates, with their advanced knowledge and strong commitment, are making enormous contributions to the nursing field and to health care in general. Most importantly, the authors point to the distinction between the MSN degree, which "allows you to be part of the change," and the Doctor of Nursing Practice (DNP), which equips you "to *be* [*sic*] the change." In other words, MSNs are qualified to carryout important, necessary changes in the practice of health care, while DNPs are the people with the knowledge and responsibility for actually *driving* that change.

The gulf between these two roles is vast. Our experience working with Drexel DNP students suggests that no book, seminar, or dissertation is sufficient to transform the DNP candidate from a nursing practitioner into a health care *leader*. Indeed, two highly respected former Drexel professors, Smith Glasgow and Lachman (2010) documented that at least half of the DNP candidates in the Drexel DNP program did not truly see themselves as future leaders, nor did they understand the connection between their unique personality preferences and the role requirements of a leader.

Effecting such a transformation does indeed require advanced knowledge, skills, and experiences, and it also requires a significant change in one's self-image—which is the first and most important step in persuading others to see you differently as well. Even the best doctoral programs, because of their academic nature, have difficulty affecting this kind of personal transformation in their students. As a result, most DNPs do graduate with the knowledge to address complex patient care challenges and to improve the efficiency of health care delivery. Where they often have difficulty, though, is in mastering the leadership skills required to enlist others in the effort—to implement real and lasting improvement in the nursing profession and health care in general. In short, to *be* the change—which, after all, is the key reason for obtaining a DNP degree in the first place. As one second year Drexel doctoral residency student said, "Karen's ability to empower us into transformational leadership is very valuable. We need to transform and elevate our role. We have had the role of clinicians for years. Now we are moving to the executive level which requires a different type of training."

In my years of designing and leading professional development programs, I have noted that doctoral nursing students are not the only ones in need of more comprehensive leadership training, but leadership skills are especially critical in nursing, a field still dominated by women, most of whom have been socialized to cede leadership authority to men. To be sure, male DNPs need leadership skills too, but as more and more women earn DNPs, their ability to lead will have an outsized effect on the profession as a whole—how it is viewed by other health care professionals and by the general public.

I have had the privilege of working with Drexel DNP students to enhance their leadership abilities. Like Professors Smith Glasgow and Lachman, I have observed that the typical female student does not see a "disconnect" between her own personality preferences—such as the desire to be liked and avoid confrontation—and the more active role requirements of a leader. Effective leadership depends on a variety of factors, from vision and assembling the right team of people, to the integrity of personal actions and behaviors. However, developing leadership skills has to begin with self-image. We need to think of ourselves as leaders in order to have others see us as leaders.

Impression management (Kaufman & Kaufman, 2010) is the term our firm uses to describe the distinctions and tools for building and expanding the key relationships required to meet complex leadership challenges. It is the art and science of making a favorable, role-appropriate impression on others, both personally and professionally. In our work at Drexel, we discuss and dissect these tools in a classroom setting. We are confident that much more could be accomplished with one-on-one consultations.

Our recommendation for all forward-thinking DNP programs—is to treat DNP candidates as we do our executive coaching clients. To help prepare these students for leadership roles, DNP programs would do well to offer a few individualized sessions in which each candidate is profiled according to his or her unique combination of perceptual, cognitive, behavioral, and emotional traits. That analysis can then become the foundation of a customized development plan in which students identify and optimize their strengths while also focusing on areas of improvement to maximize role performance.

DNP programs would benefit by including impression management for nursing leadership into the curriculum. This will provide a proactive approach toward transforming nursing practitioners who are enrolled in DNP programs into health care leaders through detailed analysis and behavioral focus. Such an approach, when consistent with the student's professional goals and advanced knowledge, is the best possible way of transforming nursing practitioners into the leaders that our health care system so urgently needs.

■ REFERENCES

Kaufman, K. D., & Kaufman, D. R. (2010). *The Kaufman Impression Management System®*. Unpublished manuscript. Philadelphia, PA.

Smith Glasgow, M. E., & Lachman, V. D. (2010). Impression management: A key leadership skill in DrNP graduates from Drexel University College of Nursing and Health Professions. *Poster presentation before the American Association of Colleges of Nursing Doctoral Education Conference*, Captiva Island, FL, January 2010.

Primary and Secondary Contemporary Roles for Doctoral Advanced Nursing Practice

The Role of the Practitioner

Sandra Bellini and Regina M. Cusson

In their 2004 position statement, the American Association of Colleges of Nursing (AACN) declared that the future entry-level educational requirement for nurse practitioners (NPs) would be the Doctor of Nursing Practice (DNP) degree. The move has raised many controversies for both currently practicing MS-prepared NPs and NP faculty. More than a decade has passed since the publication of the position statement and the target date of 2015 for entry into DNP has arrived. What progress has been made? In 2015, the MS-entry option remains the degree of choice for the majority of NPs (Auerback et al., 2014). However, the degree has become an extremely popular option for clinicians seeking advanced nursing education. Some of the continuing controversies are: (a) whether the DNP is a degree or a role, (b) how DNP-prepared NPs are currently practicing, (c) whether DNP-prepared practice is really different from MS-prepared NP practice, (d) what effect DNP education will have on certification, and (e) whether programs conferring a DNP degree truly are at the doctoral level of scholarship. In this chapter, we explore these issues to date and discuss the potential etiologies for, and resolutions to, many of the issues impacting the future role of the NP.

■ EVOLVING ACADEMIC PREPARATION FOR THE PRACTITIONER

The academic preparation path for NPs has evolved several times since the initial establishment of the NP role. From early certificate programs, to MS-required preparation, to the more recent 2004 AACN position statement elevating future NP entry-level education to the doctoral level, nursing continues to strive for the highest education standards in order to best serve our patients and society. That said, the move to doctoral degree–only preparation for NP education raises many questions, with answers that may remain elusive for some time. In fact, in light of this second edition text, it is important to assess the extent to which progress has been made toward the AACN (2015) goal to raise entry into advanced practice registered nurse (APRN) practice to DNP preparation (AACN, 2004). At the time of writing of this second edition chapter, it is interesting to note that of the four APRN roles targeted for "elevation" of practice entry academic credentials, three organizations have endorsed the move to the DNP (all except the American College of Nurse-Midwives [ACNM] reaffirmed in 2012), but only two have clearly articulated a plan for implementation of the new practice entry require-ments. Although it is admirable progress that 50% of APRN roles will be transitioned to the DNP entry level, these transitions will not happen until 2025 for nurse anesthe-tists (American Association of Nurse Anesthetists [AANA], 2007) and not until 2030 for clinical nurse specialists (National Association of Clinical Nurse Specialists [NACNS], 2015). Since 2006, the National Organization of Nurse Practitioner Faculties (NONPF) has held the position that while they endorse the notion of the DNP, the change would be gradual and the organization holds no time frame on which to require a DNP for entry into NP practice (NONPF, 2015). As we begin our chapter, we mention as a note to the reader that the term "practitioner" is used as a broadly inclusive term throughout this chapter, pertaining to traditional APRN roles, not exclusively or specifically to the role of the certified NP.

Among a number of issues to be explored in this chapter, there is one very basic question: What does the DNP degree itself represent? Is it a degree, or is it to be synon-ymous with a particular advanced nursing role? Because AACN has made this deter-mination now more than a decade ago, what precisely is different when comparing the current *practice* of an MS-prepared NP to that of a DNP-prepared NP? What are the potential consequences to our discipline if we move too quickly to close our MS APRN programs? What about the apparent variability in curriculum and foci in DNP pro-grams? Should they all be the same? Do they need to be? Another contentious issue at present is certification. When in the educational process should DNPs become certified, in what, and by whom? Does the DNP curriculum prepare graduates to assume full-time academic faculty roles? Finally, this chapter reexamines the document that got us here: *The Essentials of Doctoral Education for Advanced Nursing Practice* (AACN, 2006) and the report of the Task Force on the Implementation of the DNP: *New White Paper on the DNP: Current Issues and Clarifying Recommendations* (2015b); are they fluid enough?

At the present time in our society, with such uncertainty in the economy, an aging population with increasingly diverse health care needs, and the health care system at a breaking point in spite of recent reforms to enhance access to health care, is this really the moment to undertake such a grand agenda on the part of our profession? Added to these societal issues are other intraprofessional issues that further complicate the pic-ture, such as uncertainty about the adequacy of the nursing workforce, the aging work-force, the nursing faculty shortage, as well as faculty nearing retirement. Or perhaps at this time in history, with a constellation of such pressing issues, this is exactly the right time.

■ THE DNP: DEGREE OR ROLE?

Unlike many sweeping changes in education, it is important to remember that the move to the DNP degree for entry into practice for future NPs did not result from poor patient outcomes with NP-managed care. On the contrary, research comparing physician-managed patient outcomes with those of their NP counterparts has consistently demon-strated comparable outcomes (Horrocks, Anderson, & Salisbury, 2002; Mundinger et al., 2000). The decision to elevate the educational requirement for NPs came as a result of a broad consensus among health professions: In order to meet the needs of health care reform, tomorrow's clinicians would need additional skill sets from those currently exist-ing in today's NP programs. Multiple publications by the Institute of Medicine (IOM, 1999, 2001) and the National Research Council of the National Academies (NRCNA, 2005) highlighted the serious nature of health care quality issues in the United States.

These publications also called on the many health care professions to align their visions and educational processes to produce clinicians with advanced skills and knowledge to address these issues (IOM, 2003). The AACN heeded this call and set about redesigning the role of the NP. This move to DNP education has evidently resonated with many. As of March 2015, a total of 264 DNP programs have been established in 48 states and the District of Columbia, with reports of an additional 60 programs in the planning stages (AACN, 2015). The Commission on Collegiate Nursing Education (CCNE) began accrediting DNP programs in 2008, with 158 programs currently accredited and 33 additional programs seeking accreditation (AACN, 2015). Program growth has been robust with more than 18,000 enrolled DNP students and more than 3,000 DNP graduates in 2014 (AACN, 2015).

The NP of tomorrow, as articulated by AACN (2006), will need expertise and leadership ability in areas such as quality assessment, outcomes evaluation, evidence-based practice, health policy, systems leadership, and health information technologies—topics identified in the IOM papers—in addition to the current required competencies for NPs. If the goals of health care reform are to be met, the existing research–practice gap, cited as existing for as long as 17 years in some studies, needs to be closed (Balas & Boren, 2000). Important research findings generated at the bench need to be implemented in a far more timely fashion at the bedside. Research findings establish the evidence on which clinical practice guidelines are founded. By integrating the most recent research findings into clinical practice and reducing variation in practice, adherence to evidence-based practice guidelines can improve patient outcomes as much as 28% (Heater, Becker, & Olson, 1988; Melnyk, 2015). It can be argued that NPs, as frontline care providers, are ideally positioned to contribute toward that goal. Therefore, DNP programs need to have strong emphasis on advancing the evidence base for practice within their curricula.

When discussion of the DNP degree first emerges in conversation, one of the more common controversies that can quickly come to light is whether the DNP is a role or a degree. To be clear, the DNP is a terminal practice degree (AACN, 2006), designated as the educational level for several advanced nursing practice–registered nurse (APRN) roles, including certified nurse-midwife, certified registered nurse anesthetist, clinical nurse specialist, and NP (APRN Joint Dialogue Group Report, 2008). That said, the AACN endorses the notion that although all APRNs must be DNPs, not all DNPs will be APRNs. Although the DNP will be required for APRN practice, MS-prepared academic nurse educators as well as nurse administrators from practice settings also seek the degree.

What do nurses think about the role of the DNP-prepared nurse? A recent study by Udlis and Mancuso (2015) was designed to examine nurses' perception ($N = 340$) of the roles that DNP-prepared nurses engage in (Udlis & Mancuso, 2015). They found that nurses' understanding of the DNP degree as a terminal degree was clear, but that there was ambiguity regarding potential overlap between PhD and DNP roles and the DNP's ability to unite the nursing profession, even though DNPs would be able to describe how nurses contribute to health care. Respondents felt that DNPs were prepared as leaders in clinical practice who could influence changes in health care delivery systems, policy, and interprofessional collaboration. They were less sure of the DNP's role as leaders in academia. They did appreciate that DNPs could help ameliorate the faculty shortage, but were not certain that DNPs were prepared as educators. They thought that DNP preparation provided equivalence to other entry-level doctorally prepared clinicians and that the DNP degree would enhance outcomes, as well as lead to improved position, salaries, and professional regard. They did not think that employers would prefer a DNP-prepared graduate over an MS-prepared practitioner. Clearly, there is work to be done in articulating and examining the contributions that DNP-prepared nurses are making in health care and education, although reports in the literature are scarce to date.

The curriculum in DNP programs, as described by the AACN, should focus on advanced nursing practices and issues relevant to advanced nursing practice. In a departure from previous guidance, the AACN supports the eligibility of DNP graduates as nursing educators in the academic setting, because they possess a terminal degree in nursing (AACN, 2015). The AACN (2015) continues to recommend that DNP programs offer courses in educational pedagogy beyond the expected courses in the curriculum. This recommendation is also mentioned in the 2006 AACN document for PhD graduates, whose doctoral education focuses on research rather than the process of education. There has been support for the DNP-prepared graduate to enter academia on graduation and for the need of clinical practice and nursing education to work more closely together to change the way we educate nurses (Benner, Sutphen, Leonard, & Day, 2010; Danzey et al., 2011). DNP-prepared educators who are active in clinical practice and comfortable with collaboration can make a valuable contribution to bridging the academic–practice gap.

Conversely, an alternative argument regarding academic preparation and qualifications for teaching various curriculum contents could be raised. Specifically, are DNP graduates who are not APRNs qualified to teach APRN/DNP students? If so, what content is appropriate? What is not? A similar issue may arise in the years to come, as more research-focused faculties obtain BSN–PhD degrees that do not include APRN education. Are they qualified to teach APRN/DNP students? Suffice it to say that faculty composition and roles as we know them are likely to change and evolve over the next several years and that diversity of preparation can enhance faculty roles (AACN, 2015). The allocation of teaching assignments will need to be based on subject matter expertise and the needs of the students. In any event, coursework in the knowledge and process of teaching could benefit all educators, regardless of their specific degree focus, would undoubtedly benefit students, and should therefore be encouraged for all doctoral students.

■ THE ARRIVAL OF THE DOCTORALLY PREPARED NP: IS IT DIFFERENT FROM THE MS-PREPARED NP?

Now that the first decade of DNP-prepared NPs have arrived in the workforce, who are they, where are they, and what are they doing? Most importantly, are they practicing any differently than their MS-prepared counterparts? Perhaps, it is too soon to adequately answer this question in light of the limited numbers, but we can examine what evidence is currently available.

In 2009, Dreher and Montgomery published an editorial focusing on a recent new graduate of a DrNP program; simply defined as a DNP program encompassing a research component beyond what is typical for DNP curricula. The graduate described ways in which she saw herself as practicing differently than she had as an MS-prepared NP with many years of experience. This "doctoral advanced practice nurse" articulated a newfound confidence not only in investigating practice issues but also in the ability to investigate, evaluate, and question the evidence on which much of clinical practice is founded. Interpreted in another way, these anecdotes speak to larger concepts, such as increased leadership ability and clinical scholarship—concepts articulated in the AACN publications supporting the move to the DNP. These qualities, built on solid NP education obtained historically at the MS level, combine to give rise to the role and abilities that AACN envisioned for the DNP-prepared NP.

The following year (2010) an online article was published in the *New England Nursing News* ("The DNP: An Emerging Trend"). In this article, seven DNP graduates and current DNP students relayed similar accomplishments to those cited in the Dreher and Montgomery (2009) article. From the DNP-prepared chief nursing officer to the various NPs from a variety of practice settings, the featured subjects articulated significant perceived benefits from their additional education. The DNPs who were interviewed described increased knowledge regarding evidence-based practice, quality and outcomes evaluation research, systems leadership, the needs of the increasingly complex health care system, and the need to bridge the research–practice gap. Another theme that clearly resonated from the article was that all of the graduates and students felt that they now possessed a level of leadership ability to face the challenges of the health care system that they did not previously possess. In a more recent publication, many of these same perspectives were conveyed via a case study describing one DNP-prepared NP's practice (Paul, 2015). Despite the occasional case study or other anecdotal evidence however, the literature remains quite limited regarding what these DNP graduates are currently *doing in practice*, including how many NPs currently in practice hold a DNP degree.

Although it was assumed early on in the DNP movement that the practice setting would be home to the largest numbers of doctorally prepared NPs, it was also assumed that the academic setting would assimilate a portion of these graduates as educators in NP programs, members of faculty practice groups, as part of joint appointments bridging the academic and practice settings, and possibly as educators in undergraduate clinical courses. However, what has come to pass is that according to Loomis, Willard, and Cohen (2007), more than 50% of DNP graduates seek employment in the academic setting.

As discussed elsewhere in this chapter, the DNP as educator is a controversial issue because DNP curricula do not include courses in education as part of their core coursework. That said, DNP graduates who obtain elective coursework in educational pedagogy may arguably become quite successful in the academic setting and bring current clinical expertise, advanced educational preparation, and a wealth of experience from the practice setting to the classroom. For those DNP faculty holding joint appointments in order to remain current in the chosen NP specialization area, such an arrangement might be very rewarding. This structure allows the continuation of NP practice and opportunities for involvement in the health care setting at the systems level, as well as the connection to the academic setting. Joint appointments can also provide an opportunity for DNP-prepared NP faculty to make significant contributions to health care organizations in nontraditional ways, such as sitting on nursing leadership councils and participating in collaborative translational research studies. Joint appointments can have benefits to the educational setting as well; for example, joint appointments may provide a means to attract experienced NPs with strong devotion to the clinical practice setting to the academic setting, helping to alleviate some of the faculty shortage (Bellini, McCauley, & Cusson, 2012). In the years to come, joint appointments may become a staple in nursing faculty composition as they have been for decades in medicine.

Perhaps, as time passes and the skill set of DNP graduates becomes clearer, the ability to appreciate the increased leadership skills and clinical scholarship abilities brought to the practice arena by DNP-prepared NPs will erase any lingering resentments toward the degree. After all, the goal for DNP education is to benefit health care institutions and populations of patients by providing NPs with advanced levels of education built on their core NP education, or to educate the NP of the future—it is not to disenfranchise the NPs of today. The future role of the DNP-prepared NP will likely be oriented toward adding additional areas of expertise to current practice roles and aimed at improving patient outcomes across practice settings. DNPs will also likely lead many organizational-level performance improvement initiatives, take on leadership roles in ensuring best practices based on current evidence, and assume leadership roles in health care legislation and policy at the national level. Given the remaining timelines before the DNP-entry requirement changes indicated by AANA and NACNS however, as well as the silence on the issue from NONPF and the AANM, it may be decades yet before the role and scope of practice for DNP-prepared APRNs becomes any clearer.

The intended scope of practice for DNP-prepared NPs is an issue that needs to be settled, although it is unlikely to be resolved in the near future. A hotly debated topic currently in nursing academic circles is whether the DNP degree will broaden the current scope of practice for NPs, allowing "advanced" NP competencies traditionally held as the purview of physicians, especially in light of calls for "doctoral-level clinical practice." This idea has incited much disagreement and debate among nursing scholars as well as among physicians. In order to lend clarity regarding what is and is not intended regarding scope of practice issues pertaining to the DNP-prepared NP, perhaps the confluence and level of agreement of several documents published by key leading nursing organizations need to be raised for discussion.

First, there is no evidence put forth by the AACN in any of their documents that the intent of the DNP is to "expand scope of practice" for NPs (AACN, 2004, 2006). In fact, the question is raised and answered unequivocally for all via the AACN website (AACN, 2009). Aligned with and supported by AACN, neither the APRN Consensus Work Group nor the National Council of State Boards of Nursing (NCSBN) APRN Advisory Committee put forth any language supporting expanded scope of practice for NPs in their licensure, accreditation, certification, and education (LACE) document (APRN Joint Dialogue Report, 2008). Finally, there is also no mention of expanding the scope of practice for NPs based on doctoral-level competencies as articulated by the NONPF (2006). In contrast, all documents speak to doctoral-level education for APRNs as focusing on the concepts articulated in the *Essentials* documents and aligned with the IOM papers (IOM, 1999, 2001, 2003). These documents seem to identify the need for an APRN provider with a new, unique skill set designed to fill a current need within the health care arena, not necessarily to produce more providers with the skill sets traditionally held by physicians.

Opportunity exists at this time for nursing to say "yes, expand the scope of traditional NP practice," but perhaps not in the manner in which academicians traditionally envision. The notion that "advanced clinical skills" beyond those currently encompassed in NP practice, in light of the content of various relevant publications, although intriguing, seems rather contrary to the intent of the degree and the skill set collectively described by AACN, the NCSBN APRN Advisory Committee, and NONPF. For the purposes of clarity, perhaps nursing academics should broaden their application of the word "clinical" to include "things relevant to the practice setting" rather than the single, more traditional use of the term denoting "hands on, individual-level patient management." If the confusion relating to "expanding scope of practice" were to be disavowed, perhaps the lingering resentment of physicians and their opposition to DNP education may also abate. In any case, the domain of DNPs will likely become clearer and less controversial in the decades to come as more DNP-educated practitioners begin to demonstrate their skill set in the health care arena, presenting themselves as credible leaders and collaborative partners with a unique knowledge base rather than as competitors.

■ CLOSING MS-LEVEL NP PROGRAMS: POTENTIAL PITFALLS

Despite the 2015 goal cited by AACN (2004, 2006) as the year graduating NPs would be required to have DNP degrees to enter advanced practice, a recent study sponsored by AACN (Auerback et al., 2014) has illuminated very different data. In fact, as of 2014, approximately 70% of APRNs across specialty roles were still entering practice with an MS degree (Auerback et al., 2014). The document goes on to describe many of the barriers and facilitators to closing MS-level advanced practice programs as well as exploring the reasons that the DNP has not been received with as much enthusiasm beyond the academic world as was previously hoped for. Although it is true that the expansion of available DNP programs has grown at an impressive rate and still more programs are in the planning stages, there appears a rather clear dichotomy in viewpoints based on the data.

The debate regarding whether to close MS-level programs offering APRN education remains one that seems to be made at the individual school level. Some have already closed their MS programs, other have taken a "wait and see" pragmatic approach, and still others located in educational setting where conferral of a doctoral degree is not an option, remain committed to their MS programs. Again, the recent data from the Auerback et al. (2014) study provide important information. We know that only 30% of APRNs were entering practice with a DNP as of 2014. Additionally, estimates project increasing percentages of DNPs entering APRN practice over the next several years, but will the DNP actually reach the level of 100% as put forth by AACN? Not according to the Auerback et al. (2014) findings, which suggest that in the future, approximately 50% of APRNs will enter practice with a DNP. This is an interesting number, given the parallels to the ANA position statement from 1965 (American Nurses' Association [ANA], 1965) advocating bachelor of science in nursing (BSN) entry for nursing practice. Despite the ensuing 50 years between the publication of the ANA paper, recent data demonstrate that as of 2013, the percentage of nurses *in practice*, who held a minimum of a BSN degree was somewhere between 55% and 61% depending on the study (Budden, Zhong, Moulton, & Cimiotti, 2013; Health Services and Resources Administration, 2013). It should be noted that these data included nurses who had obtained a BSN post-RN licensure from either a diploma or associate degree program. It will be interesting to see what impact might be on the push for BSN entry should the federal government realize its stated goal of free education at community colleges (Obama, 2015). Regardless, it does not appear that DNP entry for APRNs will be accomplished with any greater success than the BSN entry argument made half a century ago.

Today, our discipline has its roots firmly established in the academic setting, with nursing now recognized as a scholarly profession rather than as an "apprenticeship" occupation as it was in past decades. Nursing, as a discipline, has a responsibility toward society to care for the sick and to promote wellness in the larger society. In light of current needs, is this really the appropriate time to advance this agenda? What will be the impact to society, to the current nursing workforce, and to the faculty workforce?

At the NP level, shortages exist and are predicted to worsen, especially in certain specialty areas, such as the national shortage of primary care providers (Pho, 2008) increasing the demand for primary care NPs (Stanik-Hutt, 2008a), the acute care NP (Howie-Esquivel & Fontaine, 2006), and the neonatal NP (Bellini, 2013). Although some of these shortages result from small numbers of students within and entering existing programs, the larger issue is anticipated increased demand for NPs in these areas consistent with sweeping national changes stemming from the Affordable Care Act (2010).

As a shortage of NPs in these areas exists, what impact will the move to the DNP have on the existing shortage? Will the added time commitment for graduate education, and therefore added expense, combine to act as a deterrent to RNs considering advanced degrees? If so, what impact will this direction have on schools of nursing if the number of applicants were to fall significantly? What will be the effect of smaller numbers of APRNs to society? For all of these reasons, some would argue that the DNP degree should remain an option rather than a requirement for advanced nursing practice at least for the foreseeable future. With some educators feeling that preparing the post-BS student as an APRN while concurrently attaining the competencies expected of the DNP-prepared NP is perhaps too much, it might give one pause to consider a possible compromise. Perhaps consideration should be given to the possibility of continuing MS-level APRN preparation for initial certification and licensure, with subsequent licensure *renewals* requiring a DNP degree perhaps in a decade or so after entering practice (Bellini & Cusson, 2012). This would allow APRNs to enter practice with an MS thus stabilizing the workforce and providing time to learn about health care systems and the role of advanced practice nurses while practicing and gaining expertise. Would this potential solution meet the needs of all parties? It might, but at least for now it appears that the 2015 plan for DNP entry into APRN is not close to being realized before the close of the year.

■ VARIABILITY AMONG DNP PROGRAMS: TO WHAT EXTENT ARE DNP PROGRAMS PRODUCING CLINICIANS WHO ARE DISTINCTLY DIFFERENT FROM MS-PREPARED NPs?

There is compelling evidence that the nursing community values DNP education to "prepare nurses to meet future health care needs" (AACN, 2015, p. 1). However, this strong support for the value of DNP education has not translated into consistency in preparation, in spite of guidance provided by AACN in the *Essentials* document (2006), as well as numerous position papers and reports in the past 10 years. AACN recognized the need for further guidance at this juncture and commissioned white papers from two AACN task forces: the Implementation of the DNP task force and the APRN Clinical Training task force. The task force for the implementation of the DNP released their white paper: *New White Paper on the DNP: Current Issues and Clarifying Recommendations* in August 2015. This new white paper provides additional recommendations on the characteristics of DNP scholarship, the DNP project, efficient resource use, and characteristics of programs, such as program length, curriculum, clinical practice, and collaboration with clinical partners. AACN's goal is to enhance consistency across programs, recognizing that significant variability currently exists.

A recent study by Udlis and Mancuso (2012a, 2012b) demonstrated considerable variation in admission criteria and program characteristics among the 137 DNP programs in existence at the time of the study. Particularly salient to this discussion is the variability in program characteristics across the United States. While some variability is to be expected, there are indications that some recommendations were not followed. For example, although credit hours were fairly consistent with AACN recommendations, the length of time for completion of the post-MS DNP program was recommended to be approximately 1 year, but the results indicated that the average length was 21 ± 5.9 months. Pertinent to the DNP nurse educator role, few schools offered courses in nursing education, perhaps in response to the original recommendation by AACN that preparation in education should not be the focus of the DNP program.

Findings from the RAND study (Auerbach et al., 2014) demonstrated that 30% of nursing schools with APRN programs do offer the BSN–DNP option, with evidence that the rate will increase to 50% within the near future (RAND Study on the DNP by 2015). Although most APRN programs continue to offer the MS degree (14% are DNP exclusively), an additional 27% plan to close their MS programs in the next few years, indicating an acceleration in the national progression to DNP-only education for APRNs. Finally, the report concluded that demand remains robust for all types of APRN preparation programs, with applications exceeding available program slots.

Now that many programs are conferring DNP degrees, what makes them "doctoral-level" rather than "master's-plus?" Undoubtedly, there are programs today that fall into both of these categories. In light of the "credit-creep" rationale mentioned by AACN as part of the reason for the move to the DNP, some programs may have simply added several courses to their current MS-level curriculum to address the DNP essentials and competencies and retitled the degree as a "doctorate," while philosophically retaining the notion the DNP programs are really "master's-plus" (AACN, 2006). Other programs have embraced the idea that a doctorate degree denotes academic expectations well beyond those expected at the master's level and have designed a truly doctoral-level curriculum. Perhaps this philosophical difference of opinion is more important than we think, and if resolved, might result in programs with more consistent levels of expectation.

The case for and against PhD-style educational rigor in DNP programs has been discussed in the literature (Sheriff & Chaney, 2007), and while both sides of the issue present strong arguments, we would have to make our decision based on a traditional risk–benefit ratio. Although the level rigor of DNP programs as perceived by some might not *necessitate* a level consistent with what is expected in a PhD program, the outcomes may offer significant benefits in terms of valuable learning experiences consistent with clinical scholarship and development of leadership abilities, thereby establishing the DNP-prepared graduate as a truly learned individual, respected in the academic setting and valuable in the practice setting. Conversely, the question that must be considered is: What is the perceived risk of traditional doctoral-level scholarship if offered to DNP students? It could hardly be argued that DNP students graduating from such rigorous programs would be considered "too scholarly"; therefore, we take the position that expected level of scholarship should be equitable, but with a distinctly different focus.

Important points to consider in this distinction are competencies to be achieved at the DNP level as designated by both AACN (2006) in their *Essentials* document and NONPF (2006). Competencies articulated by both organizations are distinctly different for MS-level programs and for DNP-level programs. Simply stated, MS-level competencies address the expectations for patient care management at the traditional APRN level, while DNP entry-level competencies speak to additional areas of expected expertise having to do with quality assessment, practice inquiry, policy, and leadership (NONPF, 2006). Perhaps going forward, BS-DNP programs might consider various curriculum design schemes whereby mastery of APRN competencies might be attained early in the program, allowing for leadership competencies to be acquired via DNP coursework later in the program. An example of this curricular structure may offer all "traditional," MS-level APRN specialty-focused content within the first 2 years of the program, while the latter years of study would be devoted to the DNP-level competencies such as systems perspectives, populations and quality focus, the development of clinical scholarship, and leadership skills. True leadership experience may be gained through an immersion experience at the DNP residency level. It is difficult to imagine that mastery of skills at the traditional APRN level could be attained at the same time that leadership expertise within that role is gained. Generally, leadership follows mastery consistent with findings from the 2010 Carnegie Report (Benner et al., 2010). To expect concurrent attainment of both sets of skills may be unrealistic, despite the proliferation of BS–DNP Programs.

■ THE CONCEPT OF SCHOLARSHIP AND THE DNP ESSENTIALS

When the AACN issued their position statement on the DNP in 2004 and later published the DNP *Essentials* in 2006, the intent was likely to articulate and define their vision of both DNP education and their intent for the DNP role that would follow. Their publications were to serve as a guiding light for nursing programs throughout the nation to establish and refine their DNP programs. In all of the AACN's well-intended and truly inspired documents, however, there may in fact have been a lost opportunity to very clearly state for posterity what the expected level of "scholarship" for DNP programs was intended to be, at least as seen in 2006.

For example, while there are many references to Boyer's model of *Scholarship* (Boyer, 1990) throughout the *Essentials* document (2006) that clearly spoke to research-focused programs such as "Scholarship of Discovery" and practice-focused programs such as "Scholarship of Application," there appears only a brief sentence regarding the final "project" for the DNP degree, which may in fact be at the root of some of the variation in levels of expected scholarship seen today in DNP programs. For the sake of clarity, while there has been much discussion and debate over the last several years regarding the appropriate level of "rigor" for DNP programs, including elsewhere in this chapter, we would like to propose an alternative parameter to evaluate DNP programs, specifically scholarship rather than rigor. As rigor tends to be synonymous with traditional research methodology in the academic setting, scholarship is a broader concept, which may actually lend some clarity to our current dilemma.

AACN (2006) states, "For practice doctorates, requiring a dissertation or other original research is contrary to the intent of the DNP" (p. 20). The paragraph goes on to offer alternative suggestions that the final project may take. Although it can be inferred that the intent was to guide and clarify, it may be that this statement and this entire section of the document have contributed toward much of the resultant confusion. Although many agree that research dissertations should be the "gold-standard" outcome measure for programs focused on scholarship of discovery, perhaps it was too soon for the AACN to seek to define the gold-standard outcome measure for programs focused on scholarship of application. AACN sought to correct these impressions most recently in their new white paper: *New White Paper on the DNP: Current Issues and Clarifying Recommendations*. The very first point addressed is "DNP Graduate Scholarship." In which they indicate that DNP scholarship, rather than focusing on generalizability (the purview of the research-based doctoral program), instead contributes to enhanced outcomes. The DNP task force concludes that graduates of both types of doctoral programs are prepared to generate new knowledge, but that the DNP graduate is prepared to generate new knowledge through "innovation of practice change, the translation of evidence, and the implementation of quality improvement processes in specific practice settings, systems, or with specific populations to improve health or health outcomes." They further propose that "Organizational and systems leadership knowledge and skills are critical for DNP graduates to develop and evaluate new models of care delivery and to create and sustain change at the organization and systems levels." Neither type of knowledge generation should be viewed as superior since "the application and translation of evidence into practice is a vital and necessary skill that is currently lacking in the healthcare environment and nursing profession." Thus, the DNP task force sends a strong message that DNP scholarship is the generation of new knowledge and is a highly prized commodity lacking and sorely needed in our current health care system. The task force then goes on to provide recommendations for the DNP project that are far more directive and prescriptive than previous guidance, in an effort to enhance consistency and dispel uncertainty about the final product of the DNP program. Although many will appreciate these new recommendations, schools that have followed a different path will be challenged to carefully study the recommendations and decide how their current process meets the recommendations for the generation of new knowledge that enhances practice outcomes.

■ DO WE NEED ADDITIONAL CERTIFICATION TO INDICATE "DOCTORAL ADVANCED PRACTICE NURSING"?

Another controversial area concerning NP certification and the DNP degree is certification. When in the educational process should NPs be allowed to sit for initial certification in their specialty area? Historically, NPs have been eligible to sit for certification following successful completion of their APRN programs, having achieved an MS degree. As NP education moves to the doctoral level, the APRN Consensus Work Group and the NCSBN APRN Joint Dialogue Group Report (2008) will serve as guides for current graduate programs to align their plans for LACE. As of the writing of this chapter, a DNP is not required to sit for any advanced practice certification examinations; all remain available with a minimum of an MS degree, despite the initial 2015 timeline endorsed by AACN. Whether the DNP will be required to sit for NP certification exams in the future remains unclear at this time in large part due to NONPF's position that the transition to the DNP "will be gradual" (NONPF, 2006), or more recently that the transition to DNP should not take another 10 years (NONPF, 2015), while failing to state exactly how long the transition should indeed take. The most recent "unified statement" put forth from NONPF in partnership with the NP faculty specialty organizations (Nurse Practitioner Roundtable, 2008) clearly stated that the DNP is a degree, it is not a role and further that it would be inappropriate to attempt to validate an academic credential with a certification exam, which inherently tests role competencies and knowledge.

Furthermore, while all NP programs will produce graduates with DNP competencies, the specialty-specific NP competencies tested in program-specific certification exams will continue to be developed by the specialty-practice organization (APRN Joint Dialogue Report). In other words, while additional competencies will be expected of DNP graduates, the "specialty competencies" will probably remain as they are, with the exams requiring a DNP rather than an MS, assuming this evolves in the future, which is not appearing as likely as it has in the past (Auerback et al., 2014). In light of the fact that research has demonstrated that outcomes of care delivered by NPs currently holding MS degrees are at least equivalent to those of MDs (Horrocks et al., 2002; Mundinger et al., 2000), this rationale is appropriate.

The approach taken by the APRN Joint Dialogue Report group, the NCSBN, AACN, and many other nursing organizations 5 years ago seemed to indicate a clear path and commonality of purpose. Although evidently intended to serve as the collective voice of authority in speaking to the uncertainties of a profession moving forward, not all prominent leaders in nursing agreed with the content areas anticipated for future DNP certification exams.

For example, some schools of nursing, in conjunction with the Council for the Advancement of Comprehensive Care (CACC), have endorsed the notion that DNP-prepared NPs should sit for certification exams as "Diplomats in Comprehensive

Care" (Mundinger, 2008) via an exam prepared and administered by the American Board of Comprehensive Care. The CACC has made the argument that the intent of having DNPs sit for and successfully pass an exam very similar in content to the exam taken to license MDs is to "assure the public of quality and reliable standards for these new clinical nurse experts" (Mundinger, 2008, p. 4), or the DNP-prepared NP. This position has raised the ire of the American Medical Association, as well as many within nursing. If the underlying assumption for this certification exam is that without it, the "assurance of quality to the public" (Mundinger, 2008, p. 4) would be in question, the idea seems inconsistent with previous research findings (Horrocks et al., 2002; Mundinger et al., 2000), which have shown that NPs (most with MS preparation) and MDs provide equivalent care. Although still popular in some circles, the idea that DNP-prepared NPs would be designated by this additional certification has been "debunked" in a 2008 statement from the American Academy of Nurse Practitioners as unnecessary and potentially disenfranchising to the large numbers of MS-prepared NPs in the workforce (Stanik-Hutt, 2008a, 2008b). At the time of writing of this second edition text, the CACC certification endorsed in 2007 appears to have stalled. The website for the CACC (abcc.dnpcert.org/#), while active and containing information about the CACC exam option for DNP graduates from "across the life span" programs only, simply lists application status as "coming soon." Given the lack of momentum on this front since 2007, it is unlikely that CACC will be required, or even available, in the near future.

■ *THE ESSENTIALS:* STILL RELEVANT?

The AACN *Essentials* were published following tremendous effort on the part of the DNP Essentials Task Force in 2006. They have served as the foundation on which all DNP programs have been developed and by whose criteria today's programs are accredited. The AACN reaffirmed in April 2013 at the DNP Summit that the 2006 DNP *Essentials* should guide the DNP curriculum. Outcomes expectations are outlined in the *Essentials* and should serve as the basis for evaluation of DNP graduate competencies, however the extent to which these outcomes are aligned with the *Standards for Accreditation of Baccalaureate and Graduate Nursing Programs* from the Collegiate Commission on Nursing Education (CCNE, 2013) is somewhat open to interpretation. Student learning objectives should be clearly tied to expected outcomes per the *White Paper* (AACN, 2015), but specifically, whose outcomes? The space between the DNP *Essentials* (2006) and the AACN *White Paper* (2015b) and the *Standards for Accreditation of Baccalaureate and Graduate Nursing Programs* (CCNE, 2013) leaves plenty of latitude for academic freedom in both curriculum design and outcomes measures; not nearly as prescriptively defined as those from AACN (2015).

But are they still current? Are they fluid enough to be adapted in the ever-changing climates of health care and higher education? What about the decision by the AACN not to recognize ethics as an essential unto itself (it was previously Essential #3 in the last 1996 AACN's *Essentials of Master's Education for Advanced Nursing Practice*, which is also currently in revision)? If, in fact, DNP programs include ethical issues at the advanced practice level that are threaded throughout the curriculum and include topics considered nontraditional for clinicians, then this may be a solid decision on their part. Although it is imperative to include traditional ethics content for clinicians, such as ethical treatment of patients, it would also be pertinent to include ethics related to participation in research, business ethics, and the role of ethical principles such as "justice" as it relates to health care economics and reform. Topics such as these are important to include, as the DNP graduate is expected to bring a higher, broader level of understanding of the complexity of issues and leadership to the practice setting. If, however, ethics are not truly being incorporated in the light of competing priorities, perhaps the decision not to recognize ethics as a separate essential was not a wise one.

Opinions on these controversies concerning the *Essentials* may vary. What *is* evident, however, is that the content areas addressed in the *Essentials* (e.g., health policy, leadership, quality, advocacy) are still very much relevant. Indeed, they dominate the national news media and inspire national debate. Rather than asking are the *Essentials* fluid enough, perhaps what nursing needs to ask is: "As a discipline, are we creative enough to envision what the *Essentials do not* say?" Myopia is a dangerous condition, regardless of its context.

■ SUMMARY

The move to require a DNP for entry into NP practice by 2015 has raised many controversies; yet, while some strides have been made, the goal remains largely unmet as of 2015. Among the continuing controversies are: whether the DNP is a degree or a role, how DNP-prepared NPs are currently practicing, whether DNP practice really is different from MS-prepared NP practice, what effect DNP education will have on certification, and whether programs conferring a DNP degree truly are at the doctoral level of scholarship. In this chapter, we have explored these issues to date. As with the rest of the nursing profession, we continue to await the arrival of large numbers of DNP–NPs (and other DNP–APRNs) for the future. What will be their contribution to health care, to patient outcomes, to faculty roles and to nursing? Additionally, as time passes and demographics of faculty compositions change to an obvious tipping point, where DNP-prepared educators serve as the primary educators and directors of DNP education, we likely can and should anticipate future paradigm shifts in relation to the content, design, and level of scholarship expectations for DNP students. Although this remains to be seen to a large extent, the potential impact of the DNP–practitioner role appears very promising indeed.

■ CRITICAL THINKING QUESTIONS

1. *What strengths do preparation as a DNP bring to the advanced practice practitioner role? In what ways do you think NP practice will change once the majority of NPs are prepared at the DNP level?*
2. *What is the role of teachers of various educational backgrounds in the education of the DNP practitioner? Should the majority of DNP educators be practicing clinicians? Explain.*
3. *Do you anticipate that outcomes should be different from MS-prepared practitioners? What outcomes can be expected from DNP-prepared practitioners?*
4. *Do you think that attaining competency as an NP is necessary before becoming a change agent? How will DNP student practitioners gain the skills to become change agents in clinical practice if they cannot practice as NPs until they complete their DNP education?*
5. *Should DNP students be encouraged to develop original scholarly work through the scholarship of application? Would this approach better prepare NPs with the skills to demonstrate enhanced patient outcomes resulting from their care? In what way?*

6. *Should NPs and MDs take the same certification exams? What are the advantages and drawbacks of this approach to determining competencies?*

7. *Are the AACN's* Essentials *relevant and futuristic enough to provide guidance in the development of the practitioner going forward? Should an essentials document be futuristic?*

8. *Should ethics be added as an essential? Discuss ways to incorporate ethics appropriately throughout the curriculum.*

9. *Should PhD and DNP students be educated together? Are there areas where each should be educated separately? What areas should be shared?*

10. *What level of rigor should exist in a DNP program? Should it be similar to the PhD program?*

■ REFERENCES

American Academy of Nurse Practitioners, American College of Nurse Practitioners, Association of Faculties of Pediatric Nurse Practitioners, National Association of Nurse Practitioners in Women's Health, National Association of Pediatric Nurse Practitioners, National Conference of Gerontological Nurse Practitioners, National Organization of Nurse Practitioner Faculties. (2008). Nurse practitioner DNP education and certification, and titling: A unified Statement. Retrieved from http://c.ymcdn .com/sites/www.nonpf.org/resource/resmgr/imported/DNPUnifiedStatement0608.pdf

American Association of Colleges of Nursing. (1996). *The essentials of master's education for advanced practice nursing.* Washington, DC: Author.

American Association of Colleges of Nursing. (2004). *AACN position statement on the practice doctorate in nursing.* Washington, DC: Author.

American Association of Colleges of Nursing. (2006). *The essentials of doctoral education for advanced nursing practice.* Washington, DC: Author.

American Association of Colleges of Nursing. (2009). DNP frequently asked questions. Retrieved from http://www.aacn.nche.edu/dnp/about/frequently-asked-questions

American Association of Colleges of Nursing. (2015). DNP fact sheet. Retrieved from http://www .aacn.nche.edu/media-relations/fact-sheets/dnp

American Association of Colleges of Nursing. (2015a). AACN releases findings of the national study of the practice doctorate. Retrieved from http://www.aacn.nche.edu/news/articles/2014/ dnp-study

American Association of Colleges of Nursing. (2015b). *New white paper on the DNP: Current issues and clarifying recommendations.* Report of the Task Force on the Implementation of the DNP. Retrieved from http://www.aacn.nche.edu/news/articles/2015/dnp-white-paper

American Association of Nurse Anesthetists. (2007). AANA announces support of doctorate for entry into nurse anesthesia practice by 2025. Retrieved from http://www.aana.com/newsandjournal/ News/Pages/092007-AANA-Announces-Support-of-Doctorate-for-Entry-into-Nurse-Anesthesia -Practice-by-2025.aspx

American College of Nurse-Midwives. (2012). Position statement: Midwifery education and the doctor of nursing practice (DNP). Retrieved from http://www.midwife.org/ACNM/files/ ACNMLibraryData/UPLOADFILENAME/000000000079/Midwifery%20Ed%20and%20 DNP%20Position%20Statement%20June%202012.pdf

American Nurses' Association. (1965). *A position paper.* New York, NY: Author.

APRN Joint Dialogue Group Report. (2008). *Consensus model for APRN regulation: Licensure, accreditation, certification & education.* Consensus Work Group & the National Council of State Boards of Nursing APRN Advisory Committee.

Auerback, D., Martsolf, G., Pearson, M. L., Tayloer, E. A., Zaydman, M., Muchow, A.,...Dower, C. (2014). *The DNP by 2015: A study of the institutional, political, and professional issues that facilitate or impede establishing a post-baccalaureate doctor of nursing practice program.* Washington, DC: RAND.

Balas, E. A., & Boren, S. A. (2000). *Managing clinical knowledge for health care improvement* (pp. 65–70). Stuttgart, Germany: Schattauer Verlagsgesellschaft.

Bellini, S., & Cusson, R. M. (2012). The DNP for entry into advanced practice: The controversy continues as 2015 looms. *Newborn and Infant Nursing Reviews, 12*(1), 12–16.

Bellini, S., McCauley, P., & Cusson, R. M. (2012). The DNP graduate as faculty member. *Nursing Clinics of North America, 47*(4), 547–556.

Bellini, S. (2013). State of the state: NNP program update 2013. *Advances in Neonatal Care, 13*(5), 346–348.

Benner, P., Sutphen, S., Leonard, V., & Day, L. (2010). *Educating nurses: A call for radical transformation.* San Francisco, CA: Jossey-Bass.

Boyer, E. L. (1990). *Scholarship reconsidered: Priorities of the professoriate.* Princeton, NJ: Carnegie Foundation for the Advancement of Teaching.

Budden, J. S., Zhong, E. H., Moulton, P., & Cimiotti, J. P. (2013). Highlights of the National Workforce Survey of Registered Nurses. *Journal of Nursing Regulation, 4*(2), 5–14. Retrieved from https://www.ncsbn.org/JNR0713_05-14.pdf

Collegiate Commission on Nursing Education. (2013). Standards for accreditation of baccalaureate and graduate nursing programs. Retrieved from http://www.aacn.nche.edu/ccne-accreditation/Standards-Amended-2013.pdf

Danzey, I., Ea, E., Fitzpatrick, J., Garbutt, S., Rafferty, M., & Zychowicz, M. (2011). The doctor of nursing practice and education: Highlights, potential and promise. *Journal of Professional Nursing, 27,* 311–314.

Dreher, H. M., & Montgomery, K. (2009). Let's call it "doctoral" advanced practice nursing. *The Journal of Continuing Education in Nursing, 40*(12), 530–531.

Health Services and Resources Administration. (2013). The U.S. nursing workforce: Trends in supply and education. Retrieved from http://bhpr.hrsa.gov/healthworkforce/reports/nursingworkforce/nursingworkforcefullreport.pdf

Heater, B., Becker, A., & Olson, R. (1988). Nursing interventions and patients outcomes: A meta-analysis of studies. *Nursing Research, 37,* 303–307.

Horrocks, S., Anderson, E., & Salisbury, C. (2002). Systematic review of whether nurse practitioners working in primary care can provide equivalent care to doctors. *British Medical Journal, 324,* 819–823.

Howie-Esquivel, J., & Fontaine, D. (2006). The evolving role of the acute care nurse practitioner in critical care. *Current Opinion in Critical Care, 12,* 609–613.

Institute of Medicine. (1999). *To err is human: Building a safer health system.* Washington, DC: National Academies Press.

Institute of Medicine. (2001). *Crossing the quality chasm: A new health system for the 21st century.* Washington, DC: National Academies Press.

Institute of Medicine. (2003). *Health professions education: A bridge to quality.* Washington, DC: National Academies Press.

Loomis, J., Willard, B., & Cohen, J. (2007). Difficult professional choices: Deciding between the PhD and the DNP in nursing. *The Online Journal of Issues in Nursing, 12*(1), 6.

Melnyk, B. (2015). Important information about clinical practice guidelines: Key tools for improving quality of care and patient outcomes. *Worldviews on Evidence-based Nursing, 12*(1), 1–2.

Mundinger, M. (2008). Certification is the answer: What is the question? *Clinical Scholars Review, 1*(1), 3–4.

Mundinger, M., Kane, R., Lenz, E., Totten, A., Tsai, W.-Y, Cleary, P., . . . Shelanski, M. L. (2000). Primary care outcomes in patients treated by nurse practitioners or physicians: A randomized controlled trial. *Journal of the American Medical Association, 283*(1), 59–68.

National Association of Clinical Nurse Specialists. (2015). National Association of Clinical Nurse Specialists endorses requiring doctor of nursing practice degree for clinical nurse specialists. Retrieved from http://www.nacns.org/docs/PR-DNP-Statement1507.pdf

National Organization of Nurse Practitioner Faculties. (2006). *Practice doctorate nurse practitioner entry-level competencies.* Washington, DC: Author.

National Organization of Nurse Practitioner Faculties. (2015). The doctor of nursing practice NP preparation: NONPF perspective. Retrieved from http://c.ymcdn.com/sites/www.nonpf.org/resource/resmgr/DNP/NONPFDNPStatementSept2015.pdf

National Research Council of the National Academies. (2005). *Advancing the nation's health needs: NIH research training programs.* Washington, DC: National Academies Press.

Nurse Practitioner Roundtable. (2008, June). *Nurse practitioner DNP education, certification and titling: A unified statement.* Washington, DC: Author.

Obama, B. (2015). Building American skills through community colleges. Retrieved from https://www.whitehouse.gov/issues/education/higher-education/building-american-skills-through-community-colleges

Paul, F. (2015). The doctor of nursing practice-prepared clinical expert. *Clinical Scholars Review, 8*(1), 80–83.

Pho, K. (2008, March 13). Shortage of primary care threatens health system. *USA Today*, A.11.

Sheriff, S., & Chaney, S. (2007). Should DNP programs follow the same rigorous coursework as PhD programs? *The Journal for Nurse Practitioners*, 3(10), 704–705.

Stanik-Hutt, J. (2008a). Who will provide primary health care? Nurse practitioners. *USA Today Forum*. Retrieved from http://www.acnpweb.org/files/public/USA_Today_Primary_Care_03 -27-08.pdf

Stanik-Hutt, J. (2008b). Debunking the need to certify the DNP degree. *The Journal for Nurse Practitioners*, 4(10), 739.

New England Nursing News. (2010). The DNP: An emerging trend: Doctor of nursing practice graduates and students share why they chose to pursue a DNP and how it has influenced their careers. Retrieved from http://news.nurse.com/article/20100111/NE01/101110008

Udlis, K., & Mancuso, J. (2012a). Doctor of nursing practice programs across the United States: A benchmark of information. Part 1: Program characteristics. *The Journal of Professional Nursing, 28*, 265–273.

Udlis, K., & Mancuso, J. (2012b). Doctor of nursing practice programs across the United States: A benchmark of information. Part ll: Admission criteria. *The Journal of Professional Nursing, 28*, 274–283.

Udlis, K., & Mancuso, J. (2015). Receptions of the role of the doctor of nursing practice-prepared nurse: Clarity or confusion? *The Journal of Professional Nursing, 31*, 274–283

Reflective Response

Lucy N. Marion

In Chapter 5, "The Role of the Practitioner," the authors presented an interesting and lively continuing debate about Doctorate of Nursing Practice (DNP) educational issues. These issues include the DNP role versus the degree, the future of the master of science (MS) versus DNP practice degrees and respective levels of practice, the level scholarship for DNP practice project versus the DNP dissertation, and traditional certification within the DNP and certification at the end of the program. The authors also addressed the scope of practice changes and qualifications to teach in nursing education programs.

After reading Chapter 5 in this edition, I felt that the data and references painted a truly positive picture for the DNP future. The authors captured the important DNP-related papers and surveys conducted by the major professional organizations and challenged relevance of documents such as the American Association of Colleges of Nursing (AACN) *Essentials*. In this comprehensive and useful chapter, the authors provide much of the history and current status of the DNP and its issues. However, the interpretation was less optimistic, perhaps somewhat impatient, about the progress of the new nursing degree that started in earnest in about 2001—only 15 years ago.

Chapter 5 validated our early vision for anticipated struggles and trust in future leadership to tackle issues as they arose. Three decade-old publications described the hopes for the new DNP and the issues we faced or expected to face (Marion et al., 2003; Marion, O'Sullivan, Crabtree, Price, & Fontana, 2005; O'Sullivan, Carter, Marion, Pohl, & Werner, 2005). National Organization of Nurse Practitioner Faculties (NONPF) Board members wrote these articles during very exciting times when NONPF, along with other organizations, took much of the early leadership in defining DNP/NP parameters (NONPF, 2004). Later, the NONPF DNP Task Force led national forums, webinars, and conferences, and appointed more task forces to prepare first DNP/NP competencies. I was honored to represent NONPF on the first AACN DNP Task Force, with Dr. Elizabeth Lenz as chair, and on the Council for the Advancement of Comprehensive Care (CACC), with Dr. Mary Mundinger as chair (AACN, 2004). In 2005, I shepherded the development of the first DNP program in Georgia at the Medical College of Georgia (now Augusta University) and over time served as consultant to several DNP planning committees across the nation. Augusta University now offers only BSN to DNP for all NP concentrations and plans to transition the Nursing Anesthesia

Program to DNP within 2 years. With others achieving similar goals, each forward step has required careful attention to the challenges presented in Chapter 5.

Although the authors described AACN as being largely responsible for the DNP movement, a much larger group of organizational and individual participants were active in mainstreaming the DNP rather than to be a "fringe" degree. Societal forces such as complexity of health care, changing demographics, increase in doctoral degrees among other health professionals, and the rapidly emerging need for nurse practitioners (NPs) to provide much of the nation's primary care, set the stage for change in advance practice nursing education. These forces caused the stampede to create DNP programs, growing in number from four clinical nursing doctorates (NDs) in 2000 to 20 in 2006, to 120 in 2010, and to 264 in 2015 (AACN, 2015). In spite of the cries of folly (Dracup, Cronenwett, Melies, & Benner, 2005) concerning the new DNP, many issues have been resolved: the accreditation process is complete, the number of PhD students has increased instead of a dreaded decrease, and DNP graduates do get meaningful jobs and advance within their employing institutions. With almost half of APRN educational programs offering DNP degrees, we probably have reached the tipping point. Now DNP faculty are educating their stakeholders on how maximize DNP contributions to the triple aim of accessibility, affordability, and quality health care.

Of the several important and well-documented DNP issues addressed, I will target educational rigor, differences in practice capability with MS and DNP programs, the potential of DNPs as educators, and the closing of MS APRN programs. Not surprisingly, lack of standardization (Marion, 2015) or setting the appropriate methods and rigor for applying evidence to practice and practice change, standardization, continues to be a major challenge for DNP education today. Curricula for medicine, dentistry, pharmacy, and other professions include applied research methodologies as a foundation for evidence-based health care, and many require a scholarly project. Some disciplines have the option of a dual practice/research (PhD) degree with a dissertation. Nursing, on the other hand, has had challenges in envisioning the role of the DNP graduate in applied scholarship. Early efforts in creating a Doctorate of Nursing Science and other such non-PhD nursing degrees resulted in PhD look-alikes (AACN, 2009). The ND did not flourish. Could this reticence to embrace a nursing practice doctorate reflect perceptions of low prestige and usefulness of such scholarship? Do/will our DNP programs prepare the learner to conduct selected types of research? And to generate funding to support those activities? Time will tell, but DNP students and graduates can further develop their expertise in research through joint and dual degrees, postdoctoral research fellowships, and research team membership. In my view, the DNP is the degree for improving practice and patient outcomes through evidence-based practice change. Also, the DNP-prepared scholar serves best as clinical expert on research design teams, research interventionist, and intervention delivery specialist. A DNP dissertation with PhD-level research methodological rigor can detract from the primary purpose of the practice doctorate.

The authors addressed the question: Is DNP practice better than/different from MS practice? In the early years of the previous decade, open forums with advanced practice nurses and faculty discussed the viability and usefulness of the DNP, and the participant themes provided guidance for next steps (Fontaine, Stotts, Saxe, & Scott, 2008). We heard the need for synthesis of content, more evidence-based practice, and more chronic disease management, genomics, ethics, informatics, cutting-edge pharmacology, systems leadership, and so on. Strong themes were later incorporated in the AACN's *Essentials* (2006) and NONPF competencies (2016). The ensuing DNP education provides vision, structure, and additional credits to meet the new demands of a highly complex system undergoing radical design change. The few available studies indicate that DNP practice is different from the MS, as would be expected—albeit mostly in the systems arena, which can be measured by standard health services research methods. Specifying comparative effectiveness in direct patient care and determining the questions and analyses to answer the effectiveness questions will require a complex design and methods. The answers are likely to emerge from qualitative inquiry, big data gleaned from CMS and other insurance data, more comprehensive surveys, and perhaps from APRN relicensure data.

The DNP-prepared faculty workforce has had a major impact on nursing education in most parts of the country. According to the RAND study (Auerbach et al., 2015), approximately half of DNP graduates are in educational settings. Doctorally prepared nurses are relatively rare (AACN, 2006), and those with practice doctorates are welcome in most educational settings. Whether the DNP graduate is qualified to teach is just one aspect of the question: Can or should any nursing faculty member, including PhD graduates, be expected to teach without gaining minimal competencies to teach? The authors describe how DNP programs could add education courses to the curriculum, and some programs have done so with tracks, graduate certificates, and graduate degrees in education. More often the clinician is employed without preparation in pedagogy and curriculum, and the nursing program then is held accountable for extensive faculty orientation and development to ensure quality teaching. This costly problem is exacerbated when clinical faculty members decide to return to the clinical setting (due to lower income and lack of preference after all) following extensive faculty development efforts. Most doctorally prepared faculty members do not have a solid foundation in education and indeed the profession should address this need.

The question of *who* is qualified to teach DNP students is interesting. Overall, many nursing programs generally accept that credentialed professionals with requisite skills and teaching ability can teach selected components of the curriculum to any level of nursing students. The issue of PhD APRN faculty as qualified to teach clinical content to DNP students has not yet been addressed, but the question is being asked. Interprofessional teaching and learning are targets for many health science centers if not already in practice. For example, a physician's assistant who performs a screening test or treatment proficiently several times each day should be considered qualified to teach that skill to an NP student. Similarly, a DNP/NP faculty member should be able to teach health assessment to medical students. The DNP faculty member is not usually expected to teach all components of the entire DNP curriculum, and the wide range of topics necessitates different types of faculty. Of course, nursing programs must stay within the limits of accreditation standards, most of which are not yet evidence based, but are the product of collective wisdom of educators and will likely change as we gather more data on competency process and outcomes.

Finally, the authors discussed the closing of MS APRN programs by the AACN sanctioned year of 2015. This aspiration was not reached for several reasons including the growing demand for primary care APRNs from health care reform and increasing demand for complex care outside of acute care settings; different APRN groups' time frames for closure; and program leaders' inability to accommodate this time frame. State regulatory boards and accreditation and certification bodies are not obligated to follow the AACN membership vote or NONPF guidance. With budget challenges for many nursing programs and parent institutions, administrators are fearful that closing traditional MS APRN programs will reduce tuition generation. However, programs with the DNP as entry to APRN practice will be able guide others in the transition. Some creative partnership models have already emerged and more will follow (AACN, 2006). One negative consequence of program conversion from MS to DNP has been the shortage of fully qualified, doctorally prepared faculty to teach at the DNP level. A potentially positive consequence could be that large, efficient interprofessional coalitions are created to teach more students with better-prepared faculty. The authors rightfully point to uncertainty found in recent AACN and NONPF documents about a date for APRN programs to be at the doctoral level. In my view, that date should be set with transitional supports as needed.

The authors of Chapter 5 have courageously undertaken topics that are still controversial and have provided reasonable questions or solutions. My comments are a reflection of my perspectives and are intended to complement the work to date.

■ REFERENCES

American Association of Colleges of Nursing. (2004). AACN position statement on the practice doctorate in nursing. Retrieved from http://www.aacn.nche.edu/dnp/pdf/dnp.pdf

American Association of Colleges of Nursing. (2006). *The essentials of doctoral education for advanced nursing practice*. Retrieved from http://www.aacn.nche.edu/dnp/pdf/essentials.pdf

American Association of Colleges of Nursing. (2009). *Annual report: Advancing higher education in nursing*. Washington, DC: Author. Retrieved from http://www.aacn.nche.edu/media/pdf/AnnualReport09.pdf

American Association of Colleges of Nursing. (2010). Fact sheet: The doctor of nursing practice (DNP). Retrieved from http://www.aacn.nche.edu/Media/FactSheets/dnp.htm

American Association of Colleges of Nursing (2015). DNP fact sheet. Retrieved from http://www.aacn.nche.edu/media-relations/fact-sheets/dnp

Auerback, D., Martsolf, G., Pearson, M. L., Tayloer, E. A., Zaydman, M., Muchow, A., . . . Dower, C. (2015). *The DNP by 2015: A study of the institutional, political, and professional issues that facilitate or impede establishing a post-baccalaureate doctor of nursing practice program*. Santa Monica, CA: RAND.

Dracup, K., Cronenwett, L., Meleis, A., & Benner, P. (2005). Reflections on the doctorate of nursing practice. *Nursing Outlook, 53*(4), 177–182.

Fontaine, D., Stotts, N., Saxe, J., & Scott, M. (2008). Shared faculty governance: A decision-making framework for evaluating the DNP. *Nursing Outlook, 56*, 167–173.

Marion, L. (2015). Raising the bar: Ready or not? In *Special topics conference: Pushing the envelope in NP education*. Washington, DC: National Organization of Nurse Practitioner Faculties.

Marion, L., O'Sullivan, A., Crabtree, K., Price, M., & Fontana, S. (2005). Curriculum models for the practice doctorate in nursing. *Topics in Advanced Practice Nursing Journal, 5*(1). Retrieved from http://www.medscape.com/viewarticle/500742

Marion, L, Viens, D., O'Sullivan, A. L., Crabtree, K., Fontana, S., & Price, M. M. (2003). The practice doctorate in nursing: Future or fringe? *Topics in Advanced Practice Nursing eJournal, 3*(2). Retrieved from http://www.medscape.com/viewarticle/453247

National Organization of Nurse Practitioner Faculties. (2004). Updated statement from the NONPF board of directors on the practice doctorate. Retrieved from http://www.nonpf.com/displaycommon.cfm?an=1&subarticlenbr=16

National Organization of Nurse Practitioner Faculties. (2016). NP competencies. Retrieved from http://www.nonpf.org/?page=14

O'Sullivan, A., Carter, M., Marion, L., Pohl, J., & Werner, K. (2005). Moving forward together: The practice doctorate in nursing. *The Online Journal of Issues in Nursing, 10*(3), Manuscript 4. Retrieved from http://search.proquest.com/docview/229520175?pq-origsite=gscholar

CHAPTER SIX

The Role of the Clinical Executive

Barbara Wadsworth, Tukea L. Talbert, and Robin Donohoe Dennison

■ SUPPLY, DEMAND, AND PREPARATION OF A CLINICAL EXECUTIVE—WHY IS IT IMPORTANT?

Over the past decade, there has been emerging evidence of the connection between organizational performance and leadership (Frearson, 2002; Hallinger & Heck, 1996; Muijs, Harris, Lumby, Morrison, & Sood, 2006). The Institute of Medicine (IOM) Committee on the Quality of Health Care in America has issued a mandate to the American health care community to bring "state-of-the-art" health care to all Americans (Fasoli, 2010, p. 25). Fasoli indicates that nursing has reached a point of inflection, a tipping point, and the nursing role must evolve in order to remain fully engaged in health care. Of even greater importance, the nurse leader must be prepared to change and create health care policies, create and implement evidence-based practice guidelines, and embrace and represent quality nursing practice at every level of the organization and of society. Now is the time to ensure that the right people are in key leadership positions, and that those individuals are well prepared to face the dynamic environment and challenges of the health care milieu. Organizational performance during this turbulent time in health care will be contingent on the effectiveness of the leadership team.

The American Association of Colleges of Nursing (AACN) in its position statement (2004) puts forth that the transformation in the health care delivery system will require clinicians to design, evaluate, and constantly improve the context in which care is delivered. The AACN strongly believes that nurses with doctoral preparation that encompasses clinical, organizational, economic, and leadership skills are most likely capable of critiquing scientific findings and subsequently developing programs of care that significantly impact health care and that are economically feasible. The AACN adopted the Doctor of Nursing Practice (DNP) position statement in October 2004 calling for a transformational change in the education necessary for professional nurses who will practice at an advanced level of nursing practice, *The Essentials of Doctoral Education for Advanced Nursing Practice* (AACN, 2006). The AACN recognizes the practice demands affiliated with an increasingly complex health care system amid a major health care reform that has gotten new momentum from the President Obama administration. One can conclude that these demands comprise a new strain with a different genotype that is placing new pressure on the preparation of those nurses in senior leadership positions and on their level of preparation.

In this chapter, the following areas are discussed: an operational definition of the clinical executive; the AACN's *Essentials of Doctoral Education for Advanced Nursing Practice*; a comparison of the AACN's *Essentials for Master's Education for Advanced Practice Nursing* with *The Essentials of Doctoral Education for Advanced Nursing Practice*; a comparison of the DNP degree with the master of science in nursing (MSN) and master of science in nursing and master of business administration (MBA); and the position of the American Organization of Nurse Executives (AONE) regarding the DNP degree requirement for nurse executives. The objectives of this chapter are to give readers the opportunity to have a more in-depth view of the demand for a different level and type of education beyond the master's degree for clinical executive leadership; the results of a DNP education; and the potential challenges of making the DNP a requirement for nurse executives.

■ DEFINITION OF A CLINICAL EXECUTIVE

Webster (2000) defines an executive as, "capable of, or concerned with, carrying out duties, functions... or managing affairs in a business or organization; empowered and required to administer" (p. 497). One cannot fully respect the role of the clinical executive without acknowledging the context in which it occurs. The clinical executive must oversee all aspects of clinical practice in health care organizations. The nursing practice within any organization is a "24/7" accountability for processes, structures, and outcomes of care delivery (Fasoli, 2010). The responsibility of the clinical executive is ever changing and growing, and the expectations on those in the role are greater. For the purposes of this chapter, the authors agree that senior-level nursing leadership (chief nursing officer [CNO], chief nursing executive, and vice president [VP] of nursing) in a health care setting is a form of advanced nursing practice as evidenced by the differentiation option offered by the DNP degree, which is the eighth option beyond the seven core essentials.

■ AACN *ESSENTIALS OF DOCTORAL EDUCATION FOR ADVANCED NURSING PRACTICE*

The AACN (2006) identified seven core competencies for the DNP along with two additional differentiated competencies for nurses who choose to focus more on an advanced practice administrative role (i.e., clinical executive role) or an advanced practice–focused role (nurse anesthetist, nurse practitioner, midwife, clinical nurse specialist). The seven core essentials are: (a) scientific underpinnings for practice; (b) organizational and systems leadership for quality improvement and systems thinking; (c) clinical scholarship and analytical methods for evidence-based practice; (d) information systems/technology and patient care technology for the improvement and transformation of health care; (e) health care policy for advocacy in health care; (f) interprofessional collaboration for improving patient and population health outcomes; (g) clinical prevention and population health for improving the nation's health (8a—practice-focused) individual, family, and population-focused advanced nursing practice competencies for improving patient care processes and outcomes; and (8b—executive/administrative) systems or organization-focused advanced nursing practice competencies for improving patient care processes and outcomes.

The authors of this chapter strongly believe that the DNP degree offers an expansive educational experience very different from that of the administrative tract of the master's of science degree. This belief hinges on some of the following benefits from the DNP degree that includes extensive literature on leadership theory that encompasses the process of leadership and more specifically leadership in health care; mentoring opportunities with other leaders in advanced practice roles as part of residency/practicum; the differentiated option to focus more on students' desired specialization in the program; and the capstone project, which is a work in progress throughout the program. The capstone project serves as the student's population focus. Throughout the program, the chosen population focus will undergo several analyses that include cost-benefit analyses/return on investment, statistical analyses, utilization-focused evaluations, and extensive literature reviews, especially if students have interventional studies as part of their capstone projects.

■ THE DNP CLINICAL EXECUTIVE PRACTICA: A CRITICAL ELEMENT

Although all aspects of the DNP educational experience are important, additional focus will be spent on the practicum experience and the capstone project. The practicum experiences for each student are designed around the student's choice for specialization (administrative/executive or practice focused). The second author's (TT) practicum took place at Dartmouth Hitchcock Medical Center in Lebanon, New Hampshire, with the VP of nursing. During the experience, the VP of nursing along with other members of the senior leadership team undertook a restructuring of the organizational chart. The change, as you can imagine, was enormous. It not only was going to impact the hospital, but also had implications for change for other hospitals that were part of an alliance with Dartmouth. The VP of nursing was able to articulate the communication plan at every level of the facility and to those hospitals outside the physical boundaries of Dartmouth. The ability to participate in this monumental event at that hospital was vastly different from any of the clinical experiences in the MSN program experienced by this author 10 years before the DNP program.

During the practicum at Dartmouth, as a doctoral student, the second author functioned as a consultant and generated questions that might be posed by stakeholders and various team members within and outside the organization. During the residency, students are expected to exhibit critical thinking and participate in scholarly discussions. The key objective during the residency hours (practicum) is that the students drive the learning experience by being active participants who are not simply in an organization solely to shadow their mentors. Each course has course objectives that provide guidelines for students' practicum experiences; however, the students also create unique objectives for each practicum experience, which results in ownership of the process and outcome of the residency. Although there were other practicum experiences (see Figure 6.1), the Dartmouth experience demonstrated the practice of an effective leader dealing with a very toxic change in a major health care organization. The overall focus of this practicum therefore was on the process of leadership and leadership style, and its effect on organizational culture.

A second practicum occurred at the University of Texas MD Anderson Cancer Center in Houston, Texas, one of the top oncology health care facilities in the nation. The focus of this residency revolved around my (TT) capstone project, which actually was a quasi-experimental pre- and post-test design study that investigated psychological distress among patients undergoing hematopoietic stem cell transplants. During this time,

Site	Experience	Purpose/Focus
Dartmouth-Hitchcock Medical Center: Lebanon, NH	Worked with the VP of Nursing for a week to observe, listen, learn, and participate on a project to alter the organizational structure at facility. This experience was beneficial because it focused on the importance of communication, identification of all the stakeholders to make change and the importance of changes in the organizational infrastructure and its subsequent impact on the decision making, span of control, and the re-alignment of staff, lines of authority, and potentially to changes in the organizational culture.	• Met requirements for leadership course early in program that focused on effective use of self to impact change; the process of leadership, constituency, and organizational development • The final product included a paper titled "Leadership: The Pathway to Excellence" • This paper addressed stakeholder involvement with change and leadership effectiveness and the ability of the individual to lead during tumultuous times in health care.
MD Anderson Cancer Center: Houston, TX	Worked with a combination of nurse leaders at the cancer center for a 1- to 2-week experience to identify practices incorporated to protect immuno-suppressed hematopoietic stem cell transplantation patients from environmental bacteria/germs.	A portion of student's course research was to identify the effectiveness of traditional versus nontraditional interventions to prevent infection among stem cell patients post transplantation. MD Anderson is a premier cancer center that conducts more than 500 stem cell transplants annually so it provided a good sample size for evaluation.

FIGURE 6.1 Student's practica experiences.

this second author was able to examine protocols and isolation practices used by experts in hematopoietic stem cell transplants. This practicum provided insight on current versus traditional practices for isolation and outcomes associated with various isolation interventions. The overall focus of this practicum was to evaluate the impact of leadership on the development of practice policies, standards, processes, and patient outcomes.

Throughout the DNP program, each student works with a patient population for which she must identify an evidence-based health care intervention to implement. Other critical components associated with the intervention and/or practice change includes cost-effective analyses, program evaluation, literature review in search of best practices, and identification of stakeholders that may influence the practice change and/or be affected by the change.

Another key focus of the DNP program is program evaluation. Several options for evaluation are introduced to students, which include utilization-focused evaluation, and formative and summative evaluations. In comparison to the master's of science in nursing

(MSN) administrative track, the detail with evaluation, research, evidence-based interventions, cost-effectiveness analysis, and policy development associated with health care initiatives, interventions, and outcomes was significantly different. Each of the authors believes that with the completion of the DNP program, we acquired a new level of thinking about program development and evaluation; identification and placement of best practices into practice settings; advanced practice in health care; interpretation of patterns from large data sets; and, most importantly, leadership in health care. Overall, the DNP practicum (residency) experiences greatly enhance the learning experience of students and it enables them to view advanced practice from a macroscopic perspective, which is vastly different from the more microscopic approach experienced in the MSN administrative track.

■ COMPARISON OF *THE ESSENTIALS OF MASTER'S EDUCATION FOR ADVANCED PRACTICE NURSING* AND *THE ESSENTIALS OF DOCTORAL EDUCATION FOR ADVANCED NURSING PRACTICE*

This section highlights some of the key areas of difference between the 1996 *Essentials of Master's Education for Advanced Practice Nursing* document (which is currently under revision) from the AACN and the 2006 *Essentials of Doctoral Education for Advanced Nursing Practice* (see Figure 6.2). Figure 6.2 demonstrates some of the key differences noted between the traditional MSN educational preparation and DNP competences as defined by AACN. There are four critical differences noted:

1. The DNP competencies are more system wide and provide a macroscopic view of health care that combines all the sciences and better prepares graduates to engage in partnerships that will impact change in health care at a higher level. The student's focus reaches beyond the traditional patient setting within the organization.
2. DNP competencies are geared toward creating graduates who lead to change as opposed to assisting with change, which seems to be more the case with the MSN competencies. This competency is evident through the residency hours and the capstone projects. Students through their residency hours and capstones potentially generate new knowledge, and, in most cases, focus on adapting best practices to the clinical setting.
3. The DNP graduate demonstrates the nursing role to the community at large (even nationally) through both performance and communication, while the MSN graduate competencies focus more on communication of the nursing role on a narrower scope.
4. The DNP competencies are more population based and prepare a graduate to make change globally, while the MSN competencies are more population and community specific, thus limiting one's impact on health care to a smaller scale.

Figure 6.2 illustrates a juxtaposed comparison of each set of competencies, pointing out key differences, which are shown in boldface. Although there is a small amount of overlap with a few of the competencies, the differences stated earlier clearly indicate the variation in the level of preparation among graduates from the two programs.

The CNO's influence will likely extend to areas outside of nursing. The CNO must engage in collaborative professional relationships with many internal and external stakeholders. Many authors conclude that success at the executive level hinges on being visionary and making decisions on a macroscopic level. Hader (2010a), senior VP and CNO of Meridian Health System in New Jersey, states that the CNO's strategic plan must reach beyond the traditional scope of nursing practice. He

Master's Essentials	Doctorate of Nursing Practice Essentials	Key Differences
1. Research prepares the graduate to: access relevant data needed to address questions, analyze outcomes and initiate change, understand statistics and research methods, write and communicate effectively	**1. Scientific underpinning for practice** prepares the graduate to: integrate nursing science from all sciences/disciplines, use science to determine significance of health/health care delivery system, and evaluate outcomes **3. Clinical scholarship/analytical methods for EBP** prepares the graduate to: use analytical methods to critically evaluate existing literature and other evidence relevant to practice, use technology research methods to identify gaps in research, and to disseminate research findings to improve practice of other providers	• Macroscopic base with DNP essentials expanded to include all sciences to impact care at the highest level of nursing care • Population-based problem solving to impact health and health care system overall • DNP prepares students to evaluate large, complex data sets and recognize/interpret patterns • DNP prepares students to identify best practices and incorporate these practices into the clinical setting (translational research focus) • DNP graduate will disseminate findings of research to improve both practice and care delivery system
2. Health care policy prepares graduates to: analyze policy results, articulate concerns to appropriate political officials regarding health care consumer advocacy; interpret to consumers	**5. Health care policy for advocacy in health care prepares the graduate to:** demonstrate leadership with the development of health care polices, critically analyze policies with consideration of consumers, providers, and other disciplines, and lead implementation of policy	• MSN graduate will analyze policy results while the DNP graduate will develop health care policy and analyze results • Stronger focus on DNP essentials for systems-wide thinking and approach • MSN essentials focus on population specific focus approach as opposed to population based (large complex data set) with DNP • The DNP graduate is leading the change in most regards while the MSN graduate assists with leading the change (may initiate/catalyze, but not lead the change for policy development)

FIGURE 6.2   Comparison of essentials of master's education and doctorate of nursing practice. *(continued)*

Master's Essentials	Doctorate of Nursing Practice Essentials	Key Differences
3. Ethics prepares the graduate to: identify and analyze common ethical dilemmas; evaluate ethical methods of decision making; understand the role of ethic in the health care system	**No specific essential for ethics**	No specific essential for ethics
4. Professional role development prepares the graduate to communicate, advocate about the nursing profession including advanced practice role; functions as a change agent;	**6. Interprofessional collaboration for improving patient and population health outcomes** prepares the graduate to: partner with other professionals to analyze complex clinical issues; assume leadership roles in interprofessional team to develop practice models, guidelines, and health policy	• DNP focuses on development of partnerships and is more actively involved in defining the role of the DNP-prepared nurse • DNP graduate better able to effectively develop the partnerships based on system-wide approach, ability to be involved in collaborative relationships with others beyond the traditional organizational boundaries • DNP graduate has a greater self-knowledge and self-mastery from extensive study of leadership theory and leadership development exposure—this creates a strong foundation for effectiveness with leadership

FIGURE 6.2 Comparison of essentials of master's education and doctorate of nursing practice. (*continued*)

Master's Essentials	Doctorate of Nursing Practice Essentials	Key Differences
5. Theoretical foundations of nursing practice prepares the graduate to: critique and evaluate a variety of theories, apply and use appropriate theories to improve health care	**2. Organizational and systems leadership for QI and systems thinking** prepares the graduate to: use advanced communication skills/processes to **lead change**, employ principles of business, finance, health law **to develop plans** for practice level and/or system-wide improvement	• Key differences again continues to be the scope of practice (macroscopic-DNP versus microscopic-MSN) • DNP graduate will exhibit the ability to incorporate leadership, organizational, and systems theories to impact change with large data sets over many organizational boundaries/nationally • MSN focuses on the application of principles while the DNP will develop organizational- wide improvements for application • The MSN continues to have a limited focus on population and/or community-focused/ specific issues while the DNP focuses on national trends to address health care issues across several boundaries and geographic areas
6. Human diversity/social issues prepares the graduate to confront subcultural influences on human behavior, including ethnic, racial, gender, and age differences; deliver multicultural competent advance nursing care	**No specific essential**	No specific essential— although these concepts are embedded in the DNP essentials

FIGURE 6.2   Comparison of essentials of master's education and doctorate of nursing practice. (*continued*)

Master's Essentials	Doctorate of Nursing Practice Essentials	Key Differences
7. Health promotion/ disease prevention: prepares students to: • use epidemiological, social, and environmental data to draw conclusions regarding health status of client populations (i.e., families, individuals, groups, and communities) • Develop and monitor comprehensive, holistic plans of care that address the health promotion and disease prevention of client populations	**7. Clinical prevention and population health for improving the nation's health** prepares student to: • analyze epidemiological, biostatistical, environmental and other appropriate data related to population health • Develop, implement, and evaluate interventions to improve health status/access patterns and/or address gaps in care within a community	• DNP clearly has a broader scope of practice • Continues to analyze health endpoints of large data sets/make changes that reach beyond traditional boundaries • MSN impact much more limited • Both the DNP and MSN essentials incorporate principles of epidemiology while the DNP does also integrate biostatistics as a means to analyze and interpret data and identify trends
No specific competency	**4. Information systems/ technology and patient care technology for the improvement and transformation of health care** prepares the graduate to: access, use, and evaluate data to alter health care system	No specific MSN competency for this essential
Was excluded from VII Core Essentials but included in III additional Advanced Practice Essentials: advanced health/physical assessment, advanced physiology/ pathophysiology, and advanced pharmacology	**8. Advanced nursing practice** prepares the graduate for direct care roles or an indirect care role	DNP essentials enhances discussion of essentials for doctoral advanced nursing practice. Student is expected to meet competencies in either advanced practice focus or aggregate/systems/ organizational focus

FIGURE 6.2 *(continued)* Comparison of essentials of master's education and doctorate of nursing practice.

DNP, Doctor of Nursing Practice; EBP, evidence-based practice; MSN, master of science in nursing; QI, quality improvement.

notes that the key stakeholders in the health care organization that include the chief medical officer (CMO), chief financial officer (CFO), chief executive officer (CEO), and board of trustee members. The inability to think and function on a macroscopic level will greatly limit the level of effectiveness of decision making and subsequently the organizational success. Nurse executives exert a great deal of power from the perspective of title and capacity to influence. Nurse executives generally have the majority of the workforce under their span of control, due to their position and the fact that nurses generally are one of the largest sectors of the health care workforce within health care organizations. This opportunity to influence many people who ultimately provide the delivery of care at the bedside is not a position to be understated. It is critical that the individuals in these roles are well prepared for the challenge and are capable of making a difference in health care outcomes.

Our view is that the DNP clinical executive tract is unique in that this degree prepares nurses to be better leaders in a very challenging, dynamic health care arena. Nurses in the role of the clinical executive are no longer invited to the table solely based on their clinical insight, but more so for their ability and capacity to lead organizations based on their leadership competencies. Many of these key competencies are outlined in the AACN's *Essentials for Doctoral Education for Advanced Nursing Practice* document and they include organizational and systems leadership, health care policy for advocacy in health care, and inter professional partnerships for improving patient and population health outcomes.

■ NURSE EXECUTIVE PREPARATION: THE DNP VERSUS OTHER DEGREE OPTIONS

In terms of reviewing options to prepare the contemporary nurse executive (aside from the DNP or DrNP at one school), the options include: an MSN degree with an administrative focus and a master's of business administration (MBA); some colleges offer a combination of the MSN/MBA as a concurrent option.

Curriculum and course descriptions were obtained and reviewed from an online search of the following institutions: Indiana Wesleyan University (MBA); University of Texas Tyler (MSN/MBA); and hard copies were obtained from the University of Kentucky (DNP) and Eastern Kentucky University (MSN).[1] Through a juxtaposed comparison, some of the following initial conclusions can be made: The MSN with an administrative focus appears to be more focused on a microperspective of leadership development, preparing a novice leader or someone with leadership aspirations; the MBA seems to offer a broader base of courses to better equip the nurse executive, because it includes management concepts, managerial economics, ethics, law, and some leadership courses as well; the MSN/MBA option seems to be the most broad in that it has a good blend of the financial competencies along with some basic entry-level leadership development courses. Overall, any of these three options would be feasible pathways to prepare novice leaders or individuals pursuing a leadership career. In comparison, the post-master's DNP degree with a clinical executive option offers a much more in-depth preparation for advanced leadership roles, such as the clinical executive who may serve as the VP of nursing, CNO, chief operating officer, and/or the chief nurse executive. With the DNP, one satisfies the requirements of a doctorate, which prepares the individual on a different graduate level (a doctorate) in comparison to the MBA and the MSN options (i.e., a master's degree). Although being a doctorally prepared nurse executive does not always confer credibility, it does confer the unique competence of the individual who holds the degree (Gerrish, McManus, & Ashworth, 2003).

When further comparing these different degree programs, the DNP degree appears to offer a more in-depth overview of leadership and focus on reaching leadership capacity through self-knowledge and self-mastery. The key benefits revolve around the well-designed, focused residency hours; the extensive overview of leadership literature from diversified author-based sources; the initiation of the capstone project at the inception of the DNP program; the liberty to take elective courses outside the College of Nursing, which included Geriatric Policy and the College of Business courses for this chapter's second author; research principles and courses required for a doctoral degree; and the exposure to theory on health policy development. In concert with the aforementioned benefits, the student is prepared to constantly ask why, always seek new knowledge through research and evidence-based practice, and to design programs and policy with the ability to evaluate these initiatives clinically and financially. DNP graduates demonstrate the importance of always asking the best next question(s). They recognize that while one may not always have the answers, it is the question that may be more important because it highlights an aspect of a complex situation that may have been missed. Students have a sharpened sense of critical thinking outside the scope of nursing, which forces the doctoral clinical executive scholar to examine how health care is truly integrated both horizontally and vertically.

The DNP degree is an option that prepares nurse executives to perform at a higher level. We are not suggesting that the other degree options reviewed are inferior, because they are not. The authors believe that they offer a very sound preparation for one interested in leadership, while the DNP offers an advanced level of preparation for someone who desires more knowledge and preparation. The DNP is not more of the same, but a newer version or model of preparation for the nurse executive who functions as the senior nurse leader in organizations with other members of the executive team. The primary difference in the DNP is best described by Hader who states, "The curriculum and expectations of academic performance in the clinical doctorate programs are far more extensive than those in a traditional graduate program" (2010b, p. 6). The focus of the DNP program is uniquely different and, in theory, does create a different type of graduate with the ability to think outside traditional boundaries and develop collaborative partnerships to move organizations forward successfully.

■ AMERICAN ORGANIZATION OF NURSE EXECUTIVES: NURSE EXECUTIVE COMPETENCIES

At this time, the AONE has not endorsed the proposal that the DNP should be a requirement for either the clinical nurse executive or practice-focused nurse in advanced nursing practice roles. In their position statement, AONE (2007) supports the DNP as a terminal degree option for practice-focused nursing. They believe, however, that master's nursing degree programs in both generalist and specialty courses of study should remain intact. The Professional Practice Policy Committee of AONE concludes that questions and concerns that have been voiced regarding patient outcomes, salary compensation, and financial impact on organizations have not been fully identified, investigated, or addressed as they relate to the DNP requirement.

Having said the aforementioned, AONE considers nurse leadership as a subspecialty within nursing practice that requires competence and proficiency unique to the executive role. They believe that there are five core competencies that are common to nurses in executive practice regardless of their educational level or title (AONE Nurse Executive Competencies, 2005). These five competencies are: (a) communication and relationship building; (b) knowledge of the health care environment; (c) leadership; (d) professionalism; and (e) business skills. These core leadership competencies align with specific core essentials of the AACN's *Essentials of Doctoral Education for Advanced Nursing Practice*, such as interprofessional collaboration, organizational and systems leadership, and clinical scholarship. AONE recognizes that their competencies are core competencies and are not exhaustive of all areas of expertise for the nurse executive. They believe that the core competencies establish the standard for executive practice and can be used as a guideline for educational preparation of nurses seeking knowledge in executive practice.

The authors agree with the position of AONE in that there needs to be more evidence to support making the DNP a requirement for those nurses functioning in clinical leadership advanced nursing practice roles. The authors, DNP graduates themselves, aver that this degree is scholarly, uniquely different from a graduate-level preparation for leadership, and is an educational process that prepares the nurse executive to think and function at an advanced level as evidenced by the positions held by these individuals and their accomplishments in these roles. Having said this, it is necessary to address some key questions before concluding that the DNP must be a requirement for any nursing leadership roles. In addition to the questions posed by AONE, other questions need to be addressed as well. First, one must determine for what level of nurse leadership should the doctorate be required. It is the belief of the authors that it would be illogical to require all nurses in leadership to be doctorally prepared. As stated by Jones (2010), this becomes a scope of practice and a level of accountability issue. It connects back to the level of preparation offered by the DNP that has been highlighted as producing graduates able to function at a macroscopic level. The nurse executive at the most senior level in the organization needs to see the big picture that often times transcends traditional organizational boundaries. Second, what impact, if any, would such a requirement have on MSN programs? This issue is also raised by AONE in their position statement. Some colleges have or are moving in the direction to eliminate MSN tracks as they create DNP degree options as part of their academic offerings. Third, what impact would the potential elimination of MSN programs have on the supply of nurses? AONE recognizes that nurses may choose other disciplines to acquire a master's degree, which may result in outward migration from the nursing profession. Overall, the reduction of the number of MSN programs or their elimination may result in some unintended consequences that may have long-term effects on the nursing profession and particularly on providing a steady pool of highly educated clinical nurse executives at a variety of levels. Does the MSN in nursing administration or health systems leadership benefit a mid-level manager/executive? We believe such preparation is highly beneficial for new directors.

■ FUTURE PERSPECTIVES

Future considerations regarding the DNP degree need to include three key components. (a) The nursing profession must find a way to ensure that the degree can withstand the test of time through evidence to support its benefits. Since the inception of the DNP degree, there is growing evidence of its impact as demonstrated by successful graduates of the program functioning as effective clinical executives. Key indicators, as highlighted by AONE, that need to be further investigated include the financial impact of increasing salary expectations of doctorally prepared executives and the corresponding financial impact on organizations, patient satisfaction with holders of this degree, and specific degree-related patient outcomes as evidenced by organizations' performance with core measures established by the Centers for Medicare and Medicaid (CMS) and Hospital Consumer Assessment of Health-care Providers and Systems (HCAHPS) scores. (b) The profession must carefully examine the scope of practice and the level of accountability of nurses who would benefit most from a DNP degree. Jones (2010) indicates that executives at the top level of nursing administration are accountable for the executive level of patient services. She further states that executives will be expected to function at a macro level with decision making and actions that impact patients and others within the organization. Mid-level managers have a narrower focus and span of control within organizations and are more likely to function at a microlevel by virtue of the organizational chart and structure of organizations. The nurse executive will work across both microsystem and macrosystem levels that include groups both internal and external to the organization. As stated earlier, one of the unique qualities of the DNP degree is its preparation of the nurse executive to think and function on a macrosystem level. (c) Investigators must continue to monitor the market and demand for DNP graduates. Many authors have noted the turbulence, variability, and increasing complexity of the health care environment (AACN Fact Sheet, 2010; Fasoli, 2010; New, 2010; Schaffner & Schaffner, 2009). All of these factors continue to add momentum to the demand for preparation beyond a graduate level. One other significant finding is that employers have quickly recognized the contributions that DNP graduates are making in the practice setting (Waxman & Maxworthy, 2010). This last point is further supported by early studies that show the DNP is perceived as a viable advanced education option and enables students to make viable contributions to the nursing profession (Loomis, Willard, & Cohen, 2006). In closing, the supply is present and the demand continues to create a need for clinical executives who are prepared beyond a master's level. Based on the aforementioned data, the DNP is necessary and should continue to be an option for nurses seeking a clinical executive specialty in advanced nursing practice.

■ A PIONEER'S PERSPECTIVE: A GRADUATE FROM THE NATION'S FIRST DNP PROGRAM

As the second author of this chapter (TT) and a member of the first DNP graduating class in the United States (at the University of Kentucky), I recall a moment in time that I shall not forget. One of the members of my doctoral capstone committee asked me what was most beneficial about the DNP program. My response at that time was that I had a better understanding of myself and my personal leadership style. Although this may sound somewhat trivial, it was and continues to be, for me, a profound realization. This realization continues to facilitate my personal leadership journey and development, because I better understand what makes me successful as a leader. It also illuminates and highlights what skill sets are necessary to improve my leadership. Through reflection and my current practice, other responses to that question would include the increased confidence and competence to create a culture of collaboration by navigating through departmental and organizational borders by using focused evaluations, evidence-based practice, and influencing others beyond the traditional boundaries of the nursing component of health care. One could also say that health care today has an entirely different look; it is something that stretches beyond the physical and sometimes human boundaries of the health care facility. Successful clinical executives must be willing and equipped to see the new paradigm and context in which health care is practiced. As a graduate of a DNP program (TT), I am able to see the difference and the shift in the health care paradigm, and understand that it requires one to think and function at a different, more advanced level.

■ SUMMARY

Nurses in the clinical executive role are no longer invited to the table solely based on their clinical insight but more so for their ability and capacity to lead organizations based on their leadership competencies. The nursing profession can lead the "way to knowing" and the capacity to lead by continuing to offer the DNP as a credible degree option for nurses seeking to expand their leadership skill set and knowledge to be better prepared to function in the increasingly turbulent health care environment.

In summary, because there are other strategies necessary to prepare nurses for clinical executive roles, the nursing profession cannot solely depend on a new degree. They must be proactive in developing a framework that ensures ongoing development of leaders in executive roles that can be incorporated in the context in which they practice. These frameworks must include organizational charts that are aligned with the corporate strategic plan and that create the propensity for nurse leaders to have the capacity to lead and be involved in decision making at every level. The frameworks must provide ongoing opportunities for professional development, mentoring opportunities, and, last but not least, succession planning. Leadership development should not be by default or a second thought, but by design. It must be part of the culture established and supported by the nurse executive in collaboration with the other executive team members. It is too soon to say that a DNP should be required for individuals in clinical executive advanced nursing practice roles. However, it is not too soon to reexamine the process in which nurse executives are prepared for their leadership roles. Because leadership development is a process, it cannot be learned in a day or by completing another degree. The DNP degree offers an innovative educational experience that superbly prepares the nurse executive, but it is only the beginning of the process of leadership development. Nurse executives must be proactive and create organizational cultures that cultivate empowerment, ongoing professional development, and succession planning so that no leader is left behind and organizations advance from good to great.

Over the past 7 years, the number of DNP programs has grown to more than 289 with 125 achieving accreditation by CCNE (AACN, 2015a). The emphasis on DNP learning, and the significance of the eight DNP essentials focus development of the student on assuring competency in navigating complex health care environments, including advocating, leading, and advancing the nursing profession. Nurse executives must possess leadership skills and educational competency that is significantly valued by others, which assures them a seat at the table with responsibility to contribute and participate. DNP education preparation although evolving, is the foundational piece needed for the future.

The interest and affinity for a DNP versus a PhD are clearly different. The distinction is directly related to the type of work and the intent of the individuals' impact once the degree is achieved. PhD nurses focus on new knowledge and research that advances science as compared with DNP nurses who are focused on research integration and changing practice through translation of evidence (Rodriguez, 2016). Nurse executives are far more focused on implementing change through leading practices that result in higher clinical quality, improved outcomes, and are patient focused than conducting actual research. A DNP provides the needed academic advancement to meet the demands of the executive role and fully prepares the nurse leader to contribute in a meaningful way.

In August 2015, the AACN provided updates to their position statement on the DNP following a RAND study (Auerbach et al., 2014) completed at their request.

The AACN reports universal agreement and support for the DNP confirming that this educational preparation prepares nurses to meet future demands of health care (Auerbach et al., 2014). The recommendations are intended to clarify several key elements of DNP education, including the curriculum, the DNP project, and the program length. A noteworthy change includes the DNP capstone requirement, clearly stating the need for clinical scholarship and the importance of the project; however, requiring standardization and clarity with scope, implementation, impact, dissemination, and faculty oversight (AACN, 2015b; Alexander, 2016). The authors assert that the DNP final project for the nurse executive should be focused on quality improvement science.

The DNP program growth and numbers of graduates speaks to the importance and relevance to nurse executives. With a growing number of DNP students, more than 4,000 students in 2 years and a growth in graduates from 2,443 in 2013 to more than 3,000 students in 2014 (AACN, 2015a), the interest, willingness to engage in lifelong learning, and commitment speaks volumes to the perceived benefits and value of the education. Swanson and Stanton (2013) report that current CNOs acknowledge value and believe that the DNP is relevant and is necessary to their practice. As we continue to focus on terminal degrees and competency, the DNP is a highly sought after degree that will assure better preparation for the leadership needed. It will be important to continue to evaluate the impact and to hear from employers about the value they see and experience in their organizations.

■ CRITICAL THINKING QUESTIONS

1. *Because leadership can be developed through learning and practice, what do you believe would be the essential content and experiences in a DNP program for a nurse either in or desiring to be in a clinical executive position?*
2. *As it is the opinion of some that DNP programs should be for advanced practice nurses only, do you believe that the clinical executive's indirect role in influencing patient outcomes falls within the role of the DNP?*
3. *Do you believe that having a doctoral degree would positively affect a clinical executive's authority and influence with physicians? With other administrators? With other nurses?*
4. *Many clinical executives have earned a PhD but are not actively engaged in research. Considering the differences in coursework and focus between PhD and DNP programs, which do you believe would be the most appropriate in development of the required skill set of a clinical executive?*
5. *Considering the health care environment where you live and/or are employed, do you feel that it is desirable and/or possible to require nurses in clinical executive positions to hold a DNP?*
6. *What do you see as the advantages and disadvantages of MSN, MBA, and DNP preparation of clinical executives?*
7. *What would be the appropriate criteria to evaluate the effect of a DNP for clinical executives?*
8. *In your opinion, should the nursing profession address the issue of doctoral preparation for nurse executives and possibly establish a precedent and/or standard of preparation for other executives in top leadership roles? Why or why not?*
9. *What were your personal reasons for choosing a DNP program, and what track do you believe best meets your rationale for choosing a DNP program?*
10. *What do you believe are some of the current pitfalls with the preparation of nurse executives and how do you believe the DNP clinical track could address these issues/concerns?*

■ **NOTE**

1. Websites for each program are as follows: Indiana Wesleyan University MBA: http://www.indwes .edu/Adult-Graduate/MBA; University of Texas Tyler MSN/MBA: http://www.uttyler.edu/ academics/graduate/coordinated-msn-mba-online-degree-online.php; University of Kentucky DNP Clinical Leadership: http://www.mc.uky.edu/Nursing/academic/dnp/default.html; and Eastern Kentucky University MSN in advanced rural public health nursing with a concentration in administration: http://onlinenursingprograms.eku.edu/nursing-degree-online-options

■ **REFERENCES**

Alexander, S. (2016). Scholarship in clinical practice: An update on recommendations for doctor of nursing practice programs. *Clinical Nurse Specialist, 30*(1), 58–61.

American Association of Colleges of Nursing. (1996). The essentials of master's education. Retrieved from http://www.aacn.nche.edu/education-resources/MasEssentials96.pdf

American Association of Colleges of Nursing. (2004). AACN position statement on the practice doctorate in nursing October 2004. Retrieved from http://www.aacn.nche.edu/publications/position/ DNPEssentials.pdf

American Association of Colleges of Nursing. (2006). *The essentials of doctoral education for advanced nursing practice*. Retrieved from http://www.aacn.nche.edu/DNP/pdf/Essentials.pdf

American Association of Colleges of Nursing. (2015a, June). Fact sheet: The doctor of nursing practice (DNP). Retrieved from http://www.aacn.nche.edu/media-relations/fact-sheets/DNPFactSheet .pdf

American Association of Colleges of Nursing. (2015b, August). The doctorate in nursing practice: Current issues and clarifying recommendations. Retrieved from http://www.aacn.nche.edu/ aacn-publications/white-papers/DNP-Implementation-TF-Report-8-15.pdf

American Association of Colleges of Nursing. (2010, March). Fact sheet: The doctor of nursing practice (DNP). Retrieved from http://www.aacn.nche.edu/Media/FactSheets/dnp.htm

American Association of Colleges of Nursing. (2016). Retrieved from http://www.aacn.nche.edu/ media-relations/fact-sheets/dnp

American Organization of Nurse Executives. (2005). Nurse executive competencies. *Nurse Leader, 3*(1), 50–56.

American Organization of Nurse Executives. (2007). Consideration of the doctorate of nursing practice. Retrieved from http://www.aone.org/resources/doctorate-nursing-practice

Auerbach, D. I., Martsolf, G., Pearson, M. L., Taylor, E. T., Zaydman, M., Muchow, … Dower, C. (2014). *The DNP by 2015: A study of the institutional, political, and professional issues that facilitate or impede establishing a post-baccalaureate doctor of nursing practice program*. [RAND Report, Sponsored by the AACN] Retrieved from http://www.aacn.nche.edu/dnp/DNP-Study.pdf

Fasoli, D. R. (2010). The culture of nursing engagement: A historical perspective. *Nursing Administration Quarterly, 34*(1), 18–29.

Frearson, M. (2002). *Tomorrow's learning leaders: Developing leadership and management for post-compulsory learning: 2002 survey report*. Retrieved from http://lsda-acting.com

Gerrish, K., McManus, M., & Ashworth, P. (2003). Creating what sort of professional? Master's level nurse education as a professionalising strategy. *Nursing Inquiry, 10*(2), 103–112.

Hader, R. (2010a). Success in the "C-suite." *Nursing Management, 41*(3), 51–53.

Hader, R. (2010b). Who's the doctor, anyway? *Nursing Management, 41*(5), 6.

Hallinger, P., & Heck, R. H. (1996). Reassessing the principal's role in school effectiveness: A review of the empirical research. *Educational Administration Quarterly, 32*(1), 27–31.

Indiana Wesleyan University College of Adult & Professional Studies. (2016). Retrieved from http:// www.mbastudies.com/universities/USA/Indiana-Wesleyan-University-College-of-Adult-and -Professional-Studies

Jones, R. A. (2010). Preparing tomorrow's leaders: A review of the issues. *The Journal of Nursing Administration, 40*(4), 154–157.

Loomis, J. A., Willard, B., & Cohen, J. (2007). Difficult professional choices: Deciding between the PhD and the DNP in nursing. *The Online Journal of Issues in Nursing, 12*(1), 6.

Muijs, D., Harris, A., Lumby, J., Morrison, M., & Sood, K. (2006). Leadership and leadership development in highly effective further education providers: Is there a relationship? *Journal of Further and Higher Education, 30*(1), 87–106.

New, N. (2010). Optimizing nurse manager span of control. *Nurse Leader, 7*(6), 46–48, 56.

Rodriguez, E. S. (2016). Considerations for the doctor of nursing practice degree. *Oncology Nursing Forum, 43*(1), 26–29.

Schaffner, M., & Schaffner, J. (2009). Leadership amid times of economic challenge. *Gastroenterology Nursing: The Official Journal of the Society of Gastroenterology Nurses and Associates, 32*(1), 50–51.

Swanson, M. L., & Stanton, M. P. (2013). Chief nursing officers' perceptions of the doctorate of nursing practice degree. *Nursing Forum, 48*(1), 35–44.

Waxman, K. T., & Maxworthy, J. (2010). Doctorate of nursing practice and the nurse executive: The perfect combination. *Nurse Leader, 8*(2), 31–33.

CHAPTER SIX

Reflective Response

Patricia S. Yoder-Wise and Karen A. Esquibel

Wadsworth, Talbert, and Dennison pose some questions and insights related to the Doctorate of Nursing Practice (DNP) preparation for clinical nurse executives. They compare master's preparation (in nursing and in business administration) with DNP. Although they briefly address the PhD, they omit comparison of the DNP with the PhD degree and how each of those degrees might contribute to the excellence of clinical nurse executives. They also discuss briefly the position of the American Organization of Nurse Executives and address its core competencies for clinical nurse executives. However, they omit addressing the position of the American Nurses Association and its scope and standards document governing nursing administration. These competencies and standards are the basis of the American Association of Colleges of Nursing's (AACN) *Essentials of Doctoral Education for Advanced Nursing Practice*, Essential VIII: systems or organizations focused on advanced nursing practice competencies for *improving patient care processes and outcomes*. The emphasis on "patient care" is vital to the future of health care and the authors are clearly enthusiastic supporters of this degree.

Although this chapter focuses on DNP preparation, as it should, no mention is made of the huge numbers of nurses in administrative positions who are not even prepared with a baccalaureate degree in nursing. This diversity in the educational qualifications for someone who has the ultimate accountability for the nursing care of patients creates an overwhelming challenge to address before the refinement of the question: Should a nurse executive possess a master's or doctorate? can be resolved.

Wadsworth, Talbert, and Dennison make an excellent case for why clinical executives need solid educational preparation. The idea that nurses in those positions have "'24/7' accountability for processes, structures and outcomes" (see Definition of a Clinical Executive) and that these positions often encompass multiple professional groups is an important consideration. The authors point out the value of the *practica* and the *final scholarly project* in shaping the contributions the graduate can make. Although these two experiences are similar to clinical intensives and capstone work at the undergraduate level and the practica and thesis options at the master's level, the richness of the backgrounds that learners bring to the doctoral level study provides a higher level experience. In short, every nurse learns through clinical experiences and focused work. If an individual is learning to be a nurse, that level of insight differs greatly from what a nurse, often with multiple years of experience, brings to doctoral level study.

But what about the difference between the PhD and the DNP? We appreciate the distinction in why nurse leaders choose different programs. If nurse leaders did not continue to contribute to our ongoing body of knowledge, we would have less substantive backing in the application of that knowledge. Both of these graduates (the DNP and the PhD) see the macroscopic perspective, but they see it through a different lens.

PhD programs tend to be more similar than varied. The same is not true for DNP programs. The range of what comprises the DNP programs is between high-level application and final scholarly project consisting of work we might call intense quality improvement and, at the other end, considerable theoretical perspectives and final scholarly project, some projects that would be difficult to differentiate from dissertations. As is always true in nursing, our diversity is one of our greatest benefits and one of our greatest liabilities. On the positive side, there is a greater flexibility with tailoring the DNP to the local needs. Program variability can also be viewed as a negative when curricula are varied and there is a lack of consistency and sometimes rigor in the final scholarly project. Until we have some better description of what best comprises a DNP program, it is difficult to compare that type of programming with other degree programs. We anticipate this programmatic variability to decrease in future years in part because of individual programs' endeavors and in part because of the work of AACN to make clear the expectations of final scholarly project experiences.

One final point about the value or preference for a PhD or a DNP, or for that matter between the DNP and one of the master's programs: The numbers of nurses prepared at the master's and doctoral levels continue to be relatively small in comparison to the 3.1 million registered nurses. Rather than worrying about which is better, we should worry about how we move nurses toward graduate education more quickly and consistently. As the authors point out, "Organizational performance during this turbulent time in health care will be contingent on the effectiveness of the leadership team" (see Supply, Demand, and Preparation of a Clinical Executive—Why Is it Important?).

This chapter addresses the advanced role of the clinical executive with a focus on those positions that head nursing services in clinical agencies. Yet, many DNP programs have students enrolled in the leadership component who are in other roles, such as informaticist and clinical educators (professional development). DNP programs that are inclusive of these leaders have the potential for great impact because today's health care truly does "take a team."

The authors pose several excellent questions related to DNP education for nurse leaders. As more DNP graduates emerge from the expanding number of programs, major medical centers and systems will likely expect that the chief nurse executive hold a doctoral degree. In those organizations, many others will likely be prepared at that level. However, we know from past studies about the profile of nurses in clinical leadership positions; they are often prepared at the baccalaureate, or less, level. This fact suggests that we are unlikely to quickly advance a new educational expectation for nurse leaders. That said, we would be remiss if we did not strongly encourage increased education for nurses at every level.

Two key points resonate for us. One is that nurses are not invited to the table based solely on clinical insight; those extending invitations today look for those who are capable leaders. The second point is that ongoing development is critical for anyone in a leadership position. Whether a nurse is prepared with an MSN or a DNP is not the critical question. The question is, What is the plan for ongoing professional development to remain relevant to the rapidly changing world? Thus, if we are not learning and improving, we no longer are standing still. We are falling behind.

Finally, with the push to place nurses on boards (frequently thought of as hospital boards), nurses prepared in DNP programs are better educated to take on those roles by virtue of their education and clinical experiences than those of us without this added focus that is emerging in many DNP programs. Programs that produce clinical leaders through strengthening their leadership abilities and through inculcating the skill of continued professional development have the best opportunity to create key leaders for tomorrow's big challenges.

The Role of the Educator

Ruth A. Wittmann-Price, Roberta Waite, and Debra L. Woda

■ NURSING FACULTY SHORTAGE

Nursing education is in more of a precarious position today than it was at the first writing of this chapter in 2011. As the great basketball coach John Wooden stated, "Failure is not fatal, but failure to change might be." Even though nursing education has changed, progressed, and added innovation, the desperate need for *qualified* nurse educators is actually worsening by overtaxing current resources without an adequate succession plan. The world of doctoral nursing education is being built around the pillars of nursing practice and nursing research, with only secondary attention given to nursing education other than to profess the shortage of nurse educators.

Agreement about nurse educators' qualifications has come to somewhat of a consensus in the past 5 years with leading nursing organizations (American Association of Colleges of Nursing [AACN] and National League for Nursing [NLN]) recognizing that a doctoral nursing degree alone does not unquestionably qualify a nurse to teach and function effectively in academia. Lack of knowledge about nursing education and/ or academia is well documented in nursing literature and can be verified by asking any nurse educator who has entered academia from practice to recount his or her story (Aquadro & Bailey, 2014; Cranford, 2013; Singh, Pilkington, & Patrick, 2014). Both organizations, AACN and NLN, recognize and address the nurse educator shortage, but neither offers a concrete solution, nor are there any easy solutions to offer. AACN (2016a) honors its original vision that academic nurse educators be doctorally prepared and have preparation in educational methods and pedagogies (AACN, 2008). In addition, AACN views the master's-prepared nurse educator as an individual who is eligible to teach families and students in the clinical setting (AACN, 2016a).

The NLN recognizes the need for nursing education courses in both master's and doctoral curricula for nurses who teach either in academia or a clinical learning environment. The NLN urgently articulated the need for qualified nurse educators in the following manner (2010):

> There is growing apprehension among deans and directors that advanced practice graduates who work as full- and part-time faculty but are not educated in pedagogy, evaluation, and educational theory cannot engage meaningfully in nursing education research or make evidence-based contributions

to nursing education reform. Schools of nursing are making decisions about their master's and doctoral programs without data and without national discussion. The ability to pause and reflect about possible consequences to the nation's health care system and its global implications is critical for nursing. (p. 1)

The nursing profession is at a tipping point and must find a method to properly educate, mentor, and reward those nurses on which all other nursing relies—the nurse educator. The nurse educator shortage is well publicized, yet focus has been placed on other pressing issues, such as prelicensure nursing education moving to the baccalaureate level (Cronenwett et al., 2011; Institute of Medicine [IOM], 2010; Perfetto, 2015), increasing the advanced practice nurses to serve the growing number of insured individuals, establishing "seamless" progressive educational tracks (IOM, 2010), as well as defining and justifying the competencies and expectations of the Doctor of Nursing Practice (DNP) in relation the PhD-prepared nurse (Melnyk, 2013; Redman, Pressler, Furspan, & Potempa, 2015). All of the aforementioned initiatives are noble and effect U.S. health care changes, but without the nurse educators none of them can be actualized. Therefore, the need for nurse educators precedes the expansive need for nurses. At a basic level, the profession needs to be able to educate care providers. If there is a shortage of nurse educators, this will never be accomplished and the current rate of nurses moving into faculty roles has remained inadequate for years. South Carolina Area Health Educational Consortium (SCAHEC) predictions will be used to demonstrate the growing need for nurses and therefore nurse educators. Using a 2.3% growth rate, the number of needed RNs projected for 2028 is approximately 56,000. Today just more than 35,000 RNs provide care for South Carolinians. The estimated gap from actual RNs to needed RNs will widen as time progresses, at the current nursing educational rate (SCAHEC, 2014). These statistics are not unique either; all states in the United States are facing the same dilemma. Nationwide, states are struggling to find qualified nurse educators to educate enough nurses to care for their citizens. The concern about qualified nurse educators is starkly evident when reviewing the statistics. There is a lack of doctorally prepared faculty and the estimates predict that retirements will continue to rise at a rate that outstrips the supply of PhD-prepared faculty (Danzey et al., 2011). The deficiency of doctorally prepared faculty is highlighted by the inadequate criterion established by the Accreditation Commission for Education in Nursing (ACEN), a specialty-specific accreditation agency. In order to teach in a baccalaureate nursing program, ACEN's criterion is that 25% of faculty must have a doctorate or be active in school for a doctorate (ACEN, 2013). A quarter of a faculty group having or pursuing doctorates produce a faculty group that are not qualified to produce rigorous educational research or implement evidence-based practice in education. The second active specialty-specific accreditation agency, Commission on Collegiate Nursing Education (CCNE), does not specifically indicate a required percentage of doctorally prepared faculty. This low percentage and lack of specific criteria are telling of the long-standing need for qualified nursing faculty. Doctoral student enrollments in nursing programs have always been a small percentage of the entire group. In 2004, before the proliferation of DNP programs, only 1% of nurses were doctorally prepared (Danzey et al., 2011). Ten years later, in 2014, DNP enrollments increased at a phenomenal rate (26.2%) when compared to PhD enrollments (3.2%; Fang, Li, Arietti, & Trautman, 2015). Although the DNP has succeeded in increasing doctorally prepared nurses, their roles in relation to academia are still being vetted. Initially, some DNP programs had educational tracks developed for those master's prepared nurses who wanted to stay in a faculty role in an educational organization focused on teaching and considered a terminal degree appropriate for tenure. Yet, many DNP programs are now deleting their educational tracks, if they had one to begin with, in compliance with the original intent of the practice or clinical doctorate and CCNE standards (CCNE, 2013). CCNE accreditation standards are based on the AACN's *Essentials of Doctoral Education for Advanced Nursing Practice* (AACN, 2006) and state (2013):

> All DNP programs incorporate *The Essentials of Doctoral Education for Advanced Nursing Practice* (AACN, 2006) and additional relevant professional standards and guidelines if identified by the program. (p. 13)

AACN's (2006) *The Essentials of Doctoral Education for Advanced Nursing Practice* states:

> The DNP *Essentials* delineated here address the foundational competencies that are core to all advanced nursing practice roles. However, the depth and focus of the core competencies will vary based on the particular role for which the student is preparing. For example, students preparing for organizational leadership or administrative roles will have increased depth in organizational and systems' leadership; those preparing for policy roles will have increased depth in health care policy; and those preparing for APN roles (nurse practitioners, clinical nurse specialists, nurse anesthetists, and nurse midwives) will have more specialized content in an area of advanced practice nursing. (p. 8)

Despite this clear depiction of the DNP vision, DNP graduates are entering academia in substantial numbers, especially to teach in DNP programs (Smeltzer et al., 2015). They are filling a gap and may be no more prepared to be in a faculty role than their PhD colleagues. The 3.2% increase in PhD doctoral student enrollment may yield students with a foundational master of science in nursing (MSN) in nursing education, but the numbers are too lean, especially accounting for the upcoming faculty retirements (AACN, 2016a) and the projected need for nurse educators. Another consideration is that many colleges and universities offer MSNs in nursing education, but the quality of MSN nurse educator programs is variable. There is a wide variety of differences in the number of practicum hours, practicum productivity, and preceptor qualifications. It may be problematic that many MSN educator programs have been moved online and are educating learners for in-class or clinical teaching roles. Online learning can be enhanced if the nurse educator students' practicum hours are rich with role-modeling, quality learning experiences, and exposure to multiple teaching–learning methodologies. There are as few published specific standards for the nurse educator education as there are for other advanced nurse practice roles, not only for practicum hours but also for core curriculum inclusions.

The *NLN Nurse Educator Shortage Fact Sheet* (n.d.) further describes the need for nurse educators and the doctoral preparation of current nurse educators. The fact sheet discusses the problems of aging faculty, low compensation, and long work hours, yet the conclusion is weak and calls the nursing shortage a "critical public policy priority" (p. 6). AACN's (2016b) *Nursing Faculty Shortage Fact Sheet* describes the current shortage in terms of aging faculty and compensation, but does not discuss preparation for nurse educators. The AACN fact sheet concludes with a report of 12 financial scholarships granted over the past 10 years, which may be a start in resource allocation but much more is needed.

AACN (2006) also compares nurse educators to academic educators in other disciplines:

> As in other disciplines (e.g., engineering, business, law), the major focus of the educational program must be on the area of practice specialization within

the discipline, not the process of teaching. However, individuals who desire a role as an educator, whether that role is operationalized in a practice environment or the academy, should have additional preparation in the science of pedagogy to augment their ability to transmit the science of the profession they practice and teach. This additional preparation may occur in formal course work during the DNP program. (p. 7)

The AACN view of nursing education does not take into account the critical thinking and clinical decision-making development needed in the clinically based nursing profession. Nurse educators teach in a multitude of different realms including the classroom, online, in simulation laboratories, skills laboratories, and clinical learning environments. Each teaching environment leads to a certification or licensure that enables a student to practice competently and not just "practice specialization within the discipline" (AACN, 2006, p. 7). Promoting a safe nursing practice is not just a matter of demonstration but a condition of enhancing critical thinking and decision making through expert teaching–learning activities.

This chapter continues to discuss the plight of nurse education through a multifaceted lens that includes: (a) a discussion about nursing education for nurse educators, (b) a description of actual educational preparation in a sampling of doctoral programs, (c) recognizing the certification for nursing education, (d) briefly discussing the state of nursing education research, (e) addressing the academic expectations of nurse educators, (f) a descriptive case study of a DNP-prepared nurse educator, (g) recommendations for the future, (h) a reflective response from an expert nurse educator, and (i) critical thinking questions.

■ EDUCATING THE NURSE EDUCATOR

The NLN has set forth eight core competencies for nurse educators (NLN, 2005) that make up the standard of practice as defined by the American Nurses Association (ANA, 2010). The eight core competencies are published with task statements (Halstead, 2007) and they call for expertise in the areas of (a) teaching–learning methodologies, (b) learner assessment, (c) curriculum development, (d) evaluation strategies of learners and program outcomes, (e) quality improvement and leadership, and (f) understanding of the academic environment. NLN does not discuss at what educational level— master's, post-master's, or doctoral level—these core competencies are best attained in order to establish academically qualified nurse educators. NLN does publish nurse educator certification eligibility standards that place the minimum education for certification at the master's level (Wittmann-Price, Godshall, & Wilson, 2013).

The NLN (2010) also outlines outcomes and competencies for graduates of DNP programs, which include human flourishing, nursing judgment, professional identity, and spirit of inquiry. Within the concept of spirit of inquiry is the recommendation to develop evidence-based knowledge that contributes to nursing education (p. 41).

AACN's *The Essentials of Doctoral Education for Advanced Nursing Practice* (2006) addresses the role of DNP-prepared nurse educators:

However, individuals who desire a role as an educator, whether that role is operationalized in a practice environment or the academy, should have additional preparation in the science of pedagogy to augment their ability to transmit the science of the profession they practice and teach. This additional preparation may occur in formal course work during the DNP program. (p. 7)

The AACN (2012) also recognizes that PhD graduates are also prepared for faculty positions and states: Although a doctorate is the appropriate degree for a faculty role, the DNP program is not designed to prepare educators per se, any more than a PhD does. Graduates from all doctoral programs (PhD or DNP) who wish to be educators should have additional preparation that adds pedagogical skills to their base of clinical practice (p. 1).

The additional course work proposed to supplement DNP and PhD graduates in the realm of nursing education can be attained as a post-master's certificate. The number of courses for school-sponsored nurse educator majors/minors/certificates varies greatly, as does the content. Due to the fact that large numbers of DNP-prepared graduates are teaching in academic and clinical organizations as well as many PhD-prepared graduates, "additional preparation in the science of pedagogy" should be a mandatory minor for all nursing doctorate degrees.

The next section includes a description of several post-master's educational certificate programs to demonstrate the variety of education being afforded to both DNP and PhD graduates.

In sum, both organizations, the AACN and NLN, recognize that a graduate degree alone is not a sufficient qualification for a nurse educator. Both organizations send less conflicting messages than they did initially. Clearly, the DNP graduate is defined as the expert in nursing practice, whereas the PhD graduate is the expert in nursing research. Experts in nursing education have not been provided with a clearly assigned degree, number of courses, content of courses, or experiential experience as foundational criteria for the most innately important role in nursing—the nurse educator. With the surge in undergraduate and graduate nursing programs, who will teach the next generation?

■ NURSING PRACTICE CURRICULA TODAY

The AACN has been a driver for DNP curricular requirements because alignment with *The Essentials of Doctoral Education for Advanced Nursing Practice* is necessary for accreditation. Although this body does not support the role of the educator as a primary concentration, Agger, Oermann, and Lynn (2014) report that more than half (55%) of the new DNP graduates endeavor to occupy an academic role as an educator. Interestingly, Melnyk (2013) also purports that individuals who finish DNPs desire roles as educators; however, the emphasis of most DNP programs is on advanced practice specialization, not teaching. DNP and PhD education often lacks emphasis on teaching except for specific areas related to teaching and learning principles regarding patient teaching for DNPs. The AACN (2006) indicates that DNP graduates are expected to pursue practice leadership roles in a variety of settings such as leading quality initiatives, holding executive status in health care corporations, taking on director positions within clinical programs, and landing faculty positions accountable for implementing clinical programs and clinical teaching. Moreover, Danzey et al. (2011) report that some DNP-prepared professionals view themselves as educators and hold academic leadership roles, including dean- or director-level positions.

Undeniably, what is needed and desired by many DNP- as well as PHD-prepared professionals and what is being stipulated by an organizing body for DNPs do not conform. Given the nature of this issue, the faculty members, irrespective of the highest degree granted, ought to be equipped with proper skills for teaching and garner proficiencies to effectively fulfill their roles. Clearly, when teaching-focused courses have not been successfully completed in their graduate studies, new faculty members will require supplementary education to be adept in fulfilling an academic role (Agger et al., 2014). More progressive DNP programs that comprise primary concentrations or leadership edification focused on education provide nurses with formal foundational work including educational theory, testing, evaluation, curriculum development, and a capstone educational practicum. As such, graduates of these programs are competent to develop, execute, and evaluate nursing curriculum, in addition to being involved in the scholarship of teaching.

Several schools that offer a DNP have clearly advertised nurse educator cognates as a secondary focus or subspecialty; however, all require the applicant to have earned an MSN. To examine how they are addressing the matter of having additional pedagogical and experiential competencies to teach, a search was conducted through Google using the terms "DNP" and "nurse educator focus." A review of courses offered was assessed for the following schools: George Washington University, University of Southern Alabama, Samford University, University of St. Francis, University of Wisconsin-Madison, University of Massachusetts, and Saint Louis University. Table 7.1 highlights the number and content of courses that educational institutions provide at these schools.

When assessing a sampling of six schools of nursing specifically looking at a postmaster's certificate for nurse educators, Table 7.2 provides detailed information on the required coursework for each program. Also, each program required a BSN and MSN to enroll. Interestingly, to sit for the certified nurse educator exam, individuals must have successfully completed nine or more credit hours of graduate-level education courses.

During the search, American Sentinel University was the sole academic institution that had a primary track in education (i.e., educational leadership focus). To successfully complete this online program of study, 14 courses must be successfully completed including two onsite residencies, which typically take just over 2 years to complete.

Auerbach et al. (2015) argue that solely implementing the traditional DNP approach without incorporating other strategies will not help to resolve our faculty crisis in the nursing profession. They found that many schools are "growing their own faculty" who have successfully completed a DNP by supporting their enrollment in post-master's nurse educator programs. Taking into account the major faculty shortage, the role of DNP educators must be underscored and given equitable attention as other roles in these programs. Policies guiding credentialing require educators to intentionally examine ways to support DNP students who want and need pedagogical skills to enhance their ability to teach the science of the profession they practice. Academic institutions struggle with providing DNP degrees within the guidelines of the AACN's *Essentials of Doctoral Education for Advanced Nursing Practice* and preparing doctoral learners for the nurse educator role that so many of them assume. To date, the best resolution has been assisting students to complete additional coursework in preparation for the teaching role.

Taken together, the nursing profession remains challenged given the conundrum set before us, with having a credentialing agency dictate what is deemed appropriate for educating our students. Consequently, regulatory structures have the power to usurp control over one's profession, its own operations, and even its own destiny. As leaders, we must work toward providing exemplary academic experiences to prepare the next generation of educators, practitioners, and executives that will move our profession into the next century.

TABLE 7.1   Courses Offered in "DNP Nurse Educator Focus"

Academic Institution	Number of Courses	Course Number and Course Name
George Washington University	3	HOL 6701: Adult Learning (3 credits) HOL 6721: Assessing the Impact of Organizational Change (3 credits) HOL 6742: Design of Adult Learning Interventions (3 credits)
University of Southern Alabama	4	NU 620: Instructional Design and Technology for Nurse Educators (3 credits) NU 621: Curriculum and Outcomes Evaluation in Nursing Education (3 credits) NU 622: Nursing Education Role Synthesis (2 credits) NU 623: Nursing Education Role more at: 7.dpuf
Samford University	4	NURS 710 (3 credits) TeachingLearning Principles NURS 711 (3 credits) Nurse Faculty Role in Curriculum Development NURS 712 (3 credits) Nurse Faculty Role In Program Evaluation NURS 715 (3 credits) Nurse Faculty Role Transition
University of St. Francis	3	NURS 643 Teaching in Nursing (3 credits) NURS 644 Nursing Education Methods and Measurement (3 credits) NURS 645 Nursing Education Practicum (200 clock hours) (3 credits)
University of Wisconsin-Madison	3 required offers 4	N785 Foundations of Curriculum Development and Evaluation in Nursing Education (3 credits) N786 Foundations of Teaching and Learning in Nursing(3 credits) N787 Nursing Education Practicum (required) (3 credits) N788 Special Topics in Education in Nursing (3 credits)
University of Massachusetts	6	N/NG620 Advanced Nursing Science: Teaching and Curriculum Development for Nurse Educators (3 credits) N/NG 621B Clinical Practicum for Nurse Educators (270 Practicum hours) (3 credits)

(continued)

TABLE 7.1   Courses Offered in "DNP Nurse Educator Focus"   *(continued)*

Academic Institution	Number of Courses	Course Number and Course Name
		N/NG622 Advanced Nursing Science: Advanced Instructional Methods for Nurse Educators (3 credits)
		N623 Advanced Nursing Science: Identifying and Measuring Outcomes for Nurse Educators (3 credits)
		N624 Advanced Nursing Science: Systems Leadership for Nurse Educators (3 credits)
		N625B Advanced Nursing Science: Academic Teaching Practicum for Nurse Educators (270 Practicum hours) (3 credits)
Saint Louis University	3	NURS 557 Curriculum Development in Nursing Education (2 or 3 credits)
		NURS 558 Instructional Strategies and Evaluation for Nurse Educators (2 credits)
		NURS 559 Practicum in Nursing Education 2 (credits)

DNP, Doctor of Nursing Practice.

TABLE 7.2   Sample of Six Schools of Nursing's Post-Master's Certificate for Nurse Educators

Academic Institution	Required Courses	Course Number and Course Name
University of Nebraska	4	NRSG 691 Designing and Evaluating Learner-Centered Curricula (3 credits)
		NRSG 692 Teaching and Learning Strategies (3 credits)
		NRSG 693 Using Technology to Enhance Teaching and Learning Strategies (3 credits)
		NRSG 694 Implementation of the Educator Role: Practicum (3 credits)
Johns Hopkins University	4	Choose any 4 courses from the following:
		NR.110.540 Teaching Strategies in Nursing (3 credits)
		NR.110.543 Teaching Practicum (3 credits)
		NR.110.617 Clinical Teaching and Evaluation (3 credits)
		NR.110.637 Clinical Simulations and Other Technologies in Healthcare Education (3 credits)
		NR.110.638 Curriculum Theory and Design (3 credits)
		NR.110.641 online Teaching and Learning: Development and Instruction (3 credits)
		NR.110.730 Evaluation: From Individual to Program (3 credits)
		NR.110.830 The Evolving Roles of the Nurse Educator (3 credits)

(continued)

TABLE 7.2 **Sample of Six Schools of Nursing's Post-Master's Certificate for Nurse Educators** *(continued)*

Academic Institution	Required Courses	Course Number and Course Name
Pennsylvania State University	3	NURS 840: Nursing Education Theories and Strategies (3 credits) NURS 841: Assessment and Evaluation in Nursing Education (3 credits) NURS 842: Curriculum and Program Development in Nursing Education (3 credits) The following course is optional: NURS 843: Synthesis and Application of the Nurse Educator Role (4 credits)
Villanova University	5	NUR 8500 American Higher Education (3 credits) NUR 8950 Curriculum in Nursing Education (3 credits) NUR 8951 Principles in Measurement & Evaluation in Nursing (3 credits) NUR 8952 Teaching Strategies in Nursing (3 credits) NUR 8954 Practicum in Teaching of Nursing (3 credits)
Wesley College	4	Total 15 credits: credit allocation for each course not identified NR636: Evaluation and Classroom Methods in Nursing Education NR637: Theory and Process in Nursing Education NR638: Nursing Education Practicum NR639: Curriculum Development & Implementation
Howard University	7	NURE 700 Teaching and Learning in Nursing Education (2 credits) NURE 701 Curriculum and Instruction in Nursing Education (3 credits) NURE 705 Role Development as a Nurse Educator (2 credits) NURE 706 Nurse Educator Practicum (2 credits) NURE 703 Clinical Role Specialty for the Nurse Educator (2 credits) NURE 704 Clinical Role Practicum for the Nurse Educator (2 credits) NURE 702 Measurement and Evaluation in Nursing Education (3 credits)

■ CERTIFICATION FOR NURSE EDUCATORS

The NLN has sponsored a certification examination for nurse educators since 2005 (NLN, 2014). Certification is an expectation and/or requirement of many RN and advanced practice registered nursing (APRN) roles. Unfortunately, the certified nurse educator (CNE) certification is not mandated to practice nursing education, but such credentials should be a strong consideration for hiring, promoting, and retaining nurse educators.

The eligibility for the CNE examination has changed since the last writing of this chapter. The past eligibility criteria included having nine credits or semester hours in graduate nursing education courses, or 4 years of teaching, which, unfortunately, subscribes to the apprentice model of nursing. The criterion has changed to nine credits in nursing education courses or 2 years as a nurse educator (NLN, 2014). This change in eligibility coincides with the shortage of nurse educators. Interestingly, the CNE examination has a low first-time pass rate, approximately 62% (Susan Pyle, personal communication, NLN, September 6, 2015), when compared to other nursing certification examinations. This begs the questions, "is the nurse educator workforce ill-prepared in totality to successfully complete the examination or is the test non-specific for the current practice of nurse educators?" The CNE examination has been appropriately revised by nursing education experts since it was originally developed in 2005 and is based on a practice analysis.

There are only approximately 5,000 CNEs in the United States (NLN, personal communication, September 6, 2015) out of approximately 56,840 nurse educators (U.S. Bureau of Labor Statistics, 2014), or only 9%. This too is another example of the prolonged qualified nurse educator shortage that threatens the stability of every realm of professional nursing.

■ NURSING EDUCATION RESEARCH

Nursing education is one of the least researched areas of nursing (Zungolo, 2010). The current literature trend is to justify the output of the DNP scholar as different but equal to that of the PhD scholar (Melnyk, 2013; Redman et al., 2015). While recognizing that DNP- and PhD-prepared students and faculty yield vital clinical scholarship, there remains a vacuity in knowledge development about the nursing education. The current research examines the personal attributes of doctorally prepared nurse educators rather than emphasizing their fields of research. Focusing on demographics and retirement statistics of these nurses instead of distinguishing whether they are producing educational or clinical research has created redundancies rather than a true evaluation of nursing education knowledge development. Nor does the current research address how many nursing education courses were infused into the participants' graduate education (Hall Ellenbecker & Kazmi, 2014). The nursing educational knowledge is one of the least studied areas and nurse educators lacking coursework in the nursing education may very well be part of the reason as well as the scarcity of dedicated funding. One glaring epilogue that reflects the phenomenon of nursing research deprivation is the reliance that nurse educators have on third party companies to facilitate student learning, predict student National Council Licensure Examination (NCLEX) success, and remediate. The teaching–learning process in nursing that includes all of the previously mentioned activities should be and can be orchestrated within an educational department if adequate numbers of faculty with adequate expertise were available. The AACN (2006) expresses the need for quality nursing education research:

> Nursing education research centers on developing and testing more efficient educational processes, identifying new ways to incorporate technology in order to enhance learning, and discovering more effective approaches to promoting lifelong learning and commitment to leadership. To achieve these goals, the use of rigorous research strategies in the assessment of the teaching-learning process and outcomes at all levels of nursing education is essential from baccalaureate and graduate education through the continuous supply of well-educated nurses is critical to maintain and enhance our nation's health, especially in light of the changes in the demographics of the population. To this end, new strategies for recruiting and retaining bright young men and women from diverse educational and cultural backgrounds

into nursing must be developed and tested. In addition, new models of nursing education are needed to prepare nurses for faculty and research positions earlier in their careers. These efforts must assume top priority if nursing research is to continue to evolve. The lack of recognition and funding for this type of research has greatly impaired progress in this area. (p. 1)

■ THE DNP DEGREE AND TENURE

Tenure is another formidable issue within the discussion of the DNP-prepared nurses' role in academe. Depending on the academic's Carnegie Classification of Institutions of Higher Education (2010), many DNP-prepared nurse educators are eligible for tenure. When a college or university faculty guidelines state "terminal-degree" prepared nurse educators should be included, they must recognize that the PhD is not always the "terminal degree" for all disciplines; for example, a master's in fine arts (MFA) is a terminal degree. Although DNP-prepared faculty are teaching in graduate and undergraduate nursing programs and are publishing, presenting, appraising, and using evidence and integrated knowledge across disciplines (Boyer, 1996), along with demonstrating teaching excellence (Redman et al., 2015), they have less time to do so when compared with PhD nursing faculty (Smeltzer et al., 2015). The difference in time devoted to scholarship may be the effect of the different degree focus of the DNP, additional practice hours needed for certification maintenance, or additional teaching requirements in institutions whose mission is teaching as opposed to research. Both PhD- and DNP-prepared graduates need to increase their dissemination of research and evidence-based practice findings, specifically the PhD-graduate's findings related to rigorous research and external evidence and the DNP-graduate's findings of evidence and internal findings related to quality improvement (Melnyk, 2013).

Tenure guidelines have been questioned for quite some time in academia and may be a detriment in retention of nurse educators (Condon, 2015; Feldman, Greenberg, Jaffe-Ruiz, Kaufman, & Cignarale, 2015). It is well known that nurses arrive at academia later in life than other disciplines, thereby producing an unfair disadvantage to tenure (Condon, 2015). Nurses from practice who enter academia are many times ill prepared for the academic role and meeting tenure criteria (Gardner, 2014; Wittmann-Price, 2012).

Although DNP programs that are preparing students for educator roles are in direct conflict with the intent of the AACN, many are being assimilated into educator roles as well as leadership roles in nursing education in non-research-intensive colleges and universities (Melnyk, 2013). It is not practical to try to stop this trend while there is an intensive nursing faculty shortage, but cultivate it as a potential part-solution by infusing the appropriate mechanism to make those who choose to teach successfully. In congruence, Danzey et al. (2011) discuss the DNP degree as the potential cure for the drastic nurse educator shortage because of the proliferation of DNP graduates. Before a definitive stance can be made, more data need to be generated about the outcomes of DNP-prepared and PhD-prepared nurse educators as well as comparing the course's content within degrees rather than just comparing degree attainment. Another issue that has arisen in the literature related to nurse educators is mentorship. Mentorship is critical to nurse educators but the qualified nurse-educator shortage may be counterproductive to a mentorship model (NLN, 2006). Overworked and overstressed employees in high demand will not have the time or energy to properly mentor new employees. However, many academic organizations with adequate resources have instituted mentoring models that have been very successful and productive (McAllister, Oprescu, & Jones, 2014; Seekoe, 2014). Effective mentorship along with a foundation in nursing education would better serve the future of the profession (Schoening, 2013).

■ CASE STUDY: A DNP-Prepared Nurse-Midwife Goes Into Academia

As a Doctor of Nursing Practice (DNP) graduate who went into academia immediately on graduation, there are indeed challenges to being a DNP-prepared nurse in an educator role. My short experience has already taught me that there are a number of barriers for DNP faculty, as well. The nature of academia is often a treacherous place for practice-focused, doctorally prepared faculty. The issue is not competence, but the definition of scholarship by the larger academic community. The roles of the PhD and DNP have been adequately defined by the DNP *Essentials* (AACN, 2006) in terms of their respective roles in the generation and use of nursing knowledge and evidence, but in academia these differing roles are often more ubiquitous. The traditional perspective of original research is very linear and limited in that it is seen as the one true avenue of scholarship; this viewpoint persists whether it is verbalized or not. This is a contradiction to the more contemporary concept of evidence-based practice, which is being demanded of nurses in all realms, even education. Differing approaches to DNP education as is noted in this text do not make this easier, since curricula vary greatly from program to program. In other words, there are likely DNP-degree programs that are rigorous and others that are not. If research is being conducted within the academic realm using varied approaches to prepare nurse educators, a tug of war over who owns (or controls) the research enterprise can occur; this can accentuate problems and cause additional havoc.

Participating in evidence-based research programs that change practice in clinical or educational settings ultimately improves nursing practice and patient outcomes. The generation of this evidence promotes scholarly practice among the faculty and often incorporates the best of the DNP skill sets. However, many research endeavors cannot be accomplished without external funding for salary, as this type of scholarship cannot simply be compounded upon a normal teaching load. Often it is the perception in a respective nursing research department that implementing a new research project, or that creating new evidence, cannot be done without a research partner with a PhD. This can also be a limiting factor to the DNP faculty member when no PhD faculty have an interest in the project, and the department does not afford the resources to support grant writing (even for program grants) to the DNP-prepared nurse.

My experience is that scholarship seems mostly defined by the written or spoken word. The presentation of clinical papers and evidence-based guidelines are good avenues for DNP faculty. However, with the current faculty shortage (and the resulting need for more teaching), there is little time to undertake this avenue of scholarship, and it is difficult, at best, to carry it out consistently. This places the DNP-prepared faculty at a disadvantage because good writing skills need to be developed, and used often, in order for one to become proficient in publishing. Presentations require time and travel support in order to move toward enhancing one's reputation (and thus the department's or college's reputation, as well) as a clinical scholar at the national level. Such protected time is often not possible (or perhaps not valued?) for DNP faculty who are deemed "clinical faculty" and who are required to carry very heavy course loads and

(continued)

■ CASE STUDY: A DNP-Prepared Nurse-Midwife Goes
Into Academia *(continued)*

spend long hours in the clinical area, particularly in undergraduate nursing programs.

Scholarship for the DNP should also be defined by excellence in clinical practice—the goal of the clinically focused DNP is more proficient and expert advanced practice. However, not every school or college of nursing recognizes this as an important aspect of scholarship. Specific and current skills in clinical practice are necessary for effective clinical teaching at both the undergraduate and graduate level. Yet, academic appointments for DNP-prepared advanced practice faculty teaching at the graduate level are particularly challenging when accrediting bodies require significant practice hours for recertification, but nursing departments do not typically allot time for practice, and practice is not considered a scholarly endeavor. This issue has been largely ignored by schools that are actively seeking DNP graduates to teach in their respective DNP programs.

While tenure and promotion of doctorally prepared faculty should not be an issue, those disciplines that have practice-focused doctorates still lag behind in having access to tenure track positions, because the current system does not look favorably upon the type of scholarship these faculty produce. This barrier makes academia less attractive to DNP graduates. Until major research universities address these issues, there is little hope for parity for faculty who are doctorally prepared and active in practice. Mixed messages of valuing researchers (who do not practice), but taking for granted the immense time commitment *to practice* that advanced practice faculty require to teach competently and expertly, are not a prescription to attract the faculty in a shortage.

Another issue is the leveling of doctorally prepared faculty in academia. The DNP-prepared nurse educator is often viewed as a second-class citizen, one who is not eligible for full faculty privileges. Unfortunately, this is not only propagated by the larger academic system, but it is propagated by nurse educators and leaders who view their role as PhD-prepared nurses as the true terminal degree. This sets up an oppressive system ripe for horizontal violence (DalPezzo & Jett, 2010). Therefore, consideration of the aforementioned concerns is not only a professional mandate, but it is also an ethical imperative that the profession of nursing must address to enable uplifting of all our doctorally prepared nursing colleagues.

As a DNP-prepared nurse educator, I have experienced both career development benefits and liabilities. My chosen path has afforded me an opportunity to accomplish my passion to help educate the next generation of nurses, the individuals who will positively affect patient care. It has allowed me to use my clinical expertise in an educational setting and provide mentorship and role modeling to graduate and undergraduate students. The liabilities of being in the role include the lack of time in academia to pursue scholarly activity, and experiencing the rigidity of the system in relation to promotion and tenure. Overall, I choose to continue in this role because of the fulfillment I receive from witnessing the students' growth as they develop into the professional nurses and doctoral advanced practice nurses (whatever their role) so desperately needed in today's health care environment.

■ WHERE WE STAND NOW

The good news is that both the AACN and NLN recognize that nursing education is a different practice from other nursing roles and requires "additional education." The NLN competencies for nurse educators is established and recognized as significant and sufficient. The bad news is that neither organization, the AACN or NLN, will commit to what a full and rigorous nurse educator curriculum should look like other than making recommendations. Nursing experts are comfortable with practice models known by the very prescriptive standards the National Organization of Nurse Practitioner Faculties (NONPF) present for nurse practitioner programs, yet there is a lack of a consensus model for nurse educator education, DNP programs, as well as NONPF PhD programs. One argument is that there is a certification needed to practice as a nurse practitioner but nurse educators have a certification and as DNP programs move toward the entry level into advanced practice, their curriculum will need to demonstrate competencies. Additionally, research related to nursing education preparation in relation to faculty satisfaction and retention, student satisfaction, and program outcomes is needed in order to solidify a nurse educator curriculum. Another consideration is that few nurse educator curricula are preparing nurse educators for the divergent learners that we are now experiencing in class. A stronger interprofessional relationship with graduate education departments is needed in academia in order to promote current nurse educator curriculum relevant to today's learner (Francis Marion University Catalog, 2015–2016).

In addition, DNP-prepared faculty are pressed to keep their clinical practice current, which is an expectation of their practice-focused doctorate, but it also detracts from the time commitment it takes to complete academic achievements (teaching excellence, scholarship, and service) to succeed at a university (Wittmann-Price, 2012).

The authors' recommendations are to solidify the curricula of nurse educators that must be achieved on the doctoral level. Certification needs to be promoted for nurse educators just as it is for other advanced practice nursing roles. Understandably, there is a nursing faculty shortage, but by filling faculty positions with under- or unqualified nurse educators who cannot produce or evaluate nursing educational research, it will be a serious detriment to the future of the profession. Research generated by PhD-prepared nurse educators and evidence-based practice generated by DNP-prepared nurse educators about the practice of nursing education need to be a national priority, and is the only real solution to mitigating both the nursing and the nursing faculty shortage to care for the health care needs of the U.S. populace.

■ CRITICAL THINKING QUESTIONS

1. *What methods of evaluation can nurse leaders use to study the effectiveness of DNP graduates in the role of nurse educator?*
2. *When assessing a DNP candidate for an educational role in nursing, what criteria of assessment should be used?*
3. *Your nursing program is preparing for an accreditation visit; what role should your faculty member (e.g., a DNP teaching critical care) play in developing the accreditation report?*
4. *A faculty member with a DNP degree is being evaluated for tenure. The faculty handbook states under degree criteria, "a terminal degree in your discipline." How would you compose a letter of support for the tenure candidate?*

5. *You are a DNP faculty member on the curriculum revision team for the baccalaureate program. One of the team members has a PhD in public health and is being uncivil because you do not have a PhD. How would you educate that person in relation to your role, education, and preparation as a nurse educator?*
6. *What are some of the major differences in preparation between the DNP and PhD in preparing students for an educator role?*
7. *How do key features of the "practice environment" affect curriculum within the paradigm of nursing education?*
8. *What are some of the definitions of scholarship that are attainable in the DNP role and should be valued as tenurable?*
9. *Can you foresee that two different doctoral degrees in academia may lend themselves to establishing an environment that enhances or detracts academic collegiality?*
10. *Can you think of positive collaborations that could take place in the academic environment between nurse educators with a practice and research doctorate.*

■ REFERENCES

Accreditation Commission for Education in Nursing. (2013). 2013 standards and criteria. Retrieved from http://www.acenursing.org/accreditation-manual

Agger, C. A., Oermann, M. H., & Lynn, M. R. (2014). Hiring and incorporating doctor of nursing practice-prepared nurse faculty into academic nursing programs. *Journal of Nursing Education, 53*(8), 439–446. doi:10.3928/01484834-20140724-03

American Association of Colleges of Nursing. (2006). *The essentials of doctoral education for advanced nursing practice.* Retrieved from http://www.AACN.nche.edu/DNP/pdf/Essentials.pdf

American Association of Colleges of Nursing. (2008). The preferred vision of the professoriate in baccalaureate and graduate nursing programs. Retrieved from http://www.aacn.nche.edu/publications/position/preferred-vision

American Association of Colleges of Nursing. (2010). The researched-focused doctoral program in nursing: Pathways to excellence. Retrieved from http://www.aacn.nche.edu/publications/position-statements

American Association of Colleges of Nursing. (2012). Doctorate of nursing practice (DNP): Frequently asked questions. Retrieved from http://www.aacn.nche.edu/dnp/about/frequently-asked-questions

American Association of Colleges of Nursing. (2016a). Master's education in nursing and areas of practice. Retrieved from http://www.aacn.nche.edu/faculty/faculty-tool-kits/masters-essentials/areas-of-practice

American Association of Colleges of Nursing. (2016b). Nursing faculty shortage. Retrieved from http://www.aacn.nche.edu/media-relations/fact-sheets/nursing-faculty-shortage

American Nurses Association. (2010). *Nursing: The scope and standards of practice* (2nd ed.). Washington, DC: Author.

Aquadro, L. C., & Bailey, B. I. (2014). Removal of nursing faculty practice barriers in academia: An evidence-based model. *Journal of Nursing Education, 53*(11), 654–658.

Auerbach, D., Martsolf, G., Pearson, M., Taylor, E., Zaydman, M., Muchow, A., . . . Dower, C. (2015). The DNP by 2015. RAND Health. Retrieved from http://www.aacn.nche.edu/DNP/DNP-STUDY.PDF

Boyer, E. (1996). *Scholarship reconsidered: Priorities of the professoriate.* San Francisco, CA: Jossey-Bass.

Carnegie Classification of Institutions of Higher Education. (2010). *Carnegie Foundation.* Retrieved from http://classifications.carnegiefoundation.org/methodology/basic.php

Commission of Collegiate Nursing Education. (2013). Standards of nursing accreditation for baccalaureate and graduate nursing programs. Retrieved from http://www.aacn.nche.edu/ccne-accreditation/standards-procedures-resources/baccalaureate-graduate/standards

Condon, B. B. (2015). Politically charged issues in nursing's teaching-learning environments. *Nursing Science Quarterly, 28*(2), 115–120.

Cranford, J. S. (2013). Bridging the gap: Clinical practice nursing and the effect of role strain on successful role transition and intent to stay in academia. *International Journal of Nursing Education Scholarship, 10*(1), 1–7.

Cronenwett, L., Dracup, K., Grey, M., McCauley, L., Meleis, A., & Salmon, M. (2011). The doctor of nursing practice: A national workforce perspective. *Nursing Outlook, 59*(1), 9–17.

Danzey, I. M., Emerson, E., Fitzpatrick, J. J., Garbutt, S. J., Rafferty, M., & Zychowicz, M. E. (2011). The doctor of nursing practice and nursing education: Highlights, potential, and promise. *Journal of Professional Nursing, 27*(5), 311–314.

DelOezzo, N. K., & Jett, K. T. (2010). Nursing faculty: A vulnerable population. *Journal of Nursing Education, 49*(3), 132–136. doi:10.3928/01484834-20090915-04

Fang, D., Li., Y., Arietti, R., & Trautman, D. E. (2015). *2014–2015: Enrollment and graduates in baccalaureate and graduate programs in nursing.* Washington, DC: American Association of Colleges of Nursing.

Feldman, H. R., Greenberg, M. J., Jaffe-Ruiz, M., Kaufman, S. R., & Cignarale, S. (2015). Hitting the nursing faculty shortage head on: Strategies to recruit, retain, and develop nursing faculty. *Journal of Professional Nursing, 31*(3), 170–178.

Francis Marion University Catalog (2015–2016). *Francis Marion University Academic Catalog, 2015–2016.* Florence, SC: Francis Marion University. Retrieved from http://www.fmarion.edu/academics/Catalogs

Gardner, S. S. (2014). From learning tot to teaching effectiveness: Nurse educators describe their experiences. *Nursing Education Perspectives, 35*(2), 106–111.

Hall Ellenbecker, C., & Kazmi, M. (2014). BS-PhD programs in nursing: Where are we now? *Nursing Education Perspectives, 35*(4), 230–237.

Halstead, J. A. (2007). *Nurse educator competencies: Creating an evidence-based practice for nurse educators.* New York, NY: National League for Nursing.

Institute of Medicine. (2010). The future of nursing: Focus on education. Retrieved from http://www.iom.edu/Reports/2010/The-Future-of-Nursing-Leading-Change-Advancing-Health/Report-Brief-Education.aspx

McAllister, M., Oprescu, F., & Jones, C. (2014). Envisioning a process to support transition from nurse to educator. *Contemporary Nurse: A Journal for the Australian Nursing Profession, 46*(2), 242–250.

Melnyk, B. M. (2013). Distinguishing the preparation and roles of doctor of philosophy and doctor of nursing practice graduates: National implications for academic curricula and health care systems. *Journal of Nursing Education, 52*(8), 442–448.

National League for Nursing (n.d.). Nurse educator shortage fact sheet. Retrieved from http://www.nln.org/docs/default-source/advocacy-public-policy/nurse-faculty-shortage-fact-sheet-pdf.pdf?sfvrsn=0

National League for Nursing. (2005). Core competencies of nurse educators with task statements. Retrieved from http://www.nln.org/facultydevelopment/pdf/corecompetencies.pdf

National League for Nursing. (2006). Mentoring of nurse faculty. Retrieved from http://www.nln.org/professional-development-programs/teaching-resources/toolkits/mentoring-of-nurse-faculty

National League for Nursing. (2010). Reflection & dialogue #6—Master's education in nursing. Retrieved from http://www.nln.org/about/position-statements/nln-reflections-dialogue/read/dialogue-reflection/2010/06/02/reflection-dialogue-6—master%27s-education-in-nursing-june-2010

National League for Nursing. (2014). Certified nurse educator (CNE) 2014 candidate handbook. Retrieved from http://www.nln.org/professional-development-programs/Certification-for-Nurse-Educators/handbook

National Organization of Nurse Practitioner Faculties. (2013). NP competencies. Retrieved from http://www.nonpf.org/?page=14

Perfetto, L. M. (2015). Facilitating educational advancement of RNs to the baccalaureate: What are they telling us? *Nursing Education Perspectives, 36*(1), 34–41.

Redman, R., Pressler, S., Furspan, P., & Potempa, K. (2015). Nurses in the United States with a practice doctorate: Implications for leading in the current context of health care. *Nursing Outlook, 63*(2), 124–129. doi:10.1016/j.outlook.2014.08.003

Seekoe, E. (2014). A model for mentoring newly-appointed nurse educators in nursing education institutions in South Africa. *Curationis, 37*(1), 1–8.

Singh, M. D., Pilkington, F. B., & Patrick, L. (2014). Empowerment and mentoring in nursing academia. *International Journal of Nursing Scholarship, 11*(1), 1–11

South Carolina Area Health Educational Consortium. (2014). *Annual report.* Charleston: Medical University of South Carolina.

Schoening, A. M. (2013). From bedside to classroom: The nurse educator transition model. *Nursing Education Perspectives, 34*(3), 167–172.

Smeltzer, S. C., Sharts-Hopko, N. C., Cantrell, M. A., Heverly, M. A., Nthenge, S., & Jenkinson, A. (2015). A profile of U. S. nursing faculty in research and practice-focused doctoral education, *Journal of Nursing Scholarship, 47*(2), 178–185.

U.S. Bureau of Labor Statistics. (2014). 25-1072 nursing instructors and teachers, postsecondary. Retrieved from http://www.bls.gov/oes/current/oes251072.htm

Wittmann-Price, R. A. (2012). *Fast facts for developing a nursing academic portfolio.* New York, NY: Springer Publishing.

Wittmann-Price, R. A., Godshall, M., & Wilson, L. (Eds.). (2013). *Certified nurse educator (CNE) review manual* (2nd ed.). New York, NY: Springer Publishing.

Wooden, J. (n.d.). Retrieved from http://www.great-quotes.com/quote/834998

Zungolo, E. (2010). *The DNP and the faculty role: Issues and challenges.* Paper presented at the Second National Conference on the Doctor of Nursing Practice: The Dialogue Continues…, Hilton Head Island, SC, March 24–27.

CHAPTER SEVEN

Reflective Response

Theresa "Terry" M. Valiga

This chapter raises many questions that remain unanswered even after years of discussion, and it documents that we still are not close to resolving the many issues surrounding the preparation, role, and contributions of nurse educators. Why is this such a "thorny" dilemma? Is it because academe continues to perpetuate old, traditional ways of thinking? Is it because the purpose of the Doctor of Nursing Practice (DNP) was not crystal clear, resulting in confusion about the ideal curriculum design for such preparation? Or is it because our profession—like others—continues to fail to acknowledge the true value and worth of educators?

■ WHAT IS A "PRACTICE" ROLE? IS NURSING EDUCATION AN "ADVANCED PRACTICE" ROLE?

It seems that a first step in resolving some of the issues surrounding the educator role is to address the issue of "practice" and "advanced practice" roles in nursing. For too long, nursing has limited its perspective of the concept of "practice" to those activities in which nurses engage (a) in health care or clinical settings and (b) in providing care to patients, families, and communities. In essence, when many have used the word "practice," they equate it only with *clinical* practice.

There is no doubt that the provision of care in health care/clinical settings is a role that nurses have fulfilled for more than a century, that this role is an essential one in society, and that nurses who enact this role are highly valued, trusted, and respected. But such nurses would not be able to do what they do were it not for other nurses who "practice" in other roles.

Were it not for each of the following groups of nurses—and many others—those who "practice" in clinical roles would not be able to be as effective and valuable as they have been shown to be: nurses who provide leadership in organizational dynamics "practice" in administrative or management roles; nurses who influence the formation of health policy "practice" in policy roles; nurses who integrate nursing science with multiple information management and analytical sciences to identify, define, manage, and communicate data, information, knowledge, and wisdom "practice" in informatics roles; and nurses who prepare the workforce and the next generations of professional "practice" in educator roles.

Thus, one can argue that all nurses who "practice" need to be prepared for the particular role in which they will engage; and if they desire to practice at an advanced level, they need to pursue graduate education, integrate a specialized body of knowledge and specialized skills, and be able to articulate their unique contributions to intra- and interprofessional teams and to the profession. Given this perspective, the nurse educator role clearly needs to be defined as an "advanced practice" role and acknowledged as a critical component of the health and viability of our profession. As noted by the authors of this chapter, this is the role on which all other nursing relies, and without nurse educators, none of the initiatives related to strengthening nursing's contributions to health care can be actualized.

■ PERPETUATING TRADITIONAL WAYS OF THINKING

Not only do we perpetuate traditional ways of thinking about what "practice" means, we also perpetuate traditional ways of thinking about academic practices and standards for promotion and tenure. For example, despite the complexities of the world around us and the reality that an individual cannot be all things to all people, the academic environment continues to insist that only those who are accomplished scientists with extensive external funding and long lists of peer-reviewed publications are worthy of tenure and promotion.

Is it not possible to consider schools of nursing where some faculty are accomplished scientists and researchers, others are exceptional teachers, and others are providing internal leadership and service that helps the school develop, implement and evaluate new initiatives so they remain on the cutting edge as a school? This complementary cadre of faculty also would include individuals who are actively involved in practice and bring that expertise to the classroom, research agendas, and projects that engage the school with the community to address "grand challenges" that could enhance the health of that community.

Is it not possible that tenure could be awarded to faculty whose expertise is in education or practice and who have a sustained record of scholarly accomplishments in those areas, whose scholarly contributions have had an impact on educational or clinical practices, who have made significant contributions to the health and growth of the school and university, and who have the potential to continue such important contributions? Tenure was put in place in 1915 to protect academic freedom (American Association of [AAUP], 1940). Does it still serve that purpose?...Is it needed to protect academic freedom?...Are there other systems and resources in place to protect it? Tenure was not created, however, only for those who have active, externally funded programs of research, so why do today's environments seem to limit this honor only to such faculty? We need to think differently about the nature and various forms of scholarship (Boyer, 1990)—one that recognizes the full range of scholarly activity by faculty, questions the existence of a reward system that pushes faculty toward research and publication and away from teaching, and challenges the existing notions that faculty who have made less traditional forms of contributions to the school, the university, and their profession are not eligible for tenure.

Is it not possible to have schools with a diverse mix of ways and places where faculty were educated? PhD-prepared faculty would provide leadership in building the science of clinical nursing practice, the science of nursing education, and the science of other areas of practice. DNP-prepared faculty would provide leadership in evidence-based practice, evidence-based teaching, and evidence-based system improvements. EdD-prepared faculty would provide leadership in pedagogy, the assessment of learning, teaching innovations, curriculum development, student support systems, and faculty development; and MSN-prepared faculty would provide leadership related to clinical expertise and use that expertise to teach students in the clinical setting, lab, simulations, and classrooms.

As noted by these authors, there is substantial evidence that a doctoral degree in and of itself does not qualify a nurse to teach and function effectively in academia; that holding the PhD does not mean that an individual is prepared for an academic role; and that being an expert clinician does not guarantee that one will be an expert educator. Thus, while there is an important role in the academic environment for faculty with all types of preparation and passion, consideration must be given to the preparation needed to assume a faculty role.

■ PREPARING NURSE EDUCATORS WHO WILL HELP SHAPE THE FUTURE OF OUR PROFESSION

Just as one would never be allowed to practice as a nurse practitioner without formal course work and a supervised clinical practice, one should not be allowed to practice as an educator without formal course work and a supervised teaching practice. Yet, our current systems continue to appoint individuals to faculty positions who have never studied theories of teaching/learning, learning styles, how the brain works in relation to learning, curriculum development, program evaluation, the multiple demands of the educator role, the dynamics of academe, resolution of student-related issues, course development, effective student advisement, innovative teaching strategies, the research that does (or does not) underlie teaching practices, and so on. Indeed, it is quite likely that some faculty are not even aware of the existence of nationally endorsed nurse educator competencies (Halstead, 2007) or certification available to document one's expertise as an educator (National League for Nursing [NLN], n.d.), as mentioned by the authors of this chapter.

Is it not possible to consider schools where faculty are expected to demonstrate that they have been formally prepared for the educator role they will assume? Knowing that many graduates of their programs accept faculty roles, could not PhD programs incorporate education-focused courses and carefully designed teaching practice experiences to better prepare their graduates for the world of academe they will enter? Could those students not be allowed to conduct dissertation research that addresses gaps in knowledge related to effective educational practices? After all, if the goal of a PhD program is to help students build knowledge, skill, and an identity as a scientist/scholar, and to set them on a path of a program of research, why not allow them to develop the skills to study educational or pedagogical questions, thereby being able to advance that science?

Knowing that many graduates of DNP programs also accept faculty roles, could not those programs also integrate theory and practice experiences that would prepare them for that role, allow students to focus their capstone projects on education-focused problems, encourage them to study policies related to education, and develop the skills to lead system-wide initiatives that would improve our educational practices? After all, if the goal of a DNP program is to translate evidence into practice and be able to use evidence to transform systems, are not our educational systems in need of a stronger evidence base and in need of some significant transformation?

Additionally, MSN programs that are designed to prepare educators must acknowledge that they have a responsibility to help students develop the knowledge and skills related to *how* to teach (e.g., teaching strategies, assessment/evaluation methods, and/or curriculum development). However, they also need to help students develop a stronger foundation of *what* they are likely to teach and, therefore, courses related to the sciences that underlie clinical practice (e.g., physiology, pathophysiology, and pharmacology) and to clinical knowledge and skill (e.g., assessment, major health problems) need to be included.

As is occurring in the larger higher education community, it is time for our profession to think more clearly about the kind of preparation educators need to take on the awesome responsibilities associated with influencing how students think, how they practice, and the identities they assume as nurses, as citizens, as members of our profession, and as human beings living in a complex and highly diverse world. We want our students to value diversity and inclusiveness. Perhaps it is time that the academic world does the same.

■ WHAT DO WE MEAN BY "INCLUSION?" WHAT MEANING DOES THE CONCEPT HAVE FOR NURSE EDUCATORS?

There is extensive discussion in academe today about diversity and inclusiveness. Such discussions are essential as we engage with students and faculty from increasingly varied backgrounds, in varied living situations, speaking varied native languages, of varied race and ethnicity, and aiming toward varied goals and aspirations. However, many such discussions focus primarily on racial and ethnic diversity (and, in nursing, on gender diversity), oftentimes failing to acknowledge the many other ways in which we are different and the need to be inclusive of all those differences.

Perhaps schools of nursing need to engage in serious discussions of the extent to which those with expertise in education are valued, rewarded, embraced, and included. To what extent are such faculty—whether they hold a PhD, DNP, EdD, DrPH, or other credential—and the expertise they bring respected, supported, rewarded for demonstrating their scholarly and other contributions in nontraditional ways, and granted tenure?

Those who enact the educator role need to be appropriately prepared for it, valued, appreciated for the various forms of scholarship in which they engage, and compensated appropriately. Without such elements in place, the nursing faculty shortage described by the authors of this chapter will only exacerbate, and exceptional preparation of the workforce needed to care for diverse populations in this ever-changing, technology-enhanced, complex, challenging world.

■ CONCLUSION

The authors of this chapter are to be commended for highlighting the many conundrums that exist related to the role of the educator and the preparation for that role. It is hoped that the nursing profession will continue to address such conundrums through open discourse and open minds.

■ REFERENCES

American Association of University Professors. (1940). 1940 statement of principles on academic freedom and tenure. Retrieved from http://www.aaup.org/report/1940-statement -principles-academic-freedom-and-tenure

Boyer, E. L. (1990). *Scholarship reconsidered: Priorities of the professoriate.* Princeton, NJ: Carnegie Foundation for the Advancement of Teaching.

Halstead, J. A. (2007). *Nurse educator competencies: Creating an evidence-based practice for nurse educators.* New York, NY: National League for Nursing.

National League for Nursing. (n.d.). Certification for nurse educators (CNE). Retrieved from http://www.nln.org/professional-development-programs/Certification-for-Nurse-Educators

CHAPTER EIGHT

The Role of the DNP in Quality Improvement and Patient Safety Initiatives

Catherine Johnson

In 2010, the Affordable Care Act (ACA) was passed into law and with its passage came increased expectations that health care professionals would transform the current health care system. This transformation would be achieved through improvements in the quality and safety of patient experiences in health care systems, resulting in improved patient outcomes at a lower cost. At the same time that the ACA was passed, the Institute of Medicine (IOM, 2010) released a report titled *The Future of Nursing: Leading Change, Advancing Health,* promoting this expectation for the nursing profession. This report challenged nursing as a profession to realize the role of nurses as advocates and leaders in this transformational process. This report recognized that nurses are in the prime position, given their numbers and adaptability, to effect significant changes in health care system's development and delivery. Through their experience in developing partnerships with both patients and other health care providers, nurses were thought to demonstrate the skills and professional commitment to improve every environment in which they work. The IOM report states that nurses are:

> Poised to help bridge the gaps between coverage and access, to coordinate increasingly complex care for a wide range of patients, to fulfill their potential as primary care providers to the full extent of their education and training, and to enable the full economic value of their contributions across practice settings to be realized. In addition, a promising field of evidence links nursing to high quality care for patients, including protecting their safety. (IOM, 2010, p. 29)

At the same time, Robert Wood Johnson Foundation-Gallup Top Line Report (RWJ-Gallup, 2010) released a report, *Nursing Leadership From Bedside to Boardroom,* which provided findings from a survey of 1,504 opinion leaders, including university, insurance, corporate, health service, government, and industry thought leaders regarding their level of trust and confidence in nurses' ability to influence health care reform. Survey findings indicated that these leaders did not consider nurses to be *health care reformers*.

Nurses ranked below all other groups (government, insurance, pharma and health care executives, doctors, and patients). Neither physicians nor nurses were viewed as influential in the reform process, despite their being viewed as having the most credible health care–delivery system information. The top barrier to nurses' assuming this leadership role was the perception that physicians, not nurses, were the key decision makers in health care (RWJ-Gallup, 2010).

Survey respondents may not have viewed nurses as having a great deal of influence on health care reform; however, they did view them as having a significant influence on improving the quality of health care. This included reducing medication errors and increasing patient safety. Respondents also *wanted* nurses to have significantly more influence than they currently had in all areas queried. These opinion leaders, who have significant political influence, clearly valued the nursing profession's knowledge, skills, credibility, and respectability; yet, they seemed to be saying that clinical expertise alone is not enough to conceptualize and implement widespread health care reform.

Despite being 5 years old, these findings are congruent with the American Association of Colleges of Nursing's (AACN, 2015) *white paper* on implementing the Doctoral of Nursing Practice (DNP). AACN (2015) stressed the importance of the DNP role in strengthening the skills and competencies needed by advance practice nurses to impact health care at all levels. The doctoral advanced practice registered nurses (DAPRN) roles focus on providing evidence-based practice in primary and specialty care settings and leading continuous quality improvement (QI) at the individual and system levels (Dreher & Smith Glasgow, 2011). The executive DAPRN focuses on developing, implementing, refining, and leading effective and cost-efficient health care delivery models. These are clearly the skills needed to fill the perceived gap in nursing's ability to lead health care reform as noted in the Institute for Healthcare Improvement's (IHI, 2008) report on meeting a *Triple Aim*.

Established by the IHI (2008) and adopted by many as goals for health care reform, the goals of Triple Aim are of (a) simultaneously improving population health, (b) improving the patient experience of care, and (c) reducing per capita cost. These three aims became the organizing framework for the U.S. National Quality Strategy (NQS; Agency for Healthcare Research and Quality [AHRQ], 2012). AACN's vision of competencies for a DNP aligns perfectly with the skills needed to lead practice-based, organizational, and national initiatives that would support achievement of these important goals. Overcoming the barriers within the DNP educational programs and practice sites are the first and most vital challenge for the nursing profession. Implementing the clearly defined competencies for DNP graduates through consistently applying these DNP educational standards within DNP programs will go a long way toward meeting the mandate for nursing to assume leadership in health care reform.

The competencies described in the AACN's (2006) *Essentials of Doctoral Education for Advanced Nursing Practice* combined eight essential competencies with role-specific competencies established within specialty or functional areas of focus. These eight competencies serve as the core curriculum for BSN–DNP and post-master's DNP programs. These courses vary by program and most often include content areas focused on: translating evidence-based practice; interprofessional, organizational, and systems' leadership; patient education and health information technology; analytical methods including program evaluation, QI methods, and epidemiology; population health and clinical prevention; and health care policy. Details regarding the specific approaches to achieve these broad competencies are left to the faculty developing these courses. Textbooks and other resources provide support as they develop the depth needed in each content area to prepare DNP graduates to meet the stated competencies and assume their leadership roles.

Building on the documented credibility nurses have in assuming leadership in QI and patient safety activities, DNPs now have an increased opportunity to impact on system transformation through development and implementation of innovative and credible QI strategies and program designs. Yet specific QI strategies, approaches, and tools are often absent from DNP curriculum. Widespread confusion and debate regarding appropriate practice-based scholarship lends credence to this concern. The AACN's (2015) white paper on DNP implementation addresses this inconsistency and the need again to clarify the contrast of what is considered practice-based scholarship versus research-based scholarship. Specific recommendations are made in the white paper regarding program refinements that would assure achievement of DNP competencies and, when implemented, would provide more consistency in the DNP role. One of AACN's most important recommendations is the need to generate opportunities for faculty development in the areas of QI methods and measurements. Many PhD-prepared faculty have little knowledge or experience in developing or implementing QI activities, yet, they are expected to guide their DNP students through this process in diverse health care systems. Furthermore, they are expected to evaluate the relevance of these practice-based QI projects with little contact with the context in which they are implemented. This mismatch between the expectations for DNP leadership in QI and the inconsistency in DNP education in this area has created a missed opportunity for nursing to assume a leadership role in health care reform. Improvement of this aspect of DNP education is vital, as it will increase DNPs' opportunities to achieve the requisite skills, knowledge, and abilities needed to lead QI in the setting in which they practice.

This chapter focuses on the available strategies and programs developed in concert with the implementation of the ACA and the NQS that could be the foundation for the required DNP program development. Through federal and national foundation grant supports over the past 10 years, significant progress has been made in the development of evidence-based QI approaches. This chapter reviews three significant initiatives available to the DNP faculty and students for building learning opportunities. These include: (a) AHRQ's (2014a) tools and evidence-based practice (EBP) quality indicators; (b) Centers for Disease Control and Prevention (CDC, 2012) Program Evaluation model; and (c) IHI's (2016) Open School for QI education.

Acknowledgment is given to the Centers for Medicaid and Medicare Service, the Robert Wood Johnson Foundation, and the Kellogg Foundation for supporting the development of these national initiatives and strengthening the education of health care professionals who will lead the reform needed to meet the Triple Aim. For the nursing profession, poised to assume leadership in this transformation, a more significant and concerted effort by leaders in nursing education and practice is needed to join this national forum. This can be accomplished by strengthening the leadership role of the DNP in developing QI in all settings in which they practice.

■ NATIONAL STRATEGY FOR QI

The use of the terms *quality health care* and *QI* are pervasive in discussions related to health care reform. What do they mean, and how can they be implemented? As mentioned in the previous section, the IHI (2008) defined goals for health care reform as the Triple Aim: *improving population health, improving the patient experience of care, and reducing per capita cost*, which became the organizing framework. In response to the ACA's mandate to increase access to high-quality, affordable health care for all Americans, the Secretary of the Department of Health and Human Services (HHS, 2010) established the

National Strategy for Quality Improvement in Health Care (NQS) that would set priorities, guidelines, and standards to guide this effort. AHRQ was charged with leadership of this effort. The NQS was developed to promote quality health care to meet the needs of patients, families, and communities by guiding the actions of all those who deliver and pay for care. This strategy supports the incorporation of evidence-based research and scientific advances in practice standards for clinical care, public health, and health care delivery. Stakeholders across the health care system, including federal, state, local agencies as well as providers, patients and payers, were involved in their development. Measureable improvements in outcomes of care and in the overall health of Americans are the desired outcomes. Table 8.1 describes the NQS aims and priorities (AHRQ, 2012).

In support of improving patient safety through expanded evidence-based practice and consistent QI, the AHRQ provided health care leaders and providers with access to population-focused clinical practice guidelines, updated research, and quality reports. AHRQ's mission of "Producing Evidence to Improve Care" is well demonstrated in the depth of information and support provided to support DNP professional development in building QI programs.

An example of this support is AHRQ's (2014a) *Quality Indicators (QIs) Toolkit*, which is designed to support organizations in developing and implementing quality and patient safety improvement programs in hospitals and which are built on a common set of measurements. This approach will provide a consistent measurement across programs allowing comparability system to system. The toolkit is free of charge and measures of hospital quality and patient safety were developed through analysis of available hospital inpatient administrative data. Hospitals across the country contributed to their development and have used QIs to identify potential

TABLE 8.1   **National Quality Strategy**

Aims
Better Care: Improve overall quality by making health care more patient-centered, reliable, accessible, and safe.
Healthy People/Healthy Communities: Improve the health of the U.S. population by supporting proven interventions to address behavioral, social, and environmental determinants of health in addition to delivering higher quality care.
Affordable Care: Reduce the cost of quality health care for individuals, families, employers, and government.

To advance these aims, the NQS focuses on **six priorities** that address the most common health concerns that Americans face:

1. **Patient Safety**: Making care safer by reducing harm caused in the delivery of care.
2. **Person-Centered Care**: Ensuring that each person and family are engaged as partners in their care.
3. **Care Coordination**: Promoting effective communication and coordination of care.
4. **Effective Treatment**: Promoting the most effective prevention and treatment practices for the leading causes of mortality, starting with cardiovascular disease.
5. **Healthy Living**: Working with communities to promote wide use of best practices to enable healthy living.
6. **Care Affordability**: Making quality care more affordable for individuals, families, employers, and governments by developing and spreading new health care delivery models.

NQS, National Quality Strategy.

concerns about quality and safety, as well as to track their performance over time. The toolkit supports hospitals that want to improve their quality performances and includes *Inpatient Quality Indicators* and *Patient Safety Indicators*. Table 8.2 outlines the AHRQ (2012) QI Process which supports the development, implementation, and evaluation of QI processes.

Implementing this QI approach begins with preparing the environment through the assessment of barriers including gaps in knowledge, communication, and data sources. Applying these well-defined QIs is the cornerstone of the NQS, and AHRQ's activities are designed to bring about quality health care across the country. The use of this common lexicon of measurement makes quality "measureable" and consistent. *Inpatient Quality Indicators* include 28 provider-level indicators that can be used with hospital inpatient discharge data to provide a perspective on quality. They are grouped into four sets of indicators as described on Table 8.3.

Patient Safety Indicators include 18 provider-level indicators that screen for adverse events that patients experience as a result of interacting with the health care system. These are defined on two levels as described on Table 8.4.

DNP students and educators can make use of these national strategies to guide their DNP QI projects. An ideal DNP project could be one that works within the NQS implementing these national standards and processes within local organizations. This dissemination of nationally developed QI approaches and programs is an opportunity to increase the relevance of DNP projects within organizations as well as to support DNPs in their role as leaders in QI and patient safety. By integrating the NQS and AHRQ's coordinated QI approach with DNP QI Projects, the impact of DNP practice on health care's transformation can begin to be realized.

TABLE 8.2   **AHRQ's Quality Improvement Process**

Steps to Set Priorities, Plan, Implement, and Sustain Quality Improvement Initiatives
1. Determining readiness to change
2. Applying QIs to the hospital data
3. Identifying priorities for quality improvement
4. Implementing improvements
5. Monitoring progress for sustainable improvement
6. Analyzing return on investment
7. Using other resources
Toolkit's Five-Step Improvement Cycle Based on the Well-Known PDSA (Plan, Do, Study, Act)
1. Diagnose the problem
2. Plan and implement best practices
3. Measure results and analyze
4. Evaluate effectiveness of actions taken
5. Evaluate, standardize, and communicate

AHRQ, Agency for Healthcare Research and Quality; QIs, quality indicators.

TABLE 8.3   **AHRQ's Inpatient Quality Indicators**

Volume indicators	Indirect, measures of quality based on counts of admissions during which certain intensive, high-technology, or highly complex procedures were performed
Mortality indicators for inpatient procedures	Procedures for which mortality has been shown to vary across institutions and for which there is evidence that high mortality may be associated with poorer quality
Mortality indicators for inpatient conditions	Conditions for which mortality has been shown to vary substantially across institutions and for which evidence suggests that high mortality may be associated with deficiencies in the quality of care
Utilization indicators	Procedures whose use varies significantly across hospitals and for which questions have been raised about overuse, underuse, or misuse

TABLE 8.4   **AHRQ's Patient Safety Indicators**

Provider-level indicators	Potentially preventable complications for patients who received their initial care and the complication of care within the same hospitalization
Area-level indicators	All cases of potentially preventable complications that occur for a given population (metropolitan area, county, health plan), either during hospitalization or in a subsequent hospitalization

■ PROGRAM EVALUATION

Program evaluation is a central component to the NQS and AHRQ's QI process. This component of an organization's QI plan often focuses on improving the quality, credibility, and usefulness of the program as well as ascertaining whether the program's resources are being used efficiently. These data are therefore useful in guiding resource allocation as well as in identifying how to improve program outcomes. There is no specific standard for defining a program; however, the term often includes organizational activities, services, projects, functions, and policies. The term program evaluation is a broad term indicating a systematic approach to evaluating a program's performance in relationship to achieving its goals, objectives, and desired (and undesired) outcomes (CDC, 2012). This approach typically employs a variety of data collection methods based on specific questions about a program's effectiveness and efficiency. The scope of the evaluation can include the entire program, a program component, or individual program parts with the selection of scope depending on the desired outcome of the evaluation. Program evaluation results are used to assess its effectiveness in meeting defined goals and desired outcomes. Furthermore, results increasingly are used as evidence of overall organizational effectiveness.

Performance measurement and reporting is an increasingly important QI component and is closely related to program evaluation. Performance measurement is the systematic, ongoing monitoring and reporting of QIs that have been identified as central to the achievement of the organization's goals. AHRQ's inpatient quality indicator is an example of performance measures that can guide hospitals in developing specific performance measures. The measures are often conceptualized in systems terms; that is, they may address inputs (staffing and resources), process (program activities), and output (client's health outcomes). Participating in this national approach can be useful in comparing the individual organization's performance against peer health care organizations, as well as flagging potential problem areas in the program that may be affecting quality of care.

Program evaluations go beyond these discreet performance measures and look at this data from the context of the program as a whole. Relationships between program components across program settings and services are examined to determine how a program is performing in achieving the desired outcomes for the program participants. This analysis can identify how program performance is influenced, not just one area of service, but in combinations that could point to causal impact of several services impacting on each other. For example, analysis of relationships between process indicators (e.g., nursing staffing in the intensive care units [ICUs]) with postoperative infection rates or of mortality rates by surgery can provide important insight into the source of quality problems within specific programs within the organization (e.g., inpatient surgical service).

Performance measures can be useful to decision makers in providing ongoing, continuous indicators of program achievement in priority areas. This system can provide an early warning system to the management to facilitate identifying system deficiencies. Program evaluation data are more in depth and are based on studies conducted periodically. This assessment is based on analysis of multiple sources of data considered within an organizational context and provides an assessment of how the overall program is functioning and areas for adjustment. Both approaches to quality measurement are important in communicating to internal and external stakeholders of how the organization is performing and activities involved in improving this performance.

The CDC (2012) provided the *Self Study Guide Introduction to Program Evaluation for Public Health Programs,* which supports systematic program evaluation across public health programs across the United States. This practical tool summarizes essential elements of program evaluation, including steps and standards as well as the means to include contextual consideration and analysis. This framework describes types of program evaluations that can be selected for use. This selection is based on the age of the program and the questions being asked within the evaluation. What questions, who is asking them, and what will be done with the information are important questions to ask when determining which evaluation approach will be used (Table 8.5). The availability of time and resources also influence the selection of the evaluation design. Process and outcome evaluation designs are the most commonly used; however, cost–benefit evaluations are of particular use when determining the best use of limited resources. DNP educators and students could make use of this model in developing a standardized evidence-based approach to systematic program evaluation consistent with a DNP project.

■ PATIENT AND HEALTH CARE SAFETY

Eliminating medical errors and improving patient safety is one of the major drivers for health care transformation. Achieving a culture of patient safety requires understanding what values and beliefs are important in an organization and what attitudes and behaviors related to patient safety are supported, rewarded, and expected. Patient

TABLE 8.5   **Types of Program Evaluation**

Program Type/Purpose	Components	Measurement
Process/Implementation Evaluation: Evaluates the extent to which the program has been implemented as intended	Target population Regulatory requirements Professional standards Customer expectation	Number of participants SES of participants Performance Measures Customer Feedback
Effectiveness/Outcome Evaluation: Evaluates progress toward achieving desired outcomes	Change in participant's health Change in participant's risk or protective behaviors Change in participant's/ population's morbidity and mortality	Clinical indicators (e.g., BP) Tobacco use status Incidence and prevalence data of disease
Cost–Benefit Analyses: Comparison of single program outputs/outcomes with the costs (resources) to produce them	Performance indicator related to goal achievement Program cost in dollars	Inpatient postoperative infection rate Cost of nursing and medical staff infection control training

BP, blood pressure; SES, socioeconomic status.

safety practices developed within organizations are increasingly based on national standards related to accuracy in patient identification, communication systems among care givers, and precautions for high alert medications and procedures. The AHRQ's (2014b) Patient Safety Network provides support and guidance to practitioners in the latest evidence-based care as well as warns of hazards that pose risk to patients. AHRQ (2014c) has also developed a valid and reliable patient safety culture survey, the *Hospital Survey on Patient Safety Culture*, to help hospitals, nursing homes, primary care, and specialty practices and clinics evaluate how well they have established a culture of safety in their organizations. The AHRQ's (2014c) *User Comparative Database Report* consists of data from 653 hospitals in the United States that can used to compare patient safety cultures between organizations. Table 8.6 describes the 12 Patient Safety Composites that are measured and with their descriptions. These 12 composites can be viewed as the organizational supports needed to provide a culture supportive of patient safety practices (AHRQ, 2014c).

AHRQ has led the way in providing the means for hospitals and other health care organizations to focus on their health care safety practices. Examples of composite data that demonstrate areas of strength in the AHRQ report include:

1. *Teamwork Within Units (81% positive response)*—the extent to which staff support each other, treat each other with respect, and work together as a team.
2. *Supervisor/Manager Expectations and Actions Promoting Patient Safety (76% positive response)*—the extent to which supervisors/managers consider staff suggestions for improving patient safety, praise staff for following the patient safety procedures, and do not overlook the patient safety problems.
3. *Organizational Learning—Continuous Improvement (73% positive response)*—the extent to which mistakes have led to positive changes and changes are evaluated for effectiveness.

TABLE 8.6 Patient Safety Culture Composites and Descriptions

Patient Safety Culture Composite	Definition: The Extent to Which
Communication openness	Staff freely speak up if they see something that may negatively affect a patient and feel free to question those with more authority
Feedback and communication about error	Staff are informed about errors that happen, given feedback about changes implemented, and discuss ways to prevent errors
Frequency of events reported	Mistakes of the following types are reported: (a) mistakes caught and corrected before affecting the patient, (b) mistakes with no potential to harm the patient, and (c) mistakes that could harm the patient but do not
Handoffs and transitions	Important patient care information is transferred across hospital units and during shift changes
Management support for patient safety	Hospital management provides a work climate that promotes patient safety and shows that patient safety is a top priority
Non-punitive response to error	Staff feel that their mistakes and event reports are not held against them and that mistakes are not kept in their personnel file
Organizational learning—continuous improvement	Mistakes have led to positive changes and changes are evaluated for effectiveness
Overall perceptions of patient safety	Procedures and systems are good at preventing errors and there is a lack of patient safety problems
Staffing	There are enough staff to handle the workload and work hours are appropriate to provide the best care for patients
Supervisor/manager expectations and actions promoting safety	Supervisors/managers consider staff suggestions for improving patient safety, praise staff for following patient safety procedures, and do not overlook patient safety problems
Teamwork across units	Hospital units cooperate and coordinate with one another to provide the best care for patients
Teamwork within units	Staff support each other, treat each other with respect, and work together as a team

Areas that were identified with the potential for improvement included:

1. *Non-Punitive Response to Error (44% positive response)*—the extent to which staff feel that their mistakes and event reports are not held against them and that mistakes are not kept in their personnel file.
2. *Handoffs and Transitions (47% positive response)*—the extent to which important patient care information is transferred across hospital units and during shift changes.
3. *Staffing (55% positive response)*—the extent to which there are enough staff to handle the workload and work hours are appropriate to provide the best care for patients.

Many of the patient safety national initiatives have focused on inpatient care within hospitals with few focused on primary care practices or specialty ambulatory care. *The Physician Practice Patient Safety Assessment* (Medical Group Management Association, 2006) is a tool developed as a multidisciplinary assessment of patient safety practices in ambulatory settings. Six domains are assessed including: medications; handoffs and transitions between providers; surgery, anesthesia, and invasive procedures; personnel qualifications and competencies; practice management and culture; and patient education and communication. These domains are the areas of highest risk and potential for safety concerns, which should be the focus of the practice's patient safety program development. The tool is free and available through the IHI website (www.ihi .org/resources/Pages/Tools/PhysicianPracticePatientSafetyAssessment.aspx).

The IHI provides health professionals access to a wide range of QI and patient safety tools and related training, as well as case studies of successful program implementation in actual practice sites throughout the United States. Through its Open School, training is provided free to the public. The IHI (2016) Open School offers a basic certificate of QI and patient safety on completion of 16 required courses in the areas of improvement capacity; leadership; patient safety; person and family-centered care; and quality, cost, and value. These courses are used by medical schools and other health care professional schools in providing consistent training and access to well-conceived and tested approaches to QI. Inclusion of this curriculum in DNP programs would provide a consistent baseline of QI education within the context of interdisciplinary education and approaches. Students are encouraged to reach beyond their educational programs and join local and regional student-led quality initiatives. This model can teach the next generation of health care professionals to apply the professional goals nursing has supported within the broader health care system.

■ SUMMARY

The nursing profession is poised to provide leadership in the transformation that is needed in health care. Nurses have been acknowledged by health care leaders for their respectability and reliability, particularly in the areas of QI and patient safety. In 2006, the AACN proposed the role of a doctoral level advanced practice nurse who could meet the demand for improved patient outcomes through the development of improved patient-centered health care systems. There have been missteps and missed opportunities in the implementation of the DNP essentials related to quality improvement. There has been a significant gap between the expertise of the faculty leading DNP programs and the expertise needed to support students in the development of QI and patient safety projects in health care settings. Again AACN (2015) has called for DNP programs to reduce this gap significantly through faculty development and the use of national initiatives in QI and patient safety including consistent use of definitions, standards, and approaches in DNP education. This chapter has sought to bridge this gap by having described key national initiatives pertinent to supporting advanced education in QI and patient safety. In addition, resources were identified that are available to nursing as well as other health care professions that could and should be integrated into DNP educational processes. Underlying these efforts is the recognition that nursing, as well as all other health care professionals, must reduce the focus of discipline-specific strategies and approaches directed toward QI. In its place must be the recognition of the multidisciplinary nature of health care delivery and the development of strategies and approaches that are consistent with this reality. By joining these national multidisciplinary initiatives and adding nursing's unique perspective, health care reform and true transformation may be advanced.

■ REFERENCES

Agency for Healthcare Research and Quality. (2012). *Working for quality annual report.* Retrieved from http://www.ahrq.gov/workingforquality/reports/annual-reports/NQS2012annlrpt.htm

Agency for Healthcare Research and Quality. (2014a). Quality indicators toolkit for hospitals. Retrieved from http://www.ahrq.gov/professionals/systems/hospital/qitoolkit/index.html

Agency for Healthcare Research and Quality. (2014b). Patient safety network. Retrieved from https://psnet.ahrq.gov/information

Agency for Healthcare Research and Quality. (2014c). Hospital survey on patient safety culture. Retrieved from http://www.ahrq.gov/professionals/quality-patient-safety/patientsafetyculture/hospital/index.html

American Association of Colleges of Nursing. (2006). *The essentials of doctoral education for advanced nursing practice.* Retrieved from http://www.aacn.nche.edu/DNP/pdf/Essentials.pdf

American Association of Colleges of Nursing. (2015). *Report from the task force on implementation of the DNP.* Retrieved from http://www.aacn.nche.edu/news/articles/2015/dnp-white-paper

Centers for Disease Control and Prevention. (2012). A framework for program evaluation. Retrieved from http://www.cdc.gov/eval/framework/

Department of Health and Human Services. (2010). *The Affordable Care Act, section by section.* Retrieved from http://www.hhs.gov/healthcare/rights/law/index.html

Dreher, H. M., & Smith Glasgow, M. E. (2011). *Role development for doctoral advanced nursing practice.* New York, NY: Springer Publishing.

Institute for Healthcare Improvement. (2008). The triple aim: Care, health, cost. Retrieved from http://www.ihi.org/resources/Pages/Publications/TripleAimCareHealthandCost.aspx

Institute for Healthcare Improvement. (2016). Open school. Retrieved from http://www.ihi.org/education/ihiopenschool/Pages/default.aspx

Institute of Medicine. (2010). The future of nursing: Leading change, advancing health. Washington, DC: National Academies Press. Retrieved from http://www.thefutureofnursing.org/sites/default/files/Future%20of%20Nursing%20Report_0.pdf

Medical Group Management Association. (2006). The physician practice patient safety assessment. In Collaboration with Health Research and Educational Trust and the Institute for Safe Medication Practices. Retrieved from http://www.mgma.com/Libraries/Assets/Practice%20Resources/Tools/PPPSA/pppsa-09-booklet_e-version.pdf?ext=.pdf

Robert Wood Johnson-Gallup Top Line Report. (2010). Nursing leadership from bedside to boardroom: Opinion leaders perceptions. Retrieved from http://www.rwjf.org/en/library/research/2010/01/nursing-leadership-from-bedside-to-boardroom.html

CHAPTER EIGHT

Reflective Response

Susan Baseman

The imperative to reform health care delivery and payment in this country is clear—the trajectory of escalating costs for health care combined with an aging population and complicated by increasing concerns about quality, safety, access, inefficiency, and variation in care delivery combined to create a call to action for major delivery system reform in this country. The Patient Protection and Affordable Care Act (commonly referred to as the Affordable Care Act or ACA) is designed to address at least some of these issues. Although better known for its efforts to expand insurance coverage, the ACA includes a number of provisions that have the goal of improving the quality and efficiency of American health care.

Dr. Catherine Johnson has thoughtfully described how nurses, specifically nurses at the level of the professional practice doctorate, can and should be major forces in improving quality and patient safety in our increasingly complex health care system. She further describes the challenges of doing so in the context of a system that does not view nurses as health care reformers capable of influencing or leading work in quality improvement (QI) and safety. Dr. Johnson notes that one of these challenges is the lack of sufficient educational preparation and experience in the curriculum of Doctor of Nursing Practice (DNP) programs, which is compounded by the relative lack of experience of DNP faculty with QI work.

The description of the National Quality Strategy (NQS) and the work of the Agency for Healthcare Research and Quality (AHRQ, 2014a, 2014b) and the Institute for Healthcare Improvement (IHI, 2015) provide a strong foundation for understanding the goals, strategies, and programs relevant to the discussion of the role of the practice doctorate in the area of improving quality and safety for patients in the context of health reform. Areas of this issue that have not been fully addressed in this chapter are the challenges of translating the goals and best practice standards for quality and safety as laid out by the NQS, AHRQ, and others into practice, and the role of the DNP in making that happen (AHRQ, 2014a, 2014b; National Quality Forum, 2014).

The challenge facing health care organizations—whether they are small hospitals, large academic medical centers, physician practices, urban or rural—is one of shrinking revenues in the face in increasing requirements for meeting standards of quality and outcomes. In the current climate of value-based care, the potential rewards in the form of incentives for improved outcomes and reduced costs are downstream and hard to predict, while the operational costs of infrastructure and personnel needed to position providers to achieve these goals are front-loaded. This issue is compounded by the sheer volume of metrics, measures, and groups to whom they are to be reported, which includes federal and state governments, payers (public and private), and credentialing organizations such as The Joint Commission, the Leapfrog Group, and numerous specialty organizations that collect and publish clinical quality and outcome information benchmarked to peers, many of which are publically reported (Leapfrog Group, 2010). In many cases, the reporting of these metrics is required either by a licensing entity or by a payer, and is the price of doing business that is necessary to keep the doors open and to be able to receive reimbursement for the care provided. Increasingly, those payers are linking some of that payment to performance in those measures—either incentives for improved performance or financial penalties for performance that is below the established benchmarks (pay for performance).

Participation in the quality reporting programs of some organizations (including the AHRQ Quality Indicators program described in this chapter) is voluntary and the benefits to the provider or hospital are not directly financial, but rather consist of self-improvement, status relative to competitors, and public standing, which may or may not translate into a competitive advantage in terms of patients choosing their services over those of another provider or organization. While participation in these programs can be extremely helpful to the organization in making important improvements in quality and safety, participation can be costly in terms of the resources and effort that the collection and reporting of the data require. In many cases, the metrics themselves and the criteria for collecting them—which patients are included or excluded from the data collection, how the measures are defined, what constitutes meeting or not meeting a measure—vary significantly from program to program, even for measures that would seem to be the same—such as readmissions or complications. Thus, the work required to fulfill mandatory requirements to state and federal agencies and payers cannot be leveraged to fulfill the reporting requirements on most of the voluntary programs— each requires specific resources and staff specialized in understanding the measures specific to that program so that the data collection and reporting are accurate and applicable to that program.

Further compounding of these issues is the fact that electronic health record (EHR) systems are still in their infancy, and were designed much more specifically for inputting and archiving data on patient encounters than for creating outputs in the form of reports to meet needs for quality and safety tracking and reporting. The sheer number of different EHR systems, and the fact that virtually every installation is highly customized to the provider or organization who implements it, means that creating standardized reports on these measures is very, very challenging. Therefore, much of the data collection continues to be done through manual chart abstraction, requiring staff time and resources, none of which directly contributes to revenue, but rather is all overhead cost for the provider organization.

Where does the DNP fit into all of this? It is clear to see that the collection and reporting of quality and safety measures are complicated and require oversight by someone with highly specialized expertise, a role that would seem to describe a nurse with advanced practice credentials and experience. However, more important than collecting and reporting the data is understanding what it means and what to do about it. In my opinion, this is the role that the DNP can and should fulfill in the realm of improving quality, outcomes, and safety for patients. The range of skills required are part of the DNP's scope and expertise such as: interpreting the data, discerning trends, understanding variation in the data and what it means, how to improve, how to build and work with multidisciplinary teams, using Plan-Do-Study-Act and rapid cycle improvement change management processes, creating a culture of safety and quality, creating a culture of non-punitive reporting of errors, and translating evidence into practice—to name a few. In referring back to the chapter, this is the role of the "health reformer," and it is the one that apparently is not well associated with nurses, but one that seems tailor-made for a DNP.

So we return to Dr. Johnson's points about the need for specialized curriculum in quality improvement and patient safety in DNP programs, as well as experienced faculty and direct clinical experiences working with these measures and in conducting quality improvement initiatives in health care settings. Regardless of practice setting or specialty of the DNP, this understanding of quality and safety and how to both measure and improve are critical skills that will ensure that we will be the "health care reformers" that are so needed in this new world of evidence-based, value-based, pay-for-performance care. DNP-prepared nurses should be and can be the "health care reformers" of the future with the appropriate knowledge and skills in quality and safety. It is incumbent upon doctoral faculty to include this content in DNP curricula and require these competencies as the requisite skill set for DNP-prepared nurses irrespective of clinical specialty or focus.

■ REFERENCES

Agency for Healthcare Research and Quality. (2014a). Effective health care. Retrieved from http://effectivehealthcare.ahrq.gov

Agency for Healthcare Research and Quality. (2014b). Working for quality. Retrieved from http://www.ahrq.gov/workingforquality

Institute for Healthcare Improvement. (2015). History, 2015. Retrieved from http://www.ihi.org/about/Pages/History.aspx

Leapfrog Group. (2010). The leapfrog group announces top hospitals of the decade. Retrieved from http://www.leapfroggroup.org/news/leapfrog_news/4784721

National Quality Forum. (2014). Retrieved from http://www.qualityforum.org/Home.aspx

CHAPTER NINE

The Clinical Scholar Role in Doctoral Advanced Nursing Practice

Elizabeth W. Gonzalez and M. Christina R. Esperat

The maturity of the nursing discipline and the challenges created by the market-driven environment that we live in today make clinical scholarship more important than ever before. The professional roles of nurses today require that nursing practice be consistent with the emerging knowledge. The roles and responsibilities of nurses will continue to expand, as they become the key health care providers of the next decades. The health care system continues in its transformation, and along with it, new challenges for health care professionals to justify and validate the care they provide. Nurse leaders are increasingly expected to provide the direction and management of the outcomes of the evaluation process. To improve outcomes, clinical decision must be grounded in clinical inquiry where nurses who practice in a scholarly manner work directly and collegially with other health care providers in other settings, both in the discovery and the application of new knowledge. The integration of knowledge across disciplines and the application of knowledge to solve practice problems and improve health outcomes are alternative ways that new phenomena and knowledge are generated in nursing practice other than through research (DePalma & McGuire, 2005; Rolfe & Davies, 2009; Sigma Theta Tau International [STTI], 1999). This chapter addresses the kind of clinical scholarship that is continuing to evolve as advanced practice nurses (APNs) with practice-focused doctorates generate evidence/knowledge to guide improvements in practice and outcomes of care.

■ HOW IS CLINICAL SCHOLARSHIP DEFINED?

The scholarly practice of nurses can be traced to Florence Nightingale's work (1860/1992) during the Crimean War, in which data and statistical methods were used for clinical decision making. For several decades, nursing leaders have discussed the scholarship of practice (Benner, Tanner, & Chesla, 1996; Dickoff & James, 1968; Diers, 1995). Although discovery is central to expanding knowledge, linking discovery with application is an essential underpinning for practice disciplines (Riley, Beal, Levi, & McCausland, 2002). Therefore, the traditional belief that scholarship is primarily for the conduct of original research is a serious limitation in a practice discipline such as nursing.

Boyer (1990) inspired most disciplines to engage in robust dialogues about the meaning of scholarship in modern times. Various nurse scholars have shared opinions on what a scholar and clinical scholarship means. In writing about clinical scholarship, Diers (1995) argued that while clinical research in nursing is an accepted form of scholarly activity, clinical research and clinical scholarship are not the same. According to Diers, clinical scholarship offers an alternative way of extending knowledge about nursing practice. She conceptualized clinical scholarship in a practice profession as an intellectual activity that creates a new understanding for the practice. Clinical scholarship examines the practice itself and offers rich descriptions of the practice. Through clinical scholarship, the practitioner synthesizes practice knowledge and challenges the theories and procedures that we have learned and practiced.

Wright and Leahey (2000) argued that clinical scholarship requires an immersion in clinical practice while simultaneously finding ways to articulate, describe, and analyze what is occurring within clinical practice. Using a framework to describe the fundamental building blocks of clinical scholarship, they differentiated perceptual, conceptual, and executive skills related to the nursing of families. According to Wright and Leahey (2000), perceptual skills focus on what the nurse observes, and conceptual skills involve how the nurse makes sense of what is observed, relying on his or her conceptual grounding and personal experience. In addition, there are executive skills that include what the nurse does. Specifically, how the nurse responds (communication skills) is based on how he or she conceptually makes sense of what is happening within the individual, family, and larger systems, as well as between himself or herself and these systems. Clinical scholarship is refined through many hours of observation and participation in therapeutic conversations between nurse clinicians and families using written documentation that requires analysis of these conversations. Clinical scholarship requires intellectual maturity that comes from expertise and repeated experiences, which is reflected in careful analyses of situations and critical assessment of responses. The explanations and reflections offered by the clinical scholar are contextualized in his or her personal history and are enhanced by his or her well-supported interpretations.

Melanie Dreher (1999) argued that clinical scholarship is a value orientation about inquiry and implies a willingness to scrutinize nursing practice. Clinical scholarship is an intellectual process grounded in curiosity about why our clients respond the way they do and why we, as nurses, do the things that we do. It includes challenging traditional nursing interventions, testing our ideas, predicting outcomes, and explaining both patterns and expectations. Clinical scholarship is rooted in observation on ways in which clients respond to their problems and to their treatments. Unfortunately, the observations nurses typically have documented often have not been for the purpose of improving patient outcomes, but rather for limiting liability. It is not sufficient to observe phenomena. Observations must be interpreted by comparing them with similar phenomena (whether or not those comparisons are drawn from personal clinical experience). Comparisons can also be accomplished by using what is known based on the literature. Synthesis builds on the analysis to create an understanding of why these patterns and/or exceptions exist. Synthesis in clinical scholarship is the process of explaining or attaching meaning to the observations and the use of comparisons in examining events or situations. Clinical scholars generate an interpretation of their observations through the process of discussion with colleagues within the nursing community and with other disciplines. Another example is the review of literature and the conduct of integrative reviews of nursing research that incorporate the informed and expert clinical knowledge of the clinician (Ganong, 1987). At another level, understanding meta-analyses of the science literature provides stronger evidence of practice phenomena under consideration.

In addition to observation, analysis, and synthesis, clinical scholarship includes application and dissemination—all of which result in a new understanding of nursing phenomena. With the current explosion of knowledge, there is an expectation that relevant knowledge must be translated to benefit societies. Various nurse scholars argued that clinical scholarship requires the ability to engage in critical theoretical discourse and discern gaps in knowledge related to clinical practice (Dracup, Cronenwett, Meleis, & Benner, 2005). Knowledge of different theoretical frameworks with various assumptions and theoretical propositions is critical for clinical scholars when choosing different types of evidence and in translating evidence into clinical practice. The Doctor of Nursing Practice (DNP)-prepared nurse can discover new ways of refining or transforming practice by using or adapting constructs and concepts in existing theoretical frameworks to solve everyday problems.

The scholarship of application encompasses translation of the knowledge to solve problems for individuals, families, or society. This type of scholarship requires integration of the knowledge of best practices in achieving the best outcomes. Building on Boyer's (1990) perspective on scholarship, Palmer (1986) described the scholarship of application as a complex activity and synthesis of observations of clients and patients "a complex activity that has as its purpose, the discovery, organization, analysis, synthesis, and transmission of knowledge resulting from client-centered nursing practice" (p. 318).

According to the American Association of Colleges of Nursing (AACN, 2015), clinical scholarship is focused on generating new knowledge through innovation of practice change, the translation of evidence, and the implementation of quality improvement processes in specific practice settings, systems, or with specific populations to improve health or health outcomes. New knowledge generated by the DNP graduate can be transferred to other population or systems but is not considered generalizable (AACN, 2015).

Clinical scholarship requires that the desired outcomes are identified and systematic observation and scientifically based methods are used to identify and solve clinical problems. Additionally, scientific principles, current research, consensus-based guidelines, quality improvement data, and other forms of evidence are used to support clinical practice and clinical decisions. Evidence-based practice stresses the use of research findings as well as other sources of reliable data from quality improvements, consensus of recognized experts, and affirmed clinical experience (Stetler et al., 1998). The movement in nursing toward "evidence-based practice" has been articulated by the leaders like Melnyk and Fineout-Overholt (2005), and has been widely adopted by the DNP program. For example, the faculty at the University of Washington have developed a practice-focused doctorate that includes practice inquiry in the curriculum, addressing the appraisal and translation of evidence into practice, and evaluation with the potential for collaborative clinical research endeavors (Magyary, Whitney, & Brown, 2006). Both evidence-based practice and practice inquiry are likely to impact DNP clinical scholarship now and in the future.

The clinical scholar with a practice-focused doctorate will provide leadership for evidence-based practice with skills in translational research. Clinical scholarship is achieved by reading, by thinking, by discussing with colleagues (interdisciplinary efforts), and by mentoring to generate possible explanations on a clinical problem. Clinical scholars seek validation with fellow clinicians on their documented observations regarding patients' goal-related progress. Interdisciplinary efforts are necessary skills for the translation of research findings. The value of shared reflections on practice and experience is critical. These reflections can be developed formally through written clinical narratives (Benner, 1984). Reflection, self-scrutiny, and subsequent dialogue form the basis for personal growth and mutual learning among peers.

Despite the variations in the definition of what scholarship means, the following are common themes that describe a scholar. Clinical scholars are characterized by a high level of curiosity, critical thinking, continuous learning, reflection, and the ability to seek and use a spectrum of resources and evidence to improve the effectiveness of clinical interventions. They consistently bring a spirit of inquiry and creativity to their practice to solve clinical problems and improve outcomes (STTI, 1999).

■ HOW IS CLINICAL SCHOLARSHIP DEMONSTRATED IN DNP GRADUATES?

In an era of unprecedented accountability for the delivery of quality, cost-managed health care, the nurses are being challenged to demonstrate effective and efficient care. Well-informed consumers are demanding greater access to quality health care. Rising patient acuity, escalating complexity in health care needs, and the increasing infusion of technology in health care systems are creating daunting challenges for nurses. Additionally, nurses are practicing in environments with limited financial resources. As these challenges increase, nurses can no longer rely on traditional nursing practices or base their clinical decisions on intuition and years of clinical experience to plan and implement care required in today's patients. Responding to this challenge requires collective knowledge, clinical expertise, and commitment to base patient-care decisions on evidence and involvement of patients. Clinical scholarship is particularly important for APNs with practice-focused doctorates to provide leadership in establishing clinical excellence and informed health care policy.

The master of science in nursing (MSN) degree historically has been the degree for specialized advanced nursing practice. With the development of DNP programs, a practice-focused doctorate, the DNP degree will become the preferred preparation for specialty nursing practice. According to the National Organization of Nurse Practitioner Faculties (2006), the competencies for the DNP are similar to the MSN (with mastery of an advanced specialty within nursing practice), but the DNP competencies are formulated with more emphasis on leadership, quality improvement, health care delivery systems, and health care policy. The implementation of a model for evidence-based practice has been documented to promote clinical scholarship among clinical nurse specialists in various institutions such as Baystate Medical Center in Massachusetts, the University of Texas Medical Branch, Kaiser Permanente and California Pacific Medical Center, and the University of Iowa Hospitals and Clinics and College of Nursing (STTI, 1999). Clinical scholarship among nurse specialists provides opportunities to generate reflective thinking for improved clinical practice and heightened awareness for a new standard for evidence-based thinking (STTI, 1999). Clinical scholarship for the practice-focused doctorate should build on what has been started by clinical scholars with the MSN degree to provide leadership for evidence-based practice. This requires the application of knowledge to solve clinical problems and generate evidence through their practice to guide improvements in practice, outcomes of care, and participation in collaborative research (DePalma & McGuire, 2005; Magyary et al., 2006). Evidence-based practice should result in better outcomes leading to a better quality of life for all citizens.

DNP graduates engage in advanced nursing practice and provide leadership for evidence-based practice. This requires competence in knowledge application activities: the translation of research into practice, the evaluation of practice, improvement of the reliability of health care practice and outcomes, and participation in collaborative research (DePalma & McGuire, 2005).

The DNP *Essentials* (AACN, 2006) articulate the competence of the graduate in terms of clinical scholarship. Graduates of the program are trained to use analytic methods to determine and implement the best evidence for practice. They do so in order to design and implement processes to evaluate outcomes of practice, practice patterns, and systems of care against national benchmarks to determine variances in practice outcomes and population trends. In addition, they design, direct, and evaluate quality improvement methodologies and apply relevant findings to develop practice guidelines and improve practice and the practice environment. They are trained in the use of information technology and research methods to accomplish these. The DNP clinical scholar functions as a practice specialist/consultant in collaborative knowledge-generating research, and disseminates findings from evidence-based practice and research to improve health care outcomes (AACN, 2006).

■ HOW IS EXPERTISE IN THE USE OF EVIDENCE-BASED PRACTICE ACHIEVED?

In practice, the utilization of research evidence does not occur in vacuum. Multiple contextual factors influence the diffusion of practices that carry the weight of evidence borne of scientific inquiry. Funk, Tornquist, and Champagne (1995) identified four categories of barriers perceived by nurses to the utilization of research in clinical practice: those related to nurses' research values and skills, those related to limitations in the setting, those related to how the research is communicated, and those related to the quality of the research itself. The DNP role's impact on facilitating evidence-based practice needs to be conceived as that of successfully overcoming those barriers. Because DNP competencies are formulated at a higher level with more emphasis on leadership, quality improvement, health care delivery systems, and health care policy, the DNP-prepared nurse will be expected to provide leadership in creating working environments for evidence-based practice, with the expectation necessitating a certain level of skills and competency in translating science into practice.

In terms of nurses' research values and skills, the DNP nurse can become a role model for change and transformation not only for the workplace environment, but also for the individual nurses working in that environment. This can occur at two levels by: (a) increasing the nurse's confidence in evaluating the quality of the research evidence and (b) changing perceptions regarding the benefits of changing practice with the use of research evidence. The nurse leader who is prepared at the doctoral level can actively participate in formal or informal discussions on evaluating interventions reported in the research literature using the opportunity to increase nurses' knowledge and ability to evaluate research findings more wisely and logically. By taking on the role of an innovator, as an early adopter, the DNP nurse can create the climate for changing perceptions to one of increased respect and value for the scientific process and its outcomes.

As a leader in clinical practice, the DNP nurse can overcome limitations within the setting for practice. By allowing implementation of innovations through active support and provision of the needed structure and processes, the DNP administrator brings authority and accountability in facilitating the workplace environment for these innovations. This includes focusing on overcoming the limitations in how research is communicated. By providing the resources needed for the nurses and health care team to develop skills in reading, understanding, and evaluating research reports accurately and efficiently, the DNP administrator can promote, sustain, and maintain the implementation of evidence-based practice. In terms of barriers related to the quality of the research evidence, the DNP nurse can lead the effort to contribute further to the knowledge base by replicating investigations that evaluate the effectiveness of interventions. This requires a step beyond simply implementing and measuring the outcomes of interventions, to formally testing hypotheses regarding the impact of such interventions on nursing and health care. In effect, it requires the DNP-prepared nurse to be skilled in the conduct, use, and dissemination of translational research.

In various leadership roles, the DNP-prepared nurse is uniquely positioned to innovate and experiment with various models for increasing the utilization of research in practice settings. With administrative authority that comes with these leadership roles, the DNP-prepared nurse should have multiple options available for integrating research into the workplace environment. Whether it is increased and more effective use of existing resources or the deployment of external support and expertise, the DNP nurse can raise the organization to higher levels of application of translational science into practice. Particularly in promoting the translation of science into practice, the DNP nurse can engage in action research, which leads to the solution of everyday practical, as well as clinical, problems.

■ IS ACTION RESEARCH ORIENTED FOR DNP CLINICAL SCHOLARSHIP?

Methods to increase the quality and rate of research translation are increasingly becoming the focus of clinical practice. Leadership in clinical practice requires recognition that evidence-based practice is central to the achievement of effective and efficient health care delivery and to obtaining positive client outcomes (Mohide & Coker, 2005). Traditional approaches to building the evidence predominate in the current research enterprise. Nevertheless, there is increasing pressure upon the scientific community to look at alternative paradigms to increase the uptake of research evidence into community- and population-wide practice. Action research, one such alternative paradigm, is science designed to obtain practical results to solve a specific challenge. Engagement in action research is one in which the DNP nurse is optimally positioned, with the strong leadership skills in community-based initiatives that is one of the hallmarks of the education and preparation for DNP practice. In addition to the basic steps in traditional research of design, data collection, analysis, and communication, this alternative paradigm requires action, which is developmental in nature and has a wide range of applications in health care. This showcases the strengths and talents of the DNP nurse; it highlights the natural skills of the practitioner for practical solutions to real and actual problems in the clinical setting as they occur. In addition to skills and competencies in the application of multidimensional and multifaceted designs of participatory action research, the DNP nurse is prepared to lead communities to form collaborative partnerships with the academic scientists in community-based initiatives that aim to solve problems facing vulnerable populations (Stringer, 2007).

■ WHAT IS THE ROLE OF THE DNP CLINICAL SCHOLAR IN DISSEMINATION?

The role of the DNP nurse as clinical scholar has within it an inherent obligation and responsibility to disseminate knowledge and expertise gained from practice to various audiences. There are many reasons for engaging in the dissemination process. These include the sharing of ideas and new knowledge for the improvement of health care delivery to influencing outcomes of health care. In addition, for practical purposes, dissemination activities are essential job requirements, including requirements for promotion and tenure in any work setting. Thus, DNP preparation includes experiences aimed at developing and increasing skills in manuscript writing as well as in oral presentations in the dissemination of ideas. In leadership roles, the DNP nurse can create the climate for scholarship for those with whom she or he works. Increasingly, the endeavor to produce manuscripts for publication is carried on by writing teams that are engaged in common activities in health care delivery. Likewise, the tasks of preparing and delivering oral as well as poster presentations become less daunting and onerous if undertaken by teams of colleagues engaged in similar activities of dissemination. The DNP nurse provides the needed leadership to get the initiative started, to provide the resources for people to engage in these activities, and to encourage the work of continued and active scholarship. This also provides opportunities for mentoring and mentorship among nurses and other health care professionals who work together to achieve health care goals for groups of patients.

■ SUMMARY: THE FUTURE OF THE DNP CLINICAL SCHOLAR

Whether the creation of this degree enhances the progress of the clinical scholarship for the profession of nursing and furthers the quality of patient care depends entirely on the nursing profession's willingness to address the critical issues related to educational quality, outcomes, and standards. Focusing on the issue of the preparation of the DNP as a clinical scholar is of particular importance. At the current time, when standards of DNP education are continuing to evolve, it is critically important that the skills and competencies that have been articulated to prepare the DNP for this role be coupled with specific parameters for identifying the outcomes of this preparation relative to this role. Learning experiences in the educational and training curricula must emphasize increasing skills in the application of translational research, while at the same time the development of higher levels of competencies in the conduct of evaluation research and dissemination of critical findings must be facilitated and monitored before the DNP is granted the degree. The DNP graduate should be educated and trained for the increasingly interprofessional nature of practice within a transformed health care system. To prepare the DNP for the increased and enhanced roles in leadership, communication, and team practice, there must be opportunities for inter- and intra-professional collaboration, both between DNP and PhD nursing students as well as between DNP students and other health professions' students. Increasingly, many DNP students have found opportunities to work with students in other fields such as engineering, public health, health care administration, and business (AACN, 2015).

Nursing leaders and state and national organizations have spent considerable time and finances ensuring the public, legislators, and other members of the health care community that the educational level that nurses currently possess results in high quality care. Although it is intuitively appealing that educational requirements and standards will address the Institute of Medicine's (IOM's) concerns about patient safety and health care quality (IOM, 2000, 2001, 2003), there are inconsistencies in the educational preparation of DNP nurses that may not fulfill the promise on the quality of patient care and progress in the nursing profession. Studies relating educational preparation and quality at the entry level do support that more and different education results in higher quality

(Stanley, 2005). However, these data are not generalizable to advanced practice, and the suggestion that better patient care will result from this preparation, although intuitively appealing, must be documented based on evidence. These challenges must encourage continuous dialogue about the best educational preparation for doctorally prepared APNs who will assume the role of clinical scholars. This is critical as changes in technology, health care delivery systems, science, and changing and evolving roles for nurses all require that the nurse of tomorrow be prepared to participate in the health care system as it evolves. Additionally, employers and professional organizations should provide mechanisms for exercising leadership that support activities for clinical scholarship for DNPs. It is imperative that professional nursing groups and organizations endorse a call for more prolific clinical scholarship in this new cadre of DNPs as central to their mission and philosophy and as a rationale for a practice-focused doctorate. Furthermore, the workplace also needs to state its commitment through tangible means of support to enhance clinical scholarship.

■ CRITICAL THINKING QUESTIONS

1. *Explain the differences in the clinical scholarship of a practice-focused doctorate from a research-focused doctorate.*
2. *Describe the kind of clinical scholarship you believe is most appropriate for the practice-focused doctorate.*
3. *Explain why knowledge in theoretical frameworks is critical for clinical scholars with a practice-focused doctorate.*
4. *Why is clinical scholarship for APNs with practice-focused doctorates important?*
5. *How should clinical scholarship differ in advanced practice MSN from the DNP APN?*
6. *How does a DNP APN achieve expertise in use of evidence-based practice?*
7. *Explain the importance of action research for a clinical nursing scholar.*
8. *Explain how dissemination activities could be achieved by the DNP clinical scholar.*
9. *Discuss issues/barriers in the development of a DNP clinical scholar.*
10. *Explain the role of administrators in supporting DNP clinical scholars.*

■ REFERENCES

American Association of Colleges of Nursing. (2006). *The essentials of doctoral education for advanced nursing practice*. Retrieved from http://www.aacn.nche.edu/dnp/Essentials.pdf

American Association of Colleges of Nursing. (2015). *The doctor of nursing practice: Current issues and clarifying recommendations (Report from the Task Force on the Implementation of the DNP)*. Washington, DC: Author. Retrieved from http://www.aacn.nche.edu/news/articles/2015/dnp-white-paper

Benner, P. (1984). *From novice to expert: Excellence and power in clinical nursing practice*. Menlo Park, CA: Addison Wesley.

Benner, P., Tanner, C., & Chesla, C. (1996). *Expertise in nursing practice: Caring, clinical judgment and ethics*. New York, NY: Springer Publishing.

Boyer, E. (1990). *Scholarship reconsidered: Priorities of the professoriate*. Princeton, NJ: Carnegie Endowment for the Advancement of Teaching.

DePalma, J., & McGuire, D. (2005). Research. In A. B. Hamric, A. Spross, & C. Hanson (Eds.), *Advanced practice nursing: An integrative approach* (3rd ed., pp. 257–300). Philadelphia, PA: Elsevier Saunders.

Dickoff, J., & James, P. (1968). Symposium on theory development in nursing. A theory of theories: A position paper. *Nursing Research, 17*(3), 197–203.

Diers, D. (1995). Clinical scholarship. *Journal of Professional Nursing, 11*(1), 24–30.

Dracup, K., Cronenwett, L., Meleis, A. I., & Benner, P. E. (2005). Reflections on the doctorate of nursing practice. *Nursing Outlook, 53*(4), 177–182.

Dreher, M. (1999). Clinical scholarship: Nursing practice as an intellectual endeavor. In Sigma Theta Tau International Clinical Scholar Task Force. Clinical Scholarship Resource Paper (pp. 26–33). Retrieved from https://www.nursingsociety.org/docs/default-source/position-papers/clinical_scholarship_paper.pdf?sfvrsn=4

Funk, S. G., Tornquist, E. M., & Champagne, M. T. (1995). Barriers and facilitators of research utilization: An integrative review. *The Nursing Clinics of North America, 30*(3), 395–407.

Ganong, L. H. (1987). Integrative reviews of nursing research. *Research in Nursing & Health, 10*(1), 1–11.

Institute of Medicine. (2000). *To err is human: Building a safer health system.* Washington, DC: National Academies Press.

Institute of Medicine. (2001). *Crossing the quality chasm.* Washington, DC: National Academies Press.

Institute of Medicine. (2003). *Health professions education: A bridge to quality.* Washington, DC: National Academies Press.

Magyary, D., Whitney, J. D., & Brown, M. A. (2006). Advancing practice inquiry: research foundations of the practice doctorate in nursing. *Nursing Outlook, 54*(3), 139–151.

Melnyk, B., & Fineout-Overholt, E. (2005). *Evidence-based practice in nursing and healthcare: A guide to best practice.* Philadelphia, PA: Lippincott Williams & Wilkins.

Mohide, E. A., & Coker, E. (2005). Toward clinical scholarship: Promoting evidence-based practice in the clinical setting. *Journal of Professional Nursing, 21*(6), 372–379.

National Organization of Nurse Practitioner Faculties. (2006). Practice doctorate entry level nurse practitioner competencies. Retrieved from http://www.nonpf.com/NONPF2005/PracticeDoctorate ResourceCenter/CompetencyDraftFInalApril2006.pdf

Nightingale, F. (1860/1992). *Notes on nursing.* New York, NY: Lippincott Williams & Wilkins.

Palmer, I. S. (1986). The emergence of clinical scholarship as a professional imperative. *Journal of Professional Nursing, 2*(5), 318–325.

Riley, J. M., Beal, J., Levi, P., & McCausland, M. P. (2002). Revisioning nursing scholarship. *Journal of Nursing Scholarship, 34*(4), 383–389.

Rolfe, G., & Davies, R. (2009). Second generation professional doctorates in nursing. *International Journal of Nursing Studies, 46*(9), 1265–1273.

Sigma Theta Tau International. (1999). *Clinical scholarship resource paper.* Clinical Scholarship Task Force, Sigma Theta Tau International. Indianapolis, IN: Author.

Stanley, J. (2005). Evaluating the doctorate of nursing practice: Moving toward a new vision of nurse practitioner education. *Journal of Nurse Practitioners, 1*(4), 209–212.

Stetler, C. B., Brunell, M., Giuliano, K. K., Morsi, D., Prince, L., & Newell-Stokes, V. (1998). Evidence-based practice and the role of nursing leadership. *The Journal of Nursing Administration, 28*(7–8), 45–53.

Stringer, E. (2007). *Action research* (3rd ed.). Thousand Oaks, CA: Sage.

Wright, L., & Leahey, M. (2000). *Nurses and families: A guide to family assessment and intervention* (3rd ed.). Philadelphia, PA: F. A. Davis.

CHAPTER NINE

Reflective Response 1

Bernadette Mazurek Melnyk

The chapter by Gonzalez and Esperat clearly describes the role of the Doctor of Nursing Practice (DNP)-prepared nurse as providing leadership for evidence-based practice (EBP). This description is congruent with the American Association of Colleges of Nursing (AACN) and the DNP essentials, which have always been clear that the DNP should produce clinicians who are not researchers, but leaders in EBP (AACN, 2004, 2006). This DNP leadership role requires competency in translating research findings into practice, critically appraising a body of evidence, evaluating outcomes of practice changes, applying research in decision making, and implementing viable clinical innovations to change practice (Melnyk, 2016). Although it was never the intent of the DNP degree to prepare nurse researchers, there remains confusion in academic curricula across the United States about how to prepare the students enrolled in these programs. Many DNP programs continue to require original research for DNP capstone projects when it was never the intent for the DNP prepared nurse to conduct rigorous research as is expected for PhD graduates. One reason for this research expectation is that many faculty teaching in DNP programs are excellent PhD-prepared researchers, yet they have never developed strong knowledge and skills in EBP. As faculty cannot teach what they themselves do not know, they must be given the opportunity to develop these skills if they will be mentoring DNP students to be EBP experts (Melnyk, 2013). Unfortunately, publications have even contended that the role of DNPs should be practitioner-researchers (Vincent, Johnson, Velasquez, & Rigney, 2010).

Because DNP programs do not incorporate all of the research methodology and statistics courses required in PhD programs, DNP graduates are not sufficiently prepared to conduct rigorous original research. As a result, the research being produced by DNPs may have inherent limitations that could eventually weaken the body of nursing science. DNP programs should prepare EBP experts who can generate internal evidence through outcomes management and conduct evidence-based quality improvement initiatives. In addition, DNP graduates should be outstanding EBP mentors who facilitate system-wide cultures and environments that sustain evidence-based care. Instead of a research dissertation, DNP programs should require an EBP change project or evidence-based quality improvement project as the program's capstone requirement. However, DNPs can be valuable members of research teams, specifically in identifying gaps in EBP, bringing important clinical questions to the table for study, and assisting PhD researchers in conducting studies in real-world practice settings. They also can be instrumental in helping PhD researchers to develop interventions that will be relevant and scalable in clinical settings and key in rapidly translating research-based programs into practice once their efficacy has been established through research.

As a result of continued variability in the preparation of DNP graduates, health care systems also are confused about the role that DNP graduates should assume (Melnyk, 2013). Hospitals and health care systems who hire DNP graduates should expect that they are the best translators of research evidence into practice to enhance quality of care, improve population health outcomes and reduce health care costs. In their chapter, Gonzalez and Esperat mention that DNPs should conduct translational research. However, translational research should not be confused with EBP. Translational research is rigorous research that studies the barriers and facilitators of EBP and how best to translate research findings into practice whereas EBP is a seven step problem-solving approach to the delivery of health care that integrates the findings from well-designed studies with a clinician's expertise and a patient's preferences and values (Melnyk & Fineout-Overholt, 2015; Melnyk & Morrison-Beedy, 2012). It is only when clinicians deliver evidence-based care in an EBP culture and environment that it will sustain. Therefore, the DNP prepared nurse must not only be an expert in EBP, but they must have advanced knowledge and skills in facilitating individual behavior and organizational system change as many practicing clinicians do not consistently deliver evidence-based care and they must learn these new skills.

The DNP prepared nurse also must meet the new research-based EBP competences for practice nurses and advanced practice nurses. These advanced practice competencies include:

1. Systematically conduct an exhaustive search for external evidence to answer clinical questions
2. Critically appraise relevant pre-appraised evidence and primary studies, including evaluation and synthesis
3. Integrate a body of external evidence from nursing and related fields with internal evidence in making decisions about patient care
4. Lead transdisciplinary teams in applying synthesized evidence to initiate clinical decisions and practice changes to improve the health of individuals, groups and populations
5. Generate internal evidence through outcomes management and EBP implementation projects for the purpose of integrating best practices
6. Measure processes and outcomes of evidence-based clinical decisions
7. Formulate evidence-based policies and procedures
8. Participate in the generation of external evidence with other health care professionals
9. Mentor others in evidence-based decision making and the EBP process
10. Implement strategies to sustain an EBP culture
11. Communicate best evidence to individuals, groups, colleagues, and policy makers (Melnyk, Gallagher-Ford, Long, & Fineout-Overholt, 2014). Mentoring registered nurses and advanced practice nurses to meet the new research-based EBP competencies also should be inherent in the DNP role.

Both PhD prepared researchers and DNP prepared clinical scholars fulfill key roles in our health care system, but it is imperative that academic programs prepare each for the role they were intended to assume in our health care systems. Together, new evidence will be generated and quickly translated into practice and policy to improve the quality of health care and population health outcomes.

■ REFERENCES

American Association of Colleges of Nursing. (2004). AACN position statement on the practice doctorate in nursing. Retrieved from www.aacn.nche.edu/dnp/position-statement

American Association of Colleges of Nursing. (2006). *The essentials of doctoral education for advanced nursing practice.* Retrieved from http://www.aacn.nche.edu/publications/position/DNPEssentials.pdf

Melnyk, B. M. (2013). Distinguishing the preparation and roles of the PhD and DNP graduate: National implications for academic curricula and healthcare systems. *Journal of Nursing Education, 52*(8), 442–448.

Melnyk, B. M. (2016). The doctor of nursing practice degree: Evidence-based practice expert. *Worldviews on Evidence-Based Nursing, 13*(3), 183–184.

Melnyk, B. M., & Fineout-Overholt, E. (2015). *Evidence-based practice in nursing & healthcare. A guide to best practice* (3rd ed.). Philadelphia, PA: Wolters Kluwer.

Melnyk, B. M., Gallagher-Ford, L., Long, L. E., & Fineout-Overholt, E. (2014). The establishment of evidence-based practice competencies for practicing registered nurses and advanced practice nursesin real-world clinical settings: Proficiencies to improve healthcare quality, reliability, patient outcomes, and costs. *Worldviews on Evidence-Based Nursing, 11*(1), 5–15.

Melnyk, B. M., & Morrison-Beedy, D. (2012). *Intervention research: Designing, conducting, analyzing and funding intervention research. A practical guide for success.* New York, NY: Springer Publishing.

Vincent, D., Johnson, C., Velasquez, D., & Rigney, T. (2010). DNP-prepared nurses as practitioner-researchers: Closing the gap between research and practice. *The American Journal for Nurse Practitioners, 14*, 28–34.

CHAPTER NINE

Reflective Response 2

DeAnne Zwicker

As the beginning of my doctorate of nursing practice degree in 2007 with nearly 30 years of experience, I chose a research-based practice doctorate (DNP) program at Drexel University to better understand the research behind evidence-based practice (EBP). My review of the chapter "The Clinical Scholar Role in Doctoral Advanced Nursing Practice" by Elizabeth W. Gonzalez and M. Christina R. Esperat, was enlightening. When I started the DNP degree, EBP was rapidly becoming the norm. The Drexel program encompassed primarily research courses such as Qualitative and Quantitative Methods in Research, Philosophy, and a Dissertation. This was in contrast to the current Doctor of Nursing Practice (DNP) curriculum. The DrNP focused on understanding research principles, including limitations of research, levels of evidence, and translation of research evidence into practice. There were and still are a variety ways in which universities implement the DNP standards, many adding at least two more research-based courses and EBP. The DNP is rapidly becoming a requirement, especially for senior nursing role in practice. The DNP curriculum builds on prior research experience allowing nurses to lead the way in translation of evidence into practice. Building on that experience, the DNP is directed toward scholarship in clinical practice, testing delivery models, and practice improvement in health outcomes (AACN, 2004).

The concept of practice-based clinical scholarship has evolved over time as depicted by the authors in this chapter. Nurses are grounded in observation and gain perceptual and other necessary skills over many years of practice that enable them to grow and gain a higher level of knowledge and skills to analyze, synthesize, and interpret patient findings. This occurs at the graduate level. Also essential are critical thinking skills for the appropriate application of knowledge. Most experienced graduate level advanced practice registered nurses (APRNs) have learned how to learn to think critically and can apply their skills when complex problems occur in a fast-paced clinical setting. Accuracy in judgment using reasoning and problem-solving skills become well honed. Ultimately, clinical experience enables nurses to generalize knowledge and apply it to different situations (Grose, 2013). Building on the graduate knowledge is the next level of the DNP. Graduate nurses are inherently able to move to a higher level of implementation and facilitation of translation science.

The authors' discussion on interprofessional teams (IPT) is key. Rounds with other disciplines (medicine, psychology, social work, case manager, and others) can enhance the learning of the team members and address a holistic approach to care prioritizing needs of patients and family. This method is especially important in patients with complex needs. One study showed that an IPT managing vulnerable older adults (mean age: 80.9 years) were able to reduce the expected length of stay by 1.03 days and the incidence of complications, lower than the control group (Borenstein et al., 2015). Further research is greatly needed to evaluate the outcomes using IPT to demonstrate the effectiveness and cost saving of the collaboration.

The significant challenge, as noted in this chapter, seems unsurmountable. An example experienced in practice is a large hospice group has two different software systems, one for inpatients and a different system for outpatients in the same organization. These systems do not communicate. This creates repetitive, time-consuming extra work that results in not only information errors that may lead to an adverse event but also takes away time with patients and families. Finally, we now have had many graduates of DNP programs across the country. A presentation of what our DNP clinical scholars have achieved thus far would be welcome information of nursing's clinical scholarship success, to date, and the implications for the future. According to a RAND faculty survey (2014) the DNP has shown value added to practice and the Institute of Medicine agrees (Auerbach et al., 2014). Future research needs to focus not only on the outcomes of DNP scholars but also the value added.

■ REFERENCES

American Association of Colleges of Nursing. (2004). *Position statement on the practice doctorate in nursing.* Washington, DC. Retrieved from http://www.aacn.nche.edu/publications/position/DNPpositionstatement.pdf

Auerbach, D., Martsolf, G., Pearson, M. L., Taylor, E. A., Zaydman, M., Muchow, A., . . . Dower, C. (2014). *The DNP by 2015: A study of the institutional, political, and professional issues that facilitate or impede establishing a post-baccalaureate doctor of nursing practice program.* The RAND Corporation. Retrieved from http://www.aacn.nche.edu/dnp/DNP-Study.pdf

Auerbach, D. I., Martsolf, G., Pearson, M. L., Taylor, E. A., Zaydman, M., Muchow, A., . . . Dower, C. (2015). *A study of the institutional, political, and professional issues that facilitate or impede establishing a post-baccalaureate doctor of nursing practice program.* Santa Monica, CA: Rand Health Division/American Association of Colleges of Nursing.

Borenstein, J. E., Aronow, H. U., Bolton, L. B., Dimalanta, M. I., Chan, E., Palmer, K., . . . Braunstein, G. D. (2015). Identification and team-based interprofessional management of hospitalized vulnerable older adults. *Nursing Outlook, 64*(2), 137–145.

Grose, C. (2013). Beyond skills training revisited: The clinical education spiral. *Clinical Law Review, 19*(2), 489–515.

CHAPTER NINE

Reflective Response 3

Lydia D. Rotondo

In Chapter 9, the authors frame the discussion of the clinical scholar role in doctoral advanced nursing practice in the context of the external forces that are driving evidence-based responses to improve the delivery and outcomes of care and an evolving view of how Doctor of Nursing Practice (DNP)-prepared nurses can lead evidence-based practice (EBP) efforts. It has been well established that the reinvigorated efforts to launch a practice doctorate in nursing nearly 15 years ago were significantly influenced by the increasing complexity of the health care environment, clear evidence that the status quo in health care was no longer sustainable, and a strong sense that nurses could more fully leverage their clinical expertise and disciplinary perspective to accelerate health care transformation (American Association of Colleges of Nursing [AACN], 2006). Ten years after the publication of *The Essentials of Doctoral Education for Advanced Nursing Practice*, however, the nascent role of the DNP scholar continues to hold considerable unrealized potential. While the demand for scholarly output related to outcomes of DNP practice has dominated professional discourse, the equally compelling need for nurses with practice doctorates to explore the theoretical knowledge embedded in practice remains largely unaddressed.

The authors emphasize that increasingly, the generation and utilization of valid evidence in practice will be the cornerstone of transformational care that is patient-centered, high quality, and cost-effective. In this changing health care milieu, the term clinical scholarship has become synonymous with a form of practice inquiry that seeks opportunities to improve care, develops solutions to clinical problems, generates new understandings from clinical practice, and identifies new areas of practice inquiry (AACN, 2006, 2015). As the authors emphasize, clinical scholarship is inextricably enmeshed in clinical practice and they call on DNP-prepared nurses to provide leadership in driving clinical excellence and informing health care policy.

Gonzalez and Esperat's in-depth discussion of the definition of clinical scholarship reflects the pluralistic nature of nursing knowledge. Building on Nightingale's empirical work during the Crimean War, the authors provide an overview of the contributions of leading nurse scholars in recent decades that also recognize personal and experiential sources. In addition, the authors emphasize the fundamental connection between the discovery and application of knowledge that is crucial for practice disciplines. Their inclusion of Boyer's (1990) seminal work challenging traditional orthodoxy of knowledge development affirms the scholarly contributions of DNP practice that is evidence-based and context specific. The importance of contextualizing care as a hallmark of DNP scholarship cannot be overstated in an ever-increasing EBP health care culture. The authors stress the vital role that DNP-prepared nurses play in addressing contextual factors that impede practice innovation and research utilization in health care systems. In addition, Jutel (2008) contends that "[i]t is not that science does not have the ability to ask questions, rather it is unable to contextualize its answers at either the individual or social level. Science explains disease; it does not treat patients" (p. 418). Thus, as clinical scholars, DNPs have an opportunity to fill the research–practice gap by adapting interventions to meet patient needs and to develop new practice-centered models of knowledge production in nursing.

While the authors acknowledge the importance of theoretical discourse in clinical practice, conceptualizing the scholarly role of the DNP-prepared nurse as theorist is not discussed. This crucial aspect of clinical scholarship deserves further deliberation and debate in both practice and academe. The critical question remains. How will DNP-prepared nurses generate disciplinary knowledge? In AACN's (2015) recent publication on the practice doctorate, scholarship is defined as the process of knowledge development within a discipline. The report also states that graduates of both research and practice-focused doctoral programs are prepared to produce new disciplinary knowledge (AACN, 2015). Importantly, this more capacious view offers an unprecedented opportunity to significantly increase the scholarly productivity of all doctorally prepared nurses (less than 1% of all nurses). Exclusive focus on the role of DNP as knowledge translator, facilitator, and evaluator perpetuates a constraining paradigm that marginalizes nursing knowledge and undermines professional jurisdiction over practice (Jutel, 2008; Reed & Lawrence, 2008).

The pursuit of innovative approaches to developing theory-based practice knowledge by DNP-prepared clinical scholars will be critical to advancing a more unified worldview of clinical scholarship in nursing. Exposition of the "knowing practitioner" for whom theory and practice are inseparable could be an important area of DNP scholarly inquiry (Doane & Varcoe, 2005). Exploration of the mechanisms of knowledge generation in practice or the explication of practice inquiry methods that examine the unique interaction between nurse and patient could also be rich sources of DNP clinical scholarship (Reed, 2006; Rolfe, 2006). Finally, continued development of conceptual models that identify the distinct and shared contributions of nurse clinicians and nurse scientists to advance disciplinary knowledge will also be needed to further cultivate DNP scholarship (Velasquez, McArthur, & Johnson, 2011).

The authors provide a timely and relevant discussion of the clinical scholarship role of doctoral advanced nursing practice. With over 4,200 DNP graduates and more than 22,000 currently enrolled in DNP programs (Trautman, 2016), it is imperative that the scholarly contributions of doctoral-prepared advanced practice nurses to innovate and improve care be demonstrated and disseminated. Within the discipline, the emergence of the practice doctorate also provides exciting opportunities for scholarship through exploration of new epistemological approaches to knowledge production in nursing practice.

■ REFERENCES

American Association of Colleges of Nursing. (2006). *The essentials of doctoral education for advanced nursing practice*. Retrieved from http://www.aacn.nche.edu/publications/position/DNPEssentials .pdf

American Association of Colleges of Nursing. (2015). *The doctor of nursing practice: Current issues and clarifying recommendations*. Report from the Task Force on the Implementation of the DNP. Washington, DC: Author. Retrieved from http://www.aacn.nche.edu/aacn-publications/white-papers/DNP-Implementation-TF-Report-8-15.pdf

Doane, G. H., & Varcoe, C. (2005). Toward compassionate action: Pragmatism and the inseparability of theory/practice. *Advances in Nursing Science, 28*(1), 81–90.

Jutel, A. (2008). Beyond evidence-based nursing: Tools for practice. *Journal of Nursing Management, 16*, 417–421.

Reed, P. G. (2006). The practice turn in nursing epistemology. *Nursing Science Quarterly, 19*(1), 1–3.

Reed, P. G., & Lawrence, L. A. (2008). A paradigm for the production of practice-based knowledge. *Journal of Nursing Management, 16*, 422–432.

Rolfe, G. (2006). Nursing praxis and the science of the unique. *Nursing Science Quarterly, 19*(1), 4–8.

Trautman, D. (2016). *Opening program session*. Naples, FL: American Association of Colleges of Nursing.

Velasquez, D. M., McArthur, D. B., & Johnson, C. (2011). Doctoral nursing roles in knowledge generation. In P. G. Reed & N. B. Crawford Shearer (Eds.), *Nursing knowledge and theory innovation: Advancing the science of practice* (pp. 37–50). New York, NY: Springer Publishing.

Operationalizing Role Functions of Doctoral Advanced Nursing Practice

Role Strain in the Doctorally Prepared Advanced Practice Nurse: The Experiences of Doctor of Nursing Practice Graduates in Their Current Professional Positions—An Updated and Current View

Mary Ellen Smith Glasgow, Rick Zoucha, and Catherine Johnson

It is suggested that a role is the manifestation of behavior appropriate to an individual's position (Sveinsdottir, Biering, & Ramel, 2006). The Doctor of Nursing Practice (DNP) degree is a relatively new degree, created in 2004; therefore, the role of the doctoral advanced practice nurse (DAPRN) is not yet clearly defined in many settings (Nichols, O'Connor, & Dunn, 2014; Udlis & Mancuso, 2015). Nichols, O'Connor, and Dunn, (2014) observed that chief nursing officers (CNOs) are not well versed in the clinical outcomes of DNP practice or the population health outcomes that may be impacted by DNP-prepared providers. Udlis and Mancuso (2015) reported that confusion and disagreement about the DNP continues despite the rapid and steady growth of DNP programs. As a result, new DAPRNs may experience role stress in their new role. Psychologists, sociologists, and empirical researchers have conceptualized role stress from different perspectives (Hardy & Conway, 1978; Kahn, Wolf, Quinn, Snock, & Rosenthal, 1964; Lazarus, 1967). Hardy and Conway (1988) classified the dimensions of role stress specifically for health care professionals. These dimensions are role conflict, role ambiguity, role overload, role incompetence, and role incongruity. Among the many dimensions of role stress, most researchers have focused on the impact of role ambiguity or role conflict on personal or organizational outcomes; however, the role of the nurse has not been the focus of the research (Chen, Chen, Tsai, & Lo, 2007).

Role stress can arise from different patterns of mismatch in expectations, resources, capabilities, and values about the role (Chen et al., 2007). In an organization, an individual's role stress refers to "stress formed by the combined expectations of an individual's behavior from all circles" (Sveinsdottir et al., 2006). *Role strain* is a state of emotional arousal when an individual experiences role-related stress events, whereas role stress is external to the person in the role and results from societal demands. Role strain is conceptualized as one's perceived difficulty or angst in fulfilling role obligations. For example, a new DNP-prepared nurse executive who is unable to fulfill his or her obligations as defined by the chief executive officer (CEO) would experience role strain. The role expectations may be beyond what he or she is able to achieve or the CEO may push him to the limits of his abilities. It must be noted that role stress has not been differentiated from role strain in previous nursing studies, causing confusion as to whether results reflected perceptions external to the individual or internal responses over stressful events (Chen et al., 2007).

Role strain is in contrast to *role conflict*, where tension is felt between two or more, competing roles. Role conflict results when an individual encounters tensions as the result of incompatible roles. For instance, a mother who is employed full time as a DNP-prepared faculty member may experience role conflict because of the norms that are associated with the two roles she has. She may be expected to spend a great deal of time taking care of her children while simultaneously trying to advance her career as a teacher, scholar, clinician, and university citizen (Macionis, 2006).

Role ambiguity is defined as the lack of clarity related to one's position or role. A metasynthesis study by Jones in 2005 reviewed 14 relevant studies on role development and advanced practice nurses in the United States and the United Kingdom. Jones (2005) suggested that when advanced nursing roles were first introduced, clear role definitions and objectives needed to be developed and communicated to relevant key personnel to reduce role ambiguity. Interprofessional relationships and role ambiguity were the most important factors that enhanced or hindered performance. Variability of DNP academic programs in terms of quality, length, rigor, and competencies also contribute to role ambiguity (Udlis & Mancuso, 2012). So, when one considers the various sociopolitical issues that presently face new DAPRNs, given the relative newness of the role, they will confront an array of reactions and situations. For the purposes of this chapter, the term role strain is used as an umbrella term to discuss the perceived difficulty or angst in fulfilling role obligations experienced by DNP-prepared nurses for a variety of reasons.

In terms of role strain, organizational engagement efforts certainly play a key role in long-term solutions in the workplace. Engagement efforts require promoting job–person fit by matching individual and organizational profiles with six domains of work life: sustainable workload; feelings of choice and control; appropriate recognition and reward; supportive work community; fairness and justice; and meaningful and valued work (Shirey, 2006). Furthermore, the role for the DAPRN, irrespective of whether the individual is a nurse practitioner, midwife, anesthetist or clinical nurse specialist, clinical executive, or nurse educator, will demand a significant amount of the individual's time and attention. When one considers the multiple competing roles of the DAPRNs today (e.g., mother, father, caregiver, spouse or partner, professional, scholar, citizen), there are many demands for the DAPRNs' time in this fast-paced chaotic culture. The authors would be remiss if they failed to address the multiple roles of the DAPRN outside of his or her professional role, which can place great demands on the individual's time as well as serve as a great source of stress as the DAPRN attempts to achieve life balance and fulfill many competing demands.

■ DNP ROLE DESCRIPTIONS

In the workplace, DAPRNs (practitioners, clinical executives, or nurse educators) experience role strain for different reasons based on their respective roles. The following sections provide a descriptive overview of the prospective role strain for each role.

THE DNP-PREPARED PRACTITIONER

DAPRNs who are nurse practitioners provide expert primary health care or specialty health care to diverse populations in various health care agencies and venues. DAPRNs who are nurse-midwives, nurse anesthetists, and clinical nurse specialists also fulfill their professional roles. With health care reform, the future is bright for DAPRNs, especially if they innovate, design, or create efficient models of health care delivery. They may serve as leaders of nurse-managed clinics, private practices, convenient care clinics, or urgent care centers. They may serve as expert practitioners with additional confidence and knowledge to positively impact patient outcomes.

DAPRN's practice includes not only direct care, but also a focus on the needs of a group of patients, a target population, a set of populations, or a broad community. These graduates are distinguished by their abilities to conceptualize new care delivery models that are based in contemporary nursing science and that are feasible within current organizational, political, cultural, and economic perspectives. Graduates are skilled in working within organizational and policy arenas and in the actual provision of patient care by themselves and/or by others. For example, DAPRNs understand principles of practice management, including conceptual and practical strategies for balancing productivity with quality of care. They are able to assess the impact of practice policies and procedures on meeting the health needs of the patient populations with whom they practice. DAPRNs are proficient in quality improvement strategies and in creating and sustaining changes at the organizational and policy levels. They have the ability to evaluate the cost effectiveness of care and use principles of economics and finance to redesign effective and realistic care delivery strategies. In addition, DAPRNs have the ability to organize care in a way that addresses emerging practice problems and the ethical dilemmas that emerge as new diagnostic and therapeutic technologies evolve (American Association of Colleges of Nursing [AACN], 2006). Nichols et al. (2014) noted that CNOs are not well versed in the abilities and potential impact of the DNP. CNOs' knowledge of DNP-prepared nurses' abilities is critical to the widespread adoption and influence of DNPs in the health care system. CNO support is also necessary for the advocacy of DAPRN's scholarly release time and increased compensation expected with a higher level degree, increased knowledge, and expanded skill set.

It is clear that the DAPRNs can contribute significantly to the health and welfare of our nation; what is not clear is whether the role of the practitioner will change as a result of the DAPRN's additional knowledge and skills. If the workplace environment does not change, DAPRNs may feel frustrated in their role. They may also experience professional jealousy or other less than supportive behaviors from colleagues as a result of this relatively new role, as well as role overload based on the sheer amount of work to be accomplished.

THE DNP-PREPARED CLINICAL EXECUTIVE

The DNP clinical executive (CNOs, vice presidents, division leaders, and other executive-level nurse leaders) is called to address emergent and challenging issues for nursing practice, as well as to create opportunities that will shape and implement innovative changes in the health care system. Today, the DNP clinical executive is in short supply. Future doctoral level nurse administrators and executive leaders are also charged to improve health and health care outcomes through evidence-based practice in diverse clinical and health care settings. The DNP clinical executive emphasizes evidence-based approaches for quality and safety improvement in practice settings, applies research processes to decision making, and translates credible research findings to increase the effectiveness of both direct and indirect nursing practice. Some of the specific competencies outlined in the AACN's essentials document for the DNP clinical executive include the abilities to use sophisticated, conceptual, and analytical skills in evaluating the links among clinical, organizational, fiscal, and policy issues; establish processes for interorganizational collaboration for the achievement of organizational goals; design patient-centered care delivery systems or policy-level delivery models; collaborate effectively with legal counsel and financial officers around issues related to legal and regulatory guidelines; and demonstrate advanced levels of clinical judgment, cultural sensitivity, and systems thinking (AACN, 2006). The responsibilities for the DNP clinical executive may be daunting. As the leader, the DNP clinical executive will most likely not have a DNP-prepared CEO or role models to guide him or her as he or she navigates this senior executive role. He or she may experience the loneliness associated with a senior administration position. Fellow senior administrators and physicians may feel threatened with the credentials, power, influence, and position of the DNP clinical executive who traditionally did not hold a doctorate to serve in that leadership role.

THE DNP-PREPARED EDUCATOR

Current expectations of the tripartite nursing faculty role in relation to teaching, scholarship, and service are not realistic in advancing nursing science, clinical practice, or education. Nursing faculty juggle large teaching and service loads while attempting to engage in scholarship. For those nursing faculty who are research active, the juggling act is even more pronounced. In addition, few nursing faculty, with the exception of those faculty employed at universities with an academic health center, have formal practice appointments as part of their faculty role allowing them to stay clinically current to inform their teaching. For example, many nurse practitioners, nurse-midwifery, and nurse anesthesia faculty have outside practice obligations to maintain their clinical hours/expertise for specialty certification, in addition to their full-time faculty appointments. With the introduction of the DNP educator, the profession has an opportunity to reexamine the various roles of nurse faculty and create a model that encourages the faculty to master one or two areas rather than the current "jack of all trades" approach. The authors suggest three roles for the nurse in academic positions: nurse scientist for the PhD-prepared faculty member, educator clinician, and clinician educator for both the PhD and DNP-prepared faculty. Nursing education must redefine the expectations of the nursing faculty with a primary focus on research, teaching, or clinical. The DNP educator is in a unique position to serve in the educator clinician role (e.g., 80% education and 20% practice) or clinician educator role (e.g., 80% practice and 20% education) as they are able to integrate the knowledge they present in the classroom with a clinical practice context, yet they also have the educational theory to draw on in the classroom. However, this will not be easy as the academy is an institution ensconced in tradition and may not embrace the DNP educator role as an equal. Therefore, the DNP educator may be viewed as a second-class citizen in the academy causing additional role strain as well as experience role overload from the tripartite role in academe and additional practice requirements. There is dissonance in the academy regarding the role and contributions of the DNP-prepared faculty member. According to Udlis and Mancuso (2015), DNP participants felt prepared for the demands of the faculty role and the requisite tenure, research, and scholarship requirements. PhD participants disagreed that the DNP degree prepares graduates to assume these responsibilities. Multiple areas of confusion continue to exist concerning the role of the DNP-prepared faculty member with respect to faculty scholarly and practice expectations, academic leadership potential, and tenure that need to be clarified.

■ A SUMMARY OF THE 2011 FINDINGS: "THE EXPERIENCES OF DNPs IN THEIR CURRENT PROFESSIONAL POSITIONS"

The original qualitative study sought to understand the experiences of DNP-prepared nurses who held faculty, advanced practice, or executive positions in nursing by conducting a study on the lived experience of the DNP in his or her new professional role. There were nine informants who were interviewed for this original study. There were eight women and one man. The ages ranged from 38 to 64 years, with the median age being 49 years. The majority of informants ($n = 7$) were from Pennsylvania and the remainder ($n = 2$) from New Jersey. All the informants identified their culture or race as White with five more specifically identifying themselves as either Italian American or one Polish American. All the informants received DNP degrees and all started as postmaster's students. The length of the doctoral program varied from 1.5 years to 4 years, with the average length of time being 2.8 years. The focus of the DNP program for the informants included five with a focus in nursing education, three in advanced practice, and one in clinical research. The major focus of the *current job* of the informants was one nurse-midwife, three nurse practitioners, one nurse executive, three nurse educators, and one in a dual role of nurse practitioner and nurse educator. The focus of the analysis was on both description and interpretation of the phenomena of interest. Three major themes emerged from the study: (a) *Context of the DNP Role*; (b) *Feelings of Confidence and Empowerment in the Role as a DNP*; and (c) *Finding My Way by Finding and Responding to Opportunity.*

The informants' confidence and sense of empowerment was refreshing and very much needed to effect change, as well as being consistent with the AACN's vision for the degree (AACN, 2006). They were enthusiastic about their advanced knowledge and wanted to apply that knowledge in their respective roles. However, many of them experienced role strain as they reported a lack of clarity and angst related to their new position or role. This phenomenon was consistent with the findings by Jones (2005) that clear role definitions need to be developed for new roles and communicated to all stakeholders over time to reduce role ambiguity and/or strain.

When the researchers reflected on the findings in this study, the experiences of some DNP graduates were not necessarily surprising in lieu of nursing's history. DNP graduates employed in advanced nursing practice roles have expressed concern that in some cases, the work environment is not always accepting of the DNP especially in advanced practice settings. From our history, we know that nursing practice, and to some degree education, has been slow to recognize or come to terms with the distinct differences of the associate degree (AD)-level graduate versus the baccalaureate (bachelor of science in nursing [BSN])-level graduate (Moltz, 2010). Many DAPRN's role and expectations were no different than that of the master's-level advanced practice nurse's role and expectations. One hopes that the lack of differentiation in practice roles in the clinical arena may be due to the "relative newness" of the degree; however, it may also be due to the similarities in the scope of practice of the two degrees or, sadly, an anti-intellectual mentality or propensity for professional jealousy that exist for some in the profession. If the practice arena does not distinguish the role, competencies, and expectations of the DNP versus the master of science in nursing (MSN) advanced practice nurse in the future, *nursing may very well find itself in the same position as we are with the lack of differentiation between the AD and BSN graduates in clinical practice.*

■ "THE EXPERIENCES OF DNPs IN THEIR CURRENT PROFESSIONAL POSITIONS: AN UPDATED AND CURRENT VIEW"

Due to the novel and innovative nature of the various DNP roles, the authors sought to continue to understand the experiences of DNP-prepared nurses who currently hold faculty, advanced practice, or executive positions in nursing by conducting a study on the lived experience of the DNP in his or her new professional role. This study titled "The Experiences of DNPs in Their Current Professional Positions: An Updated and Current View" was unique as there are limited studies to understand the role of the DNP in the literature. Some existing studies by Smith Glasgow and Zoucha (2011); Dreher, Smith Glasgow, Cornelius, and Bhattacharya, (2012); Nichols et al. (2014); Smeltzer et al. (2015); and Udlis and Mancuso (2015) discuss the salient role and quality of work–life issues related to the DNP and address the need for further clarity on the education, role, and expectations of the DNP-prepared nurse.

PURPOSE AND SIGNIFICANCE OF THE STUDY

The AACN member institutions voted in October 2004 to champion the DNP degree as the desired preparation for future nurses prepared for advanced nursing specialty practice, including the four most recognized advanced practice nursing (APN) roles of nurse practitioners, clinical nurse specialists, nurse-midwives, and nurse anesthetists (AACN, 2009). Additionally, the AACN offered the DNP for advanced practice preparation of the clinical executive (AACN, 2006). The AACN recommended that academic institutions that prepare nurses for advanced practice prepare them at the doctoral level, instead of the current master's level, by the year 2015 (AACN, 2009). The AACN Annual Survey of Baccalaureate and Graduate Nursing Programs revealed that 98 (25%) had a BSN-to-DNP program and 229 (57%) MSN-to-DNP programs. Overall the number of schools with a DNP has increased tenfold in the past 7 years. Sixty-three schools report planning a BSN-to-DNP and another 33 schools report offering another track (Auerbach et al., 2014).

The change in the level of desired advanced practice nurse preparation has also led to a change in educational requirements and focus on evidence-based practice as noted in *The Essentials of Doctoral Education for Advanced Nursing Practice* published by the AACN in 2006. The major emphasis of the DNP is advanced practice, as opposed to the PhD, which emphasizes research (AACN, 2006). Loomis, Willard, and Cohen (2007) found that the majority of DNP students reported considering the PhD educational route, but chose the DNP over the PhD because of their disinterest in research and desire to become clinical experts. They reported that in these DNP students, 55% identified that nursing education was their professional goal, and 61% reported that they considered eligibility to be a nursing faculty member as an advantage of the DNP degree (Loomis et al., 2007). Schools and colleges of nursing are rapidly developing more DNP educational programs, and increased numbers of students are enrolling in these new APN programs. It is imperative that research is conducted to understand this possible transition in nursing education and practice, and the potential effect on nursing as a profession. Because the role of the DNP is relatively new and many are now beginning to enter into the employment arena, there is a gap in the literature as to what actual positions these DNPs are pursuing and how they are experiencing their new roles. A research study that investigates the current role choices and experiences of DNP graduates can increase nursing knowledge about the role and experiences of the newly established position. The findings can be disseminated through publication with the intention of closing the gap in the literature and contribute to future discussions about the role and educational preparations for DNP students. The authors of this chapter conducted a qualitative study to initiate this area of inquiry.

RESEARCH DESIGN AND PROCEDURES

The following research question guided the focus and method for the study: What is the lived experience of the DNP-prepared nurse who currently holds faculty, advanced practice, or administration position in nursing? Nurses holding the DNP degree were sought for this study to explore and understand their experiences in their current professional contexts using a descriptive, interpretive phenomenological approach in the tradition of the Dutch (Utrecht) School of Phenomenology. The Dutch approach to phenomenology is both descriptive and interpretive, and was used to guide this research. The research process focused on what informants verbally expressed regarding the meaning in the context of their particular DNP role. Before beginning the interviews, the researchers bracketed their presuppositions about the role of the DNP by discussing their presuppositions with each other. The process of bracketing was done to ensure that the researchers did not influence the informants and their responses during the study (Cohen, 1995). The research process allowed the researchers to engage in dialogue and discussion with the informants to clarify, verify, and interpret the data.

INSTRUMENTS

An investigator-designed open, unstructured interview guide was used to understand the experiences of DNPs who currently hold faculty, advanced practice, or executive positions in nursing. In addition, demographic data were gathered to understand the context of the informants and assist with data analysis.

INFORMANT RECRUITMENT AND INFORMED CONSENT

Once approval was obtained from the university Institutional Review Board (IRB), informants were purposefully sought out through the snowball method in the nursing community in Pennsylvania and New Jersey. Ethical considerations related to data collection were included in the procedures that honored the privacy, feelings, and dignity of the informants and were intended to minimize any risks from the research process. The informants were informed of their rights and their willingness to participate in the study by reading and signing the informed consent. They were also informed that they had the right to withdraw from the study at any time. A voluntary, purposeful sample of eight nurses who held a DNP degree and who were currently employed either in nursing education, clinical practice, or administration in nursing were recruited for this study. Nursing education DNPs were included if they were currently employed full time in a tenure or nontenure track position at a school of nursing in a college or university setting offering a minimum of a BSN. DAPRNs were included if they were employed full time as a nurse practitioner, clinical nurse specialist, nurse-midwife, or nurse anesthetist. DNP-prepared nurse executives were included who had full-time employment as a nurse executive in a health care institution.

COLLECTION OF DATA AND METHOD OF DATA ANALYSIS

The informants were interviewed in a place of their choice providing privacy and comfort. The in-depth interviews lasted up to one and one-half hours and no second interviews were requested by any informants or researchers for confirmatory purposes. Thematic saturation of the data occurred after six interviews, and two additional informants were sought for confirmation of the data. Thematic saturation for this study meant that there were no new surprises in the data and no new themes emerged (Bowen, 2008). Trustworthiness, credibility, dependability, confirmability, and transferability of the data were achieved. The data were analyzed by one researcher and validated by a second researcher during the process of data collection and analysis.

The interviews were audiotaped and the data transcribed verbatim for analysis. Concurrent data collection and analysis occurred, allowing the data to guide the analysis and further data collection. Analysis followed the procedures outlined by scholars from the Dutch (Utrecht) school (Barritt, Beekman, Bleeker, & Mulderjif, 1984). The data analysis process called for a two-part analysis of identifying common forms and shared themes or themes. In using this method, the researchers constructed a thematic analysis of the narrative through identifying the experiential (van Kaam, 1991). Nvivo 10 qualitative data manager was used to assist with the data analysis.

FINDINGS

The findings of this study are being presented according to the process of analysis. There were eight informants who were interviewed for this study. There were eight women in the study. The ages ranged from 51 to 63 years, with the median age being 57.6 years. The majority of informants ($n = 7$) were from Pennsylvania and the remainder ($n = 1$) from New Jersey. All the informants identified their culture or race as White. All the informants received DNP degrees and all started as post-master's students. The focus of the DNP program for the informants included five with a focus in advanced practice, and three in administration/leadership. The major focus of the *current job* of the informants was one nurse-midwife, one nurse practitioner, three nurse executives, and three nurse educators, with one informant having a dual role of nurse practitioner and nurse educator.

The focus of the analysis was on both description and interpretation of the phenomena of interest. The first step was to identify *common forms* after an analysis of the narrative (Barritt et al., 1984). The following were identified for this study:

1. Dual role
2. Emerging role
3. Feeling different after the degree
4. Keeping current
5. Knowing the limits
6. Nurses/colleagues pushback

7. Open doors
8. Organizational value
9. Role confusion
10. Support from nurses/colleagues
11. Things are the same

Further and more in-depth analysis of the common forms revealed shared themes or themes from the informant's experiences in their current role as a DNP. The following are the themes:

1. The changing and evolutionary context and environment of the DNP role, supported by the following common forms:
    a. Emerging role, open doors, organizational value, support from nurses/colleagues
2. The emerging feelings of confidence and respect in the role as a DNP, supported by the following common forms:
    a. Dual roles, emerging roles, feeling different after the degree, keeping current, organizational value, support from nurses/colleagues
3. Finding a settled place in the perceived role of the DNP, supported by the following common forms:
    a. Emerging roles, keeping current in clinical practice, nurses/colleagues pushback, organizational value, role confusion, support from nurses/colleagues

Theme 1: The Changing and Evolutionary Context and Environment of the DNP Role

The first shared theme interpreted from the data was the changing and evolutionary context and environment of the DNP advanced practice or nursing role. The context for this theme can be defined as the changing and more positive work environment and context of the informants. This includes hospital, school, or college of nursing, and private and collaborative practice. Informants very clearly defined, and described the content of their professional lives as DNP-prepared nurses. The informants in this study described environments where they felt valued and appreciated. They were given more responsibility and asked to engage in work that was consistent with their academic preparation. Many in the study felt that their peers were respectful of their thoughts and ideas mainly because of their academic preparation with a doctorate. Some informants felt that their education informed their current work and really prepared them for their current role. One informant summarized her thoughts about the environment of her role when she said, "People sort of celebrated the fact that I had a doctorate around me. Other people made a big deal of it which I felt was interesting." Overall, there was a sense that the environment and context of their professional roles was positive and supportive. They felt that this would only make them better at what they do as DNP-prepared nurses in their current role. Nurse executives had greater clarity about their roles and the support of the changing environment, followed by nurse educators. DNP's in practice felt that the advanced practice community did not fully embrace their doctoral level role to the same degree as nurse executives. The informants felt that the institutions in which they were employed were very accepting of the "individual nurse" in his or her role as a DNP but were not necessarily prepared to create roles for the DNP-prepared nurse. However, despite the difference in individual acceptance versus role expectations, there appeared to be pride among peers and acceptance for their new degree.

In almost all cases, there was a general level of acceptance for the DNPs in their roles despite some instances of misunderstanding and tension. Peers in the context of the work setting were generally accepting of these individuals in their new roles, especially for the nurse executive and nurse educators.

Theme 2: The Emerging Feelings of Confidence and Respect in the Role as a DNP

The second major shared theme from this study was feelings of confidence and respect in the role as a DNP-prepared nurse. The majority of informants in the roles of advance practice, nurse administrator, and nurse educator expressed confidence in their current roles. One informant said: "It is satisfying I guess, because having the doctorate, you do feel like more of a peer with the other colleagues with doctorates on campus." Another said, "It just feels like, I guess with the DNP degree, that doors kind of opened up for me." The degree has helped many of the informants feel well prepared and confident about how they both perceive their role and how they work in their role. One informant said, "I have become more open minded and I'm not afraid to bring my ideas to the table." Another informant reported that, "I think that having a level of confidence and not being afraid to fail is important." Some informants felt that the degree and preparation have helped them feel more confident in a specific role function such as evidence-based research. This is supported when one informant said, "I do feel prepared for that—sometimes I surprise myself."

Overall, the informants in this study felt that the DNP program prepared them with a sense of confidence and empowerment for their current role. Many felt that they perform their role well resulting in feeling respected—how they interact with peers, patients, students, and others in their role. Many informants felt that they were well prepared by their academic program to do their respective jobs. For many, it means that the degree has helped them feel confident and respected. Many informants felt that because they feel confident in their role currently, they will continue to grow and feel more confident and respected in the future.

Theme 3: Finding a Settled Place in the Perceived Role of the DNP

The third major theme described by the informants in this study was finding a settled place in the perceived role of the DNP-prepared nurse. This particular theme was evident in almost all the informants' experiences as they described their current role as a DNP. This shared theme is closely linked to themes one and two for many reasons. One clear connection was the fact that many informants were involved in multiple roles in their current role or primary and secondary jobs as a DNP. As found in the original study (2011) it is as if the informants in the study were seeking to find the right fit for their new-found confidence and a sense of being respected or valued by trying out a variety of roles. One informant said, "It feels good. I think that I could do anything." One informant felt that she has always been confident as a nurse practitioner but that her doctorate is giving her confidence to do well in any setting.

Informants in this study felt that they were originally seeking a place and a fit. They felt more comfortable in their current roles. Institutions and peers have accepted them in their role and they feel settled. This settled sense can be seen in the following statement by several informants: "I think people value DNP. I think they respect it. I think that when I am at the table with physicians, I think there is a sense of the playing field a little more level." Another informant said, "I think that the best thing I could say is that I am doctorally prepared and I feel more confident and comfortable arguing my points."

The majority of the informants in this study felt that their confidence has led to the acceptance of them and their role at their places of work. In the beginning they were looking for a place to fit and now feel more accepted and settled in their current role.

In summary, theme three seems to be the theme that connected and linked the three themes together. Overall, informants in this study expressed feeling more confident, respected, and settled in their current DNP role. Nurse executives seemed to have the clearest view of their role and the most support from their context or work environment. Informants felt more settled about the future and their evolving roles in administration, education, and practice. However, they would also like the profession, schools of nursing, and employers to continue to be clear about the expectations of the DNP in advanced practice, nursing education, and nursing administration. Informants felt that their programs prepared them in a manner that has helped them to feel confident and respected in their role. *They continued to express concerns that in some cases, the work environment is not always accepting of the DNP especially in advanced practice.* For those in nursing education, the environment appeared to be supportive as time goes on when there is a mutual "settling" and "fit." Overall, the informants in this study expressed feeling confident and more settled in their role than when they started their positions.

DISCUSSION AND CONCLUSIONS OF STUDY

There has been only one published study on the lived experience of the DNP graduate (Smith Glasgow & Zoucha, 2011). The DNP graduates are truly pioneers in practice, education, and administration as they bring their advanced knowledge and skill to the table. The informants' confidence and sense of respect is needed in today's nursing environment to effect change, as well as being consistent with the AACN's vision for the degree (AACN, 2006). Overall, informants were proud about their advanced knowledge and wanted to apply that knowledge in their respective roles. When compared to the findings of the previous study in 2011 there is a perceived change and in some cases a confirmation in the perceptions of the DNP role in practice, education, and administration. Informants reported feeling that the context of their work was more supportive and conducive to confidence and respect in the role. Nurse educators and nurse leaders felt more settled and supported in their roles. There was slight improvement in the perceptions and experiences of DNP's in practice, but there was still a sense of not feeling understood or supported by their advanced practice peers. However, there was improvement when compared to the 2011 study.

When the researchers reflect on the findings in this study, it provided some hope that things were changing for the DNP in nursing education, administration, and practice over time. In this study, DNP graduates employed in advanced nursing practice roles continued to express concern that in some cases, the work environment is not always accepting of the DNP role in advanced practice settings. From our history, we know that nursing practice, and to some degree education, has been slow to recognize or come to terms with the distinct differences of educational preparation. At present, the DAPRN's role and expectations are no different than that of the master's-level advanced practice nurse's role and expectations for the informants.

Based on the findings of this study, the informants feel that DAPRNs can contribute significantly to the advancement of the profession, quality, and safety metrics, and are confident about its role in the future. It is not clear, however, whether the role of the doctoral-level advanced practice nurse will actually change as a result of the DAPRN's additional knowledge and skills. The informants have sought opportunities to use their advanced knowledge and skills. It is not clear what the outcome will be as DAPRNs push for change in the practice setting to accommodate their advanced knowledge as they attempt to find their way as DAPRNs. If the workplace environment does not change, DAPRNs may feel frustrated in their role, as they are not permitted to expand their scope concomitant with their new knowledge and skills. Based on the informants' experiences, the struggle to be accepted for one's contributions is not new in nursing's history and will require more change agents to advance the profession (Dunphy, Smith, & Youngskin, 2009; Udlis & Mancuso, 2012).

The informants in the educator role felt accepted by colleagues, and felt a better fit and more settled in their role in comparison to the 2011 study. The positive news is that the informants saw themselves as more confident and respected in their role and attributed this to their educational preparation. DNP graduates in the educator role are well suited to integrate the classroom content and the practice context as called for in the recent Carnegie Foundation study, *Educating Nurses: A Call for Radical Transformation* (Benner, Sutphen, Leonard, & Day, 2009). DNP educators are in a unique position to serve as faculty members, as they are able to integrate the knowledge they present in the classroom with a clinical practice context. One hopes that the academy will value their connection to practice, which is sorely needed and find a way to use and recognize their clinical expertise (Benner et al., 2009; Udlis & Mancuso, 2015).

In this study, nurse executives continue to feel the most valued and accepted—they expressed feeling more confident and respected in their respective roles. This may be attributed to an evolving and changing environment that is more accepting of the educational preparation and competencies of the DNP. High-performing organizations closely scrutinize leadership capacity and embrace talent (Wells & Hejna, 2009). These organizations look to doctoral level nurse executives to shape their institution through their leadership and to address emergent and challenging issues for nursing practice as well as create opportunities that shape and implement innovative changes in the health care system (AACN, 2006; Upenieks, 2003). One must note that the doctoral-level nurse executive is in a unique position in health care institutions; he or she is usually one of a few nurse executives among a group of senior, non-nurse leaders. These nurse executives also have the power to shape DNP practice and roles at their own institutions (Nichols et al., 2014).

■ SUMMARY

In summarizing this chapter, the study informants spoke to the need for continuing evolution of the three distinct roles of the DNP graduate: advanced practice, educator, and executive in the educational and practice environment and the need for role clarity. Although there are core courses necessary for all DNP graduates, there is specialized knowledge required for each of the distinct roles. With the increase in DNP programs across the nation, a critical mass of DNP graduates may have a sufficiently strong voice in the education and practice settings to effect change with respect to role function and expectations. We will see if this critical mass of graduates can achieve at a national level for themselves; like the MSN-prepared advanced practice nurses were able to accomplish to truly transform the landscape of nursing practice by creating a new role highly valued by society. Ultimately, will the DNP-prepared nurse have similar success and achieve or surpass the AACN's vision of the DNP degree (AACN, 2006, 2009). The authors assert that DNP graduates will need to differentiate their practice from MSN graduates in order to substantiate their value to the profession, health care community, and public, or else the forces of role strain may occur or persist. Health care reform and other market forces will also drive the need for the DNP going forward as we see a growing need for innovation and evidence to improve care. The role of the DNP-prepared faculty member in the academy will need to be closely examined and evaluated. A very small cadre of DNP-prepared faculty are seeking the PhD as they have become more interested in nursing science and the generation of new knowledge. Given decrease in PhD students nationally, PhD-prepared faculty retirements, the existing nursing faculty shortage, and current work-life issues, the U.S. doctoral nursing faculty may need to revise DNP curricula to meet the needs of the academy. Time will tell.

■ CRITICAL THINKING QUESTIONS

1. *Please address factors that may contribute to role ambiguity and role stress.*
2. *How does variability in DNP programs contribute to role ambiguity specifically? Should there be standardization?*
3. *Discuss how job fit is a key factor in organizational engagement.*
4. *Discuss the multiple competing roles of the DNP graduate.*
5. *Discuss the role strain experienced by the DAPRN.*
6. *Discuss the role strain experienced by the DNP executive.*
7. *Discuss the role strain experienced by the DNP educator.*
8. *How can the results of this study, "The Experiences of DNPs in Their Current Professional Positions: An Updated and Current View," assist new DNP graduates in acclimating to their new roles? What can the profession learn from the informants' experiences?*
9. *How can DNP graduates differentiate themselves from MSN graduates in their roles?*
10. *How will health care reform and other market forces impact the role of the DNP-prepared nurse in his or her respective roles?*

■ REFERENCES

American Association of Colleges of Nursing. (2006). *The essentials of doctoral education for advanced nursing practice.* Retrieved from http://www.aacn.nche.edu/DNP/pdf/Essentials.pdf

American Association of Colleges of Nursing. (2009). Fact sheet: The doctor of nursing practice (DNP). Retrieved from http://www.aacn.nche.edu/Media/FactSheets/dnp.htm

Auerbach, D. I., Martsolf, G., Pearson, M. L., Taylor, E. A., Zaydman, M., Muchow, A., . . . Dower, C. (2014). *The DNP by 2015: A study of the institutional, political, and professional issues that facilitate or impede establishing a post-baccalaureate doctor of nursing practice program.* Santa Monica, CA: RAND Health.

Barritt, L., Beekman, T., Bleeker, H., & Mulderij, K. (1984). Analyzing phenomenological descriptions. *Phenomenology and Pedagogy, 2*(1), 1–17.

Benner, P., Sutphen, M., Leonard, V., & Day, L. (2009). *Educating nurses: A call for radical transformation.* Stanford, CA: The Carnegie Foundation for the Advancement of Teaching.

Bowen, G. (2008). Naturalistic inquiry and the saturation concept: A research note. *Qualitative Research, 8*(1), 137–152.

Chen, Y., Chen, S. H., Tsai, C. Y., & Lo, L. Y. (2007). Role stress and job satisfaction for nurse specialists. *Journal of Advanced Nursing, 59*(5), 497–509.

Cohen, M. Z. (1995). The experience of surgery: Phenomenological clinical nursing research. In A. Omery, C. Kasper, & G. Page (Eds.), *In search of nursing science* (pp. 159–174). Thousand Oaks, CA: Sage.

Dreher, H. M., Smith Glasgow, M. E., Cornelius, F., & Bhattacharya, A. (2012). A report on a national study of doctoral nursing faculty. *Nursing Clinics of North America, 47*(4), 435–453.

Dunphy, L. M., Smith, N. K., & Youngkin, E. Q. (2009). Advanced practice nursing: Doing what has to be done—Radicals, renegades, and rebels. In L. A. Joel (Eds.), *Advance practice nursing: Essentials for role development* (2nd ed., pp. 2–22). Philadelphia, PA: F. A. Davis.

Hardy, M. E., & Conway, M. E. (1978). *Role theory perspectives for health professionals* (1st ed.). New York, NY: Appleton-Century-Crofts.

Hardy, M. E., & Conway, M. E. (1988). *Role theory perspectives for health professionals* (2nd ed.). Norwalk, CT: Appleton & Lange.

Jones, M. L. (2005). Role development and effective practice in specialist and advance practice roles in acute care hospital settings: Systematic review and meta-synthesis. *Journal of Advanced Nursing, 49*(2), 191–209.

Kahn, R. A., Wolfe, P., Quinn, R., Snock, J., & Rosenthal, R. (1964). *Organizational stress: Studies in role conflict and ambiguity.* New York, NY: Wiley.

Lazarus, R. S. (1967). *Psychological stress and the coping process.* New York, NY: McGraw-Hill.

Loomis, J. A., Willard, B., & Cohen, J. (2007). Difficult professional choices: Deciding between the PhD and the DNP in nursing. *The Online Journal of Issues in Nursing, 12*(1). Retrieved from http://search .ebscohost.com/login.aspx?direct=true&db=cin20&AN=2009526632&site=ehost-live

Macionis, J. J. (2006). *Society the basics* (8th ed.). Upper Saddle River, NJ: Pearson.

Moltz, D. (2010). Nursing tug of war. *Inside Higher Education.* Retrieved from http://www.insidehighered .com/news/2010/01/07/nursing

Nichols, C., O'Connor, N., & Dunn, D. (2014). Exploring early and future use of DNP prepared nurses within healthcare organizations. *The Journal of Nursing Administration, 44*(2), 74–78.

Shirey, M. (2006). Stress and burnout in nursing faculty. *Nurse Educator, 31*(3), 95–97.

Smeltzer, S., Sharts-Hopko, N. C., Cantrell, M. A., Heverly, M. A., Jenkinson, A., & Nhenge, S. (2015). Work-life balance of nursing faculty in research- and practice-focused doctoral programs. *Nursing Outlook, 63*(6), 621–631.

Smith Glasgow, M. E., & Zoucha R. (2011). Role strain in the doctorally prepared advanced practice nurse. In H. M. Dreher & M. E. Smith Glasgow (Eds.), *Role development for doctoral advanced nursing practice* (pp. 213–226). New York, NY: Springer Publishing.

Sveinsdottir, H., Biering, P., & Ramel, A. (2006). Occupational stress, job satisfaction, and working environment for Icelandic nurses: A cross-sectional questionnaire survey. *International Journal of Nursing Studies, 43*, 875–889.

Udlis, K. A., & Mancuso, J. M. (2012). Doctor of nursing practice programs across the United States: A benchmark of information: Part I: Program characteristics. *Journal of Professional Nursing, 28*(5), 265–273.

Udlis, K. A., & Mancuso, J. M. (2015). Perceptions of the role of the doctor of nursing practice-prepared nurse: Clarity or confusion. *Journal of Professional Nursing, 31*(4), 274–283.

Upenieks, V. V. (2003). What constitutes effective leadership? Perceptions of magnet and nonmagnet nurse leaders. *The Journal of Nursing Administration, 33*(9), 456–467.

Van Kaam, A. (1991). *Formation of the human heart.* New York, NY: Crossroads.

Wells, W., & Hejna, W. (2009). Developing leadership talent in healthcare organizations. *Healthcare Financial Management, 1*, 66–69.

CHAPTER TEN

Reflective Response

Rita K. Adeniran

DNPs: This is our time. The evolving healthcare environment provides a unique opportunity to make a positive difference in health and healthcare. The future of DNPs is in our hands.

—Rita K. Adeniran

The passage of the Patient Protection and Affordable Care Act (ACA) on March 23, 2010, ushered the beginning of a new era of health care delivery in the United States. As the various provisions of ACA move through the multiple implementation stages of the law, the landscape of the U.S. health care system is witnessing transformation (Nichols, O'Connor, & Dunn, 2014). These transformations have tremendously increased the complexity, uncertainty, volatility, and ambiguity (CUVA) that seems to have plagued the U.S. health care delivery system for decades (Blumenthal, Abrams, & Nuzum, 2015; Larkin, Swanson, Fuller, & Cortese, 2016; Leopardo, 2013; Nair, 2011). It is within CUVA that Doctor of Nursing Practice (DNP)-prepared nurses are uniquely positioned to play a role that will distinguish them from nondoctoral-prepared advanced practice nurses and other members of the interprofessional care team.

It is worth noting that DNP programs in the United States continue to proliferate in response to the increased recognition of the value of nurses prepared at the doctoral level to lead and work side by side with other members of the interprofessional care team in addressing many of the nation's long-standing health and health care problems (Institute of Medicine, 2010; Lathrop & Hodnicki, 2014; Nichols et al., 2014). DNP-prepared nurses pursue roles in academia, clinical practice, health policy, and administration. Indeed, all roles that provide a platform for advancing and positively influencing all aspects of the nation's health and health care system.

I would argue that DNP-prepared nurses are not, and will not be bogged down or pressured by what has been described as role strain, because to some degree, role strain is associated with most new roles, distinctive job positions, and many forms of transition that are related to professional advancement (Cantwell, 2014; Carte, 2014; Cranford, 2013; Gallagher, 2005). DNP nurses have the capacity and ability to manage and allocate energies to reduce role strain to tolerable proportions and maximize role adjustment as they work to lead and deliver health care services that minimize CUVA, and meet the changing needs of health care consumers, population health, and organizational priorities.

Many stakeholders in the health care community (Lathrop & Hodnicki, 2014; Nichols et al., 2014) have called for health care providers to acquire the highest level of scientific knowledge and practice expertise to ensure optimal outcomes for patients and population health. For that, and many other reasons, it becomes important to distinguish the knowledge and practice scope of advanced practice nurses based on their educational preparation. There is a clear difference between master's and doctoral prepared advanced practice nurses. In accordance with the American Association of Colleges of Nursing (AACN) position statement, creating a culture and workforce for nursing research; one hallmark of distinction between master's- and DNP-prepared nurses is in that, master's programs prepare nurses to evaluate research findings, and to evaluate and implement evidence-based practice guidelines; while, practice-focused, doctoral educational programs prepare graduates for the highest level of nursing practice. Moreover, the DNP degree is widely recognized as one of two terminal degrees of the nursing profession, and is a preferred pathway for nurses seeking preparation at the highest level of their practice (American Association of Colleges of Nursing, 2015). DNP-prepared nurses have acquired the highest level of practice expertise integrated with the ability to translate scientific knowledge into complex clinical interventions tailored to meet individual, family, community, population health, and illness needs. DNP-prepared nurses use advanced leadership knowledge and skills to appraise the translation of research into practice and collaborate with scientists to launch and advance new health policy opportunities that evolve from research, translation, and evaluation processes (American Association of Colleges of Nursing, 2006).

Equipped with the added knowledge and skills gained from doctoral education, DNP-prepared nurses, regardless of roles, whether practitioner, clinical executive, nurse educator, or policy advocate, DNPs are prepared to mitigate CUVA, drive change, leverage innovation, and play an active role in improving quality outcomes for individual patients, populations, organizations, and the American public as a whole.

As a DNP-prepared nurse myself, I read and interpreted the contents of Chapter 10 of this book, titled "Role Strain in the Doctorally Prepared Practice Nurse: The Experiences of Doctor of Nursing Practice Graduates in Their Current Professional Positions—An Updated and Current View" with mixed feelings. Although I could not agree more with the information contained in the chapter's introduction, descriptions of the three (practitioner, clinical executive, or nurse educator) advanced practice nurse's experiences and roles, along with the report of the previous and updated views of DNPs' experiences in their professional positions, I nevertheless, feel obligated to offer additional thoughts for consideration. I understand that the findings reflect the voice of the participants in the study; however, I believe that DNPs are doing much more than what was found, reported, and discussed in Chapter 10 from the research study.

It was no surprise to learn from the study findings and discussions in Chapter 10, that gaining additional knowledge and skills from DNP-preparation enhanced informants' confidence; an experience that I personally relate to, post the completion of my DNP educational program. However, confidence is only one of the many essential ingredients necessary, and was acquired from my DNP educational preparation. DNP-prepared nurses have acquired varied competencies, including but not limited to leadership, scientific, practice, and health care policy, and are working in varied roles, positively impacting the health, and health care of the nation.

I posit that the success of DNP-prepared nurses in all roles have hinged on their abilities to make change happen. DNP's leverage their knowledge, skills, and competencies in setting direction, creating alignment, and gaining commitment toward advancing and achieving optimal outcomes for individual patient, family, community, population health, and in their various organizational settings (McCauley, 2014). Using the direction, alignment, and commitment (DAC) framework (McCauley, 2014), I succinctly share how I believe that DNP-prepared nurses are using their competencies to mitigate CUVA, and make positive change happen in health care.

Set Direction: Leveraging knowledge and skills gained from DNP foundational competencies outlined in the AACN DNP essentials, specifically Essentials I, II, and III, DNP nurses are able to effectively set direction by operationalization, a vision and strategy to address identified organizational gaps related to their expertise. This strategy will involve providing leadership that customizes organizational goals to meet patient and population health goals. DNPs have acquired the skills to thread efficiency and productivity in their work. DNPs understand the imperative to leverage the political capital of those who already shared in the direction/vision to influence others for success.

Create Alignment: DNPs know that creating and achieving alignment starts with a good understanding of what needs to be accomplished in order to create a powerful voice for change. It encompasses bringing together the right configuration of passion and talent, to use the structure and process that is in place to enable change. DNP Essentials IV, V, and VI emphasized technology, health care advocacy and interprofessional collaboration. These competencies outlined in the DNP essentials accentuate elements that are vital to creating alignment. The DNP-prepared nurse can accelerate alignment by involving many stakeholders throughout the organization or unit in crafting an implementation plan for the direction that was set. An important aspect of alignment is congruence between the organizational goals and vision that are used to set the direction. In essence, DNPs know, among many other things that the organizational leadership strategy must align with the outcome sought by the DNP-prepared nurse.

Gain Commitment: DNPs appreciate the value of getting the buy-in of organizational leadership and the whole organization to the direction that has been set. Competencies of DNP Essentials VI, VII, and VII, such as effective communication, advanced system thinking, and ability to leverage conceptual and analytical skills are crucial for gaining commitment. DNP-prepared nurses gain commitment for their cause by connecting the directions they have set to the existing motivation of individuals in the organization. This strategy results in a contagious effect, as palpable commitment of early adopters often snowball through the entire organization or unit, intensifying and growing, including the DNP's own commitment.

■ CONCLUSION

In the fast-paced, evolving health care environment, the nursing profession has risen to the challenge by preparing nurses with terminal degrees, who hold the tools to make positive contributions in solving some of the challenges of the nation's health and health care delivery system. Knowledge and education are powerful instruments for change. DNP-prepared nurses possess practice experience, leadership competencies that include change management and knowledge of research and evidence-based practice, skills that are essential to mitigate CUVA and meet the needs of changing health care consumers in an evolving health care environment.

The DNP education is a winning strategy for nursing and society! As the U.S. health care system continues to evolve, DNPs will continue to strengthen their individual and organizations' performance to enhance outcomes for patients, population health, organizations, and society at large. The current health care system lends itself well to the much needed skills and competencies possessed by DNP-prepared nurses to meet the ever increasing number of opportunities in health and health care. DNP-prepared nurses are raising the contributions of nursing in meeting the nation's goal for health and health care.

■ REFERENCES

American Association of Colleges of Nursing. (2006). Nursing research: A scientific basis for the health of the public. *AACN Position Statement on Nursing Research*. Retrieved from http://www.aacn.nche .edu/publications/position/nursing-research

American Association of Colleges of Nursing. (2015). *The doctor of nursing practice: Current issues and clarifying recommendations—Report from the task force on the implementation of the DNP*. Retrieved from http://www.aacn.nche.edu/news/articles/2015/dnp-white-paper

Blumenthal, D., Abrams, M., & Nuzum, R. (2015). The Affordable Care Act at 5 years. *New England Journal of Medicine, 372*(25), 2451–2458.

Cantwell, S. (2014). Role strain among transitioning nurse faculty: The impact of tenure-track and years of teaching (Doctoral dissertation). Northcentral University. Retrieved from https://proxy.library .upenn.edu/login?url=http://search.ebscohost.com/login.aspx?direct=true&db=cin20&AN=109 776529&site=ehost-live

Carte, N. S. (2014). Perception of role strain among male critical care registered nurses: A quantitative descriptive approach (Doctoral dissertation). University of Phoenix. Retrieved from https://proxy .library.upenn.edu/login?url=http://search.ebscohost.com/login.aspx?direct=true&db=cin20& AN=109794738&site=ehost-live

Cranford, J. S. (2013). Bridging the gap: Clinical practice nursing and the effect of role strain on successful role transition and intent to stay in academia. *International Journal of Nursing Education Scholarship, 10*(1), 1–7.

Gallagher, M. L. B. (2005). The relationship of role strain, personal control/decision latitude, and work-related social support to the job satisfaction of distance nurse educators (Doctoral dissertation). Widener University School of Nursing. Retrieved from https://proxy.library.upenn.edu/ login?url=http://search.ebscohost.com/login.aspx?direct=true&db=cin20&AN=109846712&site =ehost-live

Institute of Medicine. (2010). The future of nursing: Leading change, advancing health. Retrieved from http://books.nap.edu/openbook.php?record_id=12956&page=R1

Larkin, D. J., Swanson, R. C., Fuller, S., & Cortese, D. A. (2016). The Affordable Care Act: A case study for understanding and applying complexity concepts to healthcare reform. *Journal of Evaluation in Clinical Practice, 22*(1), 133–140.

Lathrop, B., & Hodnicki, D. (2014). The Affordable Care Act: Primary care and the doctor of nursing practice nurse. *The Online Journal of Issues in Nursing, 19*(2).

Leopardo, M. (May 29, 2013). How the Affordable Care Act affects healthcare construction. *Becker's Hospital Review*. Retrieved from http://www.beckershospitalreview.com/hospital-management -administration/how-the-affordable-care-act-affects-healthcare-construction.html

McCauley, C. (2014). Making leadership happen. Retrieved from http://insights.ccl.org/wp-content/ uploads/2015/04/MakingLeadershipHappen.pdf

Nair, S. P. (2011). Managing ICD-10-and healthcare reform-related volatility. *Healthcare Informatics, 28*(8), 33–35. Retrieved from http://www.healthcare-informatics.com/article/ managing-icd-10-and-healthcare-reform-related-volatility

Nichols, C., O'Connor, N., & Dunn, D. (2014). Exploring early and future use of DNP-prepared nurses within healthcare organizations. *Journal of Nursing Administration, 44*(2), 74–78. doi:10.1097/ nna.0000000000000029

CHAPTER ELEVEN

The 2016 Report on a National Study of Doctoral Nursing Faculty: A Quantitative Replication Study

Mary Ellen Smith Glasgow, Frances H. Cornelius, Anand Bhattacharya, and H. Michael Dreher

The April 2007 release of Robert Wood Johnson Foundation policy briefing paper suggested that as nursing faculty retire, nursing programs will yield a dual loss from the decrease in the total number of faculty available to teach nursing students at all levels and a reduction in the number of seasoned faculty who can orient and mentor new faculty and advise graduate students. Data presented in this revised text confirm that the cycle of nursing faculty retirements has exceeded the number of new full-time faculty replacements (Fang, Li, Stauffer, & Trautman, 2016; Glasgow & Dreher, 2010). Many of these senior faculty members are doctoral faculty and funded researchers. These critical positions will need to be filled when senior faculty retire. However, as Potempa, Redman, and Anderson (2008) have indicated, there is a lack of adequate role modeling, particularly in undergraduate nursing education to foster pursuing careers as nursing professors—thus the pipeline to the nursing professoriate is in crisis. As current senior faculty contemplate concluding their formal careers, we need to focus on providing the next generation of doctoral faculty (PhD, Doctor of Nursing Practice [DNP], and now increasingly the doctorate in education [EdD] with the requisite knowledge and skills that will be needed to survive and thrive in academia.

In our previous study (Dreher, Smith Glasgow, Cornelius, & Bhattacharya, 2012) we explored:

1. Who will teach DNP students if the DNP degree does not prepare graduates for their role as expert educators in graduate nursing programs (largely in advanced practice nursing programs)?
2. With the demand for advanced practice nurse educators to maintain clinical competency to retain national certification, will future graduate advanced practice registered nurses (APRN) faculty (for both master of science in nursing [MSN] and DNP programs) be marginalized and largely excluded from tenure-track positions with their inability to also engage in seeking and securing funded research?

3. With a national and global recession and intense competition for resources, will the need for additional start-up resources for DNP programs cause PhD programs to lose resources?
4. With such tumultuous changes in doctoral nursing education, what is the current state of the quality of life of doctoral nursing faculty?

We contend that the "burning questions" of the day facing the doctoral nursing education professoriate are as follows:

- Are doctoral nursing faculty satisfied with their current role?
- Are doctoral nursing faculty concerned that DNP Program enrollment has surpassed PhD program enrollment?
- Are doctoral nursing faculty concerned about the DNP's effect on nursing knowledge development?
- Are current academic administrators actively engaged in succession planning?
- Are doctoral nursing faculty concerned about nursing faculty salaries?
- If the DNP graduate is not educated specifically for an academic role, are doctoral nursing faculty concerned about who will teach nursing students in the future?

In this 2016 study, the questions have changed. Now, with this second, replicative study, we pose a new set of questions a posteriori, as we move into the near future. This chapter focuses on a comparison of the two studies, and changes over this period in the doctoral faculty landscape, rather than an emphasis on cross-sectional reporting of the 2016 findings.

■ BACKGROUND

This follow-up study was conducted to ascertain nursing faculty's perceptions and satisfaction with doctoral nursing education since the first national study of doctoral nursing faculty published in 2012 (Dreher et al., 2012). The impetus for this study was the change in demographics of doctoral nursing faculty in addition to a surge in DNP programs from 10 in 2005 to 269 programs in 2014 (American Association of Colleges of Nursing [AACN], 2015a). The landscape has changed dramatically since two of the coauthors led the first national conference on the DNP degree in Annapolis, Maryland, in 2007 and in Hilton Head Island, South Carolina, in 2009 sponsored by Drexel University Division of Continuing Nursing Education. These two conferences included papers from a diverse set of doctoral nursing faculty who expressed concerns over:

1. Who will teach DNP students if the DNP degree does not prepare graduates for their role as expert educators in graduate nursing programs (largely in advanced practice nursing programs)?
2. With the demand for advanced practice nurse educators to maintain clinical competency to retain national certification, will future graduate APRN faculty (for both MSN and DNP programs) be marginalized and largely excluded from tenure-track positions with their inability to also engage in seeking and securing funded research?
3. With the current issues in higher education and the intense competition for resources, will the need for additional start-up resources for DNP programs cause PhD programs to lose resources?
4. With such extreme changes in doctoral nursing education, what is the current state of the quality of life of doctoral nursing faculty?

Although it is not the purpose of this chapter to explore these topics in depth, these current and persistent questions framed the need to conduct this follow-up national survey in order to determine how these issues are currently impacting the doctoral nursing faculty.

The AACN (2004) has maintained since 2004, and with the 2006 publication of *The Essentials of Doctoral Education for Advanced Nursing Practice* (AACN, 2006), that the educator role is *not* an advanced nursing practice role. We recount, however, as Wittmann-Price, Waite, and Woda (2011) wrote in Chapter 7 of the first edition of this text "to what extent did members of the AACN (composed of college and nursing school deans) fully vet the implications for including the executive role as 'advanced practice' but excluding the educator role as 'advanced practice'?" Valiga notes in her Reflective Response to this same argument in the revised chapter in the second edition,

> ...if they [nurses] desire to practice at an advanced level, they need to pursue graduate education...the nurse educator role clearly needs to be defined as an "advanced practice" role and acknowledged as a critical component of the health and viability of our profession.

Zungolo (2009) and others reported that 30% or more of DNP graduates are entering academia and reiterated that these graduates are not being formally prepared for the faculty role (Smeltzer et al., 2015). The migration of large numbers of DNP graduates into academia is occurring as predicted (Dreher et al., 2012). The prospect of a replacement of the PhD with the DNP in academia appears to be a real possibility. The impact on faculty retention, research and scholarship, student outcomes, and percent of tenure-track and tenured faculty needs to be examined.

The question whether doctoral faculty who will ultimately teach in DNP and MSN programs are at a disadvantage in the tenure system is a real one. And while Nicholes and Dyer (2012) reported that some institutions may actually tenure DNP faculty (likely institutions that are not research intensive), Meleis (2011), in a point/counterpoint in the *Journal for Nurse Practitioners*, again confirmed what probably remains the most predominant view (but not necessarily the paradigm position in the future) in nursing— that DNPs should not hold tenure-track positions. But whether this remains the future practice in nursing academia is a fundamental question. Udlis and Mancuso (2015) note that DNP participants felt prepared for the demands of the faculty role and the requisite tenure, research, and scholarship requirements; however, PhD participants disagreed that the DNP degree prepares graduates to assume these responsibilities. The role and scholarly contributions of the DNP-prepared faculty member with respect to faculty scholarly and practice expectations, academic leadership potential, and tenure needs to be addressed. If we continue to insist that only those who are accomplished scientists with extensive external funding and long lists of peer-reviewed publications are worthy of tenure and promotion, we will ostracize DNP-prepared faculty engaged in clinical practice who are generating practice evidence. This is not to say that scholarship is not important; however, should we not consider individuals for tenure who have sustained record of scholarly accomplishments, who have had an impact on educational or clinical practices, who have made significant contributions to the health of a patient population or academic program, and who have the potential to continue these important contributions (Valiga, this volume)? With the growing numbers of DNP-prepared faculty in the academy, the nursing discipline may be less visible in the academy over time if we stand firm on these traditional views of tenure and promotion.

The third question is whether the surge in DNP programs is a threat to PhD program resources? However, what is undisputable is that in 2014 with fewer resources in higher education due to significant economic pressures, the number of DNP programs

(N = 269) now outnumbers PhD programs (N = 134); DNP enrollments (N = 18,352) now outnumber PhD enrollments (N = 5,290); and the number of annual DNP graduations (N = 3,065) now exceeds PhD graduations (N = 743; AACN, 2015a, 2015b).

This doctoral enrollment and graduation trend data can neither be ignored nor marginalized. Even the data on DNPs employed full time in academic warrant more attention from the AACN/Commission of Collegiate Nursing Education (CCNE) beyond their current argument that both DNPs and PhDs need to acquire teaching pedagogy preparation for the academic role. The inequity, however, is that the PhD students are normally expected (particularly in PhD in nursing/nursing science programs because these graduates largely do enter academia) to include education content in their degree program and/or as part of a graduate assistantship but DNP programs have sent very mixed messages about the appropriateness of education courses. Quoting from the AACN 2006 essentials, "This additional preparation ['preparation in the science of pedagogy'] may occur in formal course work during the DNP program" (p. 7). However, the next paragraph states "This preparation is in addition to that required for their area of specialized nursing practice" (AACN, 2006, p. 7). In the AACN's new white paper on the DNP (2015d), it reaffirms, "Additional preparation in the nurse educator role may be included as optional coursework within the DNP program" (p. 7). Further complicating the continuing, lack of consensus on this subject in the profession, the two other nursing accrediting agencies, Accreditation Commission for Education in Nursing and the National League for Nursing's Commission for Nursing Education[1] do support a DNP degree that specifically prepares the nurse educator and recognizes the master's-prepared nurse educator as an advanced practice nursing role.

Some nursing leaders would argue that the DNP is the right terminal degree for a nurse in practice. Although some speculate that the DNP degree is drawing new nurses to doctoral education, others contend that the DNP is drawing nurses away from research careers (Terhaar, Taylor, & Sylvia, 2016). Based on these trends, there is ongoing concern whether the senior faculty replacements for research-focused doctoral programs can actually be replaced with the current pipeline of prospective faculty (Dreher & Rundio, 2013). With the DNP currently being operationalized as a mostly non-research doctorate, this development has enormous implications for our disciplinary knowledge development. The lack of education-focused curricula in DNP programs has significant implications for DNP graduates assuming faculty roles.

Finally, the central question this survey sought to answer is: With these dramatic shifts occurring in graduate nursing education, particularly doctoral education, what is the current quality of life for the average nursing faculty member who has a doctoral appointment or who supervises doctoral students even if they are not currently teaching in a DNP or PhD program? As mentioned, few studies have focused on doctoral nursing faculty experiences. However, there have been other formal attempts to gather this kind of data among nursing faculty at large. For instance, a 2004 survey of nursing faculty in Minnesota (N = 298; 54% response rate) reported that only 44% had confidence in nursing's general direction (Disch, Edwardson, & Adwan, 2004). Smeltzer et al. (2015) examined work–life balance issues as self-identified by 554 doctoral program faculty teaching in research-focused and practice-focused doctoral programs. Work–life balance mean score was 3.48 with a range of 1 to 7, with lower scores signifying better work–life balance. Factors associated with good work–life balance include higher academic rank, tenure, older age, years in education, current faculty position, and no involvement in clinical practice. "Faculty involved in clinical practice had poorer work–life balance. This finding has implications for those who must maintain a clinical practice as part of their role or to maintain certification" (p. 628). Oermann, Lynn, and Agger (2016) found similar results related to faculty practice and workload balance.

DNP-prepared faculty were more likely to leave their position due to salary and workload issues which included balancing faculty teaching demands with clinical practice and certification requirements. Since nursing is a practice discipline, this finding is particularly troublesome for advanced practice nurses. Nursing academic leaders need to create formal academic clinical partnerships and practice arrangements in an effort to increase salaries, incorporate clinical practice into faculty workload, and inform clinical teaching. In other words, formal faculty practice arrangements need to become the norm beyond academic health centers. If we do not seriously address faculty practice in academic nursing, we are at risk of marginalizing our practitioner teaching faculty. They are also at risk of work–life imbalance, stress, and/or burnout from juggling practice hours/requirements, and their teaching and academic expectations (Shirey, 2006; Smeltzer et al., 2015).

In 2007, the National League for Nursing/Carnegie Foundation National Survey of Nurse Educators: Compensation, Workload, and Teaching Practices study focused specifically on the workload of full-time nursing faculty in nonadministrative positions teaching in either undergraduate or graduate nursing programs. Many of the faculty respondents indicated that they had administrative duties as well as teaching responsibilities, resulting in a 56-hour average workweek. Furthermore, in addition to their work of full-time faculty obligations, more than 62% of these nursing faculty engaged in clinical practice work outside their full-time faculty role, averaging an additional day each week (7–10 hours). Given the current nurse faculty shortage, the question of how workload impacts job satisfaction, recruitment, and attrition remains highly relevant. In this context, it was notable that overall 45% of nursing faculty stated that they were dissatisfied with their current workload (Kaufman, 2007a, 2007b, 2007c). Although this particular survey is not annually conducted, these findings are still relevant today and consistent with Smeltzer et al. (2015) concerning poor work–life balance for faculty who practice outside their faculty role. With the rise in DNP-prepared faculty, this issue of faculty clinical practice as an integral part of faculty workload requires immediate examination and solutions.

According to AACN Report on 2014 to 2015 enrollment and graduations in baccalaureate and graduate programs in nursing, U.S. nursing schools turned away 68,938 qualified applicants from baccalaureate and graduate nursing programs in 2014 due to an insufficient number of faculty, clinical sites, classroom space, clinical preceptors, and budget constraints. Almost two thirds of the nursing schools responding to the survey pointed to faculty shortages as a reason for not accepting all qualified applicants into baccalaureate programs.

Two of the coauthors of this chapter are deans and they can both attest that in formal school of nursing searches for full-time faculty positions, there is a dearth of PhD-prepared applicants. The majority applicant pool consists of master's-prepared clinicians (many who have taught clinical nursing on an adjunct basis) or DNP-prepared applicants who rarely have full-time teaching experience. In both these cases, applicants are often surprised by the range of salary offers, but these appointments are subject to differential for the doctoral degree and full-time teaching experience. The point here is that salary issues in this nursing faculty shortage may be compounded by the constitution of the applicant pool. These findings are explored further and compared to the findings from both the 2012 and 2016 National Study of Doctoral Nursing Faculty, which are detailed in following sections. It should be noted that the AACN does produce an annual enrollment and graduation report (PhD/DNP data mentioned earlier was extracted from this report), but our review of these most recent reports has found that there are only limited data related to the doctoral faculty role.

■ METHODOLOGY

STUDY DESIGN

This prospective cross-sectional study is a follow-up from the initial "Report on a National Study of Doctoral Nursing Faculty" published in 2012 (Dreher et al., 2012). This study used the same descriptive survey conducted in 2009 via Survey Monkey to compare and contrast the current perception of doctoral nursing faculty nationally with the 2009 data about issues specific to doctoral nursing education, doctoral nursing faculty demographics, and their views on doctoral education, as well as on succession planning in nursing academia. The survey titled, "A National Survey of Doctoral Nursing Faculty and Succession Planning" (Dreher et al., 2012) remained fundamentally unchanged in the current study. Data were collected during the year 2013. Qualitative findings are not reported in this study due to the enormous number of responses that could not be included in this chapter. The study authors are seeking to publish these rich findings in the near future in "Outcomes" in *The DNP e-Newsletter*.

SAMPLING

A comprehensive list of all U.S. universities offering doctoral nursing programs (DNP and PhD) was obtained from the AACN website. An e-mail invitation was sent to the department chairs of all identified programs requesting that they and their doctoral faculty participate in a web-based survey. Individual faculty who were clearly identified as having teaching appointments in either a DNP or PhD program and who had a public e-mail, were also solicited. Participation was voluntary and open to doctoral faculty from academic institutions offering a DNP, a PhD, or both degrees in the nursing discipline. In the first study (due to the initial limited number of programs admitting students in 2009), faculty who were in the process of launching a new DNP program were included in the survey, but not in this study. In order to be classified as "doctoral nursing faculty" an individual respondent had to have met one of the following criteria: (a) had taught in a PhD or DNP program in the past 2 years or (b) had been actively engaged in doctoral student supervision (normally PhD dissertation supervision or DNP project/practice dissertation supervision). Responses were anonymous and personal identification information was not requested. Clustering or stratification was not used in the sampling frame. An electronic cover letter that included an explanation of the study, institutional review board (IRB) approval, and information on providing informed consent accompanied the e-mail sent to each prospective participant. By clicking on the Survey Monkey link to the survey available at the end of the letter, prospective participants were able to provide consent and begin.

Survey Questionnaire

The researchers developed a 32-item web survey, a National Survey of Doctoral Nursing Faculty and Succession Planning in 2009, to determine the state of nursing doctoral education from a faculty perspective. This is a follow-up study with the same population of PhD and DNP faculty (with a different sample) to ascertain the current state of doctoral nursing faculty and the future of doctoral education with respect to succession planning. The same survey (minus 1 item), was used with only minor modification to the wording of certain questions so that each first survey question could be compared statistically to the follow-up survey. Questions focusing on professional characteristics and faculty responsibilities such as faculty's tenure status, rank, years in academia, teaching role, type of university where employed, presence of an administrative appointment, funding history, retirement plans, current salary, views on doctoral education, job satisfaction, history of succession planning, and demographic data were addressed (Table 11.1). In addition, participants were also qualitatively asked: (a) Please list/discuss any issues or concerns you have with DNP education; (b) please list/discuss any issues or concerns you have with PhD education; and (c) do you have any particular concerns about your doctoral faculty role and doctoral nursing education not specifically addressed in this survey (including suggestions for questions for the next survey)? This survey had far more qualitative responses than the first study, and the authors are seeking publication of these findings as this text goes to press. Chiefly, we want to disseminate our qualitative finding to a large population of DNP-prepared nurses.

Data Analyses

Frequencies and percentages were reported for the closed-ended questions. For questions that required participants to rank order multiple items, the final ranking was derived by using a weighted score to rank each item response. Finally, separate Pearson chi-square analyses were performed to ascertain whether there were differences among faculty who were teaching in a DNP program only, a PhD program only, or in both programs on selected questions. The Fisher's Exact test was used instead of the chi-square if the frequency of responses for a particular category was low and the assumption of expected count greater than 5 in each cell was violated. Level of significance for all tests were set at alpha = 0.05. All data were entered and analyzed using Statistical Package for the Social Sciences (SPSS) for Windows, Version 23 (© SPSS, Inc., Chicago, IL, www.spss.com).

Synopsis of the 2012 Report on a National Study of Doctoral Nursing Faculty
This was the original national study of doctoral nursing faculty, including both PhD and DNP faculty. Using a national sample of $N = 624$ doctoral nursing faculty, the researchers surveyed individuals on a variety of issues including succession planning, retirement, quality of life as a doctoral faculty member, their views on the new DNP degree, and how they viewed the future of doctoral nursing education. We summarize here some of the essential questions from the 2012 study:

1. Who will teach DNP students if the DNP degree does not prepare graduates for their role as expert educators in graduate nursing programs (largely in advanced practice nursing programs)? This issue was prevalent at the beginning of the DNP degree movement, and remains unresolved.
2. With the demand for advanced practice nurse educators to maintain clinical competency to retain national certification, will future graduate APRN faculty (for both MSN and DNP programs) be marginalized and largely excluded from tenure-track positions with their inability to also engage in seeking and securing funded research? Just over half (52%) of the 2012 study sample were tenured, but declining tenure percentages among doctoral nursing faculty were projected and not just because of controversy around whether DNP faculty should be eligible for tenure-track positions.
3. With a national and global recession and intense competition for resources, will the need for additional start-up resources for DNP programs cause PhD programs to lose resources? In the 2012 study, data were collected during the end of the global recession and while uncertainty or negative predictions

TABLE 11.1 Summary Data From Study: Professional Characteristics and Faculty Responsibilities

Variable	Current Sample (N = 762[a])		2012 Study (N = 624[a])		p Value
	Frequency	Percentage	Frequency	Percentage	
Taught in a PhD/nursing research doctoral program					
Taught in PhD nursing only within past 2 years	201	26	321	51	0.001*
Taught in DNP nursing within past 2 years	343	45	127	20	
Taught in both programs	121	16	104	17	
Tenured					
Yes	357	47	363	59	0.001*
Not tenured, but on tenure track					
Yes	156	38	138	52	0.001*
Current rank is best described as					
Full professor	249	34	240	40	0.02*
Associate professor	244	33	210	34	
Assistant professor	159	22	112	18	
Clinical full professor	8	1	5	1	
Clinical associate professor	40	6	18	4	
Clinical assistant professor	29	4	15	3	
Full-time working in school/university					
Yes	709	93	579	93	0.51
Director or chair of a doctoral nursing program					
Yes, PhD program only	51	7	62	10	0.04*
Yes, DNP program only	110	14	70	11	
Yes, PhD and DNP programs	6	1	8	2	
No	595	78	476	77	

Other administrator (not director/chair of doctoral nursing program)

Yes	165	22	176	30	0.002*
Years taught full time in nursing education					0.03*
Less than 3 years	58	8	42	7	
3–5 years	67	9	32	5	
More than 5 years	637	83	538	88	
Years taught in any doctoral nursing program					0.001*
Less than 3 years	210	28	216	35	
3–5 years	194	25	98	16	
More than 5 years	358	47	297	49	
Teaching role					0.93
Doctoral students exclusively	131	18	97	16	
Graduate students exclusively	306	40	253	41	
Both graduate and undergraduate students exclusively	300	39	252	40	
Undergraduate students exclusively (but supervise PhD/DNP)	8	1	7	1	
Do not teach	17	2	12	2	
School/university can best be described as					0.006*
Public/state supported	511	67	440	70	
Private non-religiously affiliated	117	15	110	18	
Private religiously affiliated	134	18	72	12	

(continued)

TABLE 11.1 Summary Data From Study: Professional Characteristics and Faculty Responsibilities *(continued)*

Variable	Current Sample (N = 762[a])		2012 Study (N = 624[a])		p Value
	Frequency	Percentage	Frequency	Percentage	
Completed a formal postdoc					
Yes	119	16	122	19	0.14
Plan to retire					
Less than 3 years	100	13	59	9	0.05
3–5 years	147	19	109	17	
More than 5 years	515	68	456	74	
Current salary					
Less than $85,000	261	34	203	33	0.99
$85,000–$115,000	279	37	210	34	
$115,000–$200,000	163	21	128	20	
More than $200,000	16	2	12	2	
Prefer not to answer	43	6	65	11	

DNP, Doctor of Nursing Practice.

*p < 0.05.

[a]Frequency and percentage are reported for available data for each variable. Some faculty did not answer every question and "no responses" were left off. For majority of the questions, 762 responses were received.

of the impact of the DNP degree on PhD resources were prevalent, it was surmised that in the follow-up study these projections (and whether they actually occurred) would be based on a longer track record of direct faculty experience.

4. With such tumultuous changes in doctoral nursing education, what is the current state of the quality of life of doctoral nursing faculty? In the 2012 study, more than half (54%) of the doctoral nursing faculty were very satisfied with their current faculty position. When "moderately satisfied" responses were 32%, this level of satisfaction rose to 86% which is extremely high. This number was very comparable to the 70% who were mostly optimistic about the future of doctoral nursing education (versus the 25% who were either ambivalent or pessimistic).

■ CURRENT COMPARATIVE RESULTS

The survey received a total of $N = 817$ responses. Of these, 55 responses either did not meet the eligibility criteria or had more than 10% of their responses missing; consequently they were excluded from the final analysis for a total sample size of 762 eligible responses. The maximum margin of error associated with the estimation of proportions from the survey responses was 4%.

PROFESSIONAL PROFILE OF THE DOCTORAL FACULTY PARTICIPANTS

Table 11.1 represents the comparison of the professional profile of the survey respondents in the current study with that of 2012. The professional profiles of the respondents are similar in both surveys with some notable exceptions in the type of program the faculty are teaching, preference for tenure and tenure track, years taught in doctoral nursing, and timeline for retirement. As evident from the table, the number of respondents teaching in a DNP program exclusively doubled from 20% in the 2012 survey to 45% in the current survey while those teaching exclusively in a PhD program halved from 51% to 26%. Faculty teaching in both programs remained steadfast across the two samples. Another area of difference is in the proportion of tenured faculty in the current survey. While every three out of five respondents in the 2012 survey indicated to be tenured, this proportion dropped to less than half in the current sample ($N = 357, 47\%$). Continuing with this trend, the number of faculty currently not tenured but on tenure track also seems to have declined in the current sample compared to the previous one. Although more than one half ($N = 138, 52\%$) of the respondents in 2012 who were not tenured indicated to be on tenure track, that number has shrunk to one in five in the current sample ($N = 156, 20\%$). Differences were also noted in the number of years of teaching full time in nursing and in a doctoral program with a higher proportion of faculty moving from less than 3 years of experience in 2012 to 3 to 5 years of experience in the current survey, a trend to be expected given this survey was conducted 3 years following the first one. Finally, a higher percentage of faculty in the current survey indicated a desire to retire within the next 3 years compared to the previous survey in 2012. These data support the statistically significant finding indicating the number of full professors in the survey declined from 40% to 45%. In all other professional areas, the two samples were similar.

DOCTORAL EDUCATION IN NURSING—THE DNP AND PhD

Like the survey in 2012, participants were asked about their support for the doctoral nursing education, the impact of DNP programs on PhD programs in nursing, and the future of doctoral education in general. In response to the question, "Which statement best supports your current view of doctoral nursing education?" Among all participants in the 2012 study (n = 548), less than half the respondents supported the DNP "enthusiastically" (41%). In the 2016 survey, however, this percentage has moved up with more than half the participants. There was a statistically significant growth in overall support for the DNP (enthusiastically, moderately, or reluctantly) from 79% to 92%, with a direct "I do not support the DNP" declining from 16% to 5% (see Figure 11.1). When comparing the support for the DNP among faculty who either teach only in DNP or PhD programs or both, we found statistical differences based on teaching program. DNP-only faculty were far more "enthusiastic" about the DNP (68%) than PhD-only faculty (22%), with faculty teaching in both programs still not predominately enthusiastic (43%). Overall support for the DNP by teaching program was 93% by DNP faculty, 74% by PhD faculty, and 84% for faculty teaching in both programs (see Figure 11.2).

With regard to the question "Which response best reflects your view if the DNP will negatively impact current PhD resources?" results in the current survey were similar to the one in 2012; however, the inclusion sample for 2012 and 2016 was modified for analysis in this chapter. In the 2012 study, all study participant responses were analyzed, regardless of whether or not there was an actual PhD program at their institution for actual comparison. In the 2012 study, the predominant response among DNP-only faculty was evenly split between 44% "unclear if DNP will negatively impact current PhD

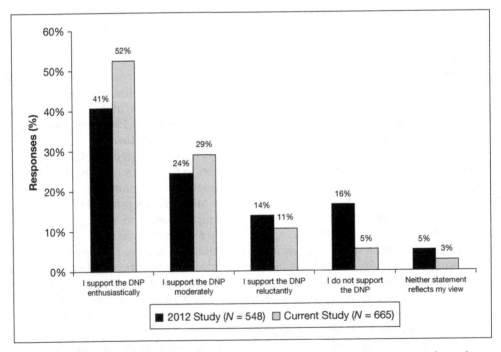

FIGURE 11.1 Comparison of level of support for the DNP between the current samples with the sample from the study published in 2012. A 2 × 3 table with chi-square analysis showed statistically significant difference (p = .001) between the two studies for their support for the DNP.

DNP, Doctor of Nursing Practice.

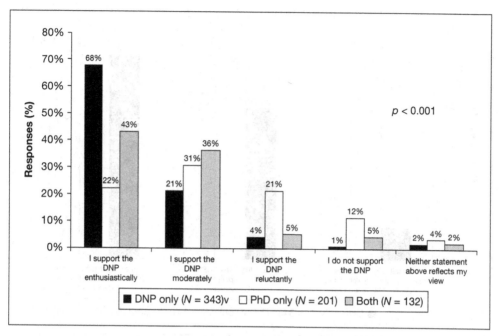

FIGURE 11.2   Comparison of distribution of PhD faculty (*N* = 201), DNP faculty (*N* = 343) and those who teach in both programs (*N* = 121) in their level of support for the DNP (*N* = 665).
DNP, Doctor of Nursing Practice.

resources" and 44% thinking that the "DNP will not impact current PhD resources." In 2016, this changed to 52% "will not impact current PhD resources" and 39% "unclear" (Figure 11.3). Among the PhD-only teaching faculty in 2012, "unclear" was 47%, followed by 38% thinking that the "DNP will negatively impact current PhD resources." In 2016, "unclear" remained stable at 49%, as did "negatively impact" at 37%. In 2012, among the combined DNP/PhD teaching faculty the percentages were 38% "unclear" closely followed by 31% "will not impact current PhD resources" and 28% "will negatively impact current PhD resources. In comparison to 2016, those changes were 38% versus 43% "unclear," 31% versus 14% "will not impact" to 22% versus 28% "will negatively impact current PhD resources."

In the current 2016 study, in a reanalysis, we decided to eliminate participants in both studies who had only a DNP program but no PhD program. In 2012, this was very prevalent as many institutions had a new DNP program and no PhD. Conversely, in 2016, we can only account for two schools that have a PhD but no DNP. We hypothesized that only schools with both programs would have doctoral faculty who were fully informed whether the DNP would impact PhD program resources or not. Novel as that question was to us, analysis of the 2012 versus 2016 study (Figure 11.4) indicated no statistical differences between the two studies. However, in 2016, it is still interesting to note that 37% of doctoral teaching faculty (who either teach in a PhD program where by inference there is also a DNP program, or who teach in both programs where both programs are obviously offered), indicated that PhD resources would be negatively impacted by the DNP in 2012 and that only decreased to 31% in the 2016 study.

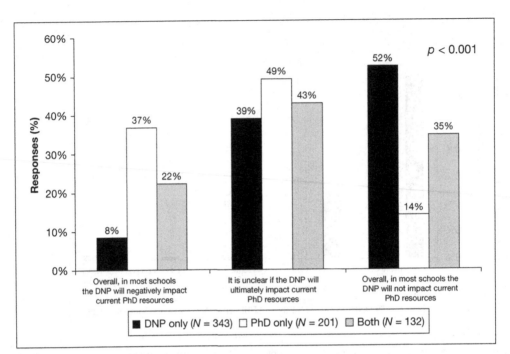

FIGURE 11.3 Comparison of distribution of PhD faculty (*N* = 201), DNP faculty (*N* = 343), and those who teach in both programs (*N* = 121) in their perception of the DNP's impact on PhD program resources (*N* = 665).

DNP, Doctor of Nursing Practice.

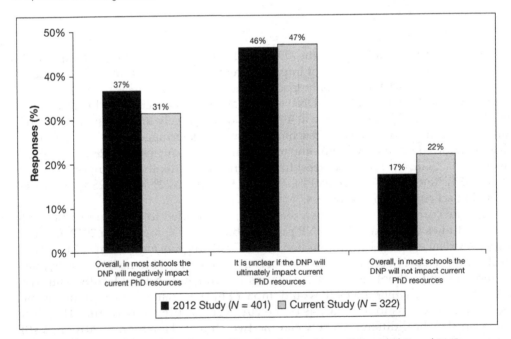

FIGURE 11.4 Comparison of distribution of faculty who teach in a PhD and PhD and DNP program from the current study (*N* = 322), with those from the 2012 study (*N* = 401) in their perception of DNP's impact on PhD program resources. Chi-square analysis showed no statistically significant difference (*p* = .18) between the two studies in their perception of DNP's impact on PhD resources.

DNP, Doctor of Nursing Practice.

NURSING FACULTY IN DOCTORAL EDUCATION

As in 2012, this section of the survey consisted of multiple-choice questions intended to illustrate the participants' perception related to the availability of adequately qualified nursing faculty and nurse scientists for the future. To the question, "Do you think there is going to be an adequate supply of nursing faculty qualified to teach in DNP programs in the next 5 years?" almost equal number of respondents in the current survey stated "Yes" ($N = 290$, 38%) and "No" ($N = 296$, 39%) while in 2012, half the respondents had selected "No" ($N = 304$, 50%). This decline from 50% to 39% likely indicates the increase in number of DNP programs, and this program expansion could not have taken place without an adequate supply of faculty to teach DNP courses. To the next question, "Do you think there is going to be an adequate supply of nurse scientists to replace the retiring nurse scientists in the next 5 years?" responses in the current survey were similar to the one in 2012, wherein the majority of respondents selected "No" ($N = 468$, 61%) just as they had done in 2012 ($N = 406$, 65%). This finding indicates that this is a very protracted problem that could likely worsen in the near future with the reported stagnant PhD enrollments and graduates (Fang et al., 2016).

PROFESSIONAL GROWTH AND WORK SATISFACTION

This section of the survey aimed to understand the academic and administrative aspirations of the faculty teaching in doctoral programs. Again, the same questions that were asked in 2012 were also asked in the current survey. The first question we asked related to work satisfaction was "How satisfied are you with your current faculty position?" To this, majority had responded as "very satisfied" ($N = 331$, 54%) in 2012; however, there was a slight drop in percentage in the current survey results with less than half ($N = 345$, 45%) indicating as feeling "very satisfied." We consider this decline, if not statistically significant, at least an impactful finding. Satisfaction is likely very closely tied to salary and this will be analyzed in the next section.

This question was followed by "Rank 1–5 the following items in order of priority (#1 is the most important to you) if you could request them to improve your faculty work life." From the 2012 study, the weighted scores indicated that "higher salary" was the topmost priority (29%), followed by "internal resources for scholarships" (23%), "reduced teaching load" (21%), "improved climate for intellectual discourse" (16%), and "higher quality students" (11%; see Figure 11.5). From 2012 to 2016 (Figures 11.5 and 11.6), the fourth and fifth rated items from 2012 ("Improved Climate for Intellectual Discourse" and "Higher Quality Students," respectively) dropped out of the top five and were replaced by a tie for fourth between "Better Academic Nursing Leadership" at 18% and "More Input Into Decision Making" (18%), but "Better Academic Nursing Leadership" was rated the highest by participants more often ($N = 75$ vs. $N = 40$). The stability of salary, resources, and teaching load between the two studies is continuing confirmation that these remain critical issues for doctoral nursing faculty, especially salary that dropped from 29% to 22% in the follow-up study, but due to weighted responses many more respondents rated higher salary as the leading factor of concern in the slightly larger 2016 study (2012, $N = 159$ vs. 216, $N = 215$).

SALARY ANALYSES

Salary data were further analyzed to provide a better picture of compensation in nursing academia based on roles. Low salaries among doctoral nursing faculty continue to

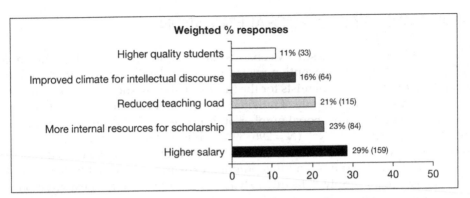

FIGURE 11.5 Weighted response in percentage in order of priority (higher percentage = more important) to improve faculty work life. Number in parenthesis indicates number of respondents who ranked the particular item first as most important from the 2012 study.

Reprinted with permission from *Nursing Clinics of North America*.

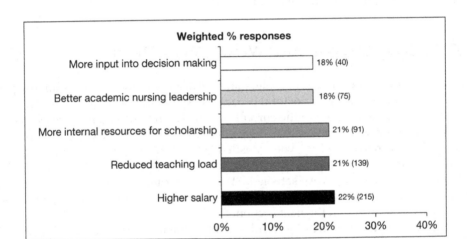

FIGURE 11.6 Weighted response in percentage in order of priority (higher percentage = more important) to improve faculty work life. Number in parenthesis indicates number of respondents who ranked the particular item first as most important from the 2016 study.

be the critical factor in job satisfaction in both studies, and thus warranted extra consideration and analyses in this study. Salary ranges of respondents who reported themselves as doctoral faculty only (no administrative role) are presented in Figure 11.7. Comparison of salaries for department chairs and other administrators are also presented in Table 11.2. Finally, although it has been previously noted that qualitative analysis is not reported in this study, we should note that in the preliminary analysis of those data one respondent reported, "I was stunned to find my salary in the bottom tier and found that so disheartening I had trouble finishing the survey," and we decided to report full salary ranges in Figure 11.7.

In the current survey, in analyzing data from Figure 11.7, 40% of respondents reported their annual salary to be less than $85,000 while the second largest range was 28% at greater than $105,000, just slightly larger than the 27% reporting a salary of between $85,000 and $105,000. These are annual salaries and it is unknown whether these are academic year or calendar year salaries. It is nonetheless surprising that in

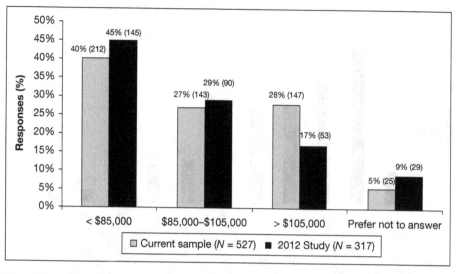

FIGURE 11.7 Salary distributions of respondents who are doctoral teaching faculty only (non-administrators) in the current study compared to the 2012 published study. Chi-square analysis showed statistically significant difference ($p = .001$) between the salary distributions between the two studies.

TABLE 11.2 **Salary Comparison Among PhD Chairs, DNP Chairs, Chairs of Both Programs, and Other Administrators (Excludes Teaching-Only Faculty; $N = 332$)[a]**

Variable (Annual Salary)	Chairs of PhD Programs ($N = 51$)	Chairs of DNP Programs ($N = 110$)	Chairs of Both Programs ($N = 6$)	Other Academic Nursing Administrator ($N = 165$)
	Frequency (%)	Frequency (%)	Frequency (%)	Frequency (%)
Less than $85,000	6 (12)	38 (35)	3 (50)	17 (10)
$85,000–$105,000	16 (31)	25 (23)	2 (33)	32 (19)
More than $105,000	27 (53)	41 (37)	1 (17)	102 (62)
Prefer not to answer	2 (4)	6 (5)	0 (0)	14 (9)

DNP, Doctor of Nursing Practice.

[a]Salary data were reported for available responses only, $p < .001$.

the current 2016 study the percent of faculty earning greater than $105,000 has dropped from 28% to 17% and the percent earning in the range $85,000 to $105,000 has dropped from 29% to 27%. Analyzing these changing salary ranges, it is difficult to discern just where the actual salary ranges have migrated except perhaps those oblique changes that are accounted for in the small percent who chose not to answer this question (down to 5% from the previous 9% in the 2012 study). Figure 11.8 identified the mode salary in 2016 as less than $75,000 (21.8%), followed by that in the range $75,000 to $84,999 at 18.4% and the third highest range being $95,000 to $104,999. Although PhD-only faculty

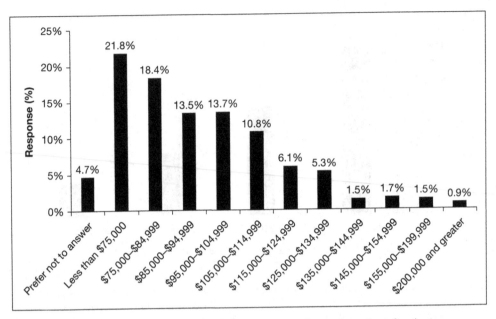

FIGURE 11.8 Salary distributions of respondents who are doctoral teaching faculty (non-administrators; N = 527).

salaries versus DNP-only salaries were not analyzed, it is likely that PhD salaries are higher if a higher salary is associated with higher rank and total years of teaching and doctoral teaching experience.

Table 11.2 presents the distribution of annual salaries for faculty that are chairs of PhD and DNP programs and administrators. As seen in the table, in the current data, among those in academic nursing administration excluding chairs of DNP or PhD programs, a higher percentage made more than $105,000 annually (N = 102, 62%). In contrast, 53% of PhD chairs reported making more than $105,000 annually while only 37% of DNP chairs made more than $105,000 annually. The salary distributions in the current data show that in general, compensation for PhD and DNP chairs and administrators have gone up slightly from 2012 where the percent of administrators more than $105,000 annually were 54% (administrators, not DNP or PhD chairs), 42% (PhD chairs), and 32% (DNP chairs).

"How confident are you in the leadership of the administrator of the doctoral program you teach in?" Most respondents chose "mostly confident" as their choice (N = 392, 63%) in 2012. In the current survey, more than half (N = 435, 57%) indicated "mostly confident." Again, similar to 2012 when one out of 10 responses expressed "lack of confidence" in their doctoral program administrator (N = 59, 10%), in the current survey that number crept marginally higher (N = 104, 14%). We were also curious to learn whether aspirations of the faculty for becoming a chair/director of a doctoral nursing program had changed since the 2012 survey. To the question of whether they agreed with the statement "I am not an academic nursing administrator but I have aspirations to become a director/chair of a doctoral nursing program," findings from the current survey were quite different from 2012. In 2012, the most frequent response was "No" (N = 275, 49%), followed by "does not apply, I am already in that position" (N = 173, 31%). Only, one fifth of the respondents said "Yes" (N = 52, 9%) to have aspiration to become a director/chair of a doctoral nursing program at that time. In the current survey however, close to half of the respondents (N = 330, 43%) said "yes" to having such aspirations.

SUCCESSION PLANNING AND FUTURE VISION

Consistent with the survey in 2012, the final section of this survey was intended to address issues surrounding succession planning in doctoral education and their views related to ability of graduates from DNP programs to lead scholarship and research in nursing through high-quality work. To the question regarding conversation surrounding succession planning, once again the findings from this 2016 survey differed considerably from that of 2012. In 2012, more than half of the responses indicated that discussion surrounding succession planning was either "visible" (N = 231, 37%) or "very visible" (N = 123, 20%) at their work. Less than one tenth of the respondents indicated that there was no discussion about succession planning at all at their workplace (N = 57, 9%). In sharp contrast, in the current survey, close to half the respondents (N = 327, 43%) indicated that succession planning was "not very visible" at all in the workplace. The final question in this section asked their current view on "How possible is it going to be for future doctoral nursing faculty, particularly those teaching in DNP programs to be tenure track, pursue substantive scholarship and maintain clinical hours for certification?" Once again, responses to this question were similar in the current survey to that of 2012. In the current survey, the most common responses were "More challenging than it has been in the past" (N = 317, 42%) and "near impossible" (N = 208, 27%). These responses are similar to the ones in 2012 when most respondents selected "more challenging than it is today" (N = 274, 44%) or "nearly impossible" (N = 154, 25%). Finally, "What best reflects your point of view about the future of doctoral nursing education?" were mostly "optimistic" among faculty teaching in DNP-only (82%), in PhD-only (70%), and in both programs (76%).

■ DISCUSSION

The landscape of doctoral nursing faculty has undergone some significant changes since 2012. The number of doctoral nursing faculty that are teaching exclusively in PhD programs has declined by 50% and the majority of doctoral nursing faculty (45%) are now teaching exclusively in DNP programs. The number teaching in both PhD and DNP programs remains stable. This shift is not surprising given the tremendous growth in the number of DNP programs since 2006. The AACN (2015b) reports that in 2014 an additional 23 new DNP programs were introduced, raising the total to 269 schools, resulting in an enrollment growth of "26.2%, with 18,352 students enrolled in DNP programs nationwide" while "enrollment in PhD nursing programs increased by 3.2% over the previous year with 5,290 students currently enrolled" (pp. 23–24). As in 2012, the majority of respondents were teaching at public/state-supported universities.

As noted previously, the number of tenured/tenure-track faculty has dropped since the 2012 survey. The drop in tenure rates for this sample in comparison to the previous sample could be attributed to retirement. Of more notable concern was the significant drop (22%) in the number of tenure-track doctoral faculty since 2012. In 2012, we noticed this trend and voiced our concern that doctoral nursing faculty may become predominantly untenured and on a non-tenure track (NTT). This seems to be becoming a reality and would have clear negative implications for individual doctoral faculty and programs in colleges and universities where tenured faculty overwhelmingly comprises the bulk of leadership in the academy. Research has demonstrated that NTT faculty report greater dissatisfaction with personal interaction with colleagues, complain of disenfranchisement within academia, and a perception of being second class citizens (Kezar, 2012; Ott & Cisnerso, 2015). An analysis of our data has indicated that the number of doctoral faculty who reported they were not tenured and not on the tenure track doubled since 2012, with 249 (33%) reporting this. This trend has been also noted in the literature as Kezar and Maxey (2013) report that between 1969 and 2009, the number of NTT positions has grown from 22% to 67% while the tenured positions have dropped from 78% to 33%. This trend has raised concerns in the academy. Cross and Goldenberg (2009) predicted that the "growth of non-tenure-track faculty numbers constitutes an erosion of the tenure system," warning that the lack of attention to this trend may lead to "erosion in academic freedom" (p. 11). Certainly, as mentioned earlier in this chapter, if DNP faculty members are going to be excluded from the tenure ranks and the current trend toward a predominantly NTT university faculty, we conclude there is going to be another disruptive trajectory in the history of the nursing discipline, where an important segment of the workforce is marginalized, well documented by Melosh in her 1982 *The Physician's Hand: Work Culture and Conflict in American Nursing*.

As for an overall forecast of the future of tenure, much has been written about this recently in the general literature (Dobbie & Robinson, 2008; Ehrenberg & Zhang, 2004; Ott & Cisneros, 2015), and we can attest that our own institutions' hiring for recent years has focused more heavily on NTT hires, and furthermore, doctoral faculty teaching appointments with DNP preparation have increasingly been among NTT faculty. At our respective graduate nursing programs, the philosophy surrounding the teaching of an individual doctoral course has been more "Who is the best expert and who is best qualified to teach this specific course?" rather than the particular tenure status of the individual.

Data from this study indicate that continuing concerns about salaries among doctoral nursing faculty are well grounded, especially because the nursing faculty shortage has not abated and significant and rising percentages of senior nursing faculty are exiting the profession due to retirements. While the total percent of faculty making between $85,000 and $105,000 has grown from 46% in 2012 to 55% in 2016, the percent making less than $85,000 a year has only decreased from 45% to 40% and the mode salary for doctoral faculty, non-administrators in 2016 is less than $75,000 a year (21.8%). Administrative salaries among non-DNP or PhD chairs has risen where the majority (62%) make more than $105,000 a year, but disparities at that same salary range exist between PhD (53%) versus DNP department/program chairs (37%). Whether this disparity is more due to seniority and/or rank needs additional analyses. We contend that the salary concerns are real barriers to recruiting a younger generation of nursing faculty. The role of gender in nursing faculty salaries as compared to male-dominated professions such as business, law, pharmacy, and engineering faculty salaries also needs to be seriously examined. The rising percentage of respondents who indicated that there was no visible or an absence of succession planning in their organization doubled from 9% in 2012 to 18% in 2016. What are the origins of this increase? Is it because academic nursing departments are struggling with this issue or is it being ignored?

In 2012, the data indicated that some 26% of doctoral faculty planned to retire within the next 5 years and 53% within the next 10 years. In 2016, doctoral faculty plan retire within the next 5 years has risen to 32% heightening the need for succession planning. A notable shift from the previous survey is the increased number of respondents who report having aspirations to become a director/chair of a doctoral nursing program, rising from 9% in 2012 to close to half of the respondents (N = 330, 43%). However, another way to look at these data is to note that also in 2012, 49% of the respondents had no wish to go into academic nursing administration and that has only marginally improved in 2016 at 44%. Our concern remains that there are limited leadership development programs for the doctoral faculty who could be recruited and prepared to assume these roles. In addition, there must be real tangible benefits to being an academic nursing administrator, and we are very aware of many schools of nursing that give these individuals only very modest stipends, and many doctoral faculty may prefer the flexibility of their full-time teaching roles. Moreover, with the decline in tenure-track hires that most nursing schools are seeing, will directors and department chairs of the future be NTT faculty? This is very likely to be a trend among DNP program directors and chairs if they are going to be institutionally classified as NTT faculty. Again, if the PhD chair is tenured and the DNP chair is not, what kind of signal does this send to the profession?

In 2012, the enthusiasm for the DNP degree, still a relatively new doctorate, was at 43%, but when combined with "moderately" (22%), the percentage rose to 65%. Still, at that time, a substantial number (30%) did not support the DNP or only supported it reluctantly. We found it interesting that of the 231 faculty (37%) who reported that they taught in a DNP program (or taught in both DNP and PhD programs), 7% did not support the DNP degree and another 14% only supported the DNP reluctantly (chi-square $p < 0.001$; see Figure 11.3). This presented an ethical issue of an individual faculty member who was teaching in a program with which he or she philosophically disagreed or did not support. This had significant implications, particularly when doctoral workload has to be distributed equally. We expressed concern that the merit of assigning faculty to teach courses or supervise DNP projects or practice dissertations (whatever the final work product is called), might be questioned—especially when their motivations to teach and advise these students may lack enthusiasm. In 2016, enthusiasm for the DNP degree among doctoral faculty who taught DNP exclusively was at 68%, but when combined with "moderately" (21%), that percentage rises rose to 89%. For faculty who taught both DNP and PhD, the enthusiasm was reported at 79%.

In 2012, the question of resources indicated that there were differing points of view between DNP and PhD faculty. Among PhD faculty, 38% believed that DNP programs would negatively impact PhD resources, but among DNP faculty only 9% agreed. These numbers remained essentially the same in the 2016 survey with 8% of DNP-only faculty and 37% PhD-only faculty picked that DNP "will" negatively impact current PhD resources. In 2012, 31% of doctoral faculty who taught both in DNP and PhD programs believed that DNP "will not" negatively impact current PhD resources, while in 2016, the number increased slightly to 35% and we think this is perhaps a more reliable finding, as these faculty have experience teaching in both programs and likely have the benefit of watching this trend, over time. Sixty-five percent were either unclear or certain the DNP has had a negative impact on their PhD program resources and whether or not this perception or belief has been impacted by declining PhD enrollments is unknown. The decline in higher education funds in the United States in the past several years is real and many state-funded doctoral programs, particularly PhD/research programs where full-funded students are common (perhaps less common in nursing), may have impacted these findings. Ketefian and Redman (2015) express this concern stating that not only will the PhD and DNP programs compete for resources but will also have significant implications for faculty workload and other areas as well. This question does need more investigation and its impact on the discipline, if this is true, needs to be ascertained.

The professional growth and work satisfaction section of the survey indicated a drop from 54% to 45% among doctoral nursing faculty who are very satisfied with their current faculty position. When combined with those reporting being "moderately satisfied" (35%), the level of satisfaction rises to 80%, which is extremely high. This number is very comparable to the 70% who are mostly optimistic about the future of doctoral nursing education (vs. the 25% who are either ambivalent or pessimistic), which is amazingly the exact percentage (70%) who expressed optimism about doctoral nursing education in 2012! When a separate analysis was done on 2016 survey between programs, the percentage of those teaching in PhD programs who responded "very satisfied" was 56% and percentage of those teaching in DNP programs was 52%. For those teaching in both programs the percentage was 57%. These numbers across programs seem consistent, but overall they do not appear to be exceptionally high. What is interesting is that when these same faculty were queried about how future doctoral nursing faculty in their own institutions will view the quality of their work life, the 54% ("very satisfied") declines to 17%, and the 86% ("very" and "moderately" satisfied) declines to 69%. This indicates that the current doctoral nursing faculty do not think that future doctoral nursing faculty will have the same quality of work life that they currently enjoy.

As in 2012, doctoral faculty rank higher salaries as their chief concern. Internal resources for scholarship and reduced teaching load ranked second and third in priority, followed by improved climate for intellectual discourse and higher quality students. Salary issues are well known among nursing faculty, but what constitutes "internal resources for scholarship" is unclear. While the authors of this survey considered this item might include, for example, grantsmanship support, editing services, and adequate travel support for professional meetings, it is clear that individual respondents may have thought this meant something different.

Most faculty members (57%) felt very confident in their PhD or DNP department chairs, representing only a slight drop from 63% of respondents in 2012. This stability may be related to the slight increase (6%) in enthusiasm and optimism expressed for the future of doctoral education in general, rising to a high of 76%, and a decrease in the perception that the DNP will negatively impact PhD resources—perhaps an indication of trust in administration decision making although not a resounding display of confidence. Clearly diminishing grants and other funding streams will also negatively impact PhD resources and remain a concern for doctoral faculty. In this current environment, it is essential that the individuals serving in academic nursing administrator roles, are adequately prepared to merit and sustain faculty confidence.

Perhaps our greatest concern arising from the findings in this survey was that the percentage of respondents who thought it would be more challenging than it is today (42%) or nearly impossible (27%) for future doctoral faculty, particularly those teaching in DNP programs, to have the time to pursue substantive scholarship to achieve success on the tenure track and maintain the requisite number of hours for certification remains consistent with those in 2012. Combined, this percentage is 69%, and is exactly what was reported in 2012. Despite the earlier high optimism percentages, the additional data reflect another concurrent, persistent pessimistic view among current PhD and DNP faculty. This is of particular concern since, as mentioned earlier, there are now more DNP programs, students, and graduations compared to the PhD (AACN, 2015c). Will these trends eventually impact nursing academia? Who actually will comprise the majority of nursing faculty in the future? It is likely that DNP-prepared faculty will constitute the majority ranks of nursing faculty period, and this was projected by 60% ($N = 459$) of respondents. Seventeen percent did not think that the DNP degree would predominate in nursing academic (over the PhD), and 23% were uncertain. The numbers alone seem to project that DNP degree will become more common than the PhD in academia. Already the AACN indicates that during the period from 2009 to 2010 some 24% of DNP graduates were employed in a nursing faculty position (Fang, Tracy, & Bednash, 2009–2010). Ketefian and Redman (2015) point out that there is a

> mismatch between the DNP educational preparation and the employment the graduates are seeking. The stated goal of the DNP is advanced practice to improve patient care, but the majority are taking faculty positions for which their education has not prepared them. (p. 369)

In the 2016 survey, 51% of respondents did not think that the DNP degree itself prepared individuals for the full-time faculty role ($N = 391$), while 49% ($N = 371$) agreed that it does—clearly a split opinion. Nevertheless, the migration of large numbers of DNP graduates into academia, both in DNP graduate education and undergraduate programs, is a trend that must be studied and addressed. We even addressed this question whether the respondents agreed that the DNP degree was appropriate for undergraduate nursing education and 45% ($N = 340$) said "yes" and 45% ($N = 265$) said "no." While the CCNE has stated it will not accredit such programs, the prospect of a replacement of the PhD with the DNP in academia appears to be a future possibility. Ketefian and Redman (2015) urge that this trend continues as a means to address the national faculty shortage; the DNP program content and accreditation must be revised in order to align with these real trends in the membership of academic nursing administration (Ketefian & Redman, 2015).

■ SUMMARY

The findings from this second survey have raised additional questions and considerations that warrant further exploration. Clearly, doctoral nursing education is at a crossroads with the robust increase in enrollment of DNP programs and the generally flat enrollment of PhD programs, as well as the negative effects of senior PhD-prepared faculty retirements on the current system. With these and other market forces, doctoral faculty are faced with some critical challenges that require reflection and innovation—namely the DNP-prepared faculty member in academia, a decrease in tenure-track and tenured positions, the lack of integration of faculty practice into the faculty role, lack of recognition of the faculty role, confusion over the scholarship expectations for DNP-prepared faculty, perceived lack of relevance of the PhD degree to practitioners, and the continued concern over low nursing faculty salaries (Oermann et al., 2016; Smeltzer et al., 2016). Doctoral faculty will need to grapple with these serious issues that have the ability to slow nursing's progress in the academic and clinical environment. The U.S. doctoral nursing faculty has the potential to significantly contribute to nursing knowledge, transform nursing education and practice, and positively impact health and health policy with a healthy combination of practice-focused and research-focused doctoral nursing faculty (Glasgow & Dreher, 2010). To achieve this goal, the doctoral nursing faculty need to be appropriately prepared for their role, valued for the educator/faculty role, appreciated for the various forms of scholarship in which they engage, and compensated appropriately. Without such elements in place, the nursing faculty shortage will only exacerbate, and exceptional preparation of the nursing workforce needed to care for diverse populations, generate practice knowledge, and drive innovation in this ever-changing, complex, challenging world will not be realized (Dreher & Rundio, 2013; Valiga, this volume).

■ CRITICAL THINKING QUESTIONS

1. *Do you consider the academic role an attractive career option for you?*
2. *What skills or abilities are you aiming to acquire during your respective doctoral nursing degree?*
3. *What are some of the notable trends in doctoral nursing education between the 2012 and 2016 survey do you find impactful?*
4. *Do you think a doctoral degree is valuable to the nursing profession or to the respective individual or both? Why or why not?*
5. *The DNP is still a new doctoral degree. What do you think about its short history?*

6. *What are the critical elements that you believe a DNP degree or PhD degree in nursing can contribute to the health care?*
7. *How important are salary concerns for your career?*
8. *Do you think the DNP degree is clearly understood by potential employers or not?*
9. *From the results of the 2016 study, what are some of the issues that lack consensus in the profession?*
10. *What would you ask on the next survey that is different from what has been asked in 2012 and 2016?*

■ NOTE

1. "Actually there are more [than three nursing accreditation agencies] if you consider the specialty accrediting agencies for nurse anesthetists and nurse midwives" (personal communication, Dr. Judith Halstead, May 1, 2016).

■ REFERENCES

American Association of Colleges of Nursing. (2004). AACN position statement on the practice doctorate in nursing. Retrieved from www.aacn.nche.edu/DNP/pdf/DNP.pdf

American Association of Colleges of Nursing. (2006). *The essentials of doctoral education for advanced nursing practice.* Retrieved from www.aacn.nche.edu/DNP/pdf/Essentials.pdf

American Association of Colleges of Nursing. (2015a). Report on 2014–2015 enrollment and graduations in baccalaureate and graduate programs in nursing. Retrieved from http://www.aacn.nche.edu/media-relations/fact-sheets/nursing-faculty-shortage

American Association of Colleges of Nursing. (2015b). New AACN data confirm enrollment surge in schools of nursing. Retrieved from www.aacn.nche.edu/faculty/news/2015/enrollment

American Association of Colleges of Nursing. (2015c). DNP fact sheet. Retrieved from www.aacn.nche.edu/media-relations/fact-sheets/dnp

American Association of Colleges of Nursing. (2015d). *New white paper on the DNP: Current issues and clarifying recommendations.* Report from the Task Force on the Implementation of the DNP. Retrieved from http://www.aacn.nche.edu/aacn-publications/white-papers/DNP-Implementation-TF-Report-8-15.pdf

Cross, J. G., & Goldenberg, E. N. (2009). *Off-track profs: Nontenured teachers in higher education.* Cambridge, MA: MIT Press.

Disch, J., Edwardson, S., & Adwan, J. (2004). Nursing faculty satisfaction with individual, institutional, and leadership factors. *Journal of Professional Nursing, 20*(5), 323–332.

Dreher, H. M., & Rundio, A. (2013). *The "big tent" for educating advanced practice nurses: Issues surrounding MSN, DNP, and PhD preparation in advanced practice nursing: Essentials of role development* (3rd ed.). Philadelphia, PA: F. A. Davis.

Dreher, H. M., Smith Glasgow, M. E., Cornelius, F., & Bhattacharya, A. (2012). A report on a national study of doctoral nursing faculty. *Nursing Clinics of North America, 47*(4), 435–453.

Dobbie, D., & Robinson, I. (2008). Reorganizing higher education in the United States and Canada: The erosion of tenure and the unionization of contingent faculty. *Labor Studies Journal, 33*(2), 117–140.

Ehrenberg, R. G., & Zhang, L. (2004). Do tenured and tenure-track faculty matter? Working Paper National Bureau of Economic Research, Cambridge, MA. Retrieved from http://www.nber.org/papers/w10695.pdf

Fang, D., Li., Y., Stauffer, D. C., & Trautman, D. E. (2016). *2015–2016 Salaries of instructional and administrative nursing faculty in baccalaureate and graduate programs in nursing.* Washington, DC: American Association of Colleges of Nursing.

Fang, D., Tracy, C., & Bednash, G. D. (2010). *2009–2010 enrollment and graduations in baccalaureate and graduate programs in nursing.* Washington, DC: American Association of Colleges of Nursing.

Glasgow, M., & Dreher, H. M. (2010). The future of oncology nursing science: Who will generate the knowledge? *Oncology Nursing Forum, 37*(4), 393–396.

Kaufman, K. (2007a). Headlines from the NLN—More findings from the NLN/Carnegie National Survey: How nurse educators spend their time. *Nursing Education Perspectives, 28*, 296–297.

Kaufman, K. (2007b). Compensation for nurse educators: Findings from the NLN/Carnegie National Survey with implications for recruitment and retention. *Nursing Education Perspectives, 28*, 223–225.

Kaufman, K. (2007c). Headlines from the NLN—Introducing the NLN/Carnegie National Survey of Nurse Educators: Compensation, workload, and teaching practice. *Nursing Education Perspectives, 28*, 164–169.

Ketefian, S., & Redman, R. W. (2015). A critical examination of developments in nursing doctoral education in the United States. *Revista Latino-Americana de Enfermagem, 23*(3), 363–371. doi: 10.1590/0104-1169.0797.2566

Kezar, A. (2012). *Improving contingent faculty relations: Changing campuses for the new faculty majority.* New York, NY: Routledge.

Kezar, A., & Mexey, D. (2013). The changing academic workforce. *Trusteeship Magazine, AGB Press.* Retrieved from http://agb.org/trusteeship/2013/5/changing-academic-workforce

Meleis, A. I. (2011). Should DNPs occupy tenure track faculty positions? Rational against. *The Journal for Nurse Practitioners, 7*(4), 280–281.

Melosh, B. (1982). *The physician's hand: Work culture and conflict in American nursing.* Philadelphia, PA: Temple University Press.

Nicholes, R. H., & Dyer, J. (2012). Is eligibility for tenure possible for the doctor of nursing practice-prepared faculty? *Journal of Professional Nursing, 28*(1), 13–17.

Oermann, M. H., Lynn, M. R., & Agger, C. A. (2016). Hiring intentions of directors of nursing programs related to DNP- and PhD-prepared faculty and roles of faculty. *Journal of Professional Nursing, 32*(3), 173–179.

Ott, M., & Cisneros, J. (2015). Understanding the changing faculty workforce in higher education: A comparison of full-time non-tenure track and tenure line experiences. *Education Policy Analysis Archives, 23*(90). doi:10.14507/epaa.v23.1934

Potempa, K. M., Redman, R. W., & Anderson, C. A. (2008). Capacity for the advancement of nursing science: Issues and challenges. *Journal of Professional Nursing, 24*(6), 329–336.

Robert Wood Johnson Foundation. (2007). Charting nursing's future. Retrieved from www.rwjf.org/files/publications/other/nursingfuture4pdf

Shirey, M. (2006). Stress and burnout in nursing faculty. *Nurse Educator, 31*(3), 95–97.

Smeltzer, S., Sharts-Hopko, N. C., Cantrell, M. A., Heverly, M. A., Jenkinson, A., & Nhenge, S. (2015). Work-life balance of nursing faculty in research and practice-focused doctoral programs. *Nursing Outlook, 63*(6), 621–631.

Smeltzer, S., Sharts-Hopko, N. C., Cantrell, M. A., Heverly, M. A., Jenkinson, A., & Nhenge, S. (2016). Assessment of the impact teaching demands on research productivity among doctoral nursing program faculty. *Journal of Professional Nursing, 32*(3), 180–192.

Terhaar, M. F., Taylor, L. A., & Sylvia, M. L. (2016). The doctor of nursing practice: From start-up to impact. *Nursing Education Perspectives, 37*(1), 3–9.

Udlis, K. A., & Mancuso, J. M. (2015). Perceptions of the role of the doctor of nursing practice-prepared nurse: Clarity or confusion. *Journal of Professional Nursing, 31*(4), 274–283.

Zungolo, E. (2009). *The DNP and the faculty role: Issues and challenges.* Paper presented at the Second National Conference on the Doctor of Nursing Practice: The Dialogue Continues…, Hilton Head Island, SC.

CHAPTER ELEVEN

Reflective Response

Nancy C. Sharts-Hopko

A shortage of doctorally prepared nurses able to meet the profession's multifaceted clinical, educational, leadership, and scientific agendas led to the Institute of Medicine's (IOM, 2010) recommendation that the number of doctorally prepared nurses be doubled by 2020. The authors of Chapter 11 note the confusion that persists around the role of the Doctor of Nursing Practice (DNP) versus the research doctorate (PhD) in nursing. When the DNP degree was initially proposed in the United States, its purpose was to prepare clinical nursing leaders with the knowledge and skills to transform systems of care. As it has turned out, approximately 40% of DNP graduates each year assume academic positions (Fang, Li, Arietti, & Bednash, 2014); this is actually the same proportion of PhD graduates whose primary employment is in an academic institution, but the number of DNP graduates annually is now far greater than the number of PhD graduates.

Altman, Butler, and Shern (2016) recently reported on results to date of implementation of the IOM report. They specifically identified concern about the relative stagnation in the preparation of nurses with PhDs compared to DNPs. They noted that the annual number of PhD graduates is insufficient to replace retirees. A major contributing factor is the shorter length of study required for a DNP degree. Altman et al. indicated that greater emphasis on PhD program expansion and on incentives for students to pursue PhD degrees is needed. Of course, this is contingent on having sufficient faculty with research doctorates to teach and mentor them.

It is anticipated that in the foreseeable future, most doctorally prepared faculty members in most schools of nursing will hold DNP degrees. Although there is no question that these new faculty members are urgently needed in the face of the worsening nursing faculty shortage, it is imperative that consideration be given to what this trend means for the discipline of nursing.

In 2006, the Carnegie Foundation for the Advancement of Teaching commissioned a collection of essays on the future of doctoral education, and the greatest emphasis in the collection was placed on research doctorates. It is particularly germane at this time to reflect on the specific contribution of PhDs to a discipline. Golde (2006) emphasized that the aim of PhD education is to prepare the stewards of the discipline; that is to say that PhD holders are responsible for the discipline's integrity. Disciplinary stewards should be capable of conserving the most important ideas from the past, generating new knowledge, and transforming knowledge that has been generated and conserved by relating it to ideas in other fields. Stewards of a discipline are entrusted with its care now and in the future; they preserve the essence of the field while taking risks to move the discipline forward. Disciplinary stewardship entails ensuring the preparation of new generations of scholars who understand the discipline's development from its origins, as well as the wise application of major precepts now and in the future.

In recent years, education about evidence-based practice has, to a great extent, replaced education about the conduct of research in nursing at the baccalaureate and master's degree levels (American Association of Colleges of Nursing [AACN], 2008, 2011). The value and relevance of work that is regarded as theoretical may be ignored or discounted at these levels. Some leaders in evidence-based practice believe that it is counterproductive to teach the research process to baccalaureate and master's degree students (Melnyk, 2014). This phenomenon, coupled with the shift in the doctoral preparation of faculty that was noted earlier, will result in students of the future having little or no exposure to the process of knowledge generation that is a hallmark of PhD preparation. There will be little incentive for students to consider earning a research doctorate because they will have had little exposure to role models, and it is possible that they will be unfamiliar with the contributions of nurse scientists. It is likely that they will have heard that earning a PhD takes much longer than a DNP, which further diminishes likelihood that they will entertain the option of a PhD.

Education for evidence-based practice emphasizes the examination of recent research to determine best clinical practices (LoBiondo-Wood & Haber, 2013). One of the unanticipated consequences of this trend is the danger of what has been termed *disciplinary amnesia* (Vannini, 2008). Disciplinary amnesia is the disappearance of important concepts, constructs, or theories from a field of study in response to redefinitions or to barriers imposed by the discipline. Barriers may be associated with, for example, sociopolitical or economic trends, or cultural shifts within the discipline. The loss of knowledge is problematic because it can undermine the process of building the discipline and promote inefficiency when, years later, lost knowledge is hypothesized anew and precious human and financial resources are expended on its rediscovery. Numerous current examples in nursing come to mind for which historical antecedents are plentiful, such as, patient-centered care or social determinants of health.

Given these factors of the shift in the preparation of doctorally prepared faculty and the emphasis in nursing education on evidence-based practice at the expense of knowledge generation and theory building, the ability of the discipline of nursing to fulfill its scientific mission in the future is of concern, as Smith et al. have noted. Moreover, if PhDs are recruited into academia, despite barriers such as salary that Smith et al. identified, they may find themselves in institutions or teaching appointments in which they are encumbered with heavy teaching loads that jeopardize their ability to contribute substantially to the generation of knowledge through research (Smeltzer et al., 2014).

■ IMPLICATIONS

All doctorally prepared nurses have much to contribute to the clinical, educational, leadership, and scientific agendas of the discipline of nursing. The translation of knowledge generated by the conduct of research into practice is of critical importance in ensuring safe, cost-effective, accessible, and high-quality health care for the public. Clearly, though, nurse scientists prepared with a PhD degree are an increasingly scarce resource. Several strategies with the potential to encourage nurses to earn PhDs, and to recruit and retain them in academic settings follow.

Undergraduate and graduate students must be exposed to nurses with research and clinical doctorates. Educational preparation for evidence-based practice need not mean that the process of knowledge generation be ignored. Students need to understand the theoretical underpinnings of the discipline of nursing and how they shape the unique contribution of nurses today in order for them to imagine PhD education as a career possibility. Students need to know who on their faculties are nurse scientists and the focus of their research. Relevant work of nurse scientists can be woven into course readings and classroom discussions throughout their educational preparation.

Nurses with research and clinical doctorates need to be deployed in ways that maximize their potential contributions to both research and evidence-based practice. Faculties need to confront the differences between and complementarity of these two types of doctorally prepared nurses and determine how they can best contribute to the mission of the institution. Career paths need to be tailored so that faculty with PhDs and DNPs can advance without the assertion that they are the same. All of this needs to take place within a culture of appreciation, in which faculty members value and facilitate one another's contribution to the institution's mission.

The generally longer time required to earn a PhD is the focus of projects including the Robert Wood Johnson Foundation (2016) Future of Nursing Scholars program, which was launched in 2014. The attention that PhD faculties are giving to making their programs more efficient offers hope that they may attract more applicants in the future.

■ CONCLUSION

The shortage of nursing faculty ensures that both PhD- and DNP-prepared nurses will be needed in the future. At the present time, the production of nurses with PhDs is insufficient to replace retiring PhD-prepared faculty. They can be regarded as an endangered category. Measures that could potentially support the role of PhDs as generators and conservators of knowledge and disciplinary transformers are proposed. Without actions to encourage nurses to earn PhDs, and to appropriately deploy both PhDs and DNPs in academic institutions, the long-term survival of nursing as an academic discipline is in jeopardy.

■ REFERENCES

Altman, S. H., Butler, A. S., & Shern, L. (Eds.). (2016). *Assessing progress on the Institute of Medicine Report the future of nursing*. Washington, DC: National Academies Press.

American Association of Colleges of Nursing. (2008). *The essentials of baccalaureate education for professional nursing practice*. Washington, DC: Author.

American Association of Colleges of Nursing. (2011). *The essentials of master's education in nursing*. Washington, DC: Author.

Fang, D., Li., Y., Arietti, R., & Bednash, G. D. (2014). *2013-2014 Enrollment and graduations in baccalaureate and graduate programs in nursing*. Washington, DC: American Association of Colleges of Nursing.

Golde, C. M. (2006). Preparing stewards of the discipline. In C. M. Golde & G. E. Walker (Eds.), *Envisioning the future of doctoral education* (pp. 3–20). San Francisco, CA: Jossey-Bass.

Institute of Medicine. (2010). *The future of nursing: Leading change, advancing health*. Washington, DC: National Academies Press.

LoBiondo-Wood, G., & Haber, J. (2013). *Nursing research: Methods, critical appraisal & utilization* (8th ed.). Maryland Heights, MO: Mosby.

Melnyk, B. M. (2014). Building cultures and environments that facilitate clinician behavior change to evidence-based practice: What works? *Worldviews on Evidence-Based Practice, 11*(2), 79–80. doi:10.1111/wvn.12032

Robert Wood Johnson Foundation. (2016). Future of nursing scholars. Retrieved from http://futureof nursingscholars.org

Smeltzer, S. C., Sharts-Hopko, N. C., Cantrell, M. A., Heverly, M. A., Wise, N., Jenkinson, A., & Nthenge, S. (2014). Nursing doctoral faculty perceptions of factors that affect their continued scholarship. *Journal of Professional Nursing, 30*(6), 493–501. doi:10.1016/j.profnurs.2014.03.008

Vannini, P. (2008). The geography of disciplinary amnesia: Eleven scholars reflect on the international state of symbolic interactionism. In N. K. Denzin, J. Salvo & M. Washington (Eds.), *Studies in symbolic interactionism* (Vol. 32, pp. 15–18). Bingley, UK: Emerald Group Publishing.

The DNP and Academic–Service Partnerships

Sandra Rader, Sandra J. Engberg, and Jacqueline Dunbar-Jacob

Nursing has a long history of collaboration between service settings and academic settings in the education of nurses. From the initial educational model of apprenticeship to the placement of formal educational programs within hospitals to the education of nurses over the past half century in universities and community colleges, the relationship between the clinical setting and the educational setting has been central to the education of the next generation of nurses. This relationship is consistent with other disciplines with a focus for a strong practice. Medicine has long situated much of its education within the clinical practice setting as have numerous other health professions. Professions such as education and social work also include practical experiences in work settings. The nature of the partnerships established between academic and service settings has varied from shared ownership to affiliation agreements designed to provide opportunities for learning. The agreements have principally focused on student education with the service personnel cooperating with academic instructors or serving as direct educators themselves.

In 2004, the American Association of Colleges of Nursing (AACN) determined that advanced practice education should move from the master of science to the Doctor of Nursing Practice (DNP) level. This was followed by the 2007 decision of the nurse anesthesia Council on Accreditation (CoA) and the 2015 statements by the National Association of Clinical Nurse Specialists (NACNS) and the National Organization of Nurse Practitioner Faculties (NONPF) to move these advanced practice specialties to the DNP levels. These decisions have expanded the possibilities for academic–service partnerships. Additional education in leadership, policy, finance, quality improvement and evaluation methodologies, translation of research as well as further advances in clinical or administrative education have made the DNP a highly contributing professional for both the academic and practice sides of the partnership. These skills provide added value for the inclusion of the DNP in academic–service partnerships.

■ MOVING FROM AFFILIATION TO PARTNERSHIP

The presence of the DNP in both practice and academic settings provides opportunities for collaborations extending well beyond the traditional affiliation for student education. Not the least of these is the opportunity to contribute to the quality and in-novation of both practice and education. For example, as a component of the University of Pittsburgh Medical Center (UPMC)/UPitt (UPMC Health System and University of Pittsburgh School of Nursing) Partnership, doctorally prepared senior staff at the UPMC serve on the school leadership team, as well as a variety of academic councils. Similarly, doctorally prepared faculty serve on the nursing leadership group, as well as on nursing and interdisciplinary committees. The benefit of this form of partnership is improvement of communication and broadening of the perspective in these critical working groups.

In this model, DNP-prepared senior staff serve on the undergraduates, masters, and DNP councils. The councils design curriculum, review specific learning activities, review student progress, and ensure that programs are addressing future health care workforce skills. In addition, the DNP staff serves as members of DNP-student projects, deliver lectures to classes, and precept students. The addition of the DNP staff from the health system provides information on the vision for practice, confirmation of edu-cational directions, and opportunity for the service partners to learn about changes in educational initiatives, and input on the positive and negative experiences of students, faculty, and clinical staff in the education of students. The educational background of the DNP staff in quality improvement, mentorship/preceptorship, and an advanced level of practice enriches the conversation between the academic and service partners.

Reciprocally, the DNP (and PhD) faculty of the school of nursing serve on a variety of practice councils. For example, faculty serve on the health system–nursing informat-ics council and evidence-based practice council for nursing. Faculty also serve on inter-disciplinary committees, such as recruitment committees, ethics committee, scientific review committee, infection control and patient safety committee, as well as the quality of patient care committees. In addition, faculty serve as consultants at selected hospitals and collaborate in selected quality initiatives. Faculty are able to bring the perspective of both education and advanced practice to the work of these councils enriched by the advanced clinical, translational, policy, and quality-improvement DNP education they received. Additionally, the shared participation means that clinical staff are aware of educational innovations and academic staff are aware of practice changes without acci-dental discovery. This makes interactions around students and educational processes more efficient and reinforces trust between the two groups.

The connection between the practice environment and the academic environ-ment that are enriched by the education of the DNP faculty member or clinical setting staff promotes a deeper level of engagement in both the academic and service environ-ments. The emphasis on personal opinion driving educational and practice decisions is replaced with a commitment to and understanding of the translation of research find-ings to education and practice along with both an appreciation for and competence to evaluate such innovations in the real world (educational/practice) settings. Further, the shared perspective of the DNP in both settings facilitates collaboration in advancing the profession.

One of the strongest areas of partnership is in the education of the next generations of DNP students. Two models of education currently exist. One of those models, sup-ported by AACN, NONPF, NACNS, and CoA, advocates for advanced practice educa-tion at the bachelor of science in nursing (BSN) to DNP level. In this model, the student has 1,000 or more hours of supervised clinical practice as well as education in systems, evidence-based practice and translation, policy, and leadership. Programs that follow this model may offer post-master's programs within the specialty track. The second, and currently more common model, offers leadership, evidence-based practice transla-tion, policy, and systems educational content as a general post-master's DNP program without a specialty focus. Thus, there may be some variation in the contribution to advanced practice innovations between the two groups. Whichever be the program, the education of the DNP is heavily dependent on a clinical partnership, which can support that level of education.

■ ACADEMIC–SERVICE PARTNERSHIPS IN THE EDUCATION OF THE DNP

The August 2015 report from the AACN Task Force on Implementation of the DNP (white paper) included a statement reaffirming the importance of academic–service partnerships in creating and sustaining progressive education and practice. The task force recommended that DNP programs follow the AACN-AONE (American Organization of Nurse Executives) task force on academic–service partnership-guiding principles when establishing partnerships (AANC Task Force on Implementation of the DNP, 2015). Partnerships should be formalized relationships based on "mutual goals, respect, and knowledge" (p. 1). As programs establish academic–service partnerships, they should consider potential partners beyond traditional health care systems. A broad range of partnerships should be considered (AACN, 2012).

Although we were unable to identify published articles that specifically addressed academic–service partnerships in relation to the DNP education or practice, such partnerships have the potential to benefit students as well as the partnership sites. A broad range of partnerships will allow DNP students to engage in practice experiences that allow them to attain and demonstrate the DNP essentials. Practice experiences for the DNP student should include more than direct patient care. They should also include indirect care opportunities that allow students to broaden their expertise in relation to the skill set defined in the DNP essentials (white paper). Having a broad range of practice partners will facilitate DNP programs' ability to provide these experiences for students. They will also help to ensure adequate numbers of high-quality direct patient care experiences for advance practice DNP students. The 2015 AACN report from the Task Force on Implementation of the DNP states that all DNP programs are required to document and validate that all graduates have met all of the DNP essential outcomes. This includes BSN to DNP and master of science in nursing (MSN) to DNP students and includes students in programs focusing on leadership and health policy, as well as direct patient care roles. In addition, the report recommends practice immersion experiences where students have the opportunity to apply, integrate and synthesize knowledge related to the DNP essentials, and to demonstrate achievement of outcomes in relation to advanced nursing practice (AANC Task Force on Implementation of the DNP, 2015). Meeting these requirements and recommendations requires access to a variety of practice settings and academic–service partnerships can help ensure this access.

Academic–practice partnerships are also important in giving DNP students access to settings where they can plan, implement, and evaluate their DNP project. According to the white paper, all DNP projects should:

- Be designed to effect health care outcomes through either direct or indirect care
- Have a micro-, meso- or macro-level systems focus or a population/aggregate focus
- Be implemented in the appropriate practice setting
- Include a plan for sustainability

- Include evaluation of process and/or outcomes that guide practice or policy
- Provide the basis for future practice-related scholarship (AANC Task Force on Implementation of the DNP, 2015)

DNP projects should demonstrate the cumulative knowledge and skills students have gained during their program (Waldrop, Caruso, Fuchs, & Hypes, 2014). Having an adequate number and range of academic–practice partnerships is important in providing DNP students with access to practice settings where they can develop, implement, and evaluate a clinical project that meets the earlier criteria.

In addition to the benefits that these partnerships afford DNP programs and their students, there are also potential benefits for the practice settings (Dunbar-Jacob, Nativio, & Khalil, 2013). Focus on the Magnet® recognition program and quality improvement initiatives, as well as the requirement for quality monitoring are among the forces driving current interest in academic–practice partnerships (Kleinpell, Faut-Callahan, Carson, Llewellyn, & Dreher, 2015). DNP programs are designed to prepare experts in specialized advanced practice. Students are prepared for practice that is innovative and evidence-based, applying credible research findings to improve health care outcomes (AACN, *The Essentials of Doctoral Education for Advanced Nursing Practice*). When the DNP student has the opportunity to collaborate with practice partners in the design, implementation, and evaluation of his or her project, the practice site as well as the student will benefit from the knowledge gained. DNP program faculty with expertise in quality improvement methodologies can partner with members of the clinical team in the design, implementation, and evaluation of quality improvement projects that improve quality and accessible patient-centered care. Faculty can also collaborate with clinical settings on the development of advanced practice registered nurses' (APRNs') residency programs. Finally, academic–practice partnerships can enhance the ability of practice sites to recruit and retain DNP-prepared APRNs.

Although we did not identify any academic–practice partnership models that were specifically designed to provide clinical experiences for DNP students, several of the models in the literature involved graduate students and could serve as effective DNP program-practice models. Thabault, Mylott, and Patterson (2015) described an academic–practice partnership between Minute Clinics and Northeastern University School of Nursing. The goals of the partnership were to recruit and retain APRNs in Minute Clinic practice sites, support academic progression, and provide teaching expertise in relation to knowledge and skills needed to lead interprofessional teams in retail and other community settings. Service and faculty partners developed an APRN postgraduate residency within the Minute Clinics, which included a two-credit online leadership course at the completion of the residency program. Tuition for the course was funded through the residency program. Preceptors as well as residents were invited to take the course.

Killeen et al. (2015) described a practitioner–teacher model in which APRNs in practice settings served as advanced practice nurses and preceptors for APRN students. In 2012, Rush University Medical Center was selected as a graduate nursing education (GNE) site. These sites, established under the Affordable Care Act, are administered by the Centers for Medicare and Medicaid Services with the goal of increasing the supply of APRNs to increase access to quality health care services. As a GNE site, Rush was able to trial new models of care that included training for nurse practitioner (NP) students. The authors described one of the models in the cardiac intensive care unit in which acute care NPs provided 24/7 patient coverage for the unit. Development of the model included the development of the practitioner–teacher model for NP training.

We also identified examples of academic-practice partnerships that could serve as models for DNP programs to develop indirect clinical experiences that will allow students to develop their expertise in relation to the DNP essential skills not focused on direct patient care. Jones, Mayer, and Mandelkehr (2009) described an academic-practice partnership developed between the University of North Carolina at Chapel Hill and the University of North Carolina Health Care System. The partnership was designed to educate graduate (master's level) students about health care quality and safety. The goal was to add a practicum experience to a course in the master's nursing curriculum focusing on quality improvement. The faculty member responsible for the course worked with the director of performance improvement and the patient safety officer in the health care system to develop a preceptor model and practical component as part of the course. During the practicum experiences, students work in teams with service-organization practice experts on quality and patient-safety initiatives in the participating organizations. The projects needed to be of importance to the partner organization but also relevant to the learning needs of the students, be something that could be completed during one semester, and be appropriate for teamwork. Student teams worked in parallel on different aspects of the project that allowed the teams to take on more complex problems than a single student would be able to attempt within the timeframe of the course. Preceptors in the practice setting were critical in connecting the teams with the organization and paving the way for the project to be carried out, as well as mentoring the students throughout the semester to keep the project on track. According to the authors, the collaboration has had positive benefits for both academic and practice settings. For the academic setting, it has provided students with an opportunity to apply course content in clinical practice, facilitating their learning. For the practice settings, all student projects resulted in recommendation that were implemented in the participating organizations. Within DNP programs, similar partnerships could allow students to engage in indirect clinical experiences designed to allow students to develop expertise in relation to the quality-improvement-related skill set defined in the DNP essentials. In addition, they could give students access to clinical sites for their final DNP projects.

Fairchild (2012) described an academic–practice partnership between a university and rural hospitals that focused on APRN students in a graduate online nursing informatics course. The partnership led to the development of an online nursing informatics service-learning course. Students worked with health care providers and nurse administrators in the partner rural health care settings to assist with various health information technology (HIT) needs. During the semester, students teams (two to three students) were assigned to the rural health setting where they worked with the personnel in the setting to identify HIT continuing-education needs and then worked via telecommunications with their rural health care partners to design, conduct, and evaluate a project related to and/or supported by informatics or HIT. For DNP programs, projects such as this would allow students to develop and demonstrate skills related to DNP essentials focusing on information systems and technology as well as interprofessional collaboration and teamwork.

In addition to these examples of partnerships identified in the literature, there may be an opportunity for academic settings with APRN-DNP programs to work with service or community partners to establish a nurse-run clinic. Nurse-run clinics can benefit the academic setting by providing a practice setting for APRN-DNP faculty and an opportunity for faculty to precept and evaluate students' clinical skills. They can provide practice sites for leadership as well as APRN-DNP students. These clinics can benefit service settings by increasing access to care. Many of these clinics provide care to underserved populations and can fill unmet health care needs (Sullivan-Marx, Bradway, & Barnsteiner, 2011; Xippolitos, Marino, & Edelman, 2011).

■ CREATING A STRONG INFRASTRUCTURE TO SUPPORT ACADEMIC SERVICE PARTNERSHIPS

Collaboration is an essential skill for nurse leaders. As nurses, we often find ourselves in the middle of communication between multiple partners. Many times, these partners are physicians or other clinical disciplines. This chapter provides an exemplar of effective collaboration and communication through educational and service organizations serving UPMC, Pittsburgh, Pennsylvania, and its surrounding academic partners. This work is in the form of an Academic–Service Partnership Council (ASPC).

The UPMC is characterized as a global health enterprise. It is made up of various entities including an insurance arm and an enterprise services arm known for its innovation and broad strategic thinking. The system is composed of more than 20 hospitals including a hospital in Palermo, Italy. There are over 400 doctors' offices, extended care facilities, and outpatient sites. This provides for expansive clinical opportunities for students at every level, particularly for the DNP level.

Partnering with schools of nursing has been a long-standing UPMC practice. The health system is closely affiliated with the University of Pittsburgh, a major academic institution with a top-ranked nursing program. This structure represented a strong foundation from which an academic–service partnership could be formed.

Beyond the University of Pittsburgh School of Nursing, there are many nursing academic institutions in the region. They represent programs with DNP, PhD, master's, baccalaureate, associate's, and hospital-based diploma degrees. The APSC began with the health system, its university affiliate, and nine other nursing programs within the region. Inviting each of them to have a seat at the table was somewhat intimidating. The first task was to create structure and work—a purpose to come together.

The council was first somewhat formal. The invitation list included academic representation in the form of deans, program directors, and faculty. Service representation included chief nursing officers, directors of nursing education, program administrators, and nurse educators. Meetings were held monthly and the journey began with the mission to create systems, which support the finest clinical experiences, the highest prepared nurses, and a focus on hiring and retaining the best nursing talent locally and nationally.

The goals were lofty and it was easy to see that relationships needed to be built to achieve these goals and for effective collaboration to occur. The first goal was to establish trust. Participants would only then feel comfortable discussing issues and opinions in front of those they traditionally competed with for students. The council began by identifying the challenges each faced. These included increasing patient complexity, faculty shortages, legislative changes, quality metrics and reimbursement implications, rapid technological changes, and preceptor development.

It was important to identify that first big project that all would have a stake in. The co-chairs included a DNP-prepared clinical education leader and a DNP-prepared chief nursing officer within the health system. The DNP leadership role in bridging the service and academic settings made exceptional use of the advanced clinical, leadership, and education competencies developed through the DNP education. It was clear that the health system lacked standardization across each clinical setting. Each academic institution held an affiliation agreement with each hospital in the health system. Each clinical site managed affiliation agreements differently and held different standards for student placement. This meant that multiple and different affiliation agreements needed to be processed even though all hospitals were part of the same health system. Further, a student who was cleared for clinical rotations at one of our hospitals may not be cleared for clinical rotations within another hospital. Standardizing the affiliation agreements and creating a "universal agreement" and a process whereby one centralized committee reviewed and made decisions regarding student background checks and clinical rotations would be the first big project of the ASPC.

Our ASPC partners were thrilled. This standardization improved efficiencies for the clinical sites and the academic institutions. Overcoming the various nuances such as how we processed the agreements and who held the clearance documents forced open dialogues on both sides. The work included a representative from the health-system corporate legal department, present at the table, who was involved. This helped to clear legal concerns in real time and with a great degree of credibility.

The success of this inaugural project opened the doors for the development of many projects to come. Today, the council creates its own annual strategic plan guiding work for the coming year. There are open discussions regarding recruitment needs of the hospitals and enrollment information from each of the participants is collected. Information is shared openly across all schools of nursing. This is something that would not have happened without the trust and collaboration built within the council. The council communicates and celebrates its academic partnership success while providing the cutting-edge industry information on an annual basis. This takes shape in the form of an annual ASPC retreat. This retreat brings together deans and faculty from each of our academic partners with nursing and education leaders from our hospitals. Topics and presenters usually include some successful key partnership projects from the year, as well as, expert presenters discussing national topics in health care. The event is sponsored by the health system as a token of thanks and appreciation for the past and future engagements.

The theme as presented by the work nationally has been "Academic–Service Partnerships: Building Bridges in a City of Bridges and Beyond." The partnership to enhance the student experience has taken shape in many ways that serve to address the challenges listed early in its development.

The issue of faculty shortages is very real to our education partners. Natural collaboration began to occur based on geographical location between various university partners and health-system hospitals. Soon, dedicated education units were born.

A dedicated education unit takes staff nurses on a hospital-based unit and pairs them with students serving as their clinical instructor as they collaboratively care for a group of patients. The nurses receive special training in providing nursing education and guidance as they work with students in their unit. This training focused on education practices, ethical–legal aspects of clinical education, teaching–learning strategies, and clinical evaluation. This model mimics the physician clinical education model and has been successfully replicated across the health system.

Another issue was finding enough student placements for the over-3,000 entry-level education clinical requirements needed by our education partners. Urban legend dictated that students from two different schools should not be in the same unit at the same time. The council challenged this practice specifically within one of the larger health-system hospitals. Students from one school were paired with students from another school in the same unit and, in some cases, within the same semi-private patient room. This soon dispelled the long-held tradition offering greater opportunity for student placement and flexibility.

Being part of a large system affords opportunity to access resources that others may not have. The UPMC is on the leading edge of health care reform as a truly integrated health care delivery and finance system. There is a team of government relations staff providing updates to the nursing leaders in the organization. It was easy to see that these same updates would be valued by the education partners. Therefore, part of the agenda on a quarterly basis includes a legislative update. The impact of health care reform, accountable care, and the expanding role of advanced practice providers is often a topic in the annual retreats.

Along with the changing landscape of health care reform, the council also works to tackle the rapid technological changes. This represented another area that was not coordinated as a health care system. This impacted how we educated faculty and students in each of our hospitals. Health-system informatics nurses were invited to the table and they developed a coordinated plan to provide electronic medical record access to faculty and students and one standardized class to educate academic partners. That has transformed into sharing electronic medical record of weekly communication updates with education partners and involving them in documentation optimization work. This provides opportunity to explain the details of meaningful use and the health care system is working to standardize and build in the electronic strategies to facilitate quality standards of care.

The UPMC has traditionally participated in student feedback surveys. The methodology for distributing the surveys, however, was not consistent between schools. There was also not a clear mechanism to communicate results. This provided minimal opportunity to determine how well the health system was serving students and no ability to trend the results. This was clearly another body of work for our council. The group developed and approved a standardized methodology. Surveys for faculty and students and preceptors are distributed at the end of every semester. Results are then shared openly and transparently across hospitals and our education partners. It is particularly important for the hospital chief nursing officers (CNOs) to see this valuable information by the unit. This gives the opportunity to assess the unit culture and influence the new-nurse success rates.

The UPMC, like many health care systems across the country, is working to increase the education level of nurses. Sharing our current status and future goals with our academic partners led to the availability of additional opportunities for nurses in the region to further their education. Our internal website includes a detailed listing of each school, admission requirements, degree requirements, availability, and cost. This supports nurses in making an informed decision in choosing an education institution that meets their individual needs.

The work of our ASPC continues. We have grown from a partnership with nine educational institutions to now involving over 15 education partners. The council continues to address the shared challenges in health care. This partnership has promoted innovation and collaboration in striving for excellence. The partnership program was initiated based on mutual potential benefits. Today, many of those benefits are realized. The council members have moved from competitors to collaborators on many levels. This has involved creating a stakeholder coalition, shared decision making, and a shared structure. The council now enjoys partnerships in clinical education and staff development. The outcomes have been beneficial to the health system and academic partners. This foundation serves as a strong springboard for clinical partnerships at all nursing education levels.

This culture of collaboration and partnership has created a fertile ground for the DNP student and graduate. The health system has opened its doors to many DNP clinical experiences and quality projects. Many of those experiences help shape innovative leadership and care models. Further, the health system enjoys the leadership and practice of many DNP nurses across its ranks. This model has served to strengthen the practice of nurses within the UPMC.

■ CRITICAL THINKING QUESTIONS

1. *What added benefit does the DNP bring to the academic–service partnership?*
2. *What can the DNP in the service setting contribute to the academic setting?*
3. *What can the DNP in the academic setting contribute to the service setting?*
4. *Given the two models of preparation of the DNP, what are the unique contributions of each to the academic–service partnership?*
5. *Where in the setting(s) is the DNP best positioned to enrich the academic–service partnership?*
6. *What are the optimal expectations for the DNP in the service setting and the DNP in the academic setting?*
7. *How does the academic–service partnership collaborate best to prepare the strongest DNP graduate?*
8. *What areas of DNP practice within the academic–service partnership are in need of evaluation?*
9. *What is the value of the DNP student project to the service and academic sides of the partnership?*
10. *How might an academic–service partnership be structured that maximizes the contributions of the DNP graduate?*

■ REFERENCES

American Association of Colleges of Nursing. (2012). AACN-AONE task force on academic-practice partnerships: Guiding principles. Retrieved from http://www.aacn.nche.edu/leading-initiatives/academic-practice-partnerships/GuidingPrinciples.pdf

AANC Task Force on Implementation of the DNP. (2015). The doctor of nursing practice: Current issues and clarifying recommendations. Retrieved from http://www.aacn.nche.edu/aacn-publications/white-papers/DNP-Implementation-TF-Report-8-15.pdf

Dunbar-Jacob, J., Nativio, D. G., & Khalil, H. (2013). Impact of doctorate of nursing practice education in shaping health care systems for the future. *Journal of Nursing Education, 52*(8), 423–427.

Fairchild, R. M. (2012). Hold that TIGER! A collaborative service-learning academic-practice partnership with rural healthcare facilities. *Nurse Educator, 37*(3), 108–114.

Jones, C. B., Mayer, C., & Mandelkehr, L. K. (2009). Innovations at the intersection of academia and practice: Facilitating graduate nursing students' learning about quality improvement and patient safety. *Quality Management in Health Care, 18*(3), 158–162.

Kleinpell, R. M., Faut-Callahan, M., Carson, E., Llewellyn, J., & Dreher, M. (2015). Evolving the practitioner-teacher role to enhance practice-academic partnerships: A literature review. *Journal of Clinical Nursing, 25*(5–6), 708–714. doi:10.1111/jocn.13017

Killeen, K. M., Rudy, D., Delaney, K. R., Kleinpell, R., Hinch, B., & Barginere, C. (2015). Academic/service integration advances APRN practice. *Nurse Leader, 139*(2), 57–62.

Sullivan-Marx, S. M., Bradway, C., & Barnsteiner, J. (2009). Innovative collaborations: A case study for academic owned nursing practice. *The Journal of Nursing Scholarship, 41*(1), 50–57.

Thabault, P., Mylott, L., & Patterson, A. (2015). Describing a residency program developed for newly graduated nurse practitioners employed in retain health settings. *Journal of Professional Nursing, 31*, 226–232.

Waldrop, J., Caruso, D., Fuchs, M. A., & Hypes, K. (2014). EC as PIE: Five criteria for executing a successful DNP final project. *Journal of Professional Nursing, 30*, 300–306.

Xippolitos, L. A., Marino, M. A., & Edelman, N. H. (2011). Leveraging academic–service partnerships: Implications for implementing the WJ/IOM's recommendations to improve quality, access and value in academic medical centers. *ISRN Nursing, 2011*, 1–4.

Reflective Response

Judy A. Beal

Academic–service partnerships are critical to advancing the recommendations of the 2010 Institute of Medicine (IOM) report on the future of nursing. The authors of the chapter present a strong and compelling case for the role that these partnerships have in building the capacity and growing enrollments in the Doctor of Nursing Practice (DNP) programs. I could not agree more with their statement that "the presence of a DNP program in both practice and academic settings provides opportunities for collaborations extending well beyond the traditional affiliation for student education." Exemplars from their university and health system provide rich details on not only how nursing leaders can leverage faculty, staff, and operations to embrace and grow DNP student experiences but also the benefits of such experiences to both partners. Not only is the education of DNP students beneficial to service partners, but it is dependent on the strong partnership with the clinical enterprise. In spite of the efforts made since 2010 by the AACN-AONE (American Association of Colleges of Nursing and American Organization of Nurse Executives) Task Force on Academic–Practice Partnership, there remains little, if any, published evidence of outcomes of such relationships. The AACN-AONE Academic–Practice Partnership Awards, given since 2014, present a glimpse of exceptional work to build and sustain relationships for a variety of goals ranging from the traditional to increase the educational opportunities, to building the workforce capacity, improving the health outcomes of communities of interest, expanding the research and scholarship, to name a few. A review of these awards and related publications can be viewed at the AACN website (www.aacn.nche.edu/leading initiatives/academic -practice-partnerships/academic-practice-partnerships-award-winners). Although the evidence for partnerships is strong, the fact remains that there are many barriers to developing and sustaining them. Along with the usual excuses of simply "not enough time", a recently more reoccurring barrier has emerged as the tsunami of retirements of senior nurse leaders in both the academy and service sectors. Turnover of these leaders can disrupt established goals and initiatives and building a new relationship takes time to develop the mutual respect that is essential to a shared vision and goals for partnership. As highlighted in this chapter, the AACN-AONE task force has provided guidelines for establishing and sustaining partnerships, a tool kit with specific strategies to do so, and exemplars of success (AACN, 2012). The values and benefits for both practice and academic leaders are summarized in a 2011 article discussing the hallmarks of best practice in academic–practice partnerships as identified by a sample of 72 deans and vice presidents of nursing. These hallmarks include: shared vision, goals, and resources; commitment to excellence and open communication; trust and respect; and mutual problem solving, to name just a few. Participants unanimously agreed that a successful partnership is framed by a strong personal as well as professional relationship that starts at the top and infiltrates the organizations (Beal et al., 2011).

The AACN has continued to focus on the need for and benefits of academic–service partnerships. In the recently published Futures Task Force Final Report to the AACN Board of Directors (AACN, 2015), AACN outlined four recommendations "regarding potential new efforts that can be implemented to support the mission of the organization and assure support for the development of a nursing workforce for the future." Two of the four recommendations speak directly to the importance of academic-practice partnerships in not only realizing overarching goal of AACN to be "the catalyst for innovation in nursing education that will improve health and health care (AACN, 2015) but also to reach the goals set forth by the IOM in 2010. Furthermore, in 2016, the AACN published a report commissioned to "examine the potential for enhanced partnership between academic nursing and academic health centers (AHCs) around the imperative to advance integrated systems of health care, achieve improved health outcomes, and foster new models for innovation" (AACN, 2016). Although intended originally as a guide for deans and CNOs in AHCs, the report has important implications equally for deans and CNOs who do not lead in AHCs. Six recommendations are posed and include:

1. Adopt the following vision: Academic nursing is a full partner in health care delivery, education, and research that is integrated and funded across all professions and missions in the AHC system
2. Implement initiatives that more fully bring nursing faculty into the clinical practice of the health system and connect the clinical service more closely to the academic mission of the school of nursing
3. Partner in preparing the nurses of the future by building a pipeline of nurses at multiple levels and creating nursing leadership development programs for faculty and practicing nurses that are jointly managed by the school of nursing and clinical practice
4. Partner in the implementation of an accountable care
5. Invest in nursing research programs and better integrate research into a clinical practice
6. Implement an advocacy agenda in support of a new era for academic nursing, which encompasses the integration of practice, education, and research (AACN, 2016)

How many times did you count the word partner in this charge? The message is loud and clear! Finally, the AACN and AONE leadership and representatives met in April of 2016 to share a vision and goals for a preferred partnership between the two organizations that would start at the national level and infiltrate all of the academia and practice. In my mind, this represents a full circle back to 2010 when the national dialogue began and demonstrates an even stronger commitment to the future of our profession. Truly, we are partners, leveraging our strengths to build a strong future. As increasingly large numbers of DNP students graduate and assume leadership roles in not only practice but also academia, we continue to embrace the role and confirm that nursing is first and foremost, like our medicine colleagues, a practice discipline. Like the authors, we at Simmons have had a long and rich partnership with the Boston-Bedford Veterans Administration (VA) hospital system. A member of NERVANA, the New England Regional Nursing Alliance, Simmons along with five other Boston-based schools of nursing have partnered with the VA to provide veteran-focused learning opportunities for our students. In 2014, NERVANA won the AACN-AONE Exemplary Academic–Practice Award. While we have significantly increased the number of clinical placements at the VA, we have also expanded program options, launched dedicated education units, developed the first Commission on Collegiate Nursing Education (CCNE)-accredited post-baccalaureate residency program, and expanded research initiatives through joint appointments of faculty nurse scientists at the VA. Most recently, we have developed a cohort model Executive Nurse Leadership DNP program for 20 nurse leaders from four of our service partners. Employees have been selected for their expanded leadership roles by our partners and many of the senior practice leaders will join the faculty in teaching roles. We are excited to be working toward a mission of a better educated workforce and the IOM goal of 50% doctorally prepared nurses by 2020. I extend congratulations to the authors who have hit the nail on the proverbial head with their chapter. The opportunities abound, the benefits exceed imagination, and the future looks bright. Although there are many such anecdotal descriptions of successful academic-practice partnerships, objective evidence of outcomes of the many innovations attempted is limited (Beal, 2012). Next steps must include published studies of outcomes that are generalizable and feasible.

■ REFERENCES

American Association of Colleges of Nursing. (2012). AACN-AONE task force on academic-practice partnerships. Retrieved from http://www.aacn.nche.edu/leading-initiatives/academic-practice -partnerships/GuidingPrinciples.pdf

American Association of Colleges of Nursing. (2015). *Futures task force final report to the AACN board of directors.* Retrieved from http://www.aacn.nche.edu/FTFReport

American Association of Colleges of Nursing. (2016). Advancing healthcare transformation: A new era for academic nursing. Retrieved from http://www.aacn.nche.edu/AACN-Manatt-Report.pdf

Beal, J. A. (2012). Academic-service partnerships in nursing: An integrative review. *Nursing Research and Practice,* 501564. Retrieved from http://DC.doi.org/10.1155/2012/501564

Beal, J. A., Breslin, E., Autsin, R., Brower, L., Bullard, K., Light, K., . . . Ray, N. (2011). Hallmarks of best academic-practice partnerships in nursing Lessons learned from San Antonio. *Journal of Professional Nursing, 27*(6), e90–e95. doi:10.1016/j.professnurs.2011.07.006

National Academies of Sciences, Engineering and Medicine (formerly the Institute of Medicine). (2010). The future of nursing: Leading change, advancing health. Retrieved from nationalacad emies.org/hmd/reports

Executive Coaching to Support Doctoral Role Transitions and Promote Leadership Consciousness

Beth Weinstock and Mary Ellen Smith Glasgow

This chapter addresses the many challenges inherent in professional work transitions. It speaks to the need for heightened leadership consciousness during times of change, and describes how executive coaching can support new leaders in making effective transitions that develop their best gifts, talents, and strengths.

As a doctorally prepared nurse, the Doctor of Nurse Practice (DNP) graduate is in a position of leadership. As the nursing profession itself becomes more and more central to our health care system, the DNP will increase its importance and scope of influence. This role expansion involves transitions and challenges for the individual DNP graduate and also for the discipline itself. Understanding the challenges and preparing to meet them will help the DNP graduate realize her or his full leadership potential.

Transitions in the work place can be personally and professionally satisfying and yet be difficult to manage. Switching roles and increasing responsibilities entails not only adjustments to new task assignments, but also to a new relationship with ourselves, and with those around us. As in a kaleidoscope, when we turn just one small part of the design, the entire structure transforms. When we move into new roles, it feels as if the world has gone on tilt until we find ourselves fully settled in the new design. Transitions need time and attention for all parts to integrate and realign with one another. This chapter sheds light on the often hidden aspects of work transitions for the DNP graduate, with the intent to help those individuals evolve as leaders in practice, education, administration, and/or clinical research.

The DNP graduate's new leadership role will require expanded ways of thinking and being, best summed up in the concept of *leadership consciousness*. Leadership consciousness is a constant and pervasive awareness that one's actions have impact that matters. This consciousness holds awareness that all behavior influences its environment, and that the influence needs to be carefully tracked. As a frame of mind and attitude, it colors all the thought and behavior. Its wisdom reminds those in leadership that success is never solely about oneself, but about a contribution reflected in the people and systems that are being led. Leadership, at the simplest level, is about the execution of defined leadership tasks. At a more complex level, it is about how we develop and embody leadership consciousness. This chapter explores the route toward leadership consciousness by mapping its many domains.

Executive coaching is a leadership development intervention that can guide the new DNP through role transitions and into greater leadership consciousness. It focuses on helping clients perform to the best of their potential, both in successfully achieving their role responsibilities, and in finding their own best way of accomplishing this goal. The process of executive coaching involves a relationship of mutual respect and engagement between the coach and coaching client (or coachee), which leads to feedback and support for the client's growth and development. This chapter defines executive coaching, describes what it entails, and clarifies how it works. It presents a case study of coaching at a college of nursing and identifies its successful outcomes, while also acknowledges the need for a body of empirically based research to establish the generalized effectiveness of leadership coaching.

■ TRANSITIONS IN PROFESSIONAL DEVELOPMENT

We are living in turbulent times. On the global front, threats to safety have generated widespread anxiety. On the home front, our economic instabilities have created fears of the future. In the midst of our domestic worries there is uncertainty about the state of national health care, which causes further worry in the general population and stress within the nursing profession. The DNP is opening new possibilities for the nursing profession and health care; however, this new degree will lead the profession into uncharted territory where there are no clear maps for moving forward. The DNP graduate and our health care system are transitioning at the same time, heightening the challenges for managing change. It is of paramount importance that attention is placed on DNP professional development during such times of transition.

The academic, corporate, and practice world is accustomed to change and transition. As doctoral-level nurses transition into leadership roles, DNPs must develop skills to negotiate the politics and hierarchies of the workplace setting. Given the shortage of DNP leaders, there will be few comparably educated role models in the discipline. As new DNPs are promoted to advanced practice, faculty, and executive positions, a broader spectrum of new competencies will be required. As the role is defined, many challenges will emerge.

With each shift, there are different skill sets for DNPs to develop. Some of these skills are grounded in content related to a nursing specialty, but many fall under the umbrella of management and leadership. It is the goal of DNPs as leaders to: (a) earn the trust of the organization; (b) be deeply engaged with professional colleagues; (c) earn legitimacy and mobilize people around a focused agenda; (d) devote considerable efforts to develop employees and build the organization's collective leadership capabilities; and lastly, (e) strive for high performance that is committed to the larger institution (Eisenstat, Beer, Foote, Fredberg, & Norrgren, 2008). Clearly, major shifts in the role from a clinician to a leader create the demand for change on many fronts for the DNP.

Role shifts create change in all our relationships, both personal and professional. They create change, as well, in how we see ourselves. There is no external promotion without an internal shift; no new leadership position is embodied without personal growth and development. This transformation can be both invigorating and also disorienting. In addition to the excitement, delights, and satisfactions of new leadership positions, transitioning into them involves a labyrinth of twists, turns, and invisible obstructions. The hidden challenges are rarely addressed, which ultimately can be detrimental. Too often, it is simply assumed that if one is competent in one job with a high degree of responsibility, the same person excels when given increased and different responsibilities. This is not necessarily true. Even extremely competent leaders need adjustment time to become firmly grounded in their new roles. Success often hinges on understanding and addressing the many factors that impede or support smooth transitions (Elsner & Farrands, 2012).

■ THE HIDDEN CHALLENGES IN PROFESSIONAL DEVELOPMENT AND ROLE TRANSITIONS

THE BOUNDARY CHALLENGE

When one gets promoted from a cohort group or achieves a higher level of status among one's peers, the shift into authority can create confusion and conflict in relationships. Peers may become resentful because they think they should have been chosen for the promotion. They may feel unseen and undervalued by the authority who determined the promotion. Their work will now be evaluated by a former peer, and this may raise the fear that personal information that is already known will be used against them. They may know the weaknesses of the promoted peer and think the promotion was unjustified. Resentment can lead to distancing in the form of complaining to other colleagues or withholding information from the new leader, which previously would have been openly shared.

Making the transition into a *boss* who remains open and available, but at the same time, can shut the door, give hard feedback when necessary, or make unpopular mandates can be a daunting task. Once in a position of authority over others, there are decisions to make that are challenging:

- How much insider information should I share with my peers?
- How do I close my door without offending people who previously had easy access to my time?
- How do I make sure my former peers feel respected and valued?
- How do I give critical feedback in a way that can be heard and processed?
- How do I demand greater work productivity?

For each individual, the boundary challenge will play out differently. No matter how it is negotiated, it will require conscious behavior designed for positive impact that can maintain good relationships, while at the same time initiate changes in those very relationships. In addition to the boundary challenge posed by supervising former peers, the DNP will likely encounter being supervised by non-nurses. Non-nurses are likely to bring different approaches to the health care domain and have varying philosophies and histories with different contexts. This change will also present a range of boundary renegotiations.

THE LONELINESS CHALLENGE

Once new boundaries are set, one may feel isolated or even lonely. New leadership positions entail shifting alliances from peers to the next level of group leadership. In the course of being coached, new leaders often report that they feel alone, unsure of whose information to trust, unclear about who to go to for input and answers, and uncertain how much personal disclosure is appropriate in their new cohort group. It takes time to find the answers to these questions and to feel securely situated.

THE COMPETENCY CHALLENGE

Competency in one professional area does not necessarily translate into all aspects of new roles or assignments. Each shift in the role involves new content-related areas of skill development and also new leadership demands. For example, one coaching client (a woman) was a top-notch teacher and a highly responsible taskmaster in all parts of her faculty responsibilities. When promoted to an academic administrative role, she was surprised to learn that part of her actual job was to spend time nurturing and maintaining relationships with her colleagues. She had formerly dismissed such activities as a waste of time, but now needed to practice the art and competency of relationship building. With awareness and determination, she learned to maintain connections with her colleagues in new ways—asking about people's children, stopping by people's desks during the day, and hosting people in her office when it was not time for a meeting. As a newly promoted executive, she gained leadership skills beyond her academic excellence and increased collaboration with her own and ancillary departments.

THE CONFIDENCE CHALLENGE

If we have been at our job long enough, we usually feel settled and confident. We know the rules of the game. We know how to speak up within our work group. We have gotten feedback about how well we perform. Just when we feel proud of accomplishments and comfortable with an existing level of responsibility, a shift in role, even when positive, can create a crisis in confidence. For example, one coaching client (a woman) who was formerly accustomed to being outspoken with her professional peers, suddenly experienced great fear about speaking up in her new leadership group. She worried that her strong voice would be seen as too aggressive. She feared exposing herself as not knowing all that others expected her to know. Struggling with these doubts, she inhibited her expressions and contributions until her confidence was once again established.

THE IDENTITY CHALLENGE

As we move into different roles, we undergo a transformation. How we see ourselves, how we feel, how we dress, how we move—all these aspects of who we have been start to shift. For some, the shift in identity is quite subtle and may take place with no noticeable attention. For others, the shift is unsettling and as tumultuous as for *Alice in Wonderland*, as she slips through the looking glass.

> Who are you?" said the caterpillar . . .
> "I-I hardly know, Sir, just at the present," Alice replied rather shyly. "At least I know who I *was* when I got up this morning, but I think I must have been changed several times since then. (Carrol, 1981, p. 34)

Changing our perception of ourselves and our external reality usually takes place slowly over time. Sometimes, we do not even notice that a shift has happened until time has passed. When we notice the shift, we may even be surprised that it has happened at all. This phenomenon is probably best expressed by writers and poets. Once we live through uncertainties and come out on the other side, we find ourselves different in ways that are sometimes hard to name or even recognize. We have shed a layer, or grown one. We connect the dots and discover a new design. We have a new pair of inner glasses that creates an altered vision of our realities. As we move through the many and diverse challenges inevitable with professional transitions and integrate our new awareness with the tasks of leadership, we move into the realm of conscious leadership.

■ MYTHS ABOUT TRANSITIONS INTO LEADERSHIP ROLES

Elsner and Farrands (2012) researched the experience of many leaders who moved from one position of great corporate responsibility into another. In their book *Leadership Transitions*, they identify what they call *myths* about leadership transitions, which are here applied to the DNP experience that follows. These myths can generate considerable distress if left unrecognized. With heightened awareness of them, however, transitions can be much smoother.

Myth 1. *The job matches the job description.* Most often, the realities of high-level positions involve work tasks and organizational complexities that were never in the job description (Elsner & Farrands, 2012). As DNPs find their place in more and more organizational settings, this is bound to be true. Time and support will be needed to gain clarity on the actual territory and boundaries of their job description and new role.

Myth 2. *Leaders in new positions need to make a mark early on in order to be seen as worthy of their appointment.* DNPs are vulnerable here in seeking to prove the utility and wisdom of both the new role and the new degree. Quick action and early visibility must be carefully considered options and not merely strategies for managing anxiety (Sanaghan, Goldstein, & Gaval, 2009). Slow is sometimes the fastest way to success even though it takes patience and faith to enter with caution, observation, and thoughtfulness.

Myth 3. *Leaders should demonstrate independence and not need help.* The nursing field is predominantly female-dominated, which may make it more collaborative than male-dominated professions. To the extent that this is true, the collaborative attitude may render this myth less powerful in nursing than in other parts of corporate America. Nonetheless, across fields, new leaders are often fearful of asking for help lest they be seen as indecisive or weak (Weinstock & Sanaghan, 2015). This issue may arise for DNP graduates who report to non-nurse supervisors who may be a physician, senior hospital executive, or academic administrator. In light of this new working relationship, DNPs may try to prove themselves prematurely.

Myth 4. *Bosses can be friends and trusted work colleagues.* It is tempting to think that the person who does the hiring or promoting can be a trusted support, mentor, and/or ally. The reality is that new DNP leaders need to determine how safe it is to share work-related concerns with their boss, in this case a supervisor. They must learn how to "manage up," identify their supervisor's style, and communicate in a way that gets heard. In some instances, the supervisor will have a different educational background and discipline, thus requiring DNPs to translate their message into language that their supervisors can easily comprehend.

Myth 5. The leader does not change: everything else does. As we have seen earlier, this is not true. Leadership roles, inevitably, involve personal as well as professional change.

Myth 6. Leaders should not show emotions at work. In many work settings, this myth is beginning to change. However, women leaders in particular need to assess their work context and determine how, when, and where it is safe to show emotion. When it is not safe, they need to learn ways to contain and manage their feelings at work.

Myth 7. New leaders should be well-situated and comfortable within 100 days. The fact is that for many new leaders, it takes up to a year to truly understand the new systems where they are working, the boundaries of their power, and the culture and politics of their organization (Elsner & Farrands, 2012). For the DNP, the challenge of becoming well-integrated into their work environment is both a challenge for the individual DNP as for the profession itself, and this will take time.

These seven myths can be landmines waiting to explode if the new leader remains unaware of and/or does not attend to them. Understanding them, hopefully, works to debunk them before they take new leaders off course.

As leaders transition from one leadership position to another, they are bound to encounter the challenges mentioned earlier. As the DNP position expands its field of influence in the nursing profession, these challenges will be amplified. Increased leadership consciousness and attention to the rich potential of each individual's leadership capacity will be even more critical.

■ LEADERSHIP CONSCIOUSNESS

The leadership role requires vision, analysis, decision making, conflict management, action, influence, and the ability to inspire others, track impact, and give rewards. These are skills that can be taught and learned in leadership training programs where methods and techniques are practiced. Embodying these skills and carrying them forth with leadership consciousness is the challenge of a great leader. Great leaders are those who infuse the discrete tasks of leadership with their authentic selves—their personal passion, unique presence, and particular way of moving through daily life.

A leadership story is told about a man named Zusia. Originally, from the Hebrew tradition, it now has many variations as a teaching tale and is adapted here as the following:

Zusia was a highly regarded member of his community who decides to climb his spiritual mountain and face his Gods. He goes with great fear and trembling in spite of his community's assurances that he, of all people, who has given so much, should not be concerned. But Zusia knows better. When he returns, he appears ashen and shaken to his core. His people inquire as to what the Gods could have said to disturb him so. Zusia tells them, "The

Gods did not ask me why like Moses I did not part the Red Sea. Nor did they ask me why like Gandhi I did not go on a hunger strike for people. Nor did they ask why like Rosa Parks I did not refuse to go to the back of the bus. They asked me, 'Zusia, why have you not been more like Zusia'?" (Hassidic Stories, 2010)

The lesson from Zusia's gods is that we must be our authentic selves. We do this by increasing our self-awareness in many domains and summon the courage to bring our true selves into our leadership tasks.

Leadership consciousness translated into the tasks of leadership will involve attention to a legacy one can be proud of, a focus on long-term gains over short-term successes, consideration of what benefits the most amount of the people, and about the wellbeing of those who inherit the earth (Barret Values Centre, 2009). Leadership consciousness speaks, in addition, to the interior life of the leader—a state of being that is mindful of and quests to merge individual meaning with community benefit. David Whyte (2007), a poet who spent a chapter of his life as an organization consultant, said "We cultivate an inner life knowing that what is most important to us must be spoken and made real in the outer world" (p. 142). The route toward developing leadership consciousness will vary for each DNP according to individual style differences, histories, cultural backgrounds, age, gender, and work contexts, but this will always involve increased awareness in the multiple domains described in the following.

■ DOMAINS OF SELF-AWARENESS THAT CONTRIBUTE TO THE DEVELOPMENT OF LEADERSHIP CONSCIOUSNESS

We, ourselves, are the instruments of change. We therefore need to know who we are and who we are not. This means insight into our gifts and talents, how to use them, what blocks their potency, and what support and guidance we need for further development. It means knowing how we differ from others, that we cannot be all things to all people, and that we have limits to our gifts and strengths. Once we are clear and accept who we are and who we are not, we can move forward to actualize our leadership potential and our leadership consciousness.

AWARENESS OF PERSONAL STYLES AND STRENGTHS

Many cultures throughout time have created systems for mapping different character types. Land-based cultures—those that are literally dependent on geography, seasonal changes, and weather—have traditionally differentiated people by how they represent qualities of the seasons and the directions of the earth. These divergent qualities, when put together, reflect balance and harmony with the environment. The ancient Celtics from Ireland and Scotland referred to the Wheel of Seeing (MacEowen, 2007) and many Native American peoples refer to the Medicine Wheel to reflect archetypal ways of being in the world (Arrien, 1993). These two different cultures, developed thousands of miles away from one another, have astonishing parallels in identifying the character types. When we translate these types into our modern way of thinking, they describe four archetypes as follows: the *Leader*, or *Warrior*, represents the North; the *Visionary* represents the East; the *Healer* represents the South; and the *Teacher* represents the West (Arrien, 1993).

In our Western culture, there are many personality templates that help identify and differentiate character type and therefore raise self-awareness. One of the most widely known and used in work settings is the Myers–Briggs Type Inventory (MBTI). It is a personality profile borrowed from Jungian theory that discerns whether we are introverts or extroverts, whether we are large systems thinkers or focused on details, whether we make decisions based on objectivity or subjectivity, and whether we move through the world creating closure or staying ever open to possibilities.

Another powerful vehicle for increasing self-awareness is the "360-degree"-feedback process (Lepsinger & Lucia, 2009). This involves a leader choosing several people within their current and past work experiences to answer—for example, the same questions about his or her strengths, competencies, or areas of weaknesses.

Thus, the "360" provides the leader with feedback on how he or she is viewed from several perspectives, revealing clear themes that speak of strengths and also areas of needed development.

Personality and character assessments help us to appreciate and value the ways in which we are unique, and appreciate and value the uniqueness of others. They lend insight into how we operate, as well as how we are experienced by others. This information is essential for any leader who values heightening self-awareness, deepening authenticity, and fortifying leadership consciousness.

AWARENESS OF HOW WE BEHAVE UNDER STRESS

Leaders need to know how they tend to operate when stressed and to determine if their behaviors are useful, or not, for accomplishing a given goal. What we do well, we tend to do more of when we are feeling stressed. If we tend to be decisive, we may become controlling. If we are good at creating collaboration and consensus, under stress we may take too much time and miss deadlines for decision making. A DNP who is generally decisive, action-oriented, and a clear communicator may become aggressive and appear to bully others under pressure. If the work task is to design and develop a team approach to solving a unit's clinical problems, this behavior under pressure does not represent good leadership. If, however, the work task requires quick action in the emergency department, then the momentary aggression may be quite appropriate and acceptable.

Some of us lose the use of our greatest strength under pressure. For example, one coaching client realized that while she was incredibly gifted as a creative and visionary force, under pressure she often became fearful, lost her very gift, and made snap decisions that were not always the best for her team. In the process of executive coaching, she increased her awareness of this tendency under stress and learned to slow down, take the time she needed, and ask for input before making her final decisions.

AWARENESS OF OUR EMOTIONAL INTELLIGENCE

In 1983, Dr. Howard Gardner, a professor of education at Harvard University, developed a landmark theory of multiple intelligences, which posited that the traditional notion of intelligence (based on the standardized IQ test) was a limited way of determining human potential (Goleman, 2012). He proposed eight different intelligences (linguistic, logical–mathematical, spatial, kinesthetic, musical, interpersonal, intrapersonal, and naturalistic) to represent a wide range of ways in which we demonstrate our mental attributes. Knowing our most and least developed intelligences provides important guidance, particularly in times of uncertainty and transition. When we become aware of an underdeveloped intelligence, we can work to strengthen it. For example, a DNP graduate who took a position in a nurse-managed health clinic was formerly a highly revered, inspiring lecturer of undergraduates. Her teaching skills were excellent. However, when she transitioned into administrative responsibilities where she needed to collaborate with peers, she was initially perceived as arrogant and unapproachable. Her interpersonal "intelligence" was underdeveloped until it improved as a result of the executive coaching process.

AWARENESS OF OUR FIT WITH THE WORK ENVIRONMENT

Regardless of our professional competencies, we need to know in what environments we can contribute and feel valued and to know those environments that are likely to stifle our creativity and productivity. We are not interchangeable parts, easily fitting into any work context. The following work story demonstrates this point. A DNP graduate (a woman) sought coaching during her first year on a critical care team when she found herself challenged with the team's expectations. Passionate about helping patients understand their medical conditions and treatments, she would finish her administrative tasks and spend time with patients and their families educating them, drawing charts, and explaining how their medications worked. Her team members did not value spending this amount of time with families and criticized her for not being committed to her other responsibilities. The DNP became worried about her team's perception of her and even began to doubt herself, but at the same time questioned whether or not she could tolerate being on a team that believed that greater boundaries between the DNP and patient made for better care. Coaching sessions helped her understand that the criticism from her team was related to a culture clash, not her professional competencies. With clear understanding about the honest differences between herself and her team members, her anxiety diminished and she learned to support her own choices while managing time in such a way that her team was satisfied.

AWARENESS OF OUR "INNER CRITIC"

We all talk to ourselves silently inside our heads. The constant commentary is referred to as *self-talk*, and learning how we talk to ourselves is an important part of self-awareness. Some people are fortunate to have high levels of self-esteem that carry them through challenges with little self-criticism; they have encouraging and positive self-talk. Many of us, however, live with the internal voice of an *inner critic* that can hold us hostage to self-doubt (Shure & Weinstock, 2009). The "inner critic" can thwart spontaneity, limit freedom of expression, and create fear about what we have said or done. When we transition into new roles, the inner critic has fertile ground to get activated. Faced with a new role, it is easy to wonder:

- "Am I doing what I should be doing?"
- "Would someone be doing this a better way?"
- "Am I looking foolish in meetings when I speak up? Or when I don't speak up?"
- "Will I learn the new job well enough to be successful?"

Although the inner critic's voice may be strong, it can be tamed. Managing it and diminishing its negative effect start with having an awareness that it exists, noting what it says and with what tone it says it, and then developing the voice of an "inner coach" that can counteract it. Developing a strong "inner coach" creates self-talk that is encouraging and compassionate, and over time will triumph over the inner critic. The coaching process can assist leaders in strengthening this new voice, which is an important asset for all leaders.

AWARENESS AS MINDFULNESS

Mindfulness is the practice of focusing attention and awareness on the present moment, noticing thoughts, feelings, and bodily sensations as they appear and disappear. The goal of mindfulness is to help us observe and accept what appears in our mind without resistance, noting that our brain produces many reactions to our circumstance that, like clouds moving across the sun, continue to move and change. Mindfulness helps us to be grounded, clear, and able to let go of attachments to our own sometimes rigid ideas in order to be alert and available for what is needed at the moment.

A story from the Buddhist tradition teaches about holding on and letting go. A variation of its many renditions is adapted here as follows:

> Two Buddhist monks belong to a sect that prohibits physical contact with women. As they cross a rushing river, they come upon a woman who is struggling to make it to the other side. One monk picks her up and carries her safely across the torrent, deposits her, and moves on. The other was troubled and asked, "How could you carry that woman? You know we can't touch women." The first monk replied, "I left the woman at the river's edge a long way back, but you are still carrying her." (Personal Evolution: Health, Fitness and Personal Development, 2010)

The second monk is caught in a moment that has already passed. The first monk, attending to what is present at the moment of choice, makes a decision to save a life and moves on to the next choice point, unattached to what is now history.

Mindfulness is a form of self-awareness that helps us notice when we are bogged down in matters that have already passed, or are lost in concerns about the future rather than attending to the present. It originates from the Buddhist tradition of meditation practice and has become a highly researched stress management technique (Varvogli & Darviri, 2011). In 1979, Dr. Jon Kabat-Zinn established an innovative "stress reduction program" at the University of Massachusetts based on Buddhist meditation techniques and has since brought mindfulness to the general public (Kabat-Zinn, 1994, 2009). His teachings have spread beyond his clinic, and there are now many programs throughout the country that teach mindfulness-based stress reduction using meditation.

Mindfulness, whether or not one actively practices meditation, is an important component of good leadership. It brings attention to what is at hand. It helps to free the mind from extraneous thoughts and emotions, and it grounds one in space and time. It is one form of consciousness and, as such, it is an important component of leadership consciousness.

The many domains of awareness lead us to expanded leadership consciousness and we attempt to use the best of our personal and professional selves for making the world a better place, reaching our organization's goals and supporting the people who report to us, all while facilitating our own inner growth.

■ EXECUTIVE COACHING

In Arthur Koestler's "Janus" (1978), he tells a story about the captain of a ship who is instructed not to read his written orders until he is out on open sea. He looks forward to the moment that will end his uncertainty and confirm for him whether or not he has been on the right course. When he finally opens the envelope, he finds that the salt air has faded his instructions beyond recognition; that he will never know if he is in the right place on the high seas or following the right course.

Executive coaching is one form of support for leaders who transition through uncharted waters without a clear map, and for those who can use assistance to find their place when the mandate is unclear. In its different forms, coaching has been used throughout human history. Cave dwellers were probably coached on how to draw pictures of their hunt on cave walls, as were young medicine women on how to find medicinal herbs. The modern world of music and sports is accustomed to using one-on-one coaching to support peak performance, but only recently has executive coaching become a resource for leaders across a wide range of fields.

The International Coaching Federation defines coaching as "partnering with clients in a thought-provoking and creative process that inspires them to maximize their personal and professional potential." This process helps clients dramatically improve their outlook on work and life, while improving their leadership skills and unlocking their potential (International Coaching Federation, n.d.).

The essential intention of executive coaching is to help leaders get unstuck from leadership challenges they face and to transfer what they learn during the coaching process into behaviors that move their organization forward (O'Neil, 2007).

We would add that its purpose is to support the person of the leader through turbulent times and to facilitate leadership consciousness period needed.

There are many variations in how executive coaching is done. Some coaches work only face to face, while others work on the phone or use modern technology like Skype. Some will collect data by surveys and interviews, whereas others will work only with the client's own identification of needs. Coaches who have an expertise in organization development may combine coaching with interventions that involve the client's team, or facilitate meetings with the coaching client and other key figures in the organization. Regardless of the specifics of the executive coach's methodology, all approaches involve the following steps:

- Identifying the client (coachee's) challenge
- Identifying specific coaching goals that will address the challenge
- Understanding the challenge in light of self-assessment
- Creating and brain-storming strategies to achieve goals
- Acting upon the strategies
- Tracking the success of the strategies, both the tangible outcomes and the client's subjective experience
- Acknowledging the successes
- Evaluating the coaching process

■ EFFECTIVENESS OF EXECUTIVE COACHING

It has been our experience that coaching is an effective intervention for leadership development. However, important questions face any organization that is considering the time and investment that it involves. In 2010, a *Forbes* article said, "Business coaching has gone from fad to fundamental," yet it is important to note that establishing empirically based research on its efficacy remains a challenge (Frankovelgia, 2010).

Although anecdotal evidence (Smith Glasgow, Weinstock, Lachman, Suplee, & Dreher, 2009; Weinstock & Sanaghan, 2015) plus a slowly emerging body of research support the value of coaching with successful outcomes (Kombarakaran, Yang, Baker, & Fernandes, 2008), questions remain about how to measure success, how to account for the subjective nature of individually reported success, whether or not external observers make the best raters of post-coaching change, and how to identify the contextual elements that contribute to beneficial coaching outcomes. A *Harvard Business Review* article reported that, "The coaching field is filled with contradictions. Coaches themselves disagree over why they're hired, what they do, and how to measure success" (Coutu & Kauffman, 2009). Researcher Graham Hill reported that, "the widespread popularity of executive coaching has been based largely on anecdotal feedback regarding its effectiveness. The small body of empirical research has been growing but conclusive outcomes are rare" (Hill, 2010, p. ii).

In 2009, the Institute of Coaching was established at Harvard's McLean Hospital to house and support rigorous research on coaching. Its mission involves the intent to establish the validity and acceptance of the coaching profession by setting rigorous criteria for both research on coaching outcomes and coaching practice standards. It awards large research grants and has begun to amass a reservoir of white papers, doctoral dissertations, peer-reviewed journal articles on coaching research and bibliographies of coaching-research journal abstracts. Its current director, Carol Kauffman, has been committed to updating research as far back as 2004 and said then that "to withstand the scrutiny of a wider public, the field needs to be able to explicitly describe what principles inform interventions, suggest theories that explain why they work and to support . . . the foundation of solid empirical research. . . . We need to broaden our personal experience to include more rigorous study and analysis of what works with whom, when, where, and how" (Kauffman, 2004, p. 2).

An increasing amount of empirical evidence on the coaching outcomes is beginning to accumulate. In 2009, the Korn Ferry Institute conducted a rigorous research venture involving a meta-analysis of 23 research studies designed to evaluate the effectiveness of executive coaching. They concluded that in retrospective accounts, executives reported beneficial outcomes and their research summary stated that, "clearly, we can conclude that coaching works in most cases" (Dai & De Meuse, 2009, p. 14).

In a 2011 article "A Critical Review of Executive Coaching Research: A Decade of Progress and What's to Come," the author stated that, "we are seeing a shift from case study and uncontrolled trials to designs appropriate to the type of research questions prompted by theory generation.... By 2021, we hope that 'researchers across the globe will have completed fifty to hundred large sample size studies' that will contribute to the field" (Fillery-Travis & Passmore, 2011, p. 10).

We concur that more research is needed to establish when and where executive coaching is worth its time, attention, and resources. The good news is that there are increasing numbers of researchers and practitioners who are passionate about addressing professional standards for coaching and collecting empirical data on successful outcomes. The International Coaching Federation, *The International Journal of Evidence-Based Coaching and Mentoring*, and the ongoing work from Harvard's Institute of Coaching will provide valuable contributions to the professionalization of the coaching field. We are therefore encouraged by the slow, but increasing number of researchers who are contributing to a growing body of literature on coaching efficacy.

■ EXECUTIVE COACHING—CASE EXAMPLE

The following is a case study of executive coaching in an academic setting that reflects many of the challenges addressed in this chapter—the tensions that arise for individual professionals when their institutions undergo changes, when those professionals transition into positions of greater authority, and when the new leader faces the tasks involved in developing not only leadership skills, but also leadership consciousness.

■ CASE STUDY I

BACKGROUND

This case example involves a nursing department at a large university that was undergoing huge expansion and the promotion of faculty with teaching excellence into positions of administrative leadership (Smith Glasgow et al., 2009). The new leaders had great competencies in their areas of clinical and academic expertise, but were new to administrative roles. The female associate dean made an extraordinary move in providing executive coaching for all of her new academic nurse administrators in order to support them individually and to create a strong team. Since 2006, nine department chairs have been, or were currently being, coached. The associate dean's wise grasp of the complexities involved in times of transition, her trust in her new department chairs, and her commitment to the development of a strong team, all contributed greatly to the success of this executive coaching project.

Like most large nursing organizations, the college had, from an administrative perspective, a very large, complex undergraduate and graduate nursing program. There were three bachelor of science in nursing (BSN) tracks, ten master of science in nursing (MSN) tracks, and one DNP program that collectively enrolled a total of 1,500 nursing students and employed 60 full-time nursing faculty members as well as 200 adjunct faculty members per term. At that time, several experienced administrators were leaving. After conducting a search, the college hired or promoted faculty who had extensive teaching experience, but minimal administrative experience. In addition to a large group leadership symposium to support leadership development for these new leaders, the associate dean decided to provide executive coaching for the entire novice group of department chairs and associate chairs.

Not surprisingly, the new leaders faced all the transition challenges discussed earlier. For those promoted from within their peer group, they had to readjust boundaries and manage the emotions that accompany authority over former colleagues. Reassigning teaching schedules and clinical placements meant delicately managing a shift in relationships. Privileged information needed to be kept from former friends and discussed only with those in the leadership group. It was no longer appropriate to freely discuss personal feelings about colleagues or about administrative decisions. For some new department chairs, this generated the loneliness that can accompany leadership positions.

One department chair was brought in from outside the institution to be in charge of a large department undergoing huge growth involving administrative and structural changes. While she was learning systems that were totally

(continued)

■ CASE STUDY I *(continued)*

unfamiliar to her, she was making decisions that affected large numbers of faculty and staff. Managing these changes meant learning to contain her own anxious emotions, discerning with whom it was safe to share high emotions while consciously working to maintain her self-confidence. Another newly appointed department chair came with a whole department that had been independent of the nursing department, but who would now report to the associate dean. She was faced with no choice but to integrate her department into a faculty group that felt more like a distant relative than immediate family. Thus, although each new department chair's story had unique elements, as a new leadership group, they faced the full range of challenges that go with leadership transitions.

■ CASE STUDY II

COACHING METHODOLOGY

As stated earlier in the description of executive coaching, there are many different approaches to coaching that vary in how they collect and analyze data, involve other key players in the institution (or not), and establish the specified number of sessions, and time frame, in which the coaching process takes place. In this academic setting, assessing the new leaders' needs and identifying their coaching goals were done with a combination of approaches. A few new leaders were given a "360-degree"-feedback survey. All were administered the MBTI. There was also a team meeting of all the new department chairs where they shared their leadership style differences that were identified using the MBTI.

All the department chairs moved through the following sequence of meetings to establish their individual coaching goals.

- The coach met alone with the associate dean to hear his or her assessment of the department chair's strengths and challenges.
- The coach met alone with the department chair to hear what he or she perceived about the primary challenges to his or her development.
- The coach, department chair, and associate dean met to share their perceptions and identify coaching goals.

Structuring these first three meetings in this way created the time and space for the department chair to identify his or her challenges separately from the associate dean's analysis of his or her strengths and challenges. If there were any discrepancies, these became important discussion points in identifying the development needs and agreeing upon goals. This process created a three-way buy-in to the coaching goals, and left no room for differing perspectives to fall between the cracks.

Four to six to 10 coaching sessions followed, lasting about an hour to an hour and a half. They were designed as individual face-to-face sessions, except

(continued)

■ CASE STUDY II *(continued)*

for an occasional shared meeting between two department chairs to discuss their different leadership styles when this exploration was relevant to their coaching goals. Department chairs were also encouraged to contact the coach between sessions should they want feedback, or time to discuss a current issue. Throughout the duration of the coaching process, the department chairs were encouraged to use the associate dean as a mentor—to feel free to ask for feedback on decisions, to stop by his or her office to ask a question, and/or to brainstorm alternative ways of handling situations. In this way, the associate dean was a positive part of the ongoing coaching process and methodology.

■ CASE STUDY III

COACHING CHALLENGES

There were common leadership development themes that emerged with the new leaders in this academic setting, and also some that were unique to the individual coaching client. The following challenges emerged during the coaching process, many of which were targeted as specific goals for individual coaching clients:

- Learning to say "no" and set boundaries
- Letting go of perfection in the service of getting things done
- Attending to relationships over task accomplishment
- Learning when it is safe to ask questions and to not need to appear as an expert
- Developing listening skills
- Creating visibility outside the nursing school and within the larger university
- Managing time
- Identifying patterns of self-sabotage and reversing them
- Managing self-care in the midst of feeling overwhelmed
- Creating strategies for stress reduction
- Modulating emotional reactivity
- Finding and developing a personal style of leadership presence

■ CASE STUDIES: Two Individual Case Examples

The following two case examples describe the specific challenges for two of the newly appointed leaders who generously allowed their stories to be told.

(continued)

■ CASE STUDIES: Two Individual Case Examples   *(continued)*

CASE 1

Dr. Flynn was promoted to the department chair after years of teaching excellence at the university. Her development needs included assertiveness, managing conflict, finding a leadership presence, performing responsibilities with greater confidence, articulating opinions within the executive nursing council, and becoming more visible within the larger university system. Dr. Flynn worked closely with Dr. Morgan, the associate chair, who had a big personality, had extensive administrative experience, but who was new to the college. Together, they inherited a complex department that channeled large numbers of students into different specializations, at a time when the structure for these programs was in flux. Dr. Flynn felt responsible for helping Dr. Morgan learn the ropes and spent many hours in this role behind the scenes. She also let Dr. Morgan be of the more visible presence. One year later, Dr. Flynn was seen only in Dr. Morgan's shadow. Coaching sessions with Dr. Flynn focused on her personal barriers to establishing autonomy and on strategies to assert her authority successfully. In the coaching process, Dr. Flynn became more comfortable with the conflict resolution. She established a separate identity and created greater visibility within the university.

CASE 2

Professor Castle was promoted to administrative leadership with a reputation as an excellent teacher and an efficient taskmaster on any given professional assignment. Extremely introverted, she liked to work with her door closed with minimal social exchange and treasured quiet time alone at her desk. She spent long days at work and looked forward to renewing herself at home after hours. Although she was liked by others and always socially appropriate, she maintained a strong personal boundary. Professor Castle was surprised to learn that her new role involved not just task accomplishment, but also informal attention to relationships, which involved verbal and visible accessibility, which, by nature, she had formerly considered a waste of time. Learning to converse casually in order to gain others' trust and comfort, making daily connections, and stopping by other peoples' offices all were aspects of leadership that had not been on her radar screen. Being more accessible, while also attending to her needs for working and being alone, became a focus for the coaching process. Professor Castle and the coach talked about ways to create greater ease with stopping by other department chair's offices, and how she could answer e-mails so they were to the point, but also made some personal references that would build connection between herself, her faculty reports, and other department chairs. They identified hours of the day she could most comfortably have an "open door policy," and other times that she would partially close her door. Over time, Professor Castle felt more comfortable with the extroverted parts of

(continued)

■ CASE STUDIES: Two Individual Case Examples   *(continued)*

her new role and learned to balance her interactive and solo work time (Smith Glasgow et al., 2009).

The themes listed earlier, from learning to say "no" to developing a personal style of leadership presence, plus the issues named in these two specific case examples, are all challenges that are likely to appear in one form or another in institutions that undergo role shifts and leadership transitions.

■ SUMMARY

The DNP is an evolving field that involves twists, turns, and transitions for both the individual as well as the professional itself. As the DNP increases its presence in our shifting health care system, its opportunities for leadership and influence abound. To optimize the DNP's position, attention to leadership development is vital. Increasing the leadership skills, and also the leadership conscious, multiplies the DNP's contributions to the general public, individual patients, and the whole nursing profession.

To date, the nursing profession has not frequently engaged the use of executive coaching to help grow its future leaders. The authors would also encourage the DNP graduate to take advantage of leadership fellowships such as the National League for Nursing LEAD Program, Leadership Development Program for Simulation Educators, and Executive Leadership in Nursing Education and Practice, American Association of Colleges of Nursing Leadership for Academic Nursing Programs (LANP), and the Johnson & Johnson/Wharton Fellows Program in Management for Nurse Executives, which many times offer individual executive coaching sessions. The AANP Leadership Program is a new 12-month program developed for nurse practitioner leaders who are currently serving in clinical, administrative, or educational roles and who demonstrate the potential to assume roles of increasing national leadership both within the AANP and throughout the nation. The AANP will recruit nurse practitioners from across the United States and provide them with experiential leadership development through both face-to-face and electronic learning opportunities. However, with the advent of the DNP's new role, it is the right time, and wise, for the DNP graduate, as well as for other leaders in the nursing world, to seek support for leadership excellence. Our experience tells us that executive coaching can help individuals manifest their talents and resourcefulness and maximize their personal and professional potential. It can inspire and support the nursing profession as it attends to its mission of creating strategies and solutions that improve and heal the human condition.

■ CRITICAL THINKING QUESTIONS

1. *What professional transitions have you already experienced in your career development? What were the challenges you faced in making those transitions?*
2. *If you were promoted into a position of authority over those who are current peers, what challenges do you think you would face?*
3. *What are the likely transition challenges that the DNP will face in the near future?*

4. *What expectations or* myths *about new leaders may inhibit smooth transitions into positions of increased authority?*
5. *How do you define leadership?*
6. *What do you consider your strengths and weaknesses as a leader?*
7. *Describe an experience of your professional "personal best." What have you accomplished professionally that you are most proud of? What leadership qualities of yours contributed to your success in this endeavor?*
8. *What does* leadership consciousness *mean to you? What role models do you have for leaders who embody leadership consciousness?*
9. *What is executive coaching? In what ways might executive coaching provide leadership development for you in your leadership position?*
10. *In the executive coaching case example described in this chapter, what interests you most? Would you have wanted a similar intervention for your professional development?*

■ REFERENCES

Arrien, A. (1993). *The four fold way*. San Francisco, CA: Harper Collins.

Barret Values Centre. (2009). Supporting leaders in building values-driven cultures "The seven levels of leadership consciousness." Retrieved from https://www.valuescentre.com/mapping-values/barrett-model/leadershipconsciousness

Carroll, L. (1865/1871/1981). *Alice's adventures in wonderland and through the looking glass*. New York, NY: Dell Bantam Books.

Coutu, D., & Kauffman, C. (2009, January). What can coaches do for you? *Harvard Business Review, 87*, 91–97. Retrieved from https://hbr.org/2009/01/what-can-coaches-do-for-you

Dai, G., & De Meuse, P. K. (2009). The effectiveness of executive coaching: What we can learn from the research literature. Retrieved from http://www.kornferryinstitute.com/reports-insights/effectiveness-executive-coaching-what-we-can-learn-research-literature

Eisenstat, R., Beer, M., Foote, N., Fredberg, T., & Norrgren, F. (2008). The uncompromising leader. *Harvard Business Review, 86*(7/8), 50–57.

Elsner, D., & Farrands, B. (2012). *Leadership transitions: How business leaders can successfully take charge in new roles*. Philadelphia, PA: Kogan Page Publishers.

Fillery-Travis, A., & Passmore, J. (2011). A critical review of executive coaching research: A decade of progress and what's to come. *Coaching: An International Journal of Theory, Research and Practice, 4*(2), 70–88. doi:10.1080/17521882.2011.596484

Frankovelgia, C. (2010, April). The key to effective coaching. *Forbes Magazine*. Retrieved from http://www.forbes.com/2010/04/28/coaching-talent-developmentleadership-managing-ccl.html

Goleman, D. (2012). Emotional intelligence and why it can matter more than IQ. New York, NY: Bantam Dell.

Hassidic Stories. (2010). Retrieved from http://hasidicstories.com/Stories/Other_Early_Rebbes/zusia.html

Hill, G. (2010). Executive coaching: Perspectives of effectiveness from executives and coaches (Master's thesis). Retrieved from http://www.google.com/url?sa=t&rct=j&q=&esrc=s&source=web&cd=1&ved=0CCUQFjAA&url=http%3A%2F%2Feprints.qut.edu.au%2F40237%2F1%2FGraham_Hill_Thesis.pdf&ei=fAahVbOnCMqu-QGpt7qYCg&usg=AFQjCNFBehmj6BfU00jURNczGv1EDM51Bg &sig2=T6x6lfYkvA1lCOH254ZCDg

International Coaching Federation. (n.d.). Retrieved from https://www.google.com/?gws_rd=ssl#q=icf+definition+of+coaching

Jimenez, J. R. (1995). Title of poem you are referencing from this book. My boat struck something deep. In R. Bly (Ed., trans.), *News of the universe: Poems of twofold consciousness*. San Francisco, CA: Sierra Club Books.

Kabat-Zinn, J. (1994). *Wherever you go there you are: Mindfulness mediation in everyday life*. New York, NY: Hyperion.

Kabat-Zinn, J. (2009). *Wherever you go there you are: Mindfulness mediation in everyday life*. New York, NY: Hachette Book Group.

Kauffman, C. (2004). De-mystifying research: An introduction for coaches. Proceedings of the Second Coaching Research Symposium (pp. 161–168). Washington, DC: International Coach Federation. Retrieved from https://www.google.com/?gws_rd=ssl#q=Demystifying+Research:+An+Introduction+for+Coaches

Koestler, A. (1978). *Janus*. New York, NY: Vintage Books.

Kombarakaran, F. A., Yang, J., Baker, M. N., & Fernandes, P. (2008). Executive coaching: It works! *Consulting Psychology Journal: Practice and Research, 60*(1), 78–90.

Lepsinger, R., & Lucia, A. D. (2009). *The art and science of 360 degree feedback*. San Francisco, CA: Jossey-Bass.

MacEowen, F. (2007). *The celtic wheel of seeing*. Novato, CA: New World Library.

O'Neil, M. B. (2007). *Executive coaching with backbone and heart: A systems approach to engaging leaders with their challenges* (p. 5). San Francisco, CA: John Wiley and Sons.

Personal Evolution: Health, Fitness and Personal Development. (2010). Buddhist monk story (para 1–4). Retrieved from http://www.endlesshumanpotential.com/buddhist-monk-story.html

Sanaghan, P. H., Goldstein, L., & Gaval, K. D. (2009). *Presidential transitions: It's not just the position, it's the transition*. Lanham, MD: Rowman & Littlefield.

Shure, J., & Weinstock, B. (2009). Shame, compassion, and the journey towards health. In M. Maine, W. Davis, & J. Shure (Eds.), *Effective clinical practice in the treatment of eating disorders* (pp. 163–177). New York, NY: Routledge.

Smith Glasgow, M. E., Weinstock, B., Lachman, V., Suplee, P. D., & Dreher, H. M. (2009). The benefits of leadership program and executive coaching for new nurse administrators: One college's experience. *Journal of Professional Nursing, 25*(4), 204–210.

Varvogli, L., & Darviri, C. (2011). Stress management techniques: Evidence-based procedures that reduce stress and promote health. *Health Science Journal, 5*, 74–89.

Weinstock, B., & Sanaghan, P. (2015). Preparing tomorrow's leaders: Leadership coaching in higher education. Retrieved from http://www.academicimpressions.com/news/leadership-coaching-higher-education?awp=0

Whyte, D. (2007). *The heart aroused: Poetry and the preservation of the soul in corporate America*. New York, NY: Doubleday.

Reflective Response 1

Margo A. Karsten

Health care reform, countless stories about the eroding ethics in leadership, lack of trust among the front line staff with administration, and a disengaged workforce are ingredients for a perfect storm. However, Weinstock and Glasgow provide a silver lining to this dark health care landscape, by articulating the importance of executive coaching for nursing leaders. They not only explored the many domains of leadership consciousness, but reinforced that executive coaching is an intervention that assists leaders, in this case Doctor of Nursing Practice (DNP) graduates, to achieve their full potential. The recognition of the impact executive coaching can have on a leader comes at a critical time in health care. Articulating the transition that health care and nursing are currently experiencing, they have highlighted the critical need to have a neutral person that a leader can candidly talk to about the various challenges that face them on a day-to-day basis.

My experience of more than 16 years of administrative practice, including over a decade as chief nurse in various medical centers and experience as a chief operating officer and chief executive officer, gives me firsthand knowledge of what it feels like to transition into various executive roles. The majority of my transitions have come from within the same facility. Learning how to manage former relationships in a new role is an art. New competencies are needed as a person accepts various roles. According to Anderson (2010), organizations are transitioning from traditional paternal forms of organizations to high involvement, empowered partnership, and collaborative learning organizations. These changes warrant a new set of competencies and behaviors. Weinstock and Glasgow captured these new competencies and behaviors in their two case studies.

These two case studies highlight the need for an objective and supportive coach. Growing into a new position can be an awkward transition. Balancing the appropriate autonomy and authority is a challenge that many new leaders struggle to accomplish. As demonstrated in the first case study, an executive coach can assist in this balancing act. The second case study demonstrates another common challenge for leaders; new leaders find themselves at times in a role with high expectations of outgoing sociability. This new expectation of building relationships and creating connections can feel like foreign territory. It has been my experience that new leaders do not understand the importance and value of creating connections with their newly acquired direct reports. Successful leader takes time to create and nurture relationships throughout the work environment. Weinstock and Smith Glasgow highlight the importance of finding the balance of being accessible to a team with an open door policy and creating office time for the leader to be alone in the their second case study. In addition to finding their balance of creating relationships and finding the balance of being available to the team, I found additional challenges in transitioning from the bedside to a management position.

The hidden challenges in professional transitions reflect a previous reality that I experienced in the acute care setting. Loneliness, wavering confidence, boundary setting, questioning my own competency, and staying true to my own identity clearly haunted me as I made my various transitions from bedside to the boardroom. Over the past 12 years, having an executive coach allowed me to overcome these hidden challenges. I believe it is an art to learn how to find your own voice and ensure that it is heard in the appropriate settings. The executive coach is the person who encourages and supports you in finding your voice and reminds you that your main responsibility is *to speak the truth*. Coaching allows professionals to become neutral and objective persons who can be a mirror to reflect their true sense of self.

As Weinstock and Glasgow mentioned, there are many different approaches to coaching. I have found that to be true in my experience as well. Each coach and client will establish how they collect and analyze data, involve other key players in the institution (or not), and establish the specified number of sessions and time frame in which the coaching process takes place. I have found that the use of a "360-degree"-feedback survey enriches the coaching experience. Thach (2002) used a "360-degree"-feedback instrument to determine the impact of executive coaching on leadership effectiveness. Two hundred and eighty one leaders participated in "360-degree" feedback before and after an average of 6 months of coaching. During the two phases of the study, the overall impact of leadership effectiveness, as perceived by direct reports, peers, and managers, was an average of 55% and 60%, respectively. I have experienced similar results when coaching was combined with a "360-degree"-feedback tool. Combining a tool that gives a leader insight into her style with an executive coach who can assist in further refining the leadership behaviors and competencies that are critical for success is a perfect formula for leadership effectiveness. Laske (2004) investigated the mental and emotional growth of six executives who were coached over 14 months. Coaches and participants' developmental and behavioral profiles were assessed before and after coaching. Three executives made significant developmental progress and were perceived to have improved their leadership effectiveness through the use of coaching. This type of developmental progress takes time and a willingness to reflect on your own personal growth opportunities.

It is important in this period of significant change that nursing leaders take the time to reflect upon their own journey. Weinstock and Glasgow provide reflective questions, which stimulate the reader to pause and become introspective about their own lives. As nursing leaders take the time to become introspective, having an executive coach at their sides will only accelerate their personal and professional growth. According to Wales (2002), coaching provides a space for profound personal development and enables leaders to understand how to translate personal insights into improved leadership effectiveness and, ultimately, organizational development. As these authors noted, executive coaching can inspire and support the nursing profession as it attends to its mission of creating strategies and solutions that improve, and heal, the human condition. I believe that creating caring, healing, and compassionate cultures for our team and patients we serve takes an incredible amount of stamina and resilience. The research and evidence is clear: executive coaching can have a profound impact on the conscientiousness of nursing leaders. This leadership intervention will help ensure we lead with our values intact.

■ REFERENCES

Anderson, J. (2010). The leadership circle. Retrieved from www.leadershipcircle.com

Laske, O. (2004). Can evidence-based coaching increase ROI? *International Journal of Evidence Based Coaching and Mentoring, 2*(2), 41–53.

Thach, E. (2002). The impact of executive coaching and 360 feedback on leadership effectiveness. *Leader Organizational Development Journal, 23*, 3–4.

Wales, S. (2002). Why coaching? *Journal of Change Management, 2*(2), 275–282.

CHAPTER THIRTEEN

Reflective Response 2

Diane S. Hupp

As health care organizations continue to increase in complexity, nurse leaders' roles only become more challenging. Priorities are competing including safety and quality, financial and regulatory issues, patient experience/satisfaction, and staff engagement. Each of these competing demands has a significant impact on the overall patient outcomes. Effective leadership is necessary to establish a vision, goals and strategies for each priority to reach optimal outcomes for our patients, staff, and organizations. An additional priority for nurse leaders today is to meet the Institute of Medicine's report *The Future of Nursing: Leading Change, Advancing Health* key recommendations including achieving higher levels of education and training through an improved education system that promotes seamless academic progression (Institute of Medicine, 2010). Weinstock and Glasgow clearly demonstrate that executive coaching can help nurse leaders, and in particular, new doctorally prepared nurse leaders, both professionally and personally, to overcome these challenges and maximize their potential.

■ PERSONAL JOURNEY

Throughout my personal tenure as a leader, I have experienced and have witnessed many of the concepts that Weinstock and Glasgow address in this chapter. In particular, leadership consciousness is the most significant attribute to impacts one's effectiveness as a successful leader. Keeping in mind that the world often appears different and broader as a new doctorally prepared nurse, leadership consciousness is not only being aware of oneself at all times but more importantly, how your words, actions, and leadership presence impact others.

As I reflect about leadership consciousness, I recall my own experiences recruiting new leaders and doctorally prepared nurses. Certain skills are essential to ensure one's success as a nurse leader. Typically, in an interview for a nurse leadership position, the candidate is concerned about being familiar with the budgetary, financial, and regulatory processes, which are all important. However, to me, these competencies can all be easily taught to a new leader. In my opinion, the candidate who stands out is the one who is able to demonstrate that he or she will be able to connect with staff and raise awareness of the culture within the department. This candidate truly possesses leadership consciousness. Sometimes, this is an intuitive skill that some leaders possess. For others, it may need to be taught. An executive coach may be a wise choice to help support the leader's development and success in this area.

■ TRANSITIONING INTO LEADERSHIP ROLES

As Weinstock and Glasgow note, it can be lonely in a new role or even a greater feeling of loneliness as one climbs the ladder of leadership. As new doctorally prepared nurses enter and transition into the complex and uncertain health care environment, confidence and competency may be challenged. Former colleagues may perceive you differently and even behave "out of character," given your new role. The new leader needs to establish boundaries while attempting to maintain positive, strong relationships with colleagues. My personal experience of transitioning into multiple new roles has provided me the ability to see the value of shared leadership and staff empowerment. However, learning to be a transformational leader who empowers front-line staff to make decisions requires "vision, influence, clinical knowledge, and a strong expertise relating to professional nursing practice" (American Nurses Credentialing Center [ANCC], 2014).

Building teams, creating trust, and dispelling the leadership myths that Glasgow and Weinstein address will all take time, commitment and perseverance on the leader's part. Most importantly, the leader must be willingly to delegate and relinquish some tasks and responsibilities. For a new doctorally prepared nurse, this transition may be difficult. From personal experience, moving into my chief nursing officer role a decade ago, I can certainly relate to these challenges. I believe one of the most crucial success factors was my executive coach.

■ SELF-AWARENESS

Emotional intelligence is an attribute that is critically important to leaders (Akerjordt & Serverinsson, 2008). As Weinstock and Glasgow discuss, the development of one's interpersonal intelligence may improve as the result of executive coaching. Coaching empowers individuals to make positive changes in their professional and personal life, while promoting the goals of the organization (Byrne, 2007). On a personal note, I recall sharing my "360" with my executive coach. My coach was supportive yet forthright in identifying my own areas of professional development. Each leader has strengths and opportunities. Sometimes, it may be difficult to see our own opportunities. However, if a leader has an executive coach whom they feel comfortable sharing their "360-degree"-assessment, self-awareness and authenticity will be enhanced.

■ VALUE OF AN EXECUTIVE COACH

As the Doctor of Nurse Practice (DNP) graduate transitions to leadership roles in this complex and transforming environment, the literature supports that an executive coach will only enhance both their professional and personal growth as a leader. My executive coach has been invaluable to me throughout the last decade. Emphasis has been placed on many of the concepts described by Weinstock and Glasgow to support my own development. Understanding and relating to one's leadership consciousness cannot be stressed enough as it is a skill necessary to be a successful leader. One's words, actions, and behaviors are on stage all of the time. Further, how you manage and react to other's words, actions, and behaviors is equally important. Critical leadership attributes of mindfulness and self-awareness, coupled with an executive coach to support one's professional and personal development, will enhance both leadership and organizational performance.

■ REFERENCES

Akerjordt, K., & Serverinsson, E. (2008). Emotionally intelligent nurse leadership: A literature review study. *Journal of Nursing Management, 16*, 565–577.

American Nurses Credentialing Center. (2014). ANCC Magnet Recognition Program. Retrieved from www.nursecredentialing.org/magnet

Byrne, G. (2007). Guest editorial: Unlocking potential—Coaching as a means to enhance leadership and role performance in nursing. *Journal of Clinical Nursing, 16*(11), 1987–1988.

Institute of Medicine. (2010). *The future of nursing: Leading change, advancing health.* Retrieved from www.iom.edu/nursing

Leveraging Technology to Support Doctoral Advanced Nursing Practice

Frances H. Cornelius, Gary M. Childs, and Linda Wilson

The past several decades have been defined by the rapid pace of change and innovation. We live and work in a technology-infused world that will become even more integrated with technology in the future. Technology is integral in our efforts to meet the challenges faced by our health care system today and in the future. The doctorally prepared advanced practice nurse (APN) must be proficient in the use of technology to assume a leadership role in efforts to improve practice, and to conduct research to improve health care, systems, and patient outcomes. The doctoral APN will be using technology in a variety of roles—practitioner (and clinical expert), educator, clinical scientist, or nursing administrator—and must be competent in information technology to be able to leverage their use in every role or setting. A strong recommendation is that the doctoral APN should possess a higher level of technical competency than expected of the master's-prepared APN.

■ OVERVIEW OF CURRENT ADVANCED PRACTICE NURSE TECHNOLOGY EXPECTATIONS

The Institute of Medicine (IOM, 1999, 2001, 2003) has led the intense scrutiny of our health care system and has focused attention on health care delivery, patient safety, and the education of health professionals. Recent reports have highlighted the need for comprehensive restructuring of the education of all health professionals, with an emphasis on evidence-based practice, quality improvement, and informatics, as well as an interdisciplinary approach to patient-centered care. Given these reports and emerging trends in the health care arena, particularly related to technology, there is a heightened awareness of the importance of essential informatics/technology competencies among nurses at all degree levels. The American Association of Colleges of Nursing (2006) supports these recommendations and has proposed that doctorally prepared nurses be poised to assume *key leadership positions* to drive these changes in order to actively participate in executive decisions that address these important issues. It is for these reasons that the doctoral APN must be prepared to take full advantage of all available technologies to support his or her practice and scholarship.

■ EXPECTATIONS FOR THE MASTER'S-LEVEL PRACTITIONER

The American Association of Colleges of Nursing (AACN, 2010) has identified competencies that are essential for master's-prepared nurses to practice effectively. Although technology is assumed to be integrated throughout all the competencies, this AACN document explicitly addresses technological competencies in *Essential V: Informatics and Healthcare Technologies,* which articulates the five broad areas that these competencies encompass. The master's-level practitioner must be proficient in: (a) patient care and other technologies to deliver/enhance care; (b) communication technologies to integrate/coordinate care; (c) data management to analyze/improve outcomes of care; (d) health information management for evidence-based care/health education; and (e) facilitation and use of electronic health records (EHRs) to improve patient care (AACN, 2010, p. 17). In addition, *Essential IV: Translating and Integrating Scholarship Into Practice* requires informatics and technology competencies as well as information management skills in order to effectively "lead continuous improvement processes based on translational research skills" bringing "evidence-based practice to both individual patients for whom they directly care and to those patients for whom they are indirectly responsible" (AACN, 2010, p. 16).

Irrespective of the practice setting of the master's-prepared nurse, proficiency in the utilization of technology is crucial to any effort to address health care needs, whether directly or indirectly. The focus at this level is *proficiency.* For the doctoral APN, the expectations are much higher.

■ RAISING THE BAR: EXPECTATIONS FOR THE DOCTORAL APN

Because the use of technologies to deliver, improve, and document care is changing rapidly in the current, dynamic health care arena, it is absolutely essential that the doctoral APN possess high-level skills—basic proficiency is insufficient. It is expected that the doctoral APN will function in a leadership role in the use of technologies to support health care delivery (Chase & Pruitt, 2006; Otterness, 2006; Porter-O'Grady & Malloch, 2008; Webber, 2008). It is important that the doctoral APN not only possesses these skills, but also takes measures to ensure that these skills are kept up-to-date.

The doctoral APN is expected to leverage the skills and knowledge of information systems and technology in both academic and health care settings with the goal of improving patient care and the health care systems charged with providing this care. To accomplish this, the doctoral APN must not only possess technological skills, but also high-level practical research skills in order to be able to contribute to the body of scientific knowledge, and further, to serve as a catalyst for change. We admit this is and will continue to be a debatable point with regard to the practice doctorate—the graduate's role in knowledge development. We assert, however, that the overly simplified adage that the Doctor of Nursing Practice (DNP) graduate will only translate and disseminate research findings is problematic if it is assumed that all doctoral graduates should contribute to the evidence base of their respective discipline. In addition, he or she must be able to manage and use effectively an increasing volume of evidence to guide practice and establish new standards of care within health care systems. Technologies explored in this chapter provide doctorally prepared nurses and those beginning doctoral studies with an understanding of how these innovations can be used effectively to support the advanced practice role and meet these expectations.

■ INFORMATICS AND TECHNICAL COMPETENCIES FOR THE DOCTORAL APN

The AACN's (2006) *Essentials of Doctoral Education for Advanced Nursing Practice* has identified specific competencies expected of a doctoral. Again, the use of technology is threaded throughout the document; however, APN, *Essential IV* clearly speaks to expected proficiencies with information systems and patient care technologies. The AACN maintains that nurses at this level are "distinguished by their abilities to use information systems/technology to sustain and improve patient care and health care systems, and provide leadership within health care systems and/or academic settings" (2006, p. 12). The doctoral APN should be able to take a leadership role in: (a) the design, selection, use, and evaluation of technologies for care; (b) analysis and identification of critical elements to assist in the selection and evaluation process of these technologies; and (c) design and implementation of mechanisms to extract data from practice information systems and databases for the purpose of evaluation and improvement in "programs of care, outcomes of care, and care systems" (2006, p. 12). A key competency involves the ability to combine information from a variety of data sources to create new information, and possibly new knowledge, to support care delivery, decision support, and care outcomes. Dreher (2010) termed the knowledge emanating out of DNP programs (by both DNP and DrNP graduates) as *practice knowledge*. This practice knowledge has the potential to contribute significantly to the body of knowledge, change practice standards, and improve patient outcomes.

INFORMATICS COMPETENCIES

It is expected that the doctoral APN would have informatics competencies at an expert level. It is expected that he or she will be a role model to others in the integration and utilization of clinical data systems to support the development of "practice wisdom," the development and application of unified nursing documentation language, the utilization of information systems to improve quality and care outcomes, as well as demonstrate advanced troubleshooting skills (Barton, 2005; Gassert, 2008; Staggers, Gassert, & Curran, 2002; Westra & Delaney, 2008).

The Technology Informatics Guiding Educational Reform (TIGER Informatics Competency Collaborative, 2009) initiative has identified three categories of informatics skills: (a) basic computer competency, (b) information literacy, and (c) information management (Gugerty & Delaney, 2009). At an expert level, it is expected that the doctoral APN would possess advanced skills using word processing, spreadsheets, and presentation software. In addition, it is expected that he or she would possess high-level skills in distance learning technologies. Essential information literacy skills include the ability to:

1. Determine the nature and extent of the information needed
2. Access needed information effectively and efficiently
3. Evaluate information and its sources critically and incorporate selected information into his or her knowledge base and value system
4. Individually or as a member of a group, use information effectively to accomplish a specific purpose
5. Evaluate outcomes of the use of information (TIGER Informatics Competency Collaborative, 2009)

Recently the TIGER Initiative Foundation issued a report, *The Leadership Imperative: TIGER's Recommendations for Integrating Technology to Transform Practice and Education*, which identifies the growing need for nurse leaders to be prepared to meet the challenges of a health care environment in which care will be "delivered remotely through the use of mobile monitoring and innovative communications . . . using online and electronic communication and telehealth strategies to enhance communication among providers and between patients and providers. As a result, nurse leaders' accountability for patient-care oversight will extend well beyond the hospital setting. To support these new models of care delivery, innovative nurse leaders will be required to integrate an ever-expanding arsenal of health IT into practice" (TIGER Initiative Foundation, n.d., p. 16). This goal will require educational preparation for the doctoral APN to step into the role of an innovative nurse leader who is capable of leading an expanded interprofessional teams of nontraditional experts to achieve the goal of a transprofessional approach to support innovation, redefine health care and improve outcomes (O'Keefe & Griffin, 2013).

KNOWLEDGE MANAGEMENT COMPETENCIES

Knowledge management competencies are integral to health care and nursing practice (Dreher, 2009a). While it is a growing expectation that nurses at all levels should possess knowledge management skills, the doctoral APN must take a leadership role in efforts to document and understand the impact of nursing care on the health of patients. It is through the use of knowledge management systems that these important data can be collected, stored, retrieved, and used to generate knowledge regarding nursing outcomes and improve patient care and safety. Integral to these efforts is the EHR, as it can provide a mechanism to record data collected at the point of care. The doctoral APN must have a good understanding of knowledge management systems in order to influence the design and management of these systems (Canadian Nurses Association [CNA], 2006; Contino, 2004; Hsia, Lin, Wu, & Tsai, 2006; Staggers et al., 2002).

In addition, the doctoral APN must champion efforts to have a standardized nursing language system that is integrated with universal clinical care terminology. A standardized nursing language makes nursing data more visible within health systems and can support the development of nursing knowledge (Coenen & Bartz, 2006). A standardized nursing language can facilitate "better communication among nurses and other health care providers, increased visibility of nursing interventions, improved patient care, enhanced data collection to evaluate nursing care outcomes, greater adherence to standards of care, and facilitated assessment of nursing competency" (Rutherford, 2008, para 1). Without a standardized language, we will not be able to realize our vision of a fully integrated health information system (HIS) that can support interdisciplinary collaboration and data sharing across settings and can provide a way for the impact of nursing care to be more visible and contribute more effectively to the body of knowledge. The doctoral APN must be knowledgeable in health information technology (HIT) and informatics and assume a leadership role to drive the transition to integrated systems that can support evidence-based practice, clinical decision making, improve outcomes and fully reflect the impact of nursing practice on these outcomes. Until this is fully realized, the impact of nursing care "will be unidentifiable for outcomes reporting and therefore invisible" (Conrad, Hanson, Hasenau, & Stocker-Schneider, 2012, p. 450)

An essential part of knowledge management entails the gathering of information and requires "information mastery" (Slawson, Shaughnessy, & Bennett, 1994). The main point of information mastery is that "the most important information is highly relevant and highly valid and takes little work to obtain" (Ebell & Shaughnessy, 2003, p. S53). The information being consumed should be related to a clinical question that is common or important in practice, deals with patient outcomes, and could lead to change of clinical practice (Ebell & Shaughnessy, 2003).

However, during a recent literature search (August 28, 2015) of the CINAHL database, a keyword search for the term information mastery only produced seven results. Another interesting observation is the majority of these results noted physicians and residents versus nurses as participants. Doctoral APNs have opportunities to address this gap and improve clinical practice using techniques such as information mastery.

∎ TECHNOLOGICAL TOOLS THAT CAN SUPPORT THE DOCTORAL APN

As technological innovation continues, the list of tools that can be used to support the doctoral APN's practice continues to grow, and can be organized into four categories: (a) reference management, (b) data collection, (c) data analysis, and (d) report generation. Specific information regarding these tools is presented in Table 14.1.

Reference management tools can be divided into two subcategories: (a) basic reference management tools and (b) integrated reference management tools. Basic reference management tools include web-based applications such as CiteULike, Connotea, and JabRef. These tools allow the user to collect, organize, and share personal bibliographies and information with colleagues. These resources permit access from any computer and can facilitate collaboration with colleagues who share a similar research interest. Zotero is similar to the other three tools; however, it offers the additional capability to cite your research sources. A key characteristic shared by these tools is that the bibliography can be accessed from any computer.

Integrated reference management tools take the basic reference management features one-step further by integrating a literature database search with reference management and the writing process. Using the advanced functionalities of tools such as

TABLE 14.1 **Selected Research Tools**

Category	Tool	Website
Reference management	CiteULike	www.citeulike.org
	Connotea	www.connotea.org
	JabRef	http://jabref.sourceforge.net
	Zotero	www.zotero.org
	Endnote®	www.endnote.com
	RefWorks©	www.refworks.com
Data analysis and report generation	PSAW (formally SPSS)	www.spss.com
	SAS	www.sas.com
	Atlas	www.atlasti.com
	NVivo	www.qsrinternational.com
	Crystal Reports	http://crystalreports.com

PSAW, Predictive Analytics Software; SAS, Statistical Analysis System; SPSS, Statistical Package in the Social Sciences.

RefWorks and Endnote, the doctorally prepared nurse can write a paper while automatically generating citations and reference lists in the correct format. These tools provide the option to easily switch style formats, such as from the *Publication Manual of the American Psychological Association* (APA) style to the American Medical Association (AMA) style, which is sometimes required when submitting papers for publication. These tools/skills are useful to the doctoral student, and can also be useful for the clinical scholar beyond graduation given the expectation of dissemination of practice scholarship.

Data collection tools can range from simple Excel spreadsheets or Access databases, to more complex EHRs, to even more sophisticated system-wide data collection systems such as a HIS. The key consideration for the doctoral APN is that it is imperative that one has a clear understanding of how these various data collection mechanisms operate, how databases are organized, and how these can be used to improve patient outcomes and knowledge generation. Collecting and managing data using electronic data collection tools can improve accuracy, completeness, and timeliness of data, consequently ensuring data integrity. All of these ones then can efficiently support enhanced clinical decisions by practitioners/clinicians when delivering patient care or by supporting the nondirect care functions of doctoral advanced nursing practice. As health care systems amass more and more health information, the use of these sophisticated tools to analyze big data repositories will drive changes in the health care landscape, ranging from improved treatments to reducing hospital admissions and improving patient outcomes (Bates, Saria, Ohno-Machado, Shah, & Escobar, 2014). The doctorally prepared APN must be able to understand and "use available health information management tools for evidence-based care/health education . . . and to improve patient care" (AACN, 2010, p. 17).

Data analysis and report generation demands yet another skill set involving the use of programs such as Predictive Analytics Software (PASW; formally Statistical Package in the Social Sciences [SPSS]) or Statistical Analysis System (SAS) for quantitative data analysis, and Atlas or NVivo for qualitative data analysis. In the past, the majority of research conducted by APNs was quantitative. It is important to note that qualitative research in primary care settings is gaining acceptance and is more widespread in the literature (Aflague & Ferszt, 2010; Doherty, 2010; King, Muzaffar, & George, 2009; Tanyi, McKenzie, & Chapek, 2009; Thrasher & Purc-Stephenson, 2007).

Products such as Crystal Reports or i-net Clear Reports permit extraction of information from multiple data sources to create reports. A good understanding of these and similar tools and of how to present information meaningfully is essential. Using tools such as these can help the doctoral APN to not only manage large data sets but to conduct high-level analysis that can generate new knowledge.

■ PROFESSIONAL ORGANIZATIONS AND INFORMATICS EXPECTATIONS OF THE DOCTORAL APN

AMERICAN ASSOCIATION OF COLLEGES OF NURSING

The AACN published *The Essentials of Doctoral Education for Advanced Nursing Practice* in 2006, and some 5 years later, it is critically apparent that the original essentials must be revisited. According to the AACN (2006) there are eight essentials comprising the following key areas: (a) scientific underpinnings for practice; (b) organizational and systems leadership for quality improvement and systems thinking; (c) clinical scholarship and analytical methods for evidence-based practice; (d) information systems/technology and patient care technology for the improvement and transformation of health care; (e) health care policy for advocacy in health care; (f) interprofessional collaboration for improving patient and population health outcomes; (g) clinical prevention and population health for improving the nation's health; and (h) advanced nursing practice. We pose the following question: Should the informatics competencies be different for students in doctoral advanced practice tracks versus students in the aggregate/systems/organizational tracks?

AMERICAN ASSOCIATION OF NURSE ANESTHETISTS

The American Association of Nurse Anesthetists (AANA) developed a task force to examine the appropriateness of the DNP degree for the nurse anesthetist. After investigation, the AANA decided to support doctoral education for entry into practice for the nurse anesthetist by the year 2025. In the AANA (2007) position statement on *Doctoral Preparation of Nurse Anesthetists*, it states their rationale: "to best position Certified Registered Nurse Anesthetists (CRNAs) to meet this ongoing challenge and remain recognized leaders in anesthesia care, the AANA believes it is essential to support doctoral education that encompasses technological and pharmaceutical advances, informatics, evidence-based practice, systems approaches to quality improvement, health care business models, teamwork, public relations, and other subjects that will shape the future for anesthesia providers and their patients" (p. 1). It should be noted, however, that the AANA was not exclusively endorsing the DNP degree, but other doctoral options for CRNAs as well.

AMERICAN ORGANIZATION OF NURSE EXECUTIVES

The American Organization of Nurse Executives (AONE) Nurse Executive Competencies (AONE, 2015) addresses technology competencies within the Business Skills Competency section under the subtitle of Information Management and Technology (AONE, 2015). The concepts included were the following: "(a) use technology to support improvement of clinical and financial performance, (b) collaborate to prioritize for the establishment of information technology resources, (c) participate in evaluation of enabling technology in practice settings, (d) use data management systems for decision making, (e) identify technological trends, issues and new developments as they apply to patient care, (f) demonstrate skills in assessing data integrity and quality, (g) provide leadership for the adoption and implementation of information systems" (p. 10).

AMERICAN ACADEMY OF NURSE PRACTITIONERS

The American Academy of Nurse Practitioners (AANP) has not specifically identified informatics competencies as an essential component in their *Discussion Paper: Doctor of Nursing Practice* (AANP, 2013). There is an implication that the APN would possess advanced skills in the roles of manager and researcher, and would effectively manage and negotiate health care delivery systems.

AMERICAN COLLEGE OF NURSE-MIDWIVES

The American College of Nurse-Midwives (ACNM) in their publication *Position Statement: Appropriate Use of Technology in Childbirth* (2014) emphasizes, "the use of technology in childbirth based on the evidence of benefit" (p. 1). Their official position is limited to the "use of appropriate technological interventions where the benefits of such technology outweigh the risks" during the childbirth process (ACNM, 2014, p. 1).

■ OTHER FACTORS INFLUENCING EXPECTATIONS OF THE DOCTORAL APN

Although professional organizations play a key role in influencing expectations of the doctoral APN, there are other entities that are also playing an important role. The TIGER Informatics Competency Collaborative was created to develop informatics competency expectations and recommendations for all practicing nurses and graduating nursing students (TIGER Informatics Competency Collaborative, 2009). They espouse that the doctoral APN will need to be competent in the following three primary areas: basic computer competencies, information literacy, and information management.

The Robert Wood Johnson Foundation (RWJF) funded the Quality and Safety Education for Nurses (QSEN) project with the broad objective of "preparing future nurses with the knowledge, skills, and attitudes necessary to continuously improve the quality and safety of the health care systems in which they work" (Cronenwett et al., 2007, p. 122). The QSEN has defined six competencies for the professional nurse. These include: professional development, patient-centered care, teamwork and collaboration, evidence-based practice, quality improvement, and safety and informatics. Within each competency "there are specific domains of knowledge that must be mastered, skills that must be developed, and attitudes that must be cultivated if a nurse is to deliver high-quality, safe, patient-centered care as a member of a health care team" (Hall, More, & Barnsteiner, 2008, p. 417).

The evidence-based practice movement has significant impact for the doctoral APNs. In the clinical expert role, it is imperative for the doctoral APN to promote the use of evidence-based practice, not only in one's own practice, but also as a catalyst for change. The doctoral APN is expected to assume a leadership role within his or her organization and, in this capacity, to spearhead the development of an evidence-driven organization. This requires an in-depth understanding of the organizational components including infrastructure, processes, and behaviors, which must be integrated into efforts to incorporate evidence into all aspects of clinical practice. "Evidence-driven practice is no longer optional and is now a fundamental leadership requisite in all clinical settings" (Porter-O'Grady & Malloch, 2008, p. 176). Recall that *Essential IV: Translating and Integrating Scholarship Into Practice* requires that the doctoral prepared APN must possess informatics and technology competencies as well as information management skills in order to effectively "lead continuous improvement processes based on translational research skills" bringing "evidence-based practice to both individual patients for whom they directly care and to those patients for whom they are indirectly responsible" (AACN, 2010, p. 16).

■ ROLE AND RELEVANCE OF THE DOCTORAL APN AND TECHNOLOGY

There are many opportunities and roles within health care for the doctorally prepared APN. According to AACN (2006), the role of the doctoral APN is specifically in the clinical setting; some DNP programs also focus on the administrator/executive role. Generally, within contemporary DNP programs, the APRN must select one of the AACN endorsed roles—either the clinical practitioner or the executive role.

In the clinical setting, the doctoral APN works as a nurse practitioner, clinical nurse specialist, nurse midwife, or nurse anesthetist. In this role, the doctoral APN is the clinical expert providing direct care to the patient. In the administrator/executive role, the doctoral APN serves in a position of nursing leadership, such as director of nursing, vice president of nursing, or any other nursing leadership role.

Although not endorsed by the AACN, some programs also acknowledge the DNP's expanded role of clinical scientist in the clinical research industry, and of nurse educator providing additional coursework to prepare students for these roles. These specially trained doctoral APNs will be uniquely prepared to meet not only the need in for these specialty roles but also the challenges associated with these roles.

In an academic setting, clinical setting, or staff development setting, the in-depth clinical expertise of the doctoral APN can contribute significantly to the education of current and future generations of health care providers. With that wealth of clinical expertise, coupled with the current and projected nursing faculty shortage, the doctorally prepared APN may be well poised to fill the gap. However, the AACN maintains that the doctoral APN is not sufficiently prepared to serve in an educator role unless there is "additional preparation in the science of pedagogy to augment their ability to transmit the science of the profession they practice and teach" (2006, p. 6). The clinical scientist APN will conduct clinical research and assist staff nurses with activities for any ongoing clinical trials/clinical research activities. Table 14.2 identifies the representative technology competencies for these specific doctoral advanced practice roles.

■ BEYOND THE DNP DEGREE: STRATEGIES FOR DEVELOPING AND MAINTAINING ESSENTIAL SKILLS

LIBRARY SEARCH SKILLS

Development of library database research-related skills among doctoral APNs is essential to success. Health care providers need to learn how to access and evaluate information used to make clinical decisions (Buus-Frank, 2004). Due to the overwhelming amount of information available and the technological skill that is required to become a thorough researcher, multiple library/research-related workshops are strongly recommended. Whether a formal component within a program or offered on an individualized one-on-one basis, this method allows the librarian to go into more depth and cover more material to build these essential competencies (Megaw & McClendon, 2003). Table 14.3 includes a selected database resource list that is highly recommended for any graduate nursing student.

Both practicing doctoral APNs and students who are entering a DNP program require training to familiarize themselves with the primary academic library they have access to and ensure their database research skills are up to date. Components of comprehensive library training include an orientation to the physical as well as the electronic

TABLE 14.2   Representative Informatics Competencies for Specific Doctoral APN Roles

AACN Endorsed Roles		Non-Endorsed Roles	
Practitioner/ Clinician	Clinical Executive	Educator	Clinical Scientist
Identify the importance of health information systems		Identify the importance of health information systems	
Demonstrate knowledge of various health information systems		Demonstrate knowledge of various health information systems	
Recognize the importance of the confidentiality of patient information		Recognize the importance of the confidentiality of patient information	
Examine information and its source critically		Examine information and its source critically	
Use technology to assist with evidence-based projects and research	Use available information technologies to manage organizational operations, and guide strategic business development	Use available evaluation and assessment technologies for curricular design/ improvements and facilitate learning	Use evidence to drive improvements in nursing practice and maintain professional standards of practice
Examine the use of technology in clinical, education, and administrative settings	Analyze available systems and financial data to determine value, utility, and significance in the current and future for achieving desired outcomes	Use an evidence-based approach to design systems that support continuous improvement in nursing education	Use available technologies to collect and analyze patient care data to identify new approaches to improve patient safety and outcomes
Use available technologies to collect, store, and examine data	Use information systems to conduct organizational assessments to enhance agility, effectively manage resources, and adhere to regulatory standards and industrial/legal responsibilities	Use an evidence-based approach to incorporate instructional technologies, such as simulation into education while collecting and refining assessment data to improve student outcomes	Apply information systems knowledge and clinical expertise to participate in the design of clinical information systems
Demonstrate how to effectively access information from various sources	Determine the type and amount of information needed	Identify and analyze appropriate student outcome measures to support curricular improvements	Demonstrate the ability to access information efficiently
Examine outcomes of the use of information	Use information to accomplish a specific purpose	Demonstrate the ability to access resources through library information systems	Use information to accomplish a specific purpose

AACN, American Association of Colleges of Nursing; APN, advanced practice nurse.
Source: TIGER Informatics Competency Collaborative (2009).

TABLE 14.3 **Selected Database Resource List**

Tool	Web Address
CINAHL (Cumulative Index to Nursing and Allied Health Literature; Ebsco Publishing)	www.ebscohost.com/cinahl
Cochrane Library (Wiley InterScience)	www3.interscience.wiley.com/cgi-bin/mrwhome/106568753/HOME
DynaMed	http://health.ebsco.com/products/dynamed
ERIC (Institute of Education Sciences—U.S. Department of Education)	www.eric.ed.gov
LexisNexis Academic (LexisNexis, a division of Reed-Elsevier Inc.)	http://academic.lexisnexis.com/online-services/academic-overview.aspx
National Guidelines Clearinghouse (Agency for Healthcare Research and Quality/U.S. Department of Health and Human Services)	www.guideline.gov
ProQuest Nursing & Allied Health Source	www.proquest.com/products-services/pq_nursingahs_shtml.html
PubMed (U.S. National Library of Medicine/National Institutes of Health)	www.ncbi.nlm.nih.gov/pubmed
TRIP Database (Turning Research into Practice)	www.tripdatabase.com
Web of Science	http://thomsonreuters.com/en/products-services/scholarly-scientific-research/scholarly-search-and-discovery/web-of-science.html
Health and Psychosocial Instruments (HaPi)	www.ebscohost.com/academic/health-and-psychosocial-instruments-hapi

library, an overview of resources and services available, and in-depth database searching. Specific skills that must be developed and maintained include:

1. Use of keyword searching, truncation/wildcard symbols, subject heading searching, Boolean logic, the use of limits (including clinical queries) in databases such as Cumulative Index to Nursing and Allied Health Literature (CINAHL), LexisNexis, and Education Resources Information Center (ERIC)
2. Creation and maintenance of personal accounts within various databases to facilitate the retention of search strategies, citation information, and establishing alerts for frequently searched topics
3. Use of the various publication styles such as APA or AMA for in-text citation style and references in writing for publication
4. Use of bibliographic management tools such as EndNote, described earlier in this chapter, to assist in organizing and managing writings
5. Ability to locate evidence-based practice information using "Clinical Queries" in various databases such as PubMed/MEDLINE, the Cochrane Library, the National Guidelines Clearinghouse (NGC), and the TRIP Database (Turning Research into Practice)

In one example of a DNP orientation, a 3-hour workshop lead by the students' primary library liaison introduces them to the topics listed earlier. The doctoral students also have a 3-hour technology update workshop during their subsequent summer residency where they receive further training in patient safety, simulation, and additional technologies. Providing research and technology-related training to develop and maintain skills is essential to success within an academic program and can assist with answering clinically related questions in the future.

EMERGING TECHNOLOGIES IMPACTING HEALTH CARE

We live in an era of rapid technological innovation. Emerging technologies are driving exponential change in health care and may have the potential to improve outcomes. Clearly, we cannot predict what impact technologies will have—whether positive or negative or perhaps a bit of both. It is, however, imperative that the doctoral APN be aware of these technologies in order to maximize the potential benefits to patients. Carsten Stahl (2011) concedes that the future is often unpredictable but believes with focused analysis one can make some reasonable predictions regarding the emerging technologies and their potential impact on health care (Table 14.4). In addition, Jayanthi (2014) also describes the positive impact that technological advances have had upon health care delivery over the past decade. "Devices like smartphones and tablets are starting to replace conventional monitoring and recording systems, and people are now given the option of undergoing a full clinical consultation in the privacy of their own homes. Technological advancements in health care have contributed to services being taken out of the confines of hospital walls and integrating them with user-friendly, accessible devices" (Jayanthi, 2014, para 2).

LIFELONG LEARNING: KEEPING SKILLS UP TO DATE LONG AFTER GRADUATION

Lifelong learning is a core value that must be embraced by the doctoral APN. New information and emerging technologies that can improve health care, health care systems, and patient outcomes are made available daily. It is an overwhelming task to keep up with the flow of information. There are several strategies and technological tools that can assist doctoral APNs in keeping up to date. These include: (a) keeping research-related skills current; (b) reference alerts, also known as Selected Dissemination of Information (SDIs); (c) Web 2.0 tools such as RSS and Twitter; (d) Web 3.0 tools, (e) personal learning environments (Dreher, 2009a, 2009b); and (f) clinical information resources. Some of the web resources to explore these strategies are included in Table 14.5.

Keeping research-related skills up to date can be challenging. Bibliographic databases such as MEDLINE are not static works. New information is added on a routine basis. In addition, valuable features such as subject headings/controlled vocabulary and interfaces that allow researchers to more easily search for new information from endless sources that rapidly change. Furthermore, databases are not just often updated sometimes completely redesigned. Bibliographic management tools receive these updates when new versions are released. Moreover, even publication styles can change (e.g., the *second printing* of the new *Publication Manual of the American Psychological Association, Sixth Edition* [updated from the previous fifth edition] was released in October 2009).

There are ways to address these needs in traditional or remote settings. Many libraries offer assistance via telephone, e-mail, and instant messaging. Other forms of contact include collaborative learning software applications, such as Webex, Zoom, or Adobe Connect, which allow information to be shared in a synchronous or asynchronous fashion via a recorded archive.

TABLE 14.4 **Key Emerging Technologies With Predicted Impact on Health Care**

Technology	Impact
Artificial intelligence Affective computing Robotics	The characteristics of intelligence, ability to perceive emotions and affects will permit expressive behavior by computers or artificial agents; sophisticated motor function will lay the groundwork for surrogate support for caregiving and reducing personnel costs while providing round-the-clock support, assistance, and services for elderly or disabled.
Bioelectronics Human–machine symbiosis Neuroelectronics	The miniaturization and complexity of these technologies will blur the boundaries between machine and human with improved monitoring and treatment capabilities. For example, less invasive, more comprehensive diagnostic capabilities; improved treatments for individuals with brain injuries, impairments, or diseases (e.g., Parkinson's or Alzheimer's); and improved prosthetics, rehabilitative and assistive devices.
Future Internet	The future Internet is expected to be more pervasive and ubiquitous, setting the stage for greater accessibility, information sharing, and interoperability, which will increase real-time data collection from expanded data collection points enhancing surveillance capabilities and information access for patients and health care providers.
Quantum computing	Much faster and more powerful computing for special purposes that will enable faster data analytics, increased capability to manage and analyze "big data" repositories as well as simulation of various phenomena to contribute toward understanding of these phenomena. Quantum computing will also enhance surveillance capabilities.
Ambient intelligence	Ambient Intelligence brings forth a novel human-technology interaction via the ability to customize, built-in adaptive environmental responsiveness to individual needs such as change in body temperature, lighting adjustment.
Virtual/augmented reality	Physical/mental immersion and synthetic sensory stimulation can provide new treatment technologies for mental health, behavioral and rehabilitative therapies and services (e.g., posttraumatic stress therapy and other disorders).
Three-dimensional (3D) bio printing	This technology will transform health care by providing the capability of creating interchangeable body parts for transplant and defect repair.
Holographic images	The use of holographic images to project instrument panels, such as keyboards or infusion pump controls, onto easily sanitized solid surfaces will significantly reduce infection transmission, reducing incidence of hospital-acquired infections.
3-D Laser scan	This technology will allow "real-time" three-dimensional imaging to accurately capture and document patient data such as wound measurements.

(continued)

TABLE 14.4   **Key Emerging Technologies With Predicted Impact on Health Care**   (*continued*)

Technology	Impact
Biometrics	This technology will provide additional security to privacy and confidentiality to health information. It will also offer functionality for conducting audit trails.
Genetics and genomics	Currently, this technology is providing valuable screening and genetic predictive information; however, in the future genetics and genomics will transform the health care system providing preventative treatment to patients for conditions/diseases they are likely to develop, and also to provide designer medications/treatments for individuals based on genetic markers.

Adapted from Carsten Stahl (2011), Huston (2013), Rabkin and Weberg (2015), and Govett (2015).

TABLE 14.5   **Selected Web Resource List**

Tool	Web Address
Active Worlds Educational Universe	www.activeworlds.com
Health Care Hashtag Project	www.symplur.com
Hootsuite	https://hootsuite.com/
Netvibes (Netvibes Incorporated)	www.netvibes.com
Scrapplet (radWEBTECH)	www.scrapplet.com/index.html
Second Life (Linden Research Incorporated)	https://secondlife.com
Twitter (Twitter Incorporated)	https://twitter.com
Wonderland (LeadingVirtually.com)	www.leadingvirtually.com

Reference alerts are very helpful in providing the busy practitioner an automated mechanism to receive notification of new publications related to a specific topic. After completing a search in a bibliographic database, users can sign up for individual accounts in order to save their searches, relevant citations, and receive current awareness alerts. Users can determine the frequency of alerts along with specifying how they would prefer to receive this type of information. Common formats include e-mail notifications and really simple syndication (RSS) feeds. Listservs can also provide an excellent platform for connecting with other professionals and staying up to date with trends.

Web 2.0 tools such as RSS feeds and Twitter provide yet another means to support lifelong learning. RSS is a mechanism by which individuals or organizations can publish and distribute content, audio, or video to the world. RSS feeds eliminate the need to constantly check to see if there is any new information available by "pushing" out information when it becomes available.

Web 3.0 tools promise to bring the best of Web 2.0 to the next level with expanded portability and mobility in addition to an improved, individualized search experience resulting from enhanced natural language search capability. The "intelligent web" will offer greater capability to provide just-in-time and just-enough information for decision support. In addition, cloud-based technologies offering hosting and software as a service (SAAS) further expand the capacity of a mobile environment and have the potential to further expand health care beyond the traditional service settings.

Twitter offers another way to receive updated information using a hybrid instant messenger transmitting 140 characters at a time to a select group. This technology can be useful to communicate with a research team, providing a mechanism to pose a question and get immediate responses. Twitter is a relative newcomer to the social networking arena, debuting in 2006, but has had a major impact on disseminating health information (Dreher, 2009b). Thirty-one percent of health professionals and 26% of U.S. hospitals are using social media, like Twitter to communicate with patients, sharing news and networking with colleagues (MacDonald, 2014). Notable examples include a surgeon sending "tweets" from an operating room when a particularly innovative surgical procedure was underway at Henry Ford Hospital in Detroit, Michigan (Cohen, 2009), and when researchers demonstrated to efficacy of using tweets to monitor disease outbreak (Nagel et al., 2013). There are many prominent and reputable "Tweeters" such as the Centers for Disease Control, Johns Hopkins University, Mayo Clinic, and World Health Organization. The Healthcare Hashtag Project provides an opportunity for health care professions to connect by serving as a community that makes it easy for health care professionals to join Twitter conversations on specific areas of interest, within a specialty or disease or just find out what health care topics are trending in real-time (www.symplur.com). Products like Hootsuite (https://hootsuite.com) can help you manage multiple social media feeds and have the capability to analyze the big data that are available in social media to identify trends. Hootsuite can also be used to monitor what is being said about your organization in social media and allow more timely intervention should negative or inaccurate information be circulating via social media.

Personal learning spaces, such as NetVibes and Scrapplet, are gaining in popularity as a means to individualize one's web experience by creating a single, personalized page that has the capability to function as an aggregator collecting and organizing RSS feeds and other information from multiple sources. Information collected from news sources such as blogs, social networks, or podcasts will be organized and presented in a uniquely customized manner and automatically updated. One particularly valuable feature is the capability to set up a "watch" dashboard to keep track of subjects of interest. One of the strengths of a personal learning environment (PLE) is that it allows the individual to manage their formal and informal learning needs (Dabbagh & Kitsantas, 2012). A personalized learning environment permits the user to access "mash-up" information. The capability of combining and remixing information, media, content, and web applications and services opens up the opportunity to perceive information in new ways by enhancing lifelong learning through a highly personalized experience.

The clinical information resource DynaMed contains an easy-to-use alert service that can be established in the product's "Recent Updates" menu. Users are able to select a general area of interest from this screen, along with having the ability to select an additional filter "Practice Changing Updates Only" that will deliver notifications to a preferred e-mail address on a daily basis. In a cohort study of updating speeds of commonly used clinical information summary resources, DynaMed was found to offer the quickest updates based on citation analysis (Banzi et al., 2011).

Clearly, there is a tremendous value to be found in these tools. The strategies and tools described in this section offer the doctorally prepared nurses not only a way to stay up to date and support lifelong learning activities essential in a dynamic health care arena, but also a way to make it both highly personalized and relevant.

■ TECHNOLOGY FOR LEADERSHIP ROLES AND RESPONSIBILITIES OF THE DOCTORAL APN

The doctoral APN's academic preparation as a clinical expert and leader with an intimate understanding of health care practitioner information needs places him or her in a position to play an important role in influencing the health care system. Important competencies to meet the challenges of this role include a broad understanding of basic information management, strong communication skills, and the ability to work collaboratively with interdisciplinary teams that include health care professionals, administrators, and HIT specialists.

INTERFACING WITH INFORMATION SYSTEMS TEAMS

In a highly complex health care system, interprofessional collaboration is essential, and it is expected that the doctoral APN will be prepared to interface effectively with the information systems team in order to help shape organizations and to drive system changes essential in supporting APN needs and the needs of evolving health care systems. This necessitates not only skills in communication and a keen understanding of organizational behavior, but it also requires a working knowledge of hospital information systems and systems life cycles in order to participate in the ongoing dialogue to improve patient outcomes. The fourth and sixth DNP essentials identify this role for the APN as critical in efforts to transform the health care system (AACN, 2006; Smith & McCarthy, 2010). As HISs and patient care technologies are becoming more and more central to health care delivery, the APN must be prepared to use these technologies, not only in practice, but also to actively participate in efforts to use these technologies to drive a transformation. Owing to the dynamic nature of health care systems, interprofessional teams are fluid and adjust to accommodate system needs. The doctoral APN must be prepared to be an active member of the team, playing "a central role in establishing interprofessional teams, participating in the work of the team, and assuming leadership of the team when appropriate" (AACN, 2006, p. 14).

INTERFACING WITH LIBRARIES FOR RESEARCH-BASED SUPPORT

Interfacing with key librarians for research-based support can be extremely beneficial. Libraries are variable, for example, in physical size, staff size, scope of subject coverage, access to resources, and classification schemes. Obtaining specific information from an institution's library related to materials/resources and available services allow beginning researchers to focus on locating data versus having to discover appropriate resources on their own. Connections to individual members of the library staff can be built and, over time, can be critical in sustaining a research career.

There may be subject-specific reference librarians who can assist with navigating the library catalog, electronic databases (e.g., MEDLINE, CINAHL), and bibliographic management tools (e.g., EndNote, RefWorks). As indicated earlier, reference librarians have considerable expertise in this area and spend a large portion of their workday providing assistance to patrons who require skills related to database searching and associated technology. Due to their focus on these types of skills, reference librarians can provide assistance to beginning, intermediate, and advanced researchers either virtually or in person.

■ EVOLVING AND EMERGING TRENDS TO ENHANCE DOCTORAL APNs

SIMULATION FOR EDUCATION AND TRAINING

There are many opportunities for the doctoral level APN to use simulation including education, clinical practice, and research. Simulation activities can include the use of human patient simulators, standardized patients (simulated patients; patient actors), hybrid simulation, task trainers, virtual reality and much more. The human patient simulator is a simulation mannequin device. There are many different vendors and levels of fidelity available with the human patient simulators. An example of a low-fidelity human patient simulator would be a simulator that would be able to portray lung and heart sounds. A high-fidelity simulator would be a simulator that would be able to demonstrate realistic body functions such as diaphoresis, crying, and seizures. The varying levels of fidelity coincide with varying levels of programmable software to be used to develop and run simulation scenarios.

A standardized patient is an actor who is trained to demonstrate realistically a selected patient condition, disease process, psychiatric disorder, or even a distraught family member. In this type of simulation, the scenario is developed very similarly to an actor's script. This script contains all the information needed by the standardized patient to act out the scenario included in the following: (a) timing of the scenario; (b) overview of the scenario; (c) opening line; (d) challenge questions; (e) position at the beginning of the scenario; (f) patient attire; (g) all questions that can be potentially asked during the scenario and the appropriate response; (h) personality or emotions to be portrayed during the scenario; (i) student or nurse items to be evaluated during the scenario; and (j) specific feedback to be provided to the simulation participant following the completion of the scenario during the feedback session.

Hybrid simulation is a simulation experience where there is a combined use of both the human patient simulator and a standardized patient. Examples of a hybrid scenario include the following: (a) a standardized patient portraying the mother of a child and the child represented by an infant human patient simulator; (b) a human patient simulator used as a patient and a standardized patient portraying a sibling or a significant other; and (c) an obstetrical patient with vaginal complications where the vaginal area is a simulator or task trainer.

Task trainers are used to evaluate skills (Aebersold & Tschannen, 2013) in all nursing programs including doctoral nursing. Virtual reality simulation is one of the newer types of simulation. Virtual reality simulation is used for education and training for a variety of health care disciplines in varied settings (Fliszar, 2014). We have also seen an increase in the use of augmented reality with simulation such as the incorporation of Google Glasses (Cass & Choi, 2015).

SIMULATION TO ENHANCE AND EVALUATE COMPETENCY

The doctoral APN (or student) can use simulation strategies to evaluate competencies in an academic educational program or in a clinical setting. Competencies for individuals, teams, and interprofessional teams can be assessed using human patient simulators, standardized patients, or task trainers. In each of these types of simulations, specific competency assessments or expected outcomes must be identified in advance. Then, depending on the type of simulation used, a competency evaluator must be identified such as the standardized patient, a faculty member, a clinical manager, or others. Simulation is a very effective tool that can be used to provide complex situations in a very safe environment.

SIMULATION FOR RESEARCH

The doctoral APN (and student) can also use simulation strategies in many types of research in the academic setting and the clinical setting. Simulation can be used to portray a limitless number of scenarios. These scenarios can be specific to a particular educational activity, an educational process, an interaction, a relationship, or a self-evaluation. A variety of research designs can also be included such as a pretest/posttest design or a posttest-only design. Simulation can also be used for a research examining a workflow or work processes to determine which is most effective (Kneebone, 2006).

■ TECHNOLOGIES THAT SUPPORT COMMUNICATION AND INFORMATION ACCESS IN MOBILE ENVIRONMENTS

Over the past decade, mobile devices (e.g., tablets and smartphones) have had an increasing presence in the health care arena. For the past decade, there has been growing recognition that had a significant impact. In 2005, Lu et al. observed that these devices had significantly improved "information access, enhanced workflow, and promoted evidence-based practice to make informed and effective decisions at the point of care" (Lu, Xiao, Sears, & Jacko, 2005, p. 409), and the momentum has continued. Mobile devices provide "real-time" access to health care information and have transformed the way information is managed in the health care arena (Siau & Shen, 2006; Ventola, 2014). It is expected these devices will be even more pervasive in health care as product and software improvements are released and HISs offer greater interoperability. The true value of these devices will not be fully realized until institutions provide seamless integration with hospital information systems permitting access to essential information at any place and any time via wireless networks.

One particular benefit of a widely dispersed, integrated system will likely be reduced medical errors resulting from improved access to vital information (Sarasohn-Kahn, 2010; Varshney, 2007; Ventola, 2014). Another major benefit will be the ability to collect and more effectively manage surveillance data in real time to more quickly identify emerging trends/or threats such as communicable diseases or biohazards. The doctoral APN must not only be proficient in the use of these technologies, but also be prepared to champion mobile initiatives as a means of "improving quality of care, enhancing patient services, increasing productivity, lowering costs, improving cash flow, as well as facilitating other critical delivery processes"(Lin & Vassar, 2004, p. 343). Critical to these efforts will be the ability to achieve full interoperability of health information. The use of integrated clinical data from all available data sources will offer improved decision support and patient care across the continuum. In addition, secondary analysis of data can support clinical research, allowing identification of trends within patient populations for research to inform evidence-based care (Cornelius, Harman, & Mullen, 2016; Soneshwar, 2013). Interoperability will expand the ability of the APN to meet *Essential IV* by providing greater capacity to translate and integrate scholarship into practice.

■ VIRTUAL WORLDS FOR EDUCATION AND RESEARCH

High Fidelity, Second Life, Active Worlds, Wonderland, and other virtual worlds offer extraordinary opportunities for education, simulation, and research. In education, a virtual world can provide an enriched learning experience, strengthen the sense of social presence, and use multilevel interaction and enriched multimedia resources employing a constructivist approach in the learning process (Wang & Hsu, 2009; Wheelock & Merrick, 2015). Virtual worlds are important to higher education because these environments: (a) offer an immersive environment where users interact and construct knowledge; (b) shift from a traditional dissemination tool to one where users create and design content to add value and meaning; and (c) provide learners an array of opportunities for interaction within a multiuser environment (Skiba, 2007).

Virtual worlds have been used in health professions education with great success. Initial endeavors suggest that virtual worlds offer extraordinary opportunities for educators to enhance learning outcomes beyond that which is provided by more conventional online or face-to-face classroom experiences. Virtual worlds offer rich opportunities for postgraduate professional development activities, continuing education, professional certification or recertification, and much more. This very flexible environment can be used to stage experiences that help students and health care professionals build cultural competency and improve communication and patient interviewing skills. In addition, virtual worlds have been used to provide very realistic disaster simulation training (Simon, 2010; Wiecha, Heyden, Sternthal, & Merialdi, 2010; Young, 2010).

Virtual worlds provide opportunities for creativity that are not limited by the laws of physics, financial constraints, or geography. Realistic environments and simulation experiences can be designed to educate and conduct research by containing costs while simultaneously expanding your reach to vast numbers of students and potential research subjects.

Although virtual worlds can be used for education, simulation, and research purposes, caution is advised. Due to the nature of massive multiplayer games, users may encounter some less-than-ideal occurrences including vandalism and other disruptions (Boulos, Hetherington, & Wheeler, 2007). One notable example mentioned in a previous work by Childs (2008) involved an online chat that was disrupted by digitally rendered, flying objects. These instances can be proactively managed effectively by using available security settings within the virtual environment. In addition, as a means to combat these malicious attacks, virtual worlds offer policing and enforce strict sanctions to offenders (Boulos et al., 2007).

■ WHAT'S ON THE HORIZON?

These are very exciting times. It is a time in which technological innovations are emerging rapidly and diffusion of these technologies is taking place at an unprecedented rate (Kittleson, 2009). Major shifts will involve: (a) a "smarter web" through parallel processing capabilities; (b) more personalization; (c) expanded portability of personalized web content via ubiquitous Internet access and cloud computing; (d) increasing data collection and analysis capabilities to work with "big data"; (e) interoperability; (f) cybersecurity; and (g) virtual and augmented reality.

A major innovation in the future will be a "smarter Internet." In the very near future, the parallel processing technology will make it possible for the Internet to "recognize" the relevance of information as it appears in real time. The convergence of "all of this data and these technologies will necessitate sophisticated algorithmic models to aid interpretation and decision making" (Newton, 2009, p. 1). The design of these models will require the input of health care professionals such as the doctoral APN.

A major benefit of expanded processing capabilities will likely be with more intelligent search tools provided by Web 3.0, which will be "smarter," functioning similar to a personal assistant who "knows" your likes and dislikes and "understands" the context of the information being sought. As a result, searches for information will deliver personalized and highly relevant information directly to your PLE, no matter where you are. Currently, the focus is upon social networking and connections to people. The shift in the future will be increased connections to information that will have limitless application for practice.

"Cloud computing" will further increase the portability of personalized web content. As more and more applications, content, and communities become web-based, we will demand access to the web anytime and everywhere. It is expected that expanded bandwidths and the capabilities of smartphones and other wireless devices globally will continue to evolve and further expand opportunities to access and use data (Newton, 2009).

Another transformative change that is anticipated with the expanded functionality of the Internet (smarter web and ubiquitous wireless network access) is the ability to use widely dispersed sensors to collect all types of data. The data collection possibilities will thus be limitless. For example, sensors can collect ". . . vital signs, energy usage, soil moisture, traffic patterns, manufacturing efficiency. . . it will all be tracked remotely and analyzed in real time and fed into the Smart Web" (Newton, 2009, p. 1). This opens the door for extraordinary research opportunities; however, consideration must be given to the privacy concerns that are bound to arise. The doctoral APN must be prepared to take a leadership role in supporting new research while championing the privacy rights of the individual.

It is reasonable to expect that all advances in technology described thus far will impact the health care system. One major impact will be on system interoperability. Currently, many hospital systems are not integrated and, consequently, system wide communication is impaired, making it difficult to provide seamless care. Improved data tracking and tightly integrated systems will transform health care by improving disease management and patient outcomes. Health care delivery will likely become more decentralized due to an extensive network-based system, high-tech equipment, and software permitting more sophisticated telehealth encounters in one's home via clinical video teleconferencing. The area of telehealth offers many opportunities (e.g., tele-intensive care unit [ICU], teledermatology, telemental health, etc.) for the doctoral APN. This innovative care delivery model coupled with interoperability will spill over to other areas of the health care system and even our personal lives, bringing new levels of "life-wide" connectivity across the life span.

One concern and limitation regarding the application and use of technology in the clinical setting are policies that prohibit the use of mobile devices. This is a very nuanced issue. There are many benefits that such devices provide in such a setting, but they can be distracting or lead to breaches in confidentiality. Policies that note specific uses versus outright bans may be an option to consider. Given the potential benefits of mobile data collection, analysis, and decision support at the point of care, it will be very short-sighted to ban the use of mobile devices.

Cybersecurity considerations will be in the forefront. The recent highly publicized security breaches at Community Health Systems and Anthem as well as reported incidents of wireless biomedical infusion pumps being "hacked" clearly convey the serious risks that currently exist and that are likely to increase in the future. These incidences substantiate the need for health professionals in leadership positions to work closely with interdisciplinary team to ensure proactive security measure are in place. In 2014, the Ponemon Institute reported that cyber attacks on health care organizations have doubled since 2010 and that patient medical records are the targets of these attacks, so the APN must be cognizant of risks, both actual and potential.

High Fidelity, Second Life, Active Worlds, Wonderland, and other virtual worlds will become more sophisticated, and we will likely see overlap between virtual worlds and the real world via technologies that enable "augmented reality" interfaces. This blend will enhance our opportunities to provide rich simulated learning experiences for students, support continuing education among our practicing professionals, and conduct research. In addition, augmented reality technology will also provide the capability to provide enhanced clinical decision support in real time at the bedside where it is needed most and will have the greatest impact upon patient outcomes.

■ SUMMARY

This chapter provided an overview of technological tools that provide opportunities to work more efficiently and effectively to deliver, improve, and document care in our health system. It is absolutely critical that the doctoral APN possess high-level skills in the use of technologies to support health care delivery in order to function effectively in a leadership role (Carsten Stahl, 2011; Chase & Pruitt, 2006; O'Keefe & Griffin, 2013; Porter-O'Grady & Malloch, 2008; Webber, 2008). The APN must be able to use technology to better manage and use an increasing volume of evidence to guide practice and establish new standards of care within health care systems. The doctoral APN must *leverage these technologies* to generate more evidence-based and practice-based scientific knowledge and serve as a catalyst for change.

■ CRITICAL THINKING QUESTIONS

1. *What weaknesses did you identify from the specialty nursing organizations' discussions of their goals for technology competency and utilization?*
2. *Perform a literature search on the TIGER. Discuss what kind of impact TIGER is making on nursing informatics and health care.*
3. *Discuss the similar and different technology needs of the doctoral APNs in various settings and roles.*
4. *Evidence-based information can be located in PubMed/MEDLINE, and in the CINAHL database using certain search methods. Perform a search of one of your professors using each one of these databases. Review the results to conceptualize the focus of their scholarship.*
5. *Describe some ways in which Twitter can be used in health care beyond what was discussed in this chapter.*
6. *Evaluate your own skill at "knowledge management." Discuss what your primary specialty area is and where you go for the most up-to-date content.*
7. *Go to the Cochrane database and browse. Retrieve a systematic review close to your specialty area and discuss its significance.*
8. *Go to Active Worlds Educational Universe at www.activeworlds.com. Register for a free citizenship and request an Avatar (a name). What kind of health care uses might there be for "Second Life"?*
9. *Identify ways in which the use of the standardized patient could be used in DNP curricula.*
10. *Identify ways in which simulation can be used to improve quality and patient safety within your institution.*
11. *Discuss whether DNP-prepared APRNs ought to have better technology proficiency skills than master of science in nursing (MSN)-prepared APRNs.*

■ REFERENCES

Aebersold, M., & Tschannen, D. (2013). Simulation in nursing practice: The impact on patient care. *The Online Journal of Issues in Nursing, 18*(2), 83. doi:10.3912/OJIN.Vol18No02Man06

Aflague, J. M., & Ferszt, G. G. (2010). Suicide assessment by psychiatric nurses: A phenomenographic study. *Issues in Mental Health Nursing, 31*(4), 248–256. doi:10.3109/01612840903267612

American Academy of Nurse Practitioners. (2013). Discussion paper: Doctor of nursing practice. Retrieved from https://www.aanp.org/images/documents/publications/doctorofnursing practice.pdf

American Association of Colleges of Nursing. (2006). *The essentials of doctoral education for advanced nursing practice*. Retrieved from http://www.aacn.nche.edu/dnp/pdf/essentials.pdf

American Association of Colleges of Nursing. (2010). Draft: The essentials of master's education in nursing. Retrieved from http://citeseerx.ist.psu.edu/viewdoc/download;jsessionid=7BDA9DDA AB1278A958B4488A661EFF50?doi=10.1.1.193.2139&rep=rep1&type=pdf

American Association of Nurse Anesthetists. (2007). AANA position on doctoral preparation of nurse anesthetists. Retrieved from https://www.aana.com/ceandeducation/educationalresources/Documents/AANA_Position_DTF_June_2007.pdf

American College of Nurse-Midwives. (2014). Appropriate use of new technology in childbirth. Retrieved from http://www.midwife.org/ACNM/files/ACNMLibraryData/UPLOADFILENAME/00000 0000054/Appropriate-Use-of-Technology-in-Childbirth-May-2014.pdf

American Organization of Nurse Executives. (2015). The AONE nurse executive competencies. Chicago, IL: Author. Retrieved from http://www.aone.org/resources/nec.pdf

Banzi, R., Cinquini, M., Liberati, A., Moschetti, I., Pecoraro, V., Tagliabue, L., & Moja, L. (2011). Speed of updating online evidence based point of care summaries: Prospective cohort analysis. *BMJ, 343*, d5856. doi:10.1136/bmj.d5856

Barton, A. J. (2005). Cultivating informatics competencies in a community of practice. *Nursing Administration Quarterly, 29*(4), 323–328.

Bates, D. W., Saria, S., Ohno-Machado, L., Shah, A., & Escobar, G. (2014). Big data in health care: Using analytics to identify and manage high-risk and high-cost patients. *Health Affairs, 33*(7), 1123.

Boulos, M. N. K., Hetherington, L., & Wheeler, S. (2007). Second life: An overview of the potential of 3-D virtual worlds in medical and health education. *Health Information & Libraries Journal, 24*(4), 233–245. doi:10.1111/j.1471-1842.2007.00733.x

Buus-Frank, M. E. (2004). What you don't know can hurt you. *Advances in Neonatal Care, 4*(1), 1–5.

Canadian Nurses Association. (2006). *Position statement: Nursing information and knowledge management*. Retrieved from https://www.cna-aiic.ca/~/media/cna/page-content/pdf-en/nursing -information-and-knowledge-management_position-statement.pdf?la=en

Carsten Stahl, B. (2011). IT for a better future: How to integrate ethics, politics and innovation. *Journal of Information, Communication and Ethics in Society, 9*(3), 140–156. doi:10.1108/14779961111167630

Cass, S., & Choi, C. Q. (2015). Google glass, HoloLens, and the real future of augmented reality. Retrieved from http://spectrum.ieee.org/consumer-electronics/audiovideo/google-glass-hololens-and-the -real-future-of-augmented-reality

Chase, S. K., & Pruitt, R. H. (2006). The practice doctorate: Innovation or disruption? *Journal of Nursing Education, 45*(5), 155–161.

Childs, G. M. (2008). Are you ready for second life: Primer for online virtual society software. *MLA News, 403*, 20.

Coenen, A., & Bartz, C. (2006). A unified nursing language system. *Nursing Outlook, 54*(6), 362–364.

Cohen, E. (2009, February 6). Surgeons send 'tweets' from operating room. *CNN*. Retrieved from http://www.cnn.com/2009/TECH/02/17/twitter.surgery/index.html

Conrad, D., Hanson, P. A., Hasenau S. M., & Stocker-Schneider, J. (2012). Identifying the barriers to use of standardized nursing language in the electronic health record by the ambulatory care nurse practitioner. *Journal of the American Academy of Nurse Practitioners, 24*(7), 443–451.

Contino, D. S. (2004). Leadership competencies: Knowledge, skills, and aptitudes nurses need to lead organizations effectively. *Critical Care Nurse, 24*(3), 52–64.

Cornelius, F. H., Harman, L. B., & Mullen, V. L. (2016). Future challenges and opportunities. In *Ethical health informatics: Challenges and opportunities* (pp. 693–719). Sudbury, MA: Jones & Bartlett.

Cronenwett, L., Sherwood, G., Barnsteiner, J., Disch, J., Johnson, J., Mitchell, P., . . . Warren, J. (2007). Quality and safety education for nurses. *Nursing Outlook, 55*(3), 122–131. doi:10.1016/j.outlook.2007.02.006

Dabbagh, N., & Kitsantas, A. (2012). Personal learning environments, social media, and self-regulated learning: A natural formula for connecting formal and informal learning. *Internet and Higher Education, 15*(1), 3–8. doi:10.1016/j.iheduc.2011.06.002

Doherty, M. E. (2010). Voices of midwives: A tapestry of challenges and blessings. *American Journal of Maternal/Child Nursing, 35*(2), 96–101. doi:10.1097/NMC.0b013e3181caea9f

Dreher, H. M. (2009a). How do RNs today best stay informed? Do we need "knowledge management"? *Holistic Nursing Practice, 23*(5), 263–266. doi:10.1097/HNP.0b013e3181b66c68

Dreher, H. M. (2009b). Twittering about anything, everything, and even health. *Holistic Nursing Practice,* 23(4), 217–221. doi:10.1097/HNP.0b013e3181aece81

Dreher, H. M. (2010). Next steps toward practice knowledge development: An emerging epistemology in nursing. In M. D. Dahnke & H. M. Dreher (Eds.), *Philosophy of science for nursing practice: Concepts and application* (pp. 355–392). New York, NY: Springer Publishing.

Ebell, M. H., & Shaughnessy, A. (2003). Information mastery: Integrating continuing medical education with the information needs of clinicians. *Journal of Continuing Education in the Health Professions,* 23(S1), S53–S62. doi:10.1002/chp.1340230409

Fliszar, R. (2014). Virtual reality. In L. Wilson & R. Wittmann-Price (Eds.), *Review manual for the Certified Healthcare Simulation Educator Exam.* New York, NY: Springer Publishing.

Gassert, C. A. (2008). Technology and informatics competencies. *Nursing Clinics of North America,* 43(4), 507–521.

Govett, J. (2015). 10 Biggest innovations in health care technology in 2015, Referral MD. Retrieved from https://getreferralmd.com/2015/02/the-10-biggest-innovations-in-health-care -technology-in-2015/

Gugerty, B., & Delaney, C. (2009). TIGER Informatics Competencies Collaborative: Final report. Retrieved from http://tigercompetencies.pbworks.com/f/TICC_Final.pdf

Hall, L. W., Moore, S. M., & Barnsteiner, J. H. (2008) Quality and nursing: Moving from a concept to a core competency. *Society of Urologic Nurses and Associates,* 28(6), 417–426.

Hsia, T.-L., Lin, L.-M., Wu, J.-H., & Tsai, H.-T. (2006). A framework for designing nursing knowledge management systems. *Interdisciplinary Journal of Information, Knowledge, and Management,* 1, 13–22.

Huston, C. (2013). The impact of emerging technology on nursing care: Warp speed ahead. *The Online Journal of Issues in Nursing,* 18(2). Retrieved from http://nursingworld.org/MainMenuCategories/ ANAMarketplace/ANAPeriodicals/OJIN/TableofContents/Vol-18–2013/No2-May-2013/ Impact-of-Emerging-Technology.html

Institute of Medicine. (1999). To err is human: Building a safer health system. Retrieved from http:// iom.nationalacademies.org/~/media/Files/Report%20Files/1999/To-Err-is-Human/To%20 Err%20is%20Human%201999%20%20report%20brief.pdf

Institute of Medicine. (2001). Crossing the quality chasm: A new health system for the 21st century. Retrieved from http://iom.nationalacademies.org/Reports/2001/Crossing-the-Quality-Chasm -A-New-Health-System-for-the-21st-Century.aspx

Institute of Medicine. (2003). *Health professions education: A bridge to quality.* Washington, DC: Author. Retrieved from https://www.nap.edu/read/10681/chapter/1

Jayanthi, A. (2014). 10 Biggest technological advancements for healthcare in the last decade. Retrieved from http://www.beckershospitalreview.com/healthcare-information-technology/10-biggest -technological-advancements-for-healthcare-in-the-last-decade.html

King, T. M., Muzaffar, S., & George, M. (2009). The role of clinic culture in implementation of primary care interventions: The case of reach out and read. *Academic Pediatrics,* 9(1), 40–46. doi:10.1016/ j.acap.2008.10.004

Kittleson, M. J. (2009). The future of technology in health education: Challenging the traditional delivery dogma. *American Journal of Health Education,* 40(6), 310–316.

Kneebone, R. L. (2006). Crossing the line: Simulation and boundary areas. *Simulation in Healthcare,* 1(3), 160–163.

Lin, B., & Vassar, J. A. (2004). Mobile healthcare computing devices for enterprise-wide patient data delivery. *International Journal of Mobile Communications,* 2(4), 343–353.

Lu, Y. C., Xiao, Y., Sears, A., & Jacko, J. A. (2005). A review and a framework of handheld computer adoption in healthcare. *International Journal of Medical Informatics,* 74(5), 409–422. doi:10.1016/ j.ijmedinf.2005.03.001

MacDonald, I. (2014, April 22). Healthcare professionals flock to Twitter: More than 75,000 doctors, nurses, pharmacists and consultants post 152,000 tweets a day. *Fierce Healthcare.* Retrieved from http://www.fiercehealthcare.com/story/healthcare-professionals-flock-twitter/2014-04-22

Megaw, A., & McClendon, J. (2003). One-shot to a full barrel. In J. K. Nims & E. Owens (Eds.), *Managing library instruction programs in academic libraries* (pp. 113–115). Ann Arbor, MI: Pierian Press.

Nagel, A. C., Tsou, M. H., Spitzberg, B. H., An, L., Gawron, J. M., Gupta, D. K., . . . Sawyer, M. H. (2013). The complex relationship of realspace events and messages in cyberspace: Case study of influenza and pertussis using tweets. *Journal of Medical Internet Research,* 15(10), e237.

Newton, T. (2009). Ten trends for 2010. Retrieved from http://www.forbes.com/2009/11/24/ ten-trends-blackberry-intelligent-investing-internet.html

O'Keefe, K., & Griffin, A. (2013). *The rise of transprofessional education: Educating for task shifting of professional development?* Paper presented at the 2nd International Conference on Faculty Development in the Health Professions, Prague, Czech Republic.

Otterness, S. (2006). Is the burden worth the benefit of the doctorate of nursing (DNP) for NPs? Implications of doctorate in nursing practice: Still many unresolved issues for nurse practitioners. *Nephrology Nursing Journal, 33*(6), 685–687.

Ponemon Institute. (2014, March). Fourth annual benchmark study on patient privacy & data security. Ponemon Institute LLC. Retrieved from https://www.privacyrights.org/sites/privacyrights.org/files/ID%20Experts%204th%20Annual%20Patient%20Privacy%20&%20Data%20Security%20Report%20FINAL.pdf

Porter-O'Grady, T., & Malloch, K. (2008). Beyond myth and magic: The future of evidence-based leadership. *Nursing Administration Quarterly, 32*(3), 176–187. doi:10.1097/01.NAQ.0000325174.30923.b6

Rabkin, A. B., & Weberg, D. (2015, April). High resolution: Laser scans improve wound care at Kaiser Permanente, California Healthcare Foundation. Retrieved from http://www.chcf.org/~/media/MEDIA%20LIBRARY%20Files/PDF/N/PDF%20Nursing20WoundCareKaiser.pdf

Rutherford, M. (2008). Standardized nursing language: What does it mean for nursing practice? *The Online Journal of Issues in Nursing, 13*(1). Retrieved from http://www.nursingworld.org/MainMenuCategories/ThePracticeofProfessionalNursing/Health-IT/StandardizedNursingLanguage.html

Sarasohn-Hahn, J. (2010). How smartphones are changing health care for consumers and providers. *California Healthcare Foundation.* Retrieved from http://www.chcf.org/~/media/MEDIA%20LIBRARY%20Files/PDF/PDF%20H/PDF%20HowSmartphonesChangingHealthCare.pdf

Siau, K., & Shen, Z. (2006). Mobile healthcare informatics. *Medical Informatics and the Internet in Medicine, 31*(2), 89–99. doi:10.1080/14639230500095651

Simon, S. (2010, April 13). Avatar II: The hospital. *Wall Street Journal,* p. R8. Retrieved from http://www.wsj.com/articles/SB10001424052748703909804575124470868041204

Skiba, D. J. (2007). Nursing education 2.0: Second life. *Nursing Education Perspectives, 28*(3), 156–157.

Slawson, D. C., Shaughnessy, A. F., & Bennett, J. H. (1994). Becoming a medical information master: Feeling good about not knowing everything. *Journal of Family Practice, 38*(5), 505–513.

Smith, M., & McCarthy, M. P. (2010). Disciplinary knowledge in nursing education: Going beyond the blueprints. *Nursing Outlook, 58*(1), 44–51. doi:10.1016/j.outlook.2009.09.002

Someshwar, P. (2013, June 13). Interoperability: Not a non-issue. *Healthcare IT News.* Retrieved from http://www.healthcareitnews.com/blog/interoperability-not-non-issue?page=1

Staggers, N., Gassert, C. A., & Curran, C. (2002). A Delphi study to determine informatics competencies for nurses at four levels of practice. *Nursing Research, 51*(6), 383–390.

Tanyi, R. A., McKenzie, M., & Chapek, C. (2009). How family practice physicians, nurse practitioners, and physician assistants incorporate spiritual care in practice. *Journal of the American Academy of Nurse Practitioners, 21*(12), 690–697. doi:10.1111/j.1745-7599.2009.00459.x

Thrasher, C., & Purc-Stephenson, R. J. (2007). Integrating nurse practitioners into Canadian emergency departments: A qualitative study of barriers and recommendations. *CJEM, 9*(4), 275–281.

TIGER Informatics Competency Collaborative. (2009). TIGER informatics competencies. Retrieved from http://tigercompetencies.pbworks.com/w/page/22247287/FrontPage

TIGER Initiative Foundation. (n.d.). The TIGER Initiative Foundation. The leadership imperative: TIGER's recommendations for integrating technology to transform practice and education. Retrieved from http://www.thetigerinitiative.org/docs/TIGERReportTheLeadershipImperative.pdf

Varshney, U. (2007). Pervasive healthcare and wireless health monitoring. *Mobile Networks and Applications, 12*(2–3), 113–127.

Ventola, C. L. (2014, May). Mobile devices and apps for health care professionals: Uses and benefits. *Pharmacy and Therapeutics, 39*(5), 356–364. Retrieved from http://www.ncbi.nlm.nih.gov/pmc/articles/PMC4029126

Wang, S.-K., & Hsu, H.-Y. (2009). Using the ADDIE model to design second life activities for online learners. *TechTrends, 53*(6), 76–82.

Webber, P. B. (2008). The doctor of nursing practice degree and research: Are we making an epistemological mistake? *Journal of Nursing Education, 47*(10), 466–472.

Westra, B. L., & Delaney, C. W. (2008). Informatics competencies for nursing and healthcare leaders. *AMIA Annual Symposium Proceedings, 2008,* 804–808.

Wheelock, A., & Merrick, S. (2015). 5 Virtual worlds for engaged learning. The International Society for Technology in Education (ISTE). Retrieved from https://www.iste.org/explore/articleDetail?articleid=395&category=In-the-classroom

Wiecha, J., Heyden, R., Sternthal, E., & Merialdi, M. (2010). Learning in a virtual world: Experience with using second life for medical education. *Journal of Medical Internet Research, 12*(1), e1. doi:10.2196/jmir.1337

Young, J. R. (2010). After frustrations in second life, colleges look to new virtual worlds; the hype is gone, but not the interest, and professors think some emerging projects may have instructional staying power. *The Chronicle of Higher Education, 56*(23), A14. Retrieved from http://go.galegroup.com/ps/i.do?p=AONE&sw=w&u=drexel_main&v=2.1&it=r&id=GALE%7CA220078213&asid=bb6dc2dae7536ad573207fee9c24bf27

CHAPTER FOURTEEN

Reflective Response 1

Victoria M. Bradley

Informatics knowledge and skills are essential for all of the roles of the doctoral advanced practice nurse (APN) as technology increasingly permeates every component of the health care delivery system. The authors provide an extensive, informative review of the technology tools available to the doctoral APN and suggest ways they can be deployed to enhance practice and transform care. I absolutely agree that at the doctoral level, advanced practitioners need a higher level of technical competency to practice and lead in this technology era. I also agree that Doctor of Nursing Practice (DNP) graduates should contribute to the evidence base of their discipline, through an ongoing measurement of both process and outcomes. I have, however, a few considerations and additions gained from my experiences as a DNP graduate with clinical informatics as my specialty.

I was delighted to see the Technology Informatics Guiding Educational Reform (TIGER) initiative reference. This is a rich resource of information for incorporating informatics into all levels of practice. Increasing knowledge about health information technology (HIT) among practicing nurses and nursing faculty is a recognized challenge and is also being addressed in a number of ways by the organizations within the Alliance for Nursing Informatics. It will be interesting to compare the results of TIGER's current project to identify international competencies for: nursing management; IT management in nursing; quality management; interprofessional coordination of care; and clinical nursing, to ones identified for the doctoral APN (Healthcare Information and Management Systems Society [HIMSS], TIGER, International Competency Synthesis Project, 2016).

In the knowledge management section, the authors recommend that the doctoral APN champion use a standardized nursing language system integrated with universal clinical care terminology. I would more specifically recommend that the data elements in the electronic health record be mapped to Logical Observation Identifiers Names and Codes (LOINC) and SNOMED Clinical Terms. Resources can be found on the National Library of Medicine site on Nursing Standards and Interoperability (International Health Terminology Standards Development Organization, 2016; U.S. National Library of Medicine, 2015). Warren, Matney, Foster, Auld, and Roy (2015) describe the background of this resource on nursing terminologies and standards. As future leaders, it is imperative that the doctoral APN understand, advocate, and contribute to the use of clinically specific vocabularies to enable data exchange and expand retrieval of health information.

One of the key roles of the doctoral APN is to support evidence-based practice. As the authors describe a paucity of articles on information mastery in nursing, there is also a gap in the field of clinical decision support (CDS). As scientific knowledge continues to grow at an amazing rate, it has become impossible for a clinician to keep up—not to mention all the distractions occurring in the clinical environment. Use of clinical information systems provides an opportunity to integrate knowledge and decision support so that they are available to clinicians when needed. I would expect the doctoral APN to make recommendations from the review of the standard of care and best evidence on how CDS could be used to improve the care delivered. For example, are there components of the assessment that are routinely being missed? If so, should the data elements be rearranged on the form or reminders given when documents are submitted with missing data fields or creation of a display that illustrates critical missing data elements, to ensure collection of complete and accurate information? How and where should data be displayed that could prevent medication errors. What alerts and reminders are helpful? Osheroff, Pifer, Teich, Sittig, and Jenders (2005) described six primary ways that decision support can be provided to clinicians: documentation forms/templates, relevant data presentations, order/prescription creation facilitators, time-based checking/protocol pathway support, reference information and guidance, and reactive alerts and reminders. Excellent resources can also be found on the Agency for Healthcare Research and Quality (AHRQ) website (AHRQ, n.d.a). The majority of this work to date relates to physicians. Mitchell et al. (2009) have found little research examining what CDS systems are available to nurses or the characteristics the systems possess in comparison with physicians. Dowding et al. (2009) found that nurses used CDS systems to record information, monitor patients' progress, or confirm a decision that they had already made. Use was influenced by how well the nurse knew the patient, their experience, and how well it fit in their workflow. These studies were, however, conducted in the National Health Service in England. Dunn Lopez et al. (2016) performed an integrative review of qualitative and quantitative peer-reviewed original research studies focusing on use of CDS by the bedside nurse. They summarized the 28 articles stating CDS had positive effects on outcomes and substantiated there is much less research in nursing than in medical decision making. We need the assistance of doctoral APNs to study, develop, and further evaluate the use of CDS systems for nursing.

In the technological tools section, I would additionally suggest workflow and mind-mapping software such as Smartdraw or Visio. In the technology drill-down study, Burnes, Glassert, and Cipriano (2008) reported that 766 unique process issues (out of 946) were required to improve and enable nurses to spend more time at the bedside to address patient care needs. One of the most common reasons for lack of adoption of clinical information systems is that the system does not support the clinician workflow. Routine consistent use of these tools may decrease the number of workarounds that evolve with implementations when changes in workflow patterns are not adequately addressed preventing negative impacts to care of the patient or to the business of the organization—for example, lost or delayed charges. Identifying current practices and mapping out the new desired state workflows to use in education and training facilitates adoption of new technology enabled best practices. Reference management and report-writing tools are nice to know but suggest prioritization of workflow tools higher in the chain of the skills required for advanced practice clinicians. A resource on workflow tools can be found at AHRQ HIT website (ARHQ, n.d.b; Carayon et al., 2010).

It was interesting to read about informatics competencies in the different nursing professional groups. In addition to the nurse executive competencies, American Organization of Nurse Executives (AONE) published a position paper on the role of the nursing informatics executive leader (AONE, 2015a, 2015b). They suggest preparation for this role would be a master's degree with recognition of the trend toward a doctorate. They describe this role as someone with vision, knowledge, and skills to leverage information technology to improve practice and outcomes and also skills to collaborate with the C-suite to create an environment where deployment of technology supports organizational decision making in today's challenging complex milieu. The American Nurses Credentialing Center (ANCC) offers Nurse Executive, Advanced Board Certification (NEA-BC), which includes informatics competencies (ANCC, 2016a). In the test content outline, under the organizational structure and compliance section it lists knowledge of management systems and information technology and skills in assessing, and evaluating technology's impact on care delivery (ANCC, 2016a, 2016b). The NEA-BC certification requires a master's or higher degree in nursing or bachelor's in nursing with master in another field. These examples provide evidence of the growing expectation of information technology competencies in nursing leadership roles.

Other examples of nurses in administrative/executive roles are chief nursing informatics (or information) officer (CNIO), VP of clinical informatics, chief information officer (CIO), or chief clinical information officer (CCIO). These nurse informaticists are experts in the field of nursing informatics, which has been recognized as a specialty by the American Nurses Association (2008) since 1992. There is, however, no advanced certification for the informatics role at present. The ANCC has a specialty certification for informatics requiring a bachelor's degree in nursing or other relevant field (ANCC, 2014). There is a need to establish competencies for the doctoral APN in informatics if this is to become a recognized advanced practice specialty. This role has many of the competencies in common with the other doctoral APN roles except that their specialty and field of research is informatics. I believe that the DNP course of study can prepare APNs in informatics.

In addition to the trends listed in the emerging technologies section and what's on the horizon section I recommend referring to Gartner, Inc. Gartner identified the top 10 strategic technology trends for organizations (Gartner, 2015a) and Top Predictions for IT Organizations and Users for 2016 and Beyond (Gartner, 2015b). For example, by 2018, two million employees will be required to wear health and fitness tracking devices as a condition of employment. Nursing will be able to access this data for their patients to help guide their care. Will nurses be one of the groups required to wear a health/fitness tracking device? Again, as there are so many technological innovations, it supports increasing the number and skill level of doctoral prepared nurses in the field of informatics. As more and more devices are integrated and more data are collected, I would like to recommend faculty and students consider use of big data for their scholarly projects. An excellent resource can be found at the University of Minnesota's School of Nursing website for big data session handouts and conference proceedings from 2013 to current year 2016. Westra et al. (2015) provide an overview of the conference and information on the critical role of big data in nursing and provide many reasons why nursing should be engaged.

The authors describe one of the key competencies of the doctoral APN as interfacing with the information systems' team. It is necessary that the doctoral APN understand what technologies are available and how these technologies can be deployed to improve the care delivery system. Stead and Lin (2009) describe four domains of information technology in health care: automation, connectivity, decision support, and data-mining capabilities. When seeking solutions for problem solving or ways to improve practice, the technology-competent doctoral APN would be able to recommend how the technology could be deployed to resolve the issue, and then conduct an evaluation to see whether the change is effective and whether any unintended consequences occur.

For example, the system can be used to calculate doses (automation) or decision support to warn a nurse if a prescribed dose is out of range based on age and/or weight. For connectivity, a device interface from a vital sign monitor to clinical documentation eliminates transcription errors, provides real time display of vital signs, and can alert clinicians when abnormal trends occur. The doctoral APN can determine what data are needed in a report or a dashboard to facilitate recognition and prioritization of issues by organizational units or by patient population. The doctoral APN does not need to be a programmer but needs to understand what the electronic health record can do for the practicing nurse, nurse managers, other members of the care delivery team, the C-suite, and consumers—and many times, just as important, what technology cannot do. By working collaboratively with the information system team, the doctoral APN can continue to discover the most effective technology strategy to meet patient care and organizational needs.

I definitely support the authors' emphasis on library search skills as critical to support lifelong learning and information mastery. I also agree with authors that mobile technology is valuable and here to stay. I concur that current implementation challenges relate to balancing advantage of convenience with disadvantages of lack of interoperability and data security risks.

There is a lot of material to be covered in the informatics arena. The authors have provided an extensive informative review of the technology tools available to the DNP student and doctoral APN and have suggested ways in which they can transform care. This review serves as an excellent foundation for further discussion and development of the informatics competencies of the doctoral APN. All levels of nursing practice require informatics competencies; the doctoral APN requires the most!

■ REFERENCES

Agency for Healthcare Research and Quality. (n.d.a). Health information technology, clinical decision support. Rockville, MD: Author. Retrieved from https://healthit.ahrq.gov/ahrq-funded-projects/clinical-decision-support-cds

Agency for Healthcare Research and Quality. (n.d.b). Health information technology, workflow assessment for health IT toolkit. Rockville, MD: Author. Retrieved from https://healthit.ahrq.gov/health-it-tools-and-resources/workflow-assessment-health-it-toolkit/workflow

American Nurses Association. (2008). *Nursing informatics: Scope and standards of practice*. Silver Spring, MD: NursesBooks.org.

American Nurses Credentialing Center. (2014). Informatics nursing. Retrieved from http://nursecredentialing.org/InformaticsNursing

American Nurses Credentialing Center. (2016a). Nurse executive, advanced, eligibility criteria. Retrieved from http://nursecredentialing.org/NurseExecutive-Advanced

American Nurses Credentialing Center. (2016b). Nurse executive, advanced test content outline. Retrieved from http://nursecredentialing.org/Documents/Certification/TestContentOutlines/Nurse-Executive-Advanced-TCO.pdf

American Organization of Nurse Executives. (2015a). *AONE nurse executive competencies*. Chicago, IL: Author. Retrieved from http://www.aone.org/resources/nurse-leader-competencies.shtml

American Organization of Nurse Executives. (2015b). *Nursing informatics executive leader: Position statement, January 01, 2012*. Chicago, IL: Author. Retrieved from http://www.aone.org/resources/informatics-executive-leader.pdf

Burnes, B. L., Gassert, C. A., & Cipriano, P. F. (2008). Technology solutions can make nursing care safer and more efficient. *Journal of Healthcare Information Management*, 22(4), 24–30.

Carayon, P., Karsh, B-.T., Cartmill, R. S., et al. (2010, October). Incorporating health information technology into workflow redesign: summary report. (Prepared by the Center for Quality and Productivity Improvement, University of Wisconsin–Madison, under Contract No. HHSA 290-2008-10036C). AHRQ Publication No. 10-0098-EF. Rockville, MD: Agency for Healthcare

Research and Quality. Retrieved from https://healthit.ahrq.gov/health-it-tools-and-resources/workflow-assessment-health-it-toolkit/links

Dowding, D., Mitchell, N., Randell, R., Foster, R., Lattimer, V., & Thompson, C. (2009). Nurses' use of computerized clinical decision support systems: A case site analysis. *Journal of Clinical Nursing, 18*, 1159–1167.

Dunn Lopez, K., Gephart, S. M., Raszewski, R., Sousa, V., Shehorn, L. E., & Abraham, J. (2016). Integrative review of clinical decision support for registered nurses in acute care settings. *Journal of the American Medical Informatics Association*, 1–10. doi:10.1093/jamia/ocw084

Gartner, Inc. (2015a). Gartner identifies the top 10 strategic technology trends for 2016. Retrieved from http://www.gartner.com/newsroom/id/3143521

Gartner, Inc. (2015b). Gartner reveals top predictions for IT organizations and users for 2016 and beyond. Retrieved from http://www.gartner.com/newsroom/id/3143718

Healthcare Information and Management Systems Society. (2016). TIGER expands integration of technology and informatics with international competency synthesis project. Retrieved from http://www.himss.org/news/tiger-expands-integration-technology-and-informatics-international-competency-synthesis-project?ItemNumber=46273&utm_source=commnews&utm_medium=email&utm_campaign=tiger

International Health Terminology Standards Development Organization. (2016). *SNOMED CT.* Copenhagen, Denmark: Author. Retrieved from http://www.ihtsdo.org/snomed-ct

Mitchell, N., Randell, R., Foster, R., Dowding, D., Lattimer, V., Thompson, C., . . . Summers, R. (2009). A national survey of computerized decision support systems available to nurses in England. *Journal of Nursing Management, 17*(7), 772–780.

Osheroff, J. A., Pifer, E. A., Teich, J. M., Sittig, D. F., & Jenders, R. A. (2005). *Improving outcomes with clinical decision support: An implementer's guide.* Boca Raton, FL: Productivity Press.

Randell, R., & Dowding, D. (2010). Organisational influences on nurses' use of clinical decision support systems. *International Journal of Medical Informatics, 79*, 412–421.

Stead, W., & Lin, H. (2009). Computational committee on engaging the Computer Science Research Community in Health Care Informatics; National Research Council. *Computational technology for effective health care: Immediate steps and strategic directions.* Washington, DC: National Academies Press. Retrieved from http://books.nap.edu/catalog.php?record_id=12572

Warren, J. J., Matney, S. A., Foster, E. D., Auld, V. A., & Roy, S. L. (2015). Toward interoperability: A new resource to support nursing terminology standards. *Computers, Informatics, Nursing, 33*(12), 515–519.

Westra, B. L., Clancy, T. R., Sensmeier, J., Warren, J. J., Weaver, C., & Delaney, C.W. (2015). Nursing knowledge: Big data science—Implications for nurse leaders. *Nursing Administration Quarterly, 39*(4), 304–310.

University of Minnesota, School of Nursing. (2016). Center for Nursing Informatics, Center Projects, Big Data. Retrieved from http://www.nursing.umn.edu/centers/center-nursing-informatics/events/2016-nursing-knowledge-big-data-science-conference

U.S. National Library of Medicine. (2015). Nursing resources for standards and interoperability. National Library of Medicine. Retrieved from http://www.nlm.nih.gov/research/umls/Snomed/nursing_terminology_resources.html

CHAPTER FOURTEEN

Reflective Response 2

Cecilia Kennedy Page

In Chapter 14, by Cornelius, Childs, and Wilson, these authors describe the competencies required for a doctoral-prepared advanced practice nurse (APN) to lead in the health care environment of the future. Grounded in the roots of patient safety movement championed by the Institute of Medicine (IOM), a renewed national commitment to the development of the information infrastructure was described as being critical to support reengineering care processes and facilitate outcome measurements for accountability (IOM, 2001). The American Association of Colleges of Nursing (AACN, 2006) acknowledges the leadership required by doctoral-prepared nurses to use information systems to evaluate programs of care, outcomes of care, and care systems. This chapter delineates the expert competencies of the Doctor of Nursing Practice (DNP) leader to meet the leadership challenges of the health care industry in technology.

Described in this chapter are the base competencies required for Informatics. The initial review of the master level practitioner and the doctoral APN are described in a narrative format. A strong correlation or comparative analysis of these two levels would have called out the cognitive maturation required for the expert level. These authors go on to describe informatics competencies for specific doctoral advanced practice nursing roles. The functional differentiation is only separated by the focus domain of the professional scope of clinical practice. All roles are required to support the AACN competencies (AACN, 2006) demonstrating the ability to provide leadership within health care systems and/or academic settings related to the use of information systems. Much of the chapter addresses the tools available to the advanced practicing nurse. In a more concise fashion, the Technology Informatics Guiding Educational Reform (TIGER, 2009) collaborative states that APNs should be competent in: (a) basic computer competencies or sources of knowledge; (b) information literacy integrating information to evidence-based practice; and (c) information management leveraging the data from sources such as the electronic health records.

What is missing in this chapter is the foundational work of informatics on the metastructures: data, information, knowledge, and wisdom (DIKW); data as the discrete entities; information as the data that has been interpreted, organized, or structured; knowledge as the information that is synthesized linking relationships; and wisdom as the use of knowledge to manage and solve human problems (American Nurses Association [ANA], 2015). In this chapter, the authors describe knowledge management competencies but without the reference to the DIKW metastructure, foundational to the nursing informatics. Each level along the continuum represents an increasing level of complexity and cognitive capability. Knowledge management reflects the interpretation, integration, and understanding of patterns of data. Doctoral preparation of the APN embraces the competency of data extraction from information systems and databases, data analysis for understanding trends, and the intuitive thinking of expert nurses to support health care practitioners in decision making.

In 2011, the IOM released the *Health IT and Patient Safety: Building Safer Systems for Better Care.* In this work, the IOM makes the argument that merely installing health IT in health organizations will not result in improved care. Health IT cannot exist in isolation for its context of use. Health IT is a part of a larger system, a sociotechnical system, and safety emerges from the interaction of various factors. Since the APN competency includes the analysis in the selection, use, and evaluation of patient care technology and health care information systems, awareness of this framework and recommendations by the IOM should be included in this chapter. Leadership in the cross-disciplinary research toward the use of health IT as a part of the learning health care system is a challenge by the IOM and key for expert leadership in nursing.

One concept mentioned by these authors that should have been elaborated is the concept of practice knowledge—identified as a key competency involving the ability to combine information from a variety of data sources to create new information and possibly new knowledge. This is fundamental to the APN who is called to design and implement processes to evaluate outcomes of practice, practice patterns, and systems of care (AACN, 2006). Use cases indicative of leveraging technology to contribute to practice knowledge would have been excellent exemplars here. For example, the attributes of data collated to create a nurse-driven protocol to enhance outcomes in a nurse-sensitive indicator (falls, catheter-associated urinary tract infection [CAUTI], etc.). Practice knowledge is possible because of data obtained, aggregated, and supported through the use of informatics.

Without question, I agree that the doctoral APN is expected to exhibit leadership that not only contributes to the body of scientific knowledge but also serves as a catalyst for change. Technology advancement with the adoption and meaningful use of the electronic health record, although forced by regulatory mandates, is one of the greatest disruptive innovations of our career lifetimes. This electronic health record is the base for knowledge management systems, as stated by these authors. Nurses must lead through this transformation and use the data to continue to build the evidence-driven organizations.

The cultural transformation influenced by the development of technology is only in its infancy in health care. Challenged by the reimbursement shifting landscape from volume-based, fee for service, to value-based payments, the health care industry will seek new and innovative models of care. Technology will be at the core. For example, as virtual care becomes commonplace in the topography of technology, roles will change and the innovative nurse leader may capitalize on carving out new roles for nurses as we study the evidence and expand our influence in health outcomes. Home monitoring in the mobile health (mhealth) and virtual visits (e-visits) will demand new competencies of nursing as new technologies produce new data sources. The field of informatics and the competencies required to facilitate the use of technological tools and information management will be the cornerstone for an effective nursing practice. The doctorate of nursing practice must continue to develop expert practitioners to lead our profession in this domain.

■ REFERENCES

American Association of Colleges of Nursing. (2006). *The essentials of doctoral education for advanced nursing practice.* Retrieved from http://www.aacn.nche.edu/dnp/pdf/essentials.pdf

Institute of Medicine. (2001). *Crossing the quality chasm: A new health system for the 21st century.* Washington, DC: National Academies Press. Retrieved from www.nap.edu

Institute of Medicine. (2011). *Health IT and patient safety: Building safer systems for better care.* Washington, DC: National Academies Press. Retrieved from www.nap.edu

Technology Informatics Guiding Education Reform. (2009). Summary report: Evidence and informatics transforming nursing: 3-year action steps toward a 10-year vision. Retrieved from http://www.tigersummit.com/uploads/TIGER_Collaborative_Exec_ Summary_040509.pdf

TIGER Initiative Foundation. (n.d.). *The leadership imperative: TIGER's recommendations for integrating technology to transform practice and education.* Chicago, IL: Author. Retrieved from https://www.himss.org/file/1309406/download?token=fmjp6TwC

Negotiation Skills for the Doctoral Advanced Practice Nurse

Vicki D. Lachman and Cheryl M. Vermey

Doctoral advanced practice nurses are creating new frontiers in the field of nursing, and as practitioners, they are contributing significantly to the overall health care system. To fulfill this role, they will encounter many situations requiring negotiation skills. The realm of negotiation falls within both strategy and tactics. This chapter focuses primarily on the strategic role of the Doctor of Nursing Practice (DNP) and provides tactical examples that may be faced in actual practice.

This chapter begins with the context of organizational culture and systems theory as the place where negotiation takes place. Discussion includes the traits of successful negotiators and the crucial elements for successful negotiation, sources of power, and the five-step process for negotiation. Since not all individuals approach negotiation from a collaborative stance, skills are required for negotiating at an "uneven table," when rank and privilege affect the strategies. The chapter ends with strategies for overcoming barriers to successful negotiation, such as the "Four Horseman of the Apocalypse," and common mistakes in negotiation.

Negotiation is a crucial skill for successful relationships (Gottman, 2011; Shapiro, 2015). In order to have the necessary collaborative relations within and between disciplines, DNPs must have the skills and strategies known to diplomats. For example, individuals who take a win-win approach to conflict resolution view conflicts as problems to be solved and seek solutions that achieve both their own goals, as well as the goals of the other person. Individuals with this orientation see conflicts as opportunities for improving relationships by reducing the tension between two people (Gottman, 2011; Katz & Patterini, 2008).Therefore, the purpose of negotiation is to resolve differences over, for example, information, values, or goals. Fisher, Ury, and Patton (2011) provide the following working definition of negotiation: "Two or more parties, with common and conflicting interests, come together to put forth and discuss explicit proposals for the purpose of reaching an agreement" (p. 10).

It is important in any negotiation to begin with common interests in order to create rapport. The purpose of negotiation is to reach an agreement that is based on a thorough discussion of each party's ideas and where an agreement is reached to meet the needs of both parties. The solution is one that assures commitment to follow through to completion by each party. This differs from compromise, which is based on both party's willingness to *settle* on an option. Compromise might best be described as "mini-lose."

■ THE ROLE OF THE DNP IN NEGOTIATION—THE STRATEGIC VIEW

Before completion of her DNP degree, Dr. Schmidt was a nurse practitioner in the stroke center of an academic medical center. Because of her years of experience in the acute care of stroke patients, she decided to do her DNP clinical practicum in a rehab unit. This rounding out of her experience with stroke patients and her evidence-base focused her to conclude that stroke rehab needs to focus on all domains—social and functional—for patients to recover a sense of self and the roles in their lives and with their families. Unfortunately, she was met with a resistance to this change. What new ideas can we offer Dr. Schmidt in negotiation?

This section addresses a system context for using negotiation skills, the organizational culture as a context for change, and how gender and culture influence the role of the DNP. Helping Dr. Schmidt understand the organizational culture in which she finds herself and using the principles from CRR Global (formally known as the Center for Right Relationships; 2011), which is a systems approach described in the following paragraphs, could help her better negotiate the change. Perhaps, because of her gender, she is more focused on maintaining a relationship than in clearly and directly arguing for change for the patient's sake (Donaldson & Frohnmayer, 2007). This compromising style was a gender difference that Holt and Devore (2005) found in a metanalysis of 36 studies of self-reported data on conflict-resolution tendencies. Thomas, Thomas, and Schaubhur (2008), in a study of gender differences in conflict, found that men scored significantly higher in competing styles at low, medium, and high levels of responsibility in the workplace. Women's style remained compromising at all employment levels.

SYSTEMS THEORY AS A CONTEXT FOR NEGOTIATION

The DNP role in negotiation requires a high level of systems thinking and an ability to apply expertise in systems theory and functioning. The role includes being a participant in the larger system and being a catalyst for system's change through negotiation. Therefore, there is a compelling leadership dimension to negotiation at this higher level.

Historically, negotiation took place within top-down, patriarchal organizational systems. The 21st century is unfolding a new dimension in systems work. The dimensions are multifaceted and include a focus on the relationships within systems; organizational theory; emotional, social, and systems intelligence (Goleman, 2012; Goleman & Boyatzis, 2008; Goleman, Boyatzis, & McKee, 2013); and seminal research on process work and deep democracy, where all voices in the system need to be heard (Mindell, 2012, 2014, 2015). Arnold and Amy Mindell's work through the Deep Democracy Institute (2009) has created a worldwide think tank for the development of leadership that emphasizes the dynamic interplay between individual and collective transformations, and the seminal and empirical research conducted on relationships (Gottman, 2007, 2011; Gottman & Silver, 2015). These new approaches focus on connections between and among members of a system, and recognizing that people are in relationships at all times, starting with themselves. In his latest research, Gottman (2011) asserts that trust is a cornerstone to relationship and an essential component of negotiation, as will be explored later in the chapter.

CRR Global (2011) has created a ground-breaking model that is used internationally for coaching within organizations and groups to unfold the power and potential of relationship systems. This new methodology for facilitating human relationships is inspired by and combines the concepts from coaching, psychology, organizational development, mediation, quantum physics, process work, and general systems theory, all of which are directly applicable to the DNP's use in negotiation. In effect, the negotiation role includes managing and leading relationship systems.

CRR Global's (2011) approach is founded on the following principles, which DNPs can use to create desired outcomes rather than focus on solving a problem. The first principle is creating a shift from "who is doing what to whom" to "what is happening here?" It creates a climate of being in the right relationship with oneself, others, and the larger organization or system in which the DNP is functioning. In this view, all parties have a voice that needs to be heard and acknowledged before a successful conclusion to any negotiation can occur. Every relationship system is characterized by various dynamic and evolving situations and human interactions. The DNP needs to be prepared to assess what is happening in the situation that creates the need for negotiation. Sometimes what is needed is to reveal that there is a system breakdown that is essential to address in order to move forward.

The second principle is that the relationship system is naturally creative and whole. In this view, there is no "they" rather there is "I, you, and we." Whenever one falls into a "they" view of a situation, the individuals risk putting themselves in the place of victim, undermining their effectiveness and ability to resolve the situation. Assuming that all parties in the relationship form something larger than the whole, this change empowers members of the system to negotiate new ways of working together effectively.

A third principle is that the DNP works with the whole system within a larger context, not just what appears on the surface. It is taking a metaview of the larger picture that is important here, much like an orchestra conductor. Think of a gestalt where the whole is greater than the sum of its parts. For example, Dr. Schmidt needs to acknowledge that all opinions need to be voiced in order to uncover the real issues under the resistance to change. She can then articulate what is going on that may be negatively impacting optimal patient outcomes and use the collective knowledge and wisdom of the group to create better solutions for ensuring that a holistic framework is used. This means that the old way of working the system needs to yield to one that is more empowered toward collective interest versus individual self-interest.

In summary, the role of the DNP in a systems context is essentially to reveal the system to itself. In contrast to "fixing" what appears on the surface, the nurse can hold up a mirror to what seems to be happening in order that others may be able to respond in ways that better meet the needs of the larger system. The metaphor for the principle is "the view of the eagle looking at the system versus the ant on the floor."

POLITICAL, CULTURAL, AND GENDER CONTEXTS WITHIN THE SYSTEM

Organizations may be viewed through various perspectives through which the DNP must practice. Bolman and Deal (2013) describe the four frames of an organization from a system's perspective, which include the structural, human, political, and symbolic/cultural frames. Structure includes buildings, departments, technology, and equipment. Human resources include the people and hierarchy within the system. However, negotiation mostly takes place within the context of the political and symbolic frames.

Bolman and Deal (2013) use the metaphor of a jungle to view the political frame. This is where the intersection of power, conflict, and coalitions takes place. A critical lens through which one views negotiation recognizes that the system is composed of various political arenas including administration, governing bodies, medical groups, ancillary personnel, and nurses at all levels of education and experience. Therefore, individuals could argue that one dimension of the DNP role is that of a politician, but not in the traditional sense. For example, titles connote power in society and organizations. The title "doctor" has historically been seen as belonging to a physician or perhaps to a university professor. The title "doctor" when describing a nurse creates both confusion and conflict related to the power and political meaning of the term. The DNP needs to be prepared to respond to this issue.

Bolman and Deal (2013) also describe a symbolic frame, which includes the organizational culture and its symbols. A metaphor here is the system as theater and includes many cues, symbols, and stories that create system norms that often resist challenge or change. A recent review of the literature (Gormley & van Nieuwerburgh, 2014) supports the positive impact of a coach approach to organizational change and is consistent with the model developed by CRR Global.

Thus, the DNP role includes viewing the system from the metaview of both political and symbolic or cultural frames. Combining acute understanding of these frames along with skill in being in the right relationship with self and others distinguishes the role of the DNP from others. For example, DNPs who are using evidence-based practice may challenge organizational ways of practice (as will be seen in the following case example).

Gender Effects in Negotiation

An examination of context would not be complete without including thoughts on the effect of gender and other measures of equity on the system and the ability of the DNP to negotiate effectively. Today 94% of nurses are still women (American Association of Colleges of Nursing, 2009). The issues of gender also apply to issues of race, ethnicity, and other considerations of equity (Harris, Moran, & Moran, 2007).

In several studies on gender differences in negotiation strategies, it was found that men tend to view bargaining situations as short term and episodic in nature, whereas women tend to view transactions with others as part of a long-term relationship (Babcock & Laschever, 2008). Consequently, saying that women adopt more flexible bargaining stances than their male counterparts can be explained by their attitude toward the length of the relationship. But this difference in negotiating behavior can also be explained as women's concern for the equity of interpersonal relationships. In another gender-related study, the results suggested that women report having obtained a good outcome when they felt they had a pleasant interaction with the other party, even though they did not resolve or even discuss the conflict between them (Donaldson & Frohnmayer, 2007). The results of these studies suggest that women need to learn that it is legitimate to say what they want, even if it conflicts with what they think the other person wants.

Another gender difference was found in Babcock and Laschever (2008) research, in which men are significantly more likely to use negotiation to promote their own interests than are women. The accumulation of this disadvantage is sharply seen in salary negotiation, where women are leaving thousands of dollars, potentially millions by the time they retire. They also sacrifice visibility, training, and career growth because they also do not seek opportunities or rewards as men do.

Holt (2010) is a seasoned executive and an executive coach, whose key focus is helping women move forward. She believes women have to break some rules and deep-seeded assumptions, such as self-promoting and a will to win are wrong. She learned that expecting to be treated fairly if you do a great job was a myth and that she needed to ask for interesting projects, promotional opportunities, and a higher salary. Gallo (2015) interviewed two experts on their perspectives in negotiating salary—myth versus reality. This article shatters some myths and provides women with six important strategies in negotiating salary. For example, the "play hardball" myth is shattered by advising to focus on the overall package and be prepared to justify the amount requested.

Sandberg (2013) has popularized the movement to put women in top spots across the organizational terrain. Her book has many supporters and critics, but the encouragement she gives women wins out (Adams, 2013; Alkon, 2015). The most controversial part of the book, which stirred feminist ire, is her discussion on the internal obstacles that hold woman back. She herself struggled with the need to be liked, which she believes interferes with women's ability to take a competing versus compromising style. She scrutinizes why women's progress in succeeding at leadership roles has stalled, enlightens on the root causes, and proposes convincing, commonsense solutions that can enable women to attain their full potential. She cautions women not to be relentlessly pleasant in negotiation and to take their rightful seat at the uneven negotiation table.

In summary, the leadership needed for successful negotiation requires the DNP to assess and balance the principles of the structural, human, political, and symbolic frames of the organization. This means going beyond the organizational structure, staff-reporting lines, and job descriptions to developing skills in the political dynamics and understand cultural norms that have an often unseen but huge impact on negotiation outcomes. The four frames also need to be balanced with an understanding of the impact of gender and diversity on the issue at hand.

RANK AND PRIVILEGE

To delve deeper in the concept of rank and privilege requires distinguishing among the rank, power, and privilege. Mindell (2012) describes rank as a way of a indicating a level of status and is the amount of power that a person has relative to others in a given situation. Privilege and power can be derived from different bases or sources, such as educational, social, economic, or cultural. Therefore, a nurse with a doctoral degree has greater inherent privilege and implied power than that of a nurse with a baccalaureate degree. At present, society and organizational structures grant physicians greater rank and privilege than that of nurses, regardless of education or other forms of standing. It will be interesting to see if this will change when there are increased numbers of DNPs, especially those functioning autonomously or specifically in clinical settings.

> Dr. Bowman completed her DNP degree, where she also received a certificate in clinical research for the four courses she completed in research. She was interested in conducting research on the "Role Strain in Family Caregivers of Persons Diagnosed with Alzheimer's Dementia," as her clinical focus was with patients with Alzheimer's disease. Up to this point, she had been the nurse collecting information for many physician-led studies. After conducting this study, she was now ready to be the primary or co-investigator of studies. She put forth research ideas and possible funding sources, but met with resistance. Apparently, members on her interdisciplinary team were having difficulty seeing her as the primary researcher and as a leader. What ideas and skills can we offer Dr. Bowman in negotiation?

The DNP needs to stand in her own integrity and awareness that she now has the experience and skills to be an effective co-investigator. Kay and Shipman (2014) speak on importance of confidence and the self-assurance needed to be a successful negotiator. Their book on the latest in neuroscience on confidence states that visits with high-power women across the globe could give Dr. Bowman a different perspective in her approach. Additional research on gender and leader identify formation for senior women (Skinner, 2014) suggests that addressing gender imbalance in senior leadership, having women role models, and defining an authentic leader voice all help mitigate the impact of male norms. It is an act of inner courage and conviction that allows the DNP to be authentic in any situation that requires the use of negotiation skills. Essential inner qualities include increasing inner awareness, being a truth teller, and standing by your own integrity.

Mindell (2014) further describes low rank as being devalued, disrespected, and excluded from influence, decision making, and other benefits that come from having high rank. Because of this norm, nurses have historically been impacted in areas of self-esteem and self-worth. A source of conflict can be the unconscious use of rank. For example, a person in a higher position, confronted with "pulling rank" or dismissing the concerns or needs of others, often becomes angry or uses denial as a defense mechanism. The DNP has two critical roles here: the first is to know and effectively use skills and strategies for negotiation; the second is to use a systems approach in resolving issues involving negotiation strategies. In the case example, Dr. Bowman was seen by her colleagues as having neither the rank nor the privilege to warrant being the primary investigator of the study. One successful outcome of her negotiation is acknowledging the contributions of her colleagues, choosing to take the first step as a co-investigator of the study, and demonstrating how research builds evidence-based practice and the importance of implementing to improve patient outcomes.

■ THE ROLE OF THE DNP IN NEGOTIATION—THE TACTICAL VIEW

Dr. Land is a recent DNP graduate and he is negotiating for a promotion to a chief nursing officer position in an academic medical center where he has been a director of cardiovascular services for 10 years. He knows his competition and all have either an MSN in nursing administration or an MBA and that they are from out of the state. He decides to leverage his DNP degree and his understanding of the organization's culture and goals, which will allow him to hit the ground running. Since many on the search committee do not understand what knowledge and skills a DNP degree can bring, he decides to provide them with two brief articles outlining the MSN and DNP curriculum differences. He also plans to use his organizational power by having one of his recommendations come from the chairperson of surgery. He knows all his years as a critical care nurse will help him think clearly under the stress of the interview. His reputation as a person of integrity and his willingness to be assertive in conflict situations, with a focus on problem resolution, will stand well for him. What ideas and skills can we offer Dr. Land in negotiation?

This section focuses on the specific tactics and strategies used in negotiation, which fit within the strategic thinking or systems framework where the DNP functions. The literature describes the traits of successful negotiators and the strategies for a win-win outcome (Hennig, 2008; Lewicki, Barry, & Saunders, 2015). Dr. Land is already applying some of the crucial traits and elements for successful negotiation, and the following section should prove helpful as he plans his next steps.

TRAITS OF SUCCESSFUL NEGOTIATORS

When we study the diplomatic styles of individuals, we are able to identify seven traits in individuals that we would rate as key in their success (Malhotra & Bazerman, 2007; Raiffa, Richardson, & Metcalfe, 2007). The first trait is having strong planning skills. Successful negotiators often state that they spend 50% or more of their time planning what will be said in their interactions. Such planning includes not only the content, but where they will meet, who else should be present, whether information should be sent before the meeting, and even what time of the day the meeting should occur. Successful negotiators want to maximize their opportunities for success; therefore, they recognize that the process and place are equally as important as the meeting's discussion.

The "ability to think clearly under stress" is the second trait of successful negotiators. Being prepared is one way to reduce the stress in any negotiation process. Two other ways are staying focused on problem-solving, not on individual personalities, and recognizing at any point you can back away from the negotiation and come back at a later time. Diplomats tend to project an air of confidence; therefore, when an attack occurs, their positive self-regard holds them in good stead.

A third trait, and often an undervalued trait, is the "ability to use common sense." The most common meaning to this phrase is good sense and sound judgment in practical matters. Taking the time to establish rapport, providing sufficient information on which to base a decision, and remembering the basics about positive interpersonal relationships are all utilizing common sense.

The individual's "verbal ability" is the fourth trait. This is the ability to state one's ideas and opinions assertively, as well as to clarify the other party's ideas and opinions (Bishop, 2013; McClure, 2007; Murphy, 2011).The abilities to manage other people's defensiveness, side-stepping issues, as well as overt hostility in a nondefensive manner are also key verbal skills. An example of the persuasion skill is that agreement is facilitated when the desirability of the agreement is stressed.

"Content knowledge" is the fifth trait found in successful negotiators. For example, if Dr. Land was going to negotiate a union contract that involves changing the role of the nurse aides in the institution, he would certainly come to the table having already investigated licensure laws, how other institutions have handled such a change, and the current attitude of the staff.

The sixth trait is "personal integrity." In truth, if one is not perceived as trustworthy and credible, the person will not be seen as an individual with integrity. Being seen as trustworthy requires that the person be honest, open instead of defensive, consistent in standards and approach, and someone who treats individuals with the respect that they deserve. Gottman (2011) cites the difficulty in specifically defining trust and uses the mathematics of game theory to help us understand that trust goes beyond a cognitive definition. It entails observable behavior represented by a trust matric that accepts each partner will bargain for his interests and will do so employing a "nice-nice" exchange in contrast to a "nasty-nasty" exchange.

The final and seventh trait of successful negotiators is "the ability to perceive and use power." Power is the ability and willingness to affect the outcome. There are multiple sources of power that are available for use in negotiation. For now, suffice to say that successful negotiators keep their eye on the outcome that they desire and use multiple sources of power to move the negotiation to the conclusion they desire (Aquilar & Galluccio, 2007).

In the case example, Dr. Land needed to be consciously aware of and apply the traits or skills of planning, thinking clearly under stress, using his common sense and verbal skills, having strong knowledge of the content or information required in the situation. To this he needed to balance his own sense of personal integrity to create a positive trusting environment with his ability to perceive and use power in an effective way. This is not "power over" but the courage and willingness to step forth and do what is needed in the situation.

THREE CRUCIAL ELEMENTS FOR SUCCESSFUL NEGOTIATION

Power, time, and information are the three interrelated variables in any negotiation process (Cohen, 2007; Thompson, 2007).Power is the capacity to get things done, to exercise control over people, events, or situations. Usually when knowledgeable people complain about power, it is for one of two reasons: (a) they do not like the way power is being used—it is often power over an individual and (b) they do not approve of the goal of the person exerting control—power should never be a goal in and of itself, but should be a means of transport to a desired outcome.

In any negotiation, the second variable of time needs consideration. Expect the most significant concession behavior in any settlement action to occur close to the deadline. It is crucial that both parties know the deadline. However, deadlines are more flexible than most people realize. DNP clinicians need to use this misunderstanding of the time dimension to negotiate for outcomes that support excellence in patient care, quality education, or crucial changes in organizational effectiveness.

Information is the third crucial element in the negotiation process. During the actual negotiating event, it is often a common strategy for one or both sides to conceal their true interests, needs, and priorities. The rationale is that information is power, particularly in situations where one cannot trust the other side fully.

It is important to gain information by asking questions every time you are given answers. A way to test the credibility of the other side is to ask questions, the answers to which are already known. The more information one has about the other person's priorities, deadlines, and real needs, the better one can bargain. A key piece of information that all negotiators want to know is: "what are the real limits of the other party?," or just "how much they will sacrifice in order to make a deal?" Very often this can be ascertained by observing the pattern of concession behavior on the part of the other side.

Turning back to the case of Dr. Land, one can see how he has used the aforementioned principles. He established his background and credentials early in a negotiation. He demonstrated the kind of expertise that is required for most negotiations by asking intelligent questions to know whether the responses are accurate. It is important for Dr. Land to remember that he brings to the table clinical and managerial expertise in a negotiation process.

For example, the search committee may state that they want their candidate to have had previous experience as a chief nursing officer, whereas, there real need is that the candidate knows how to work effectively in a complex academic medical center. The more Dr. Land can acquaint himself with the committee's needs, the better will be his position to negotiate a possible resolution for their real need. An example of using the power of identification is when Dr. Land mentions that a well-respected academic medical center had just hired their internal candidate last year and he has been very successful. If the organization has had a precedent of promoting from within, Dr. Land can use the power of precedent.

TABLE 15.1   **Five Steps in Negotiation Process**

The Negotiation Process Steps	Key Points to Include
1. Prepare	Know the facts Know what self and others want Develop the strategy Identify the "must have"
2. Develop Objective Criteria	Includes laws, policies, precedence, moral standards, and community norms as possible criteria Consider accreditation standards Seek benchmark models for comparison
3. Communicate Interests and Needs	Communication includes both clear dialog and a connection to others Body language sends messages that others will see
4. Search for Mutually Acceptable Solutions	Look for areas of agreement and common ground Be willing to accept mutually accepted options, not previously considered
5. Finalize the Agreement	Ensure clear agreement on the details Who will do what and in what time frame Distribute a summary with the agreed upon outcomes Identify areas for future discussion

Source: Cohen (2007); Fisher, Ury, and Patton (2011); and Raiffa, Richardson, and Metcalfe (2007).

The best outcomes employ a systems approach where the parties rise above individual interests to view the greater good. While holding the strategic view, it is also important to use the tactical skills needed in a negotiation process (see Table 15.1).

BARRIERS TO SUCCESSFUL NEGOTIATION

Barriers to successful negotiation are multidimensional and involve behaviors that people use, often at an unconscious level to thwart resolution. This section also includes descriptions of the "Four Horsemen of the Apocalypse" (Gottman, 2011; Gottman & Silver, 2015) and individual common mistakes (Changing Minds.org) that the DNP needs to understand to be successful in negotiating. Individuals, like Dr. Ross, need to overcome these barriers for successful negotiation.

> Dr. Ross began her academic teaching career after she completed her DNP degree last year. Prior to this, she had been a women's health NP in a busy practice connected to the academic medical center for ten years. It became quickly apparent that several of the other professors with a background in women's health were unhappy with her appointment as a track coordinator. Her initial efforts at inclusion in curriculum planning were met with stonewalling and disrespect. It appeared her questions about the present curriculum were taken as criticism, rather than her effort to understand the rationale used for inclusion of the courses. The nonverbal responses included eye-rolling, silence, or looks of shock when she suggested changes. What ideas and strategies could we offer Dr. Ross in negotiation?

THE "FOUR HORSEMEN OF THE APOCALYPSE"

Dr. John Gottman (2007, 2011; Gottman & Silver, 2015) has conducted empirical research on healthy and unhealthy marriages and his work is now being extrapolated and further validated for use in organizations (Gottman, 2007). There are four toxic behaviors that doom relationships, regardless of the setting, that are called the "Four Horsemen of the Apocalypse." These behaviors include:

1. Blame/criticism, consisting of attacking or blaming other instead of his or her own behavior
2. Defensiveness in response to being criticized, which is really another way of blaming
3. Contempt, which is the use of sarcasm, belittling, cynicism, hostile humor, and belligerence
4. Stonewalling, which includes cutting off communication, silent treatments, refusals to engage, withdrawal or in some cases just not directly expressing what you are thinking

Gottman (2011) found that 69% of all problems are perpetual, meaning that they can be managed through dialog, but resist ultimate resolution. Therefore, the role of the DNP is not to "fix" the issue, but to engage in negotiation strategies that will increase positive dialogue, reduce the negative affect during conflict, particularly the difficult challenge of working with contempt, and increase the positive effect during/after a conflict resolution. Figure 15.1 includes some antidotes that are effective in working with the Four Horsemen.

The "Four Horseman of the Apocalypse" can lead negotiators to make common mistakes (see Table 15.2). Of the 15 mistakes listed (Changing Minds.org), the most recurrent ones are accepting positions, hurrying, issue fixation, and missing strengths. Creative thinking needed for win-win solutions will not occur if others do not change their positions and not look for innovative solutions, but remain fixated on their chosen solutions. Many beginning negotiators fail to see the strengths they have, often because they are hurrying to a solution to please others.

An important role for the DNP is to first assess what is going on within the system that requires negotiation. Taking a systems view, understanding issues of rank and privilege, using the skills needed to negotiate effectively, and having a clear understanding of what gets in the way of resolution—all of these approaches arm the practitioner with the background to be an effective negotiator. It is also important to be grounded in a strong sense of self and know what values one brings to the situation. Using the approaches delineated in Figure 15.2 enables the DNP to be effective in dealing with toxic behaviors.

Based on the work of CRR Global (2011), overcoming the barriers is predicated on the principle of finding a common interest. The following questions are useful: (a) Are you willing to resolve this without blame? (b) Why is it important to resolve this? and (c) What do you agree on? A caveat: if the parties are unwilling to resolve the issue without blame, there is no point in proceeding farther. One needs to develop another strategy for resolution.

Toxic Behaviors	Strategies to Deal With Them
General Behaviors	↟ Name the behavior and educate the parties on the negative impact/destructiveness. ↟ Review what happened and discuss alternative behaviors/strategies. ↟ Increase positive behaviors and attitudes where possible with a soft approach, accepting influence, and noticing efforts to "repair" what has happened. ↟ Encourage that there are alternative ways to negotiate through a situation or conflict.
Blame/Criticism	↟ Ask are you willing to resolve this without blame? ↟ Address the behavior, not the person. ↟ Try a soft start up to lessen the impact. ↟ Look for the request behind the criticism. ↟ Encourage the use of "I want . . . , I feel . . ." statements.
Defensiveness	↟ Actively listen and clarify what the other person is hearing. ↟ Assume that 2% of what you or the other person is saying is true. Look for areas of truth behind the complaint.
Contempt	↟ Ask are you willing to resolve this without sarcasm or name calling? ↟ Allow the parties to ventilate to you. ↟ Check for emotional flooding and soothe. ↟ Encourage the use of "I want . . . , I feel . . ." statements.
Stonewalling	↟ Check for emotional flooding and soothe. ↟ Address fears of what will happen if the person speaks what is being thought or felt. ↟ Encourage moving beyond the edge that is keeping the person back and support the effort.

FIGURE 15.1 The "Four Horsemen of the Apocalypse" behaviors.
Adapted from Gottman and Silver (2015).

TABLE 15.2 **Common Mistakes That Negotiators Make**

1. *Accepting positions*: Assuming the other person won't change his or her position
2. *Accepting statements*: Assuming what the other person says is wholly true
3. *Cornering*: Giving the person no alternative but to fight
4. *Hurrying*: Negotiating in haste (and repenting at leisure)
5. *Hurting the relationship*: Getting what you want but making an enemy
6. *Issue fixation*: Getting stuck on one issue and missing greater possibilities
7. *Missing strengths*: Not realizing the strengths that you actually have
8. *Misunderstanding authority*: Assuming that authority and power are synonymous
9. *Misunderstanding power*: Thinking one person has all the power
10. *One solution*: Thinking there is only one possible solution
11. *Over-wanting*: Wanting something too much
12. *Squeezing too much*: Trying to gain every last advantage
13. *Talking too much*: Not gaining the power of information from others
14. *Thinking in absolutes*: Assuming that there are only a few possibilities
15. *Win-lose*: Assuming a fixed-pie, win-lose scenario

Adapted from Changing Minds.org. *Negotiation mistakes*. Retrieved from http://changingminds.org/disciplines/negotiation/mistakes/mistakes.htm.

■ SUMMARY

Negotiation is a complex process where individuals are seeking an agreement that all parties can make a commitment to follow through to completion. In this context, the role of the DNP includes holding a strategic or systems view of the negotiations process. How to negotiate and with whom one can negotiate is largely determined by the organizational culture in which negotiators find themselves. There are cultural and gender variables to be aware of in the process. CRR Global speaks directly to possible strategies to right the system.

The role of the DNP also requires skillful and effective use of tactical strategies for negotiation. Critical is creating a climate of trust. The five steps in the negotiation process are fraught with possible complications from the "Four Horsemen of the Apocalypse" and the common errors in negotiation. The DNP graduate, in his or her leadership role, may also be responsible for facilitating negotiation between two other individuals.

■ CRITICAL THINKING QUESTIONS

1. *Why is it important to first focus on common versus conflicting ideas in negotiation process?*
2. *What are the three principles designed to resolve conflict in a system put forward by CRR Global?*
3. *Compare your present skills to the six skills of successful negotiators. What are your strengths and areas for development?*
4. *Gottman describes the "Four Horseman of the Apocalypse." What is necessary to resolve conflicts utilizing this model?*
5. *There are five steps in the negotiation process. Why is the first step, preparation, described as the most important step?*
6. *Common mistakes in the negotiation process involve cognitive and affective errors. Of this list, where are your vulnerabilities in negotiation in your workplace?*
7. *Due to the gender differences discussed, what are the vulnerabilities of woman negotiating?*
8. *What personal values are important to bring to situations requiring negotiation for successful resolution?*
9. *Think of a situation where a person was being defensive. What was the "2%" truth in that person's position? What strategies can one use to find common ground?*
10. *Review the case examples included in this chapter. Based on your experience, what are other effective strategies?*

■ ACKNOWLEDGMENT

Authors gratefully acknowledge the support and permission from CRR Global in the use of their model and the select materials in the preparation of this chapter.

■ REFERENCES

Adams, S. (2013, March). 10 Things Sheryl Sandberg gets exactly right in 'lean in.' *Forbes*. Retrieved from http://www.forbes.com/sites/susanadams/2013/03/04/10-things-sheryl-sandberg-gets-exactly-right-in-lean-in/#3e148675466f

Alkon, A. (2015, April). Science says 'lean in' is filled with flawed advice, likely to hurt women. *Observer*. Retrieved from http://observer.com/2015/05/science-says-lean-in-is-filled-with-flawed-advice-likely-to-hurt-women

American Association of Colleges of Nursing. (2009, February). Despite surge of interest in nursing careers, new AACN data confirm that too few nurses are entering the healthcare workforce. Retrieved from http://www.aacn.nche.edu/media/NewsReleases/2009/workforcedata.html

Aquilar, F., & Galluccio, M. (2007). *Psychological processes in international negotiations: Theoretical and practical perspectives.* London, UK: Springer Publishing.

Babcock, L., & Laschever, S. (2008). *Asking for it: How women can use the power of negotiation.* New York, NY: Bantam.

Bishop, S. (2013). *Develop your assertiveness* (3rd ed.). London, UK: Kogan Page.

Bolman, L. G., & Deal, T. E. (2013). *Reframing organizations: Artistry, choice and leadership.* San Francisco, CA: Jossey-Bass.

Changing Minds.org. Negotiation mistakes. Retrieved from http://changingminds.org/disciplines/negotiation/mistakes/mistakes.htm

Cohen, H. (2007). *Negotiate this! By caring, But not T-H-A-T much.* New York, NY: Business Plus.

CRR Global. (2011). *Organization and relationship systems coaching manual.* Vallejo, CA: Author.

Deep Democracy Institute. (2009). Retrieved from http://deepdemocracyexchange.com

Donaldson, M. C., & Frohnmayer, D. (2007). *Negotiating for dummies* (2nd ed.). Hoboken, NJ: Wiley.

Fisher, R., Ury, W., & Patton, B. (2011). *Getting to yes: Negotiating agreement without giving in.* New York, NY: Penguin Books.

Gallo, A. (2015, March). Setting the record straight on negotiating your salary. *Harvard Business Review.* Retrieved from https://hbr.org/2015/03/setting-the-record-straight-on-negotiating-your-salary&cm_sp=Article

Goleman, D. (2012). *Emotional intelligence.* New York, NY: Random House.

Goleman, D., & Boyatzis, R. (2008). Social intelligence and the biology of leadership. *Harvard Business Review, 86*(9), 74–81.

Goleman, D., Boyatzis, R., & McKee, A. (2013). *Primal leadership: Unleashing the power of emotional intelligence.* Cambridge, MA: Harvard Business Review Press.

Gormley, H., & van Nieuwerburgh, C. (2014). Developing coaching cultures: A review of the literature. *Coaching: An International Journal of Theory, Research & Practice, 7,* 90–101.

Gottman, J. M. (2007). Making relationships work. *Harvard Business Review, 85*(12), 45–50.

Gottman, J. M. (2011). *The science of trust.* New York, NY: W. W. Norton.

Gottman, J. M., & Silver, N. (2015). *The seven principles for making marriage work.* New York, NY: Penguin Random House.

Harris, P. R., Moran, R. T., & Moran, S. V. (2007). *Managing cultural differences: Global leadership strategies for the twenty-first century* (7th ed.). Los Angeles, CA: Butterworth and Heinemann.

Hennig, J. (2008). *How to say it: Negotiating too Win: Key words, phrases, and strategies to close the deal and build lasting relationships.* Upper Saddle River, NJ: Prentice Hall.

Holt, J. L., & DeVore, C. (2005). Culture, gender, organizational role, and styles of conflict resolution: A meta-analysis. *International Journal of Intercultural Relations, 29,* 147–151.

Holt, M. D. (2010). Overcoming the mental barriers to equal pay. *Harvard Business Review.* Retrieved from https://hbr.org/2010/04/ovecoming-the-mental-barriers

Katz, N. H., & Pattarini, N. M. (2008). Interest-based negotiation: An essential business and communications tool for the public relations counselor. *Journal of Communication Management, 12*(1), 88–97.

Kay, K., & Shipman, C. (2014). *The confidence code: The science and art of self-assurance—What women should know.* New York, NY: HarperBusiness.

Lewicki, R. J., Barry, B., & Saunders, D. M. (2015). *Essentials of negotiation* (6th ed.). New York, NY: McGraw-Hill.

Malhotra, D., & Bazerman, M. (2007). *Negotiation genius: How to overcome obstacles and achieve brilliant results at the bargaining table and beyond.* New York, NY: Bantam.

McClure, J. S. (2007). *Civilized assertiveness for women: Communication with backbone...not bite.* Denver, CO: Albion Street Press.

Mindell, A. (2012). *Bringing deep democracy to life: An awareness paradigm for deepening political dialog, personal relationships, and community interactions.* Portland, OR: Process Work Institute. Retrieved from www.aamindell.net

Mindell, A. (2014). *The leader as martial artist.* Portland, OR: Deep Democracy Exchange.

Mindell, A. (2015). *Sitting in the fire: Large group transformation using conflict and diversity.* Portland, OR: Deep Democracy Exchange.

Murphy, J. (2011). *Assertiveness: How to stand up for yourself and still win the respect of others.* Charleston, SC: CreateSpace.

Raiffa, H., Richardson, J., & Metcalfe, D. (2007). *Negotiation analysis: The science and art of collaborative decision making*. Boston, MA: Belknap Press.

Sandberg, S. (2013). *Lean in: Women, work, and the will to lead*. New York, NY: Knopf.

Shapiro, R. M. (2015). *The power of nice: How to negotiate so everyone wins—Especially you!* New York, NY: John Wiley.

Skinner, S. (2014). Understanding the importance of gender and leader identify formation in executive coaching for senior women. *Coaching: An International Journal of Theory, Research & Practice, 7,* 102–114.

Thomas, K. W., Thomas, G. F., & Schaubhut, N. (2008). Conflict styles of men and women at six organizational levels. *International Journal of Conflict Management, 14*(2), 1–38.

Thompson, L. (2007). *The truth about negotiations*. Upper Saddle River, NJ: FT Press.

Reflective Response

Jared D. Simmer

The American Association of Colleges of Nursing (AACN) issued a position statement holding that the Doctor of Nursing Practice (DNP) degree should provide advanced clinical competencies, in addition to enhanced leadership skills to strengthen practice and health care delivery, and later developed specific doctoral competencies in 2006 (AACN, 2004, 2006). In 2008, The Robert Wood Johnson Foundation (RWJF) partnered with the Institutes of Medicine (IOM) to launch a 2-year initiative that would assess and transform the nursing profession. It focused on the following question: What roles can nursing assume to address the increasing demand for safe, high-quality, and effective health care services? How well nurses are educated and do their jobs is inextricably tied to most health care quality measures that have been targeted for improvement. Thus for nursing, health care reform provides an opportunity for the profession to position itself to help address the demand for safe, high-quality, patient-centered, and equitable health care services (IOM, 2011).

Nichols, O'Connor, and Dunn (2014) noted that it remains to be seen what roles DNPs will be expected to fill, and the competencies nurse-leaders will need in order to succeed. These authors observed that chief nursing officers (CNOs) are not well versed in the clinical outcomes of DNP practice or the population health outcomes that may be impacted by DNP-prepared providers. CNOs' knowledge of DNP-prepared nurses' abilities is critical to the widespread adoption and impact of DNPs in the health care system. The nursing profession envisions an even broader health care–centric education, and practice role for DNPs, including applying research findings to improve outcomes, policy development, project management (e.g., Quality Improvement [QI] initiatives, the Magnet® application process), nursing unit management, participation on cross-disciplinary health care teams, and risk management, to name just a few.

However, wherever DNPs find themselves, in my opinion, the most important skill set they need in order to succeed will involve their ability to act as advocates, persuade others to their point of view, anticipate and resolve conflict, manage staff, encourage collaboration, and improve clinical outcomes—all skills that have at their heart the ability to negotiate with others effectively. Although career opportunities for DNPs continue to evolve, the chapter is correct to point out that they can expect to encounter many situations requiring sound negotiation skills. However, research suggests Cavanagh (1991) and my first-hand experience confirms that rather than take advantage of opportunities to negotiate, most nurses prefer to avoid/withdraw (perhaps this also helps explain one of the reasons for high nursing turnover rates). The Dual Concerns Model illustrates the consequences of using a particular negotiating style. The negotiating style has an impact on two levels, demonstrating how an avoidant style harms both the relationship between the parties and the outcome.

To me, negotiation should not be seen as a useful skill; rather, it should be accepted as an essential skill for the simple reason that sound negotiation skills provide many benefits, both personally and professionally: a greater willingness to act assertively; the ability to be a more effective advocate for both self and others; stronger powers of persuasion, enhanced credibility, better leadership, and management skills (e.g., delegation and coaching); the capacity to prevent and manage conflict and facilitate workplace collaboration; and the confidence and the ability to work more effectively with physicians and other health professionals to improve clinical outcomes; as an added benefit, DNPs with strong negotiation skills are also better positioned to search out and secure career advancement opportunities, and insist on fair compensation for their services.

While the chapter provides a useful introduction to some of the important issues in the field, DNPs should keep in mind the important difference between "learning about a skill" (the educational process), and "learning how to use a skill" (the training process) for it is this second approach that best facilitates skill acquisition. So, I would like to add to the topics addressed in the chapter by pointing out some other negotiation

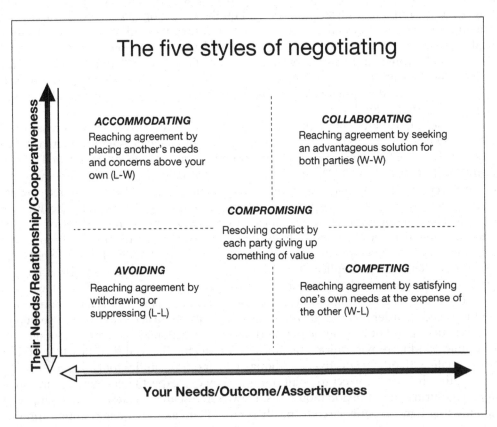

FIGURE 15.2 The dual concerns model: The five styles of negotiating.
Source: Pruitt and Carnevale (1993).

fundamentals that once mastered can lead to immediate and lasting improvements in the DNP's nurse ability to negotiate effectively:

- Self-awareness of how one reacts to conflict (because negotiation is a conflict resolution technique, how one views conflict directly affects how they approach negotiation)
- Learning to view negotiation as mutual problem-solving rather than a contest (i.e., collaboration not competition)
- Although it is true that some negotiators are born, good negotiators can also be "made" (i.e., research as well as my own experience confirm that like any other skill, negotiation can taught, oftentimes with skill improvement happening quickly and dramatically)
- Not only learning to recognize opportunities to negotiate (for instance, a staff meeting creates many opportunities to negotiate although most would not see it that way) but being aware that women are less likely to see interactions as potential negotiations, and less likely to negotiate when they do
- Awareness of gender differences, including how women tend to view the negotiation process negatively and the assumptions and behaviors that can put them at a disadvantage (fortunately, these can be ameliorated with proper awareness and training)
- It's more important for people to respect you and your abilities than it is that you go out of your way to be overly accommodating so that they "like" you
- Learning to become comfortable "asking" for things that can get your needs met (because of the way females are socialized, women are taught not to speak up; but, again, this is something that can be addressed with proper training and practice)
- Overcoming the tendency to walk away from opportunities to negotiate, even when the situation calls for it (nurses tend to be conflict avoidant, usually either because of perceived power imbalances, or because they assume that their opinions will be ignored)
- The need to understand the five styles of negotiation (compete, avoid, collaborate, compromise, and accommodate), the ability and willingness to employ each style as appropriate, self-awareness of the style or styles that are overused, and an awareness that mismatching a particular style to a given situation (e.g., acting avoidant and not speaking up when one's competency is being questioned) lead to suboptimal outcomes
- Realizing that prenegotiation preparation is the primary predictor of negotiating success, including generating a best alternative to a negotiated agreement (known as aBATNA, or the best course of action someone can take if the upcoming negotiation is unsuccessful)—having alternatives not only increases negotiating power, but improves the ability to walk away from bad deals
- Setting "asking" (what one hopes to achieve), "target" (what one expects to achieve) and "reservation" prices (the bottom line or the least one will settle for) before sitting down to negotiate
- "Framing," or how one words a proposal, can affect how willing the other side is to accept it
- The need to anticipate and prepare to overcome the "no's" one expects to hear from the other side during the negotiation
- Disabusing yourself of the notion that negotiation is something that "men do"
- Knowing that adopting a collaborative negotiation style leads to the best outcomes about 80% of the time

However, DNPs not only need to recognize how important negotiation skills are to their career success, but have to commit to take advantage of opportunities to improve their skills. There are various methodologies that can be employed to achieve this, including:

- Seeking out an effective negotiator as a mentor
- Working with a negotiation coach
- Taking a class, either in person or online
- Engaging in self-study, for instance by reading books or watching videos on negotiation-related topics
- Attending seminars
- Enrolling in a training class
- Taking a negotiation course offered by a local college or university
- Subscribing to a service that provides periodic mailings on various negotiation topics (such as Negotiation Briefings published by the Harvard Program on Negotiation)
- Signing up for online negotiation-related blogs and newsletters
- Joining negotiation-related LinkedIn groups

In conclusion, I would like to reiterate my agreement with the central theme of the chapter that negotiation is a critical competency for the DNP-prepared nurse and something that he or she will use on a daily basis. Subpar skills have many predictable negative consequences, including stunting or even terminating careers, causing difficulties in relationships, compromising one's perceived credibility and competency, creating unnecessary conflict, increasing the probability that a person has to remain underappreciated and underpaid, and harming the ability to be persuasive. Nurses can benefit personally and professionally by committing to improving their personal negotiation skills, becoming aware of their current strengths and weaknesses, taking advantage of opportunities to improve, and committing to regular putting these new skills into practice. In addition to encouraging current DNPs to improve their skills, I also strongly believe that the nursing profession could benefit greatly by including negotiation coursework in the standard DNP curriculum if for no other reason than that graduates of other programs (e.g., MBA, MHA, law schools, and master's of medical management programs) who will be competing for leadership roles in health care with DNPs have already done so.

■ REFERENCES

American Association of the Colleges of Nursing. (2004). *AACN position statement on the practice doctorate in nursing*. Washington, DC: Author.

American Association of the Colleges of Nursing. (2006). *The essentials of doctoral education for advanced nursing practice*. Washington, DC: Author.

Cavanagh, S. J. (1991). The conflict management style of staff nurses and nurse managers. *Journal of Advanced Nursing, 16*, 1254–1260. doi:10.1111/j.1365-2648.1991.tb01536.x

Institute of Medicine. (2011). *The future of nursing: Leading change, advancing health*. Washington, DC: National Academies Press. Retrieved from http://iom.nationalacademies.org/Reports/2010/The-Future-of-Nursing-Leading-Change-Advancing-Health.aspx#sthash.38nO0oh4.pdf

Nichols, C., O'Connor, N., & Dunn, D. (2014). Exploring early and future use of DNP prepared nurses within healthcare organizations. *The Journal of Nursing Administration, 44*(2), 74–78.

Pruitt, D. G., & Carnevale, P. J. (1993). *Negotiation in social conflict*. Pacific Grove, CA: Brooks/Cole.

Seeking Lifelong Mentorship and Menteeship in the Doctoral Advanced Nursing Practice Role

Roberta Waite and Deena Nardi

Doctor of Nursing Practice (DNP) programs were inaugurated by the University of Kentucky when they opened the first DNP program in 2001 (Sebastian & White, 2013). Over 250 DNP programs now exist with many more being planned (Carter & Moore, 2015). This is a relatively new role and great expectations are anticipated; however, when innovative changes such as the DNP occur, challenges as well as opportunities exist. In order to promote effective role assimilation and role development of DNPs, mentorship can play a critical role in the successful development of the next generation of nurses in advanced nursing practice, especially in today's changing climate of health care delivery. Notably, mentorship significantly influences professional career planning, professional productivity, as well as professional satisfaction.

Mentorship has existed since ancient Greek civilization (Huang, Huang, & Lynch, 1995); however, perspectives on mentorship have broadened since this time encompassing a more dynamic and fluid relationship. More contemporary perspectives assert that "mentoring has become conceptualized with respect to its relational, developmental, and contextual dimensions" (Adams, 2013, p. 38). Clearly, the underpinning of mentorship involves the social exchange theory (Bartley-Daniele, 2014). Ideally, a DNP will strive to "grow, develop, and sustain mentoring relationships that are reciprocal, communicative, and mutually beneficial;" moreover, mentorships are distinctive in "duration, intensity, and outcomes" (Bartley-Daniele, 2014, p. 30). As DNPs explore unique opportunities that stem from this interaction, it will become evident that mentoring relationships they take on will progress through the stages including initiation, cultivation, separation, and redefinition (Bartley-Daniele, 2014).

As an interactive, facilitative process intended to encourage learning and development, mentorship has the capability of minimizing transition shock of DNPs into their newfound roles. Providing support for "professional (e.g., sponsorship, exposure and visibility, coaching, protection, challenging) and psychosocial (e.g., role modeling, acceptance and confirmation, counseling, friendship) developments" helps DNPs as they enter their specialized roles and their respective professional workplaces with varying levels of confidence and experience, consequently produc-ing great variability in what they will need to achieve success (Gagliardi, Webster, Perrier, Bell, & Straus, 2014, p. 124). As such, mentees must consciously reflect on what competencies, skills, and experiences will benefit them in real-time and in the future. Insight by the mentee will be increased during mentoring interactions since emphasis is on stimulating the mentee to act with thoughtful deliberation, in conjunction with having a shared vision with the mentor. Therefore, the men-tee is motivated in a deliberate and strategic way to create a sense of purpose and nourish those shared higher goals. This unique relationship between mentee and mentor has the propensity to cultivate each mentee's capacity to succeed in their role as a DNP.

More nuanced forms of mentorship have been discussed in the literature. Thomas-MacLean, Hamoline, Quinlan, Ramsden and Kuzmicz (2010) identified differences between traditional mentoring and transformational mentoring. Traditional mentor-ship is seen as a continuation of earlier accounts of mentorship. This would translate into DNP mentors being "older, wiser, and senior" to the younger mentee that he or she would groom. Thus, there would be a hierarchical process that could value the wise sen-ior above the inexperienced junior. In contrast, transformational mentoring is "a rela-tionship between equals in which one or more of those involved is enabled to increase awareness, identify alternatives and initiate action, and develop themselves (Thomas-MacLean et al., 2010, p. e265)." As such, DNPs in a mentor–mentee relationship would share knowledge and expertise about their profession as well as mutually hone skills of mentorship to further human capacity for inner growth and development (Thomas-MacLean et al., 2010). DNPs will likely develop mentoring relationships characterizing both of these conceptualizations—traditional and transformational. In considering the aforementioned insights on mentorship, this eloquent quote embodies the essence of what should be desired:

> The greatest good you can do for another is not just to share your riches but to reveal to him his own. (Benjamin Disraeli, 1804–1881, British prime minis-ter [Ray, 2012, p. 69])

Mentorship for DNPs would benefit from deliberate decision-making processes. Forward planning by the mentee and mentor through designing appropriate interven-tions and guidance can optimize the DNPs' progression and increase their competency in the desired areas. Seeking mentorship from visionary leaders is important for DNPs as their role in promoting health and health-service delivery in the 21st century is not a replica of preparation of advanced nursing practice of the past. Mentorship is also important to help enhance consciousness about cultural diversity and promote the use of individual qualities including a personal power to solve the current-day challenges in the health care environment. DNPs will be working with interdisciplinary health care providers; therefore, they must develop and implement skills that also support strategy development to effectively address organizational issues. Taken together, building the capacity for DNPs to have a profound and positive impact on leadership and national health care policy initiatives as well as primary care services delivery is paramount and mentorship is a central ingredient in achieving these outcomes.

Even more, mentorship must be valued and supported by entities that come in contact with DNPs—for example, universities, hospital systems, professional organizations, and other health-related bodies. This investment starts with each organization; however, the culture of mentorship must permeate our greater health culture. Incentives, resources, and educational programs are all essential for the development and sustainability of nurturing a culture of mentorship. What has been written about mentorship in advanced nursing practice for those nurses who are DNPs? This chapter will examine vital elements of mentoring and their application to individuals who were recently awarded a DNP as well to those interested in mentoring DNPs. Specifically, areas to be explored include: (a) the history of mentorship in nursing; (b) mentorship models, as well as the characteristics of mentors; (c) mentoring of underrepresented groups among DNPs; (d) preparation of mentors; and (e) future trends and recommendations for the profession concerning mentorship of DNP-prepared professionals. The magnitude of concern about mentorship is heightened given the shortage of experienced leaders in the nursing profession and the lack of resources thus far attributed to support meaningful mentoring relationships.

■ HISTORY OF MENTORSHIP AND MENTEESHIP IN THE NURSING PROFESSION

The more complicated new role expectations are, the more necessary mentoring becomes.
                                              Angela Barron McBride (2008, p. 368)

EARLY HISTORY

The process of mentoring was first recorded as an important role for leaders during the Trojan War, in approximately 1,200 BCE. That is when Mentor, a family friend of the Greek king Odysseus, acted as a surrogate parent, counselor, and guide for the apprentice-king Telemachus until his father Odysseus returned from the war (Trumble & Brown, 2002). Most recently, science-based professions have used networking and mentoring to encourage and support new students and colleagues as they become enculturated to a new organization, academic setting, and/or private practice (Rosser & Taylor, 2009). One example of this goal-focused mentoring is the national STEM (acronym for science, technology, engineering, and mathematics) programs in primary, secondary, and higher education to mentor young students into science and technology-based careers (Garringer, Kupersmidt, Rhodes, Stelter, & Tai, 2015; STEM Education Coalition, 2015).

The culture of mentorship in advanced nursing practice is still in its infancy, yet nursing has been an occupation since the dawn of mankind, when early mankind probably first picked up an aloe plant and used it to soothe a wound. Nursing as a profession has a much more recent genesis; however, first recognized as such through the works of Florence Nightingale (Nightingale, 1859). Advanced nursing practice has evolved more recently as a response to regulatory requirements and rapid scientific advances and health care change, and continues to evolve as a distinct and independent health profession. Advanced nursing practice includes the four roles of advanced practice nurses (APNs) and nurses in other advanced roles. Most nurses are familiar with the four roles of nurse practitioners, clinical nurse specialists, nurse midwives, and nurse anesthetists. The health care roles of nurses with graduate and doctoral degrees and advanced interests have expanded rapidly to include other advanced roles such as informatics specialist, scientist, administrator, entrepreneur, and business owner/operator. This expanded practice and growing need for all doctorally prepared nurses makes finding and preparing mentors all the more important.

MENTORING IN PROFESSIONAL NURSING

We might consider Florence Nightingale as the first mentor of professional nurses. She mentored Linda Richards, considered the first professional nurse in the United States, who trained in 1877 at Nightingale's training school St. Thomas Hospital in London (Wayne, 2014). Ms. Richards then returned to America and established several nursing schools in the United States. Mentoring is recognized as an important facilitator of nursing scholarship, as well as socialization to the advanced nursing practice role (Chism, 2013; Robert Wood Johnson Foundation, 2012). However, in recent years, nurses in advanced roles have been faced with a paucity of mentors. This situation is due to a confluence of events, including the nursing shortage, the nursing faculty shortage, the proliferation of distance learning and online classes, new roles for doctorally prepared nurses as primary health care providers, and lack of inclusion for underrepresented nurses.

The American Association of Colleges of Nursing (AACN) emphasizes the need for mentoring/precepting/supporting new doctorally prepared nurses. They suggest that doctoral programs for nurses, including DNP programs, recruit faculty and preceptors from a wide variety of disciplines for these positions. In this way, all doctoral students have exposure to other role models and mentors when no nursing mentor is available (AACN, 2015a). The Council of Graduate Schools also reported that during exit surveys, mentoring was identified as essential for doctorate completion (Council of Graduate Schools, 2009). Nurses in doctoral advanced practice are prepared to take the lead in mentoring qualified candidates in order to establish a pipeline of competent and confident health care providers, scientists, educators, and researchers.

■ MODELS OF MENTORSHIP AND MENTEESHIP IN THE NURSING PROFESSION

A number of mentoring models have been described in the nursing literature, and most can be categorized as: traditional, group, team, peer and, most recently, e-mentoring, which would be mentoring through e-mail, teleconferencing, or the internet (Garringer et al., 2015). Traditionally, mentoring in nursing has either occurred informally or as a planned program where the individual is matched with an experienced nurse in a formal one-to-one program. Although such programs can benefit nurses, the shortage of graduate-degree nurses means that many will miss out on the opportunity to support professional growth and development of new nurses, particularly new doctoral graduates. Further, mentoring dyads do little to enhance the more collaborative atmosphere now prevalent in professional nursing and health care settings. Alternative nontraditional mentoring approaches such as team, peer, multifaceted, or group, then, can provide advantages to the traditional approach. Deciding how doctoral students and new graduates can best be supported is critical given the diverse populations and complexities in contemporary health care and the need for interprofessional collaboration (Chism, 2013). Therefore, doctorally prepared graduates may need multiple mentors to develop their new roles, or they may need several mentors in succession, as they grow into and develop new roles.

There are fewer mentorship models particularly designed for doctorally prepared nurses, but selected models have been adapted or can be adapted to meet this need. For instance, the multifaceted mentoring model was specifically developed to contribute to greater productivity of researchers, especially minority researchers, in the fields of biomedical and social sciences (Rabionet, Santiago, & Zorrilla, 2009). This multifaceted mentoring model includes establishing multi-institutional collaborations, offering systematic and continuous training based on competency development, and creating interdisciplinary research teams in which mentors and mentees work together. Attention to these three processes produces synergy and provides the solid foundation needed to foster long-standing mentor–mentee relationships.

The adaptation of this model to doctorally prepared advanced nursing practice encourages the DNP student to search for additional mentors as needed to accommodate DNP projects, objectives, practice plans, and professional goals. Fundamental to this model is the understanding that mentoring is a synergistic process in which mentors and mentees could jointly advance their commitment to scholarly pursuit; thus, mentoring is envisioned as a process of multifaceted and multi-institutional collaboration for a systematic engagement. This model also exposes students to valid perspectives from a variety of mentors, and can inspire and empower the mentee and mentors (Graves & Hanson, 2014).

When used in field supervision as "multiple mentoring" (Moran, Burson, & Conrad, 2014, p. 225), it offers a platform for researchers and clinicians from diverse disciplines to appreciate what they share and to explore what is beyond their disciplinary domains. Importantly, the multifaceted and multiple mentoring models have the potential to be replicated in various contexts, and can form a bridge to networking for future research, practice, and other scholarship for both the mentee and mentor.

■ EFFECTIVE MENTORING

MENTORING PROCESS

One example of effective mentoring is the process that the University of Rochester, School of Nursing, uses to improve the diversity of their faculty and support more minority and male enrollment in all of its nursing degree programs. Supported by the grant of New Careers in Nursing (NCIN) from the Robert Wood Johnson Foundation (2015), the mentorship process begins with the students, all of whom are second-career nurses, choosing their faculty mentor. The dean meets with NCIN students each month, each session with a special focus. The overriding theme of each session is to support and advise each other. The NCIN program has produced anther initiative, LIFT: Elevating Each Other, consisting of brown-bag luncheon sessions on leadership and diversity. Since the start of the program, seven NCIN graduates, all from underrepresented groups, have joined the faculty (Robert Wood Johnson Foundation, 2015).

Another example of effective mentoring, synthesizing the peer mentoring and multifaceted mentoring models, is the process used by the University of St. Francis College of Nursing DNP Program in Joliet, Illinois. Students in its post-master's DNP program begin their studies with mostly decades of experience as nursing leaders: many own their own businesses; others who have published, are educators, or may have served in key positions in professional organizations or in acute care hospitals. They are new again to the graduate student role, and are acculturating to the new role of DNP, but they are practicing specialists, mostly board-certified advanced practice registered nurses (APRNs), in their own right. They learn about the background, practice, and research interests of faculty at orientation, and both faculty and students are encouraged to connect and share interests with each other in preparation for the students' scholarly papers at the culmination of their programs of study. The purpose is to encourage networking, role model collegiality in doctoral advanced nurses, and build a system of mutual collaboration in scholarly projects. When planning their culminating DNP projects (i.e., scholarly initiatives), they are directed to seek out other mentors connected to their interest and practice setting to guide and provide constructive criticism. They also form or join research and practice teams as part of their doctoral course work, and several of these student–faculty and student–student partnerships have resulted in evidence-based system improvements in health care settings, have been published in peer-reviewed journals, and presented at professional conferences.

Figure 16.1 depicts this dynamic process as continuous, as the process of mentoring first moves from mutual introductions, commitment, and contract formation, through anticipatory information sharing and exchanges, to the mentor actively supporting the student's scholarship, to the final collaborative relationship. Encircling this process is the required organizational support in terms of time, recognition, and resources, which enables this relationship to develop to its potential.

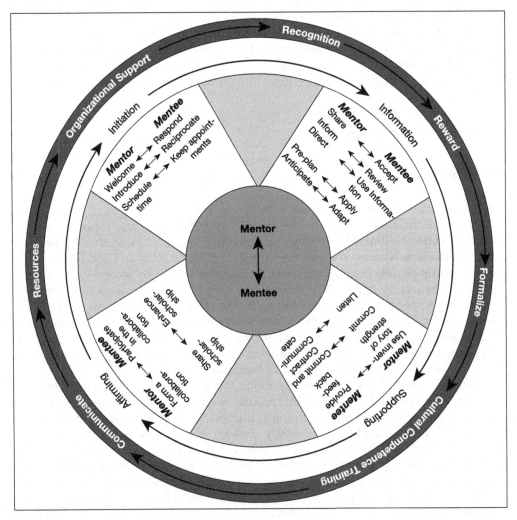

FIGURE 16.1   University of St. Francis mentoring model.

ORGANIZATIONAL AND SYSTEM SUPPORT FOR MENTORING

Anyone planning a mentoring program can learn from a wide variety of successful programs that could be adapted to doctoral education, or new careers, or research and nursing science positions. A formal program of mentorship not only requires willing participants and a plan, but also a supportive environment for the mentor and mentee alike. The mentor invests a considerable amount of time, effort, and persistence to advance and nurture the mentee. This investment ultimately benefits the organization in measurable outcomes of employee and student productivity, retention, and satisfaction. This investment needs to be recognized by the organization, but it must be supported and rewarded if it is to continue. The following are key institutional resources and supports that organizations, such as universities, schools, hospitals, and other organizations should provide to support the mentoring role of its employees. The dean or chief nursing officer can:

- See that a template for a written contract or signed agreement between mentee and mentor is developed and available for use as a guide to keep the process on target.
- Provide training on the role of a mentor, which includes cultural sensitivity training for *all* employees (e.g., administrators, staff, and faculty) to promote the value of this role to the organization. The emphasis on formal training conveys the organization's investment in diversity and the mentoring process.
- Support the mentoring process over time, since mentoring relationships develop gradually, creating mutual trust and finding mutual interests. These relationships are guided by the goals of the mentee.
- Create avenues for communicating the interests for meeting new candidates and for mentees and mentors to view the work and backgrounds of potential mentors.
- *Avoid* arbitrarily assigning mentors to newly hired employees or to new doctoral students.
- Provide logistical support, such as release time from job-related duties and functions, so the mentor can find the time to meet with the mentee, and will *not* ultimately view the role as overtime, overload, or extra work.
- Communicate the value of the mentoring role to key internal and external stakeholders This communication can be done in the form of written communication (e.g., newsletter article, posters), or formal events where mentors can be introduced to others in the organization, or in informal conversations.
- Formally recognize and reinforce effective mentoring. This recognition can come in many forms including a raise or stipend, a certificate of appreciation, or letter of support that can be added to a portfolio, or submission of the mentor's name for an award.
- Support the development of a process for mentors to identify and support each other. This process might come in the form of a support group, or list serve, or monthly meeting. The goal of the supportive process is to nurture the nurturers, and to retain the leaders among us who choose to advance and support other APNs.

Organizational support for the mentoring programs, program objectives, degree of program oversight, and ongoing relationship support, rewards for program participation, and the specific procedure used to match mentors and mentees is critical. When the organizational supports are in place, then the mentor and mentee can concentrate on creating productive relationships.

The following two cases present brief illustrations of two distinct mentoring styles, with distinctly different outcomes, depending largely upon the nature of the relationship between mentor and mentee:

■ CASE STUDY I: David: A DNP Student

David was in his last year of doctoral study, and was about to register for his culminating DNP course, which required him, as part of an interdisciplinary team in a mental health setting, to design and implement an evidence-based quality improvement program. He was having difficulty deciding on an approach to assessing the needs of the topic or population to study. His faculty advisor mentioned his difficulty to another faculty who was involved in a countywide assessment of mental health needs in uninsured patients and their families. She approached David and asked him if he would like to join her at the planning meetings and decide if he would like to participate in the project. He agreed and accompanied her to the next planning meeting, where she introduced him to several stakeholders, and directed him to sit at the table with her. During the planning discussions at the table, she would seek his opinions, and explained some constructs and history to him when needed. She asked him if he would like to develop a questionnaire and interview a group of stakeholders, and he agreed. They met in her office several times during the first few months thereafter, during which she guided him in coding, categorizing, and interpreting responses. David completed his capstone paper, which was used by the mental health center as evidence needed to fund a new program at the center. His mentor then invited him to present his study at a regional research conference. During his presentation, David pointed to his mentor and thanked her for her help. She asked him if he wanted to rewrite the paper for submission to a nursing journal, and he willingly agreed. He wrote the paper with her assistance, it was submitted to a nursing journal, was accepted, and published a year later. She incorporated the study into the literature review for a proposal she wrote a year later, which was approved and funded by the Health Resources and Services Administration division of the U.S. Department of Health and Human Services.

■ CASE STUDY II: Patricia: A PhD and New Faculty Member

Patricia returned to graduate school after 20 years of practice in acute care hospitals as a critical-care clinical nurse specialist. She had just graduated with a PhD degree, and had accepted a position as an assistant professor at a small nursing school. This would be the first time she would assume the role of a nurse educator, although she had precepted many nursing students at work. She received a short orientation to her role, and was told that the chair of the course that she was assigned to would be her mentor. She had many questions and concerns about her role and about how to identify and

(continued)

■ CASE STUDY II: Patricia: A PhD and New
   Faculty Member (*continued*)

access resources she would need to create and teach her courses. Her efforts
to contact her mentor, however, were unsuccessful. They had not established
any regular times to meet, her phone messages went unanswered, and her
e-mails were either answered late or the chair's responses were so brief as to
be useless. When she approached the chair after faculty meetings, the chair
would complain about her workload, the students, and other faculty. Patricia
reached out to other faculty, and found one who answered her questions and
helped her as she learned her new role. But even this faculty did not seem
to welcome her, or include her in any informal meetings or lunches. After
the first semester, the chair told her that the faculty who taught in the clinical course always met at her house to calculate final grades, so she would
be expected to travel across the city to her chair's home, and bring her student's graded papers with her, which she did. The meeting took most of the
day, although the actual time spent calculating students' grades was about
an hour. At the end of the meeting, she picked up what she thought was all
of her student papers, placed them in her briefcase, and traveled across the
town again to her house. Later that evening, she realized that a paper was
missing when she emptied her briefcase. She called the chair, who told her
that the paper was not there. Patricia spent a sleepless night, and then the
next morning she searched her home, car, and office but could not find the
papers. As she prepared to contact the student, another faculty called her to
tell her that the chair had the paper, but had decided to keep it for a few days
to teach Patricia to keep better track of her student's papers. Patricia finished
her semester at that nursing school, but quit at the end of the year, vowing
to never again take a teaching position in nursing. Years later, however, she
once again accepted a position as an assistant professor at a nursing school,
this time with much better results. She is now a full professor, with teaching and scholarship recognition, enjoying an academic experience, and she
makes a point of welcoming and mentoring new faculty.

■ MEETING THE NEEDS OF UNDERREPRESENTED GROUPS OF DOCTORAL ADVANCED NURSES

Professional nursing is reflective of America and its racialized society. Needless to say,
over the course of time, especially at its origin, underrepresented groups were prevented by Caucasian nurses from gaining access to professional education programs
as well as professional nursing organizations. This clearly contributed to limiting and
preventing access to leadership roles in academic programs, clinical practice, and professional organizations for racial and ethnic minority populations for a period of time.
This pattern of discrimination by a European-heritage-dominant mainstream culture
can be traced back Margaret Sanger and Ms. Nightingale, the same Nightingale who
so successfully mentored Linda Richards, a Caucasian American nurse, in 1877. Mary
Seacole, a Jamaican nurse, visited Ms. Nightingale in Scutari during the Crimean War
and offered her services as part of the nursing staff, and was refused. Seemingly un-
daunted, Ms. Seacole established a British hotel near the battlefield, where she tended to

the sick and wounded from that war (Lewis, 2013). Sanger, an early American nursing activist, "emphasized the necessity of birth control in reducing the reproduction of the 'unfit,'" reinforcing "the notion that the fertility of the poor, and by extension that of the Black race, was a proper subject of social and governmental control" (Holland, 2011, p. 19). This racialized history, nursing's tradition, and normalized values of whiteness are foundational in shaping the profession even until today with how education, practice, leadership, and mentorship are effected (Schroeder & DeAngelo, 2010).

Although increased numbers of people from minority cultures are enrolling in doctoral programs (AACN, 2015c), individual, institutional, and systemic discriminatory practices have created a system of barriers to advanced nursing practice and leadership in health care and academia. These barriers to upward mobility and practice for nurses from minority cultures challenge nursing today, and are shown in:

- Lack of mentors from underrepresented groups (i.e., gender, religion, ethnic heritage, sexual orientation—lesbian, gay, bisexual, or transgender)
- No training or insufficient training in cultural sensitivity for faculty, providers, and administrators who serve as mentors
- Lack of explicit antiracist emancipatory work in the profession of nursing especially among our leaders
- Doctoral programs that require on-campus residency, making it challenging if not impossible for many candidates with family obligations to attend
- Insufficient funding support for a doctoral study, which impedes the career advancement of many nurses who are sole financial supports of their families

Mentoring has special significance for faculty of minority status. Without such help, these faculty members can have difficulty cracking *the old girls' network* as well as exposing and challenging whiteness and its associated privileges. A mentor can be very helpful in this regard, as successful mentoring can help minority and marginalized doctoral students climb the professional ladder and aid in the dismantling of inequities encountered by underrepresented nurses seeking DNPs. For historical reasons, owing to their prominence in senior positions, middle-aged European American women predominantly have fulfilled the role of mentor in the Western world. Even though they can be capable mentors to members of underrepresented groups, there needs to be heightened critical consciousness and sensitivity when cultural differences surface in order to cultivate a fulfilling and mutually beneficial relationship.

The number of students from minority backgrounds who are enrolling in graduate and doctoral nursing programs has been slowly but steadily rising for the past 5 years, underscoring the growing need for mentors who can best understand and support this population. By 2014, students from minority backgrounds represented 39.1% of enrollments in master of science in nursing (MSN) programs, 40% of enrollments in nursing PhD programs, and 34.8% of enrollments in DNP programs (AACN, 2015c). However, just 12% of all nursing faculty are from minority backgrounds (Beard & Volcy, 2013).

Membership of minority cultures in many professional nursing organizations are also disproportionate to their total number in the population, which was 37% in 2012, and predicted to become the majority population by 2043 (AACN, 2015c). For instance, the latest survey of American Academy of Nurse Practitioners membership shows 4.9% are African American, 3.6 % are Hispanic American, and 1.5% are American Indian/ Native Hawaiian/Pacific Islander/biracial (Cook & Riley, 2014).

The AACN has examined this disparity in minority representation in advanced nursing practice. It calls for all nursing education programs to strive for ethnic and racial diversity in its faculty and students (AACN, 2015c). Meeting this goal will take a combination of collective will, focused recruiting, support, networking, and mentoring of doctoral candidates, students, and DNPs who are new to a role or position. One of the strategies to accomplish this goal is to create formal mentoring programs that embody values of inclusion, social justice, and empowerment while recruiting and supporting nurses from underrepresented groups for DNP preparation in direct health care delivery, education, and research.

One of the most successful of these formal mentoring programs is the "Bridges to the Doctorate for Minority Nursing Students" (NIGMS Minority Programs Update, 2015), which is a program begun in 2003 to increase the number of doctorally prepared minority nurses in the United States, funded through a grant of the National Institutes of Health (NIH) Bridges. The program consists of partner schools of nursing (Chicago's DePaul University, Purdue University Calumet, and the University of Illinois Chicago [UIC]) collaborating to recruit, support, and mentor MSN students into a PhD in Nursing program. Program coordinators guide and counsel students throughout the application process. Seminars and socials provide needed peer and faculty mentoring and networking time. NIH Research Training Grants support students' research and fund studies. Data show that faculty-mentoring supports as well as financial support are key to retention (L. Scott, personal communication, July 20, 2015).

No matter which model of mentoring is used, or whether mentoring is provided through a traditional or nontraditional program, doctoral advanced nursing mentors must have as their goal to increase minority representation in leadership and mentoring roles in health care as administrators, policy makers, faculty, and providers. Strategies must be developed to facilitate marketing as well as target recruitment and retention to specified populations or of nurses. For instance, ads can be placed in the journals and magazines directed to specific minority group readers, such as *Minority Nurse*. In addition, college recruiters can actively recruit and display at minority professional conferences, such as the National Black Nurses Association or the National Association of Hispanic Nurses. Mentors must advocate for closer access to doctoral programs, help with facilitation of the application process (which itself can be a barrier to access), target recruitment of minority students, and provide support for the many students who are also caring for senior parents, as well as minors in their homes. This support includes financial aid, which is considered crucial for doctoral students (Idealist, 2015).

To reiterate, effective mentoring is a process that includes the use of mutual respect, appreciation, a positive attitude, commitment, authenticity, and honesty by both mentor and mentee. The following are the tips for effective mentoring for both the mentor and mentee. These tips can be used as a guide for any doctorally prepared nurse who is planning to serve as a mentor to a colleague or student or to any nurse who is entering a new role, accepting a new position, or opening a new practice.

■ TIPS FOR MENTOR AND MENTEE

TIPS FOR THE MENTOR

- Since mentoring can occur through informal or formal processes, you do not need to wait to be appointed or asked to be someone's mentor. If you see someone who is new to a role, career, setting, position, and/or skill set, step up. Welcome, invite, introduce, and reinforce your welcome with your presence and an offer of your time or resources. Your mentoring actions will be rewarded through the growth of your colleagues in advanced nursing practice and by extension, paying it forward to someone else.

- Mentoring is a heuristic process when done well, so remember that your mentoring role will also be rewarded by your own self-growth.
- For mentoring to be worthwhile for both partners in the reciprocal relationship that is mentoring, a mentor must make a commitment to the mentoring relationship. Before stepping up and mentoring a new colleague, or before agreeing to be a mentor, first consider what time, resources, and use of self, you are able to offer to develop and support the mentoring relationship. If you do not have the time or resources, then do your prospective mentee and yourself a favor, decline the request/invitation, and find another way to use yourself as an effective resource to your colleagues.
- Conduct a self-inventory and identify the strengths and other attributes you bring to the role of mentor. You can then build upon these strengths as you experience this relationship building and career-supporting process. This self-audit process can nourish your own growth as a professional who can then integrate experience and self-reflection into evidence-based practice.
- Take time—*time* to select a colleague or student who is new to your program or organization, *time* to listen, *time* to consider what the mentee wants, and *time* to decide what information your mentee would benefit from, in order to contribute and grow in your program or organization.
- Determine if your mentee also needs or would appreciate on-site consultation.
- Negotiate with the mentee about what forms of communication would be most beneficial for both: that is, phone meetings, monthly scheduled meetings, brief e-mails, phone check-ins, as needed meetings, and/or in-person meetings at designated conferences
- Assist your mentee with setting the goals that can be met through the mentoring process, and then regularly evaluate how and if mentoring has assisted in meeting those goals.
- Clearly communicate any expectations or assumptions you have about both your role and the mentee's role to your mentee and ask for feedback. This prevents the development of misunderstandings, a barrier to effective mentoring.
- Keep all appointments and commitments.
- Be aware of the need to identify other mentors for your mentee, as their needs evolve and their skills and goals continue to evolve over time and experience.

TIPS FOR THE MENTEE

- For mentoring to be worthwhile for both partners in the relationship, the mentee must also must make a commitment to the mentoring relationship. Before agreeing to be mentored, determine what time, resources, and use of self you are able to offer, in order to contribute to the development and maintenance of a mentee–mentor relationship. If you do not have the time, inclination, or resources, then do your prospective mentor and yourself a favor, decline the invitation, and find another way to acculturate and acclimate.
- Conduct a self-inventory before you meet your mentor. Identify the strengths you bring to the organization or new position, your goals, resources, and information you will need to have in order to contribute positively to this new organization, academic setting, or professional practice.
- Communicate your needs clearly to your mentor early and often. Expect that these needs will change, but do not expect that your mentor will recognize

what they are or when they have changed, unless you have clearly communicated this information to the mentor.

- If your mentor has helped you in negotiating the system, working within the organization, or learning within an academic setting, then acknowledge the help, and thank the mentor. A simple acknowledgment in the way of a thank you is a powerful reinforcer of effective mentoring, and lays the groundwork for continuing collaboration and support in the future.
- Remember that you are a collaborative partner in the mentoring relationship, so collaborate and reciprocate.
- Keep all appointments and commitments.

Mentoring is experienced in a dynamic, dialectic relationship of give-and-take forged between mentor and mentee. Just like any other organic phenomenon, it must be nourished and protected, or it withers and dies. As these tips for mentor and mentee illustrate, if both partners in this relationship are considerate of each other's time and talents, commit to some goal setting and preparation planning, regularly clarify their interactions, and take responsibility for mishaps on their part, the relationship should flourish. The end product of this mentoring process can be improved professional skills, increased career satisfaction, and more confident doctorally prepared nurses committed to continued learning and collaborative advanced nursing practice.

■ FUTURE DIRECTIONS AND RECOMMENDATIONS

The profession of nursing plays a major role in health care today and DNP-prepared nurses are particularly vital. Specifically, DNPs will be operating in this complex health care environment and at the crux of changes occurring in health care reform and, as such, are positioned to drive change in health care through effective leadership. To successfully maneuver in this environment, mentorship is a vital and necessary resource; it is the single most influential way to successfully develop DNP students and new DNP-prepared professionals, reaping the benefits of recruitment, retention, and long-term maturation of future nurse mentors (Fox, 2015). Therefore, we can no longer wait for happenstance relationships to develop; mentorship needs to be commonplace through purpose-driven actions by individuals, organizations, and systems. Resources must be allocated to support these efforts using innovative approaches including: (a) distance or online mentoring especially for those who do not have a match with a senior mentor at their own organization/institution; (b) mentoring by teams of experts; (c) mentoring to groups of novices; (d) peer mentoring; and (e) mentoring forward (Lach, Hertz, Pomeroy, Resnick, & Buckwalter, 2013). Mentorship processes and programs must also undergo systematic evaluation to ensure their meaningfulness in impact and quality.

In order to shift the normative processes in the way we endorse change, we must have the courage and forethought to take deliberate action and invest in human capital—both mentors and mentees. Leadership development as it occurs through a mentorship supports the promotion of succession planning within the profession. DNP leaders want to expand the cadre of mature mentors and eventually replace mentor leaders through the development of new DNP students/DNP graduates. This process allows for a pool of competent DNP-prepared professionals that could be available for selection for future leadership roles. Individuals are the intellectual capital of organizations; it is therefore incumbent for organizations to place value on people and devise means of retaining their talent. Clearly, this would benefit the profession since this process leads way to a structured system of accomplishing this through succession planning, an overlooked process in the nursing profession.

■ SUMMARY

The DNP degree has sustained growth since the American Association of the Colleges of Nursing (AACN) announced their position statement on the practice doctorate in nursing in 2004. With over 100 programs in existence and graduates already having transitioned into this newfound role, strategic initiatives are required to optimize their success presently and in the long term. Mentorship, a multifaceted process that fosters development of DNP students and graduates, is a fundamental initiative that can support this endeavor. DNPs not only need mentorship that is meaningful, they will also quite often serve as mentors in their leadership capacity. The social and relational process of mentoring is optimized when concepts of authenticity, mutual respect, appreciation, an optimistic attitude, commitment, transformative complicity, cultural humility, and empowerment guide the practice of mentorship. Critical to this process also is to recognize the necessity for life-long mentorship in order to meet the needs of the DNP as they continue to develop across their career trajectory. Mentors embody this with their aspirational demeanor and requiring their mentee to continually reflect, challenge, change, and evaluate his or her practice. This process creates transformative spaces for their DNP colleagues to harness their potential. Ultimately, mentorship will be successful only with individual commitment, and organizational, and systemic support. Taken together, change that occurs will not only benefit the individual nurses by helping them in developing the capacity, the profession itself can be transformed, thereby contributing positively to the lives of our patients, their families, and communities.

■ CRITICAL THINKING QUESTIONS

1. *Conduct a personal audit of your personal and professional interest and skills: what attributes would you bring to your role as a mentor or mentee?*
2. *What are some strategies you can use to become an effective mentor?*
3. *Discuss the characteristics of an effective mentor for a doctoral student from an underrepresented group.*
4. *What are some specific obstacles to or issues about mentorship, which the mentor must be aware of and prepared to address?*
5. *Apply a systems perspective to the need for mentorship in doctoral level education for nurses and for new doctorally prepared nurses: What is the state of practice now and what needs to happen to strengthen the practice of mentorship for the future?*
6. *Compare and contrast mentorship and collegial, or peer, support in doctorally prepared advanced nursing practice. Can one role and practice evolve into another, or are they mutually exclusive?*
7. *What are some outcomes you would expect to see from an effective peer mentoring relationship between colleagues?*
8. *Conduct an audit of your organization's policy for mentoring nurses who are in, or are new to, advanced roles: Based on what you have learned from this chapter, how can you improve on, adapt, or apply that policy?*

9. *By what actions, direct or indirect, do you promote and support mentorship of colleagues or students?*

10. *Mentoring relationships can be challenged by demographic differences such as e, generations, genders, heritage, or language. How would you prepare to identify, address, and minimize effects of these differences on relationship building?*

■ REFERENCES

Adams, M. R. (2013). Growing as a leader through developing others: The effect of being a mentor principal. Dissertation, University of Nebraska, Lincoln, NE. Retrieved from http://digitalcommons.unl.edu/cgi/viewcontent.cgi?article=1169&context=cehsedaddiss

American Association of Colleges of Nursing. (2015a). AACN DNP tool kit: Template for the process of developing a DNP program. Retrieved from http://www.aacn.nche.edu/dnp/dnp-tool-kit

American Association of Colleges of Nursing. (2015b). Enhancing diversity in the workforce. Retrieved from http://www.aacn.nche.edu/media-relations/fact-sheets/enhancing-diversity

American Association of Colleges of Nursing. (2015c). The changing landscape: Nursing diversity on the rise. Policy brief. Retrieved from http://www.aacn.nche.edu/government-affairs/Student-Diversity-FS.pdf

Bartley-Daniele, P. (2014). Family nurse practitioner mentoring relationships' impact on organizational commitment. Dissertation, University of Nevada, Las Vegas, NV. Retrieved from http://digitalscholarship.unlv.edu/cgi/viewcontent.cgi?article=3242&context=thesesdissertations

Beard, K. V., & Volcy, K. (2013). Increasing minority representation in nursing. *American Journal of Nursing, 113*(2), 11. Retrieved from http://journals.lww.com/ajnonline/Fulltext/2013/02000/Increasing_Minority_Representation_in_Nursing.2.aspx

Carter, M., & Moore, P. (2015). The necessity of the doctor of nursing practice incomprehensive care for future health care. *Clinical Scholars Review, 8*(1), 13–17.

Chism, L. (2013). *The doctor of nursing practice: A guidebook for role development and professional issues* (2nd ed.). Boston, MA: Jones & Bartlett.

Cook, M., & Riley, L. (2014). The 2013–2014 national nurse practitioner practice site census. Retrieved from https://www.aanp.org/images/documents/research/2013-14nationalnpcensusreport.pdf

Council of Graduate Schools. (2009). *Exit surveys show mentoring essential to doctorate completion.* Washington, DC: Council of Graduate Schools.

Fox, D. (2015). Nursing faculty shortages: Perspectives from deans and directors of BSN programs. Dissertation, Eastern Michigan University, Ypsilanti, MI. Retrieved from http://commons.emich.edu/cgi/viewcontent.cgi?article=1984&context=theses

Gagliardi, A., Webster, F., Perrier, L., Bell, M., & Straus, S. (2014). Exploring mentorship as a strategy to build capacity for knowledge translation research and practice: A scoping systematic review. *Implementation Science, 13*, 122–132.

Garringer, M., Kupersmidt, J., Rhodes, J., Stelter, R., & Tai, T. (2015). *Elements of effective practice for mentoring* (4th ed.). Boston, MA: MENTOR. Retrieved from http://www.mentoring.org/images/uploads/Final_Elements_Publication_Fourth.pdf

Graves, C., & Hanson, D. (2014). The multiple mentoring model of student supervision: A fit for contemporary practice. *Fieldwork Issues.* Retrieved from http://www.ptsinc.net/files/8714/0147/8130/Multiple_Mentoring_Model_of_Student_Supervison.pdf

Holland, A. (2011). The place of race in cultural nursing education: The experience of white BSN nursing faculty. Retrieved from http://conservancy.umn.edu/bitstream/handle/11299/101771/Holland_umn_0130E_11739.pdf?sequence=1

Huang, A., Huang, C., & Lynch, J. (1995). *Mentoring: The Tao of giving and receiving wisdom.* San Francisco, CA: Harper Collins Publishers.

Idealist. (2015). Are you financially ready for graduate school? Retrieved from http://www.idealist.org/info/GradEducation/Resources/Financing/Ready

Lach, H., Hertz, J., Pomeroy, S., Resnick, B., & Buckwalter, K. (2013). The challenges and benefits of distance mentoring. *Journal of Professional Nursing, 29*(1), 39–48. Retrieved from http://lib.ajaums.ac.ir/booklist/22prof_nurs.pdf

Lewis, J. (2013). Biography of Mary Seacole: Women's history. Retrieved from http://womenshistory .about.com/od/nursesandnursing/a/mary_seacole.htm

McBride, A. B. (2008). Mentoring. In H. Feldman (Ed.), *Nursing leadership: A concise encyclopedia* (1st ed.). New York, NY: Springer Publishing.

Moran, K., Burson, R., & Conrad, D. (2014). *The doctor of nursing practice scholarly project: A framework for success.* Burlington, MA: Jones & Bartlett.

Nightingale, F. (1859). *Notes on nursing (Commemorative Ed.).* Philadelphia, PA: J. B. Lippincott.

NIGMS Minority Programs Update. (2015). Recent awards and fellowships. Retrieved from http:// publications.nigms.nih.gov/mpu/fall04/recent_awards.html

Rabionet, S., Santiago, L., & Zorilla, C. (2009). A multifaceted mentoring model for minority researchers to address HIV health disparities. *American Journal of Public Health, 99*(S1), S65–S70.

Ray, C. (2012). Mentoring—It's all good, right? *Seminars in Interventional Radiology, 29*(2), 69–70.

Robert Wood Johnson Foundation. (2012). *New careers in nursing mentoring toolkit: Building connections.* Washington, DC: Author. Retrieved from http://www.newcareersinnursing.org/resources/ mentoring-toolkit-and-handbook

Robert Wood Johnson Foundation. (2015). New careers in nursing program boost faculty diversity at University of Rochester School of Nursing. Retrieved from http://www.rwjf.org/en/library/ articles-and-news/2015/01/new-careers-in-nursing-program-boosts-faculty-diversity-at-unive .html

Rosser, S., & Taylor, Z. (2009). Why are we still worried about women in science? *Academe: Bulletin of the AAUP, 95*(3), 6–10.

Schroeder, C., & DeAngelo, R. (2010). Addressing whiteness in nursing education: The sociopolitical climate project at the University of Washington School of Nursing. *Advances in Nursing Science, 33*(3), 244–255.

Sebastian, J. G., & White, C. (2013). Doctor of nursing practice programs: Opportunities for faculty development. *Journal of Nursing Education, 52*(8), 453–461.

STEM Education Coalition. (2015). Retrieved from http://www.stemedcoalition.org

Thomas-MacLean, R., Hamoline, R., Kuzmicz, J., Quinlan, E., Ramsden, V. R. (2010). Querying mentorship: Primary care physicians discuss the development of a mentorship program in Saskatchewan. *Canadian Family Physician, 56*(7), e263–e272.

Trumble, W., & Brown, M. (2002). *Shorter Oxford English dictionary* (5th ed.). Oxford, UK: Oxford University Press.

Wayne, G. (2014). Florence Nightingale. The lady with the lamp. *Nurselabs.* Retrieved from http://nurse slabs.com/florence-nightingale

CHAPTER SIXTEEN

Reflective Response 1

Marlene Rosenkoetter

The authors have presented a noteworthy and in-depth discussion of the issues and conflicts surrounding the mentor–mentee relationship for Doctor of Nursing Practice (DNP) students and faculty. From my own experience, there seem to be several basic concepts that impact that relationship. The first is "willingness," namely willingness to be mentored and willingness to be a mentor. Many DNP students are well-established and highly skilled practitioners, administrators, or faculty members. Many have years of nursing experience, but are now returning at a more novice level as new doctoral students. They are faced with returning to their workplace with a degree that may not be well-received, or believed to be equivalent to the PhD. It may not provide them with PhD level or type of credentials for tenure and promotion, and may not be deemed an essential degree for advanced practice by their peers. Questions continue to remain among some advanced practice nurses regarding the appropriateness of requiring them to hold the DNP and use the title "Dr" (Miller, 2008), and it may continue to take time before the DNP is accepted by other disciplines as the equivalent of the PhD (Apold, 2008). Silva and Ludwick (2006) made a strong case for questioning the ethics of having the degree. Yet, the more experienced students may have clinical skills that exceed those of some of their nursing faculty.

At the initial point of entry into the DNP program, students may experience role shock, role ambiguity, role confusion, and role changes. The faculty member as a mentor is possibly addressing some of these same issues, having been expected to take on the role of mentoring students in a program that is clearly continuing to evolve. Students must be willing to be mentored, to be challenged, and to take responsibility for a new level of practice in their own environments. Faculty members need to be intuitive, reflective, and sensitive not only to the needs of students, but also sensitive to and aware of their own strengths and weaknesses. The DNP student will most likely need and have several mentors across the span of the educational program. There may be one in a clinical subspecialty, evidence-based practice, research, teaching, or administration, to mention a few. The key to a successful relationship seems to evolve around the most basic principles of professionalism—collaboration, collegiality, cooperation, and commitment—all of which are based on mutual trust and ethical beliefs and practices. One of the current problems is that DNP students are being prepared for advanced practice, but enter academia as faculty members. Many are not prepared for the role of teacher, mentor, researcher, or research participant. The need for mentoring becomes even more essential for these new graduates as faculty. Their levels of understanding and competence in research vary considerably, depending on the school from which they graduated. Mentoring in research involves establishing a strong relationship, understanding the knowledge base of the participants, and developing a plan to move forward.

Senior faculty can most easily assume the mentoring role, provided they are willing, receptive to the idea and, as the authors point out, have sufficient support within the school of nursing to fulfill their responsibilities. Mentoring can take many forms, not just for coursework and projects, but also in assisting the DNP student to understand the mentor role (as future mentors), what being a faculty member or administrator in advanced practice is all about, as well as how to negotiate difficult agreements, resolve conflicts, and reach consensus in meetings. To achieve this, mentors may ask students and junior faculty to join them on publications, do research, attend meetings, present papers, and participate in most any scholarly endeavor. Providing a student with the opportunity to be the first author on a publication can foster self-esteem, while experiencing the process of getting a manuscript submitted, accepted, and published. The ultimate goal in mentoring for many students is developing a long-range plan that will lead to Fellowship in the American Academy of Nursing. This needs to start early and may take years to fulfill, but can be a highly rewarding attainment in the end. This particular mentoring role may extend to both students and faculty in other schools of nursing, and even internationally.

The mentor–mentee relationship for international students becomes considerably more complex. Not only is the DNP student adjusting to a new doctoral program, but as well may be adjusting to a new culture and strange environment. This needs interactions with colleagues and interpersonal communication and commitment. It is predictable that international students will have even more challenges than native students as they progress through their programs.

Being a mentor is not as simple as forming a relationship, and the authors of this chapter clearly emphasize that. It takes interest, commitment, willingness to be available, an inclusive attitude, and the ability to be able to share rather than be possessive and protective of one's own domain. One of the most important mentor roles that I have had, which both students and other faculty appreciated, is including them on publications. This starts with providing an overview of the process, doing literature searches, reviewing the various publishing formats and online submissions, determining the different types of publications that one can submit, developing the content, and then managing the comments of the reviewers. Inexperienced faculty can be devastated by reviewer comments, especially when they feel they have "produced a masterpiece," whether in fact they have or have not. Through mentoring, students can have senior faculty input on their publications before they ever submitted for review. This, in turn, will provide the student with an opportunity to learn how to mentor early in the process.

The American Association of Colleges of Nursing's (AACN, 2006) essentials document clearly differentiates between research-focused doctoral programs and DNP programs during which students engage in advanced practice nursing and gain the ability to provide leadership for evidence-based practice. This difference needs to be clearly known by DNP students before they enter the program. Some even decide to pursue both routes simultaneously or in sequence, understanding that both degrees can help to advance the creation and translation of knowledge into practice (Edwardson, 2010). Students may initially be uninformed on both the purpose and the process for acquiring the degree. Having a temporary mentor assigned before admission can facilitate this process and help to reduce stress once the student is enrolled—and we must recognize that any doctoral program is stressful!

■ REFERENCES

American Association of Colleges of Nursing. (2006). *The essentials of doctoral education for advanced nursing practice.* Retrieved from http://www.aacn.nche.edu/DNP/pdf/Essentials.pdf

Apold, S. (2008). The doctor of nursing practice: Looking back, moving forward. *Journal for Nurse Practitioners, 4*(2), 101–107.

Edwardson, S. R. (2010). Doctor of philosophy and doctor of nursing practice as complementary degrees. *Journal of Professional Nursing, 26*(3), 137–140.

Miller, J. (2008). The doctor of nursing practice: Recognizing a need or graying the line between doctor and nurse? *Medscape Journal of Medicine, 10*(11), 253. Retrieved from http://www.medscape.com/viewarticle/582269

Silva, M., & Ludwick, R. (2006). Ethics: Is the doctor of nursing practice ethical? *The Online Journal of Issues in Nursing, 11*(2), 8. Retrieved from www.nursingworld.org/MainMenuCategories/ANAMarketplace/ANAPeriodicals/OJIN/Columns/Ethics/DNPEthical.aspx

CHAPTER SIXTEEN

Reflective Response 2

Debra A. Simons

The authors provide a compelling case regarding the importance of mentorship for successful role assimilation and professional development. The increase in Doctor of Nursing Practice (DNP) programs suggests unprecedented growth in DNP-prepared advanced practice nurses. This growth warrants the need to build collaborative partnerships and linkages between mentors and mentees. The two cases presented in this chapter provide distinct mentoring styles, mentee responses, and associated outcomes. David, a DNP student, was able to accomplish his capstone goals because he developed collaborative partnerships with *multiple mentors*. The synergy and reciprocity between the mentors and the mentee allowed mutual goals to be achieved. The transformational mentoring moved from introductions to respect networking, support of scholarship, and collaborations. In contrast, Patricia, a PhD-prepared nurse and new faculty member, received traditional dyad and assigned mentoring. She was assigned a mentor who was unresponsive to her needs. Moreover, when she reached out to another mentor, she was not welcomed. This type of mentoring can have a devastating impact on a mentee, which can result in stagnation of professional growth and stagnation in doctoral nursing practice.

The American Association of Colleges of Nursing (AACN) has perpetuated confusion within our country as well as internationally about the practice doctorate in nursing (Cronenwett et al., 2011) because a master of science and PhD degree is more readily understood globally. A new type of practice doctorate adds confusion. Some universities accept non-advanced practice nurses (APNs) in DNP programs that ultimately assume faculty positions. Therefore, students who graduate from a DNP program may not necessarily be APN, which was the original intent of the degree. The DNP degree has also expanded its vision to prepare graduates to use translational research to create clinical strategies that improve practice and health outcomes (Brown & Crabtree, 2013). The wide variety of DNP programs and graduates necessitates the need to move away from traditional mentoring to transformational mentoring using multiple mentors, as a "one-size-fits-all" approach is no longer realistic. One also needs to consider where the DNP graduate is developmentally on his or her own individual career trajectory.

As an example, my own professional role development needs have changed dramatically over time. At first, my developmental needs focused on honing my clinical knowledge and skills and later transitioned to learning the executive role and scholarship of discovery. Finding the right mentors was not a spontaneous process. It required a *willingness* on my part to seek out mentors with skills that would address my learning needs and complement my own developmental needs. My own role development continues to change in its focus and intensity.

Findings from the AACN's fall 2014 survey of nursing schools indicated that the number of students from minority backgrounds in practice-focused doctoral programs increased to 28.7% (AACN, 2015). The authors discuss the challenges of these underrepresented groups and how mentors can be especially helpful. It has been my experience that most organizations do not have formal mentoring programs complicating the problem, especially for underrepresented groups. Those individuals from underrepresented groups are also often unaware of the significance of mentoring or cannot find mentors committed to their career success (Beech et al., 2013). Innovative solutions are required to close this gap.

The author provides tips for the mentor and mentee. In order for a successful relationship between the mentor and mentee, there needs to be mutual respect and a willingness to compromise. The mentors who had the most influence in my life demonstrated a strong commitment and supported my professional goals. These mentors were not assigned but rather they were sought out through my personal motivation and self-inventory. The mentors provided guidance with respect to personal learning networks, which contributed to my personal professional growth. Thus, the mentee is also a key stakeholder in the relationship. Mentees need to be accountable, be prepared and on time, ask relevant questions, and explore issues from multiple angles. Mentors may need to put aside their own agendas unless they are mutually shared.

One of the biggest obstacles in a fruitful mentoring relationship is finding the time for the mentor–mentee relationship. Since the world is shrinking because of technology, technology is a catalyst to bring the mentor and mentee together via virtual meetings and e-mail, meeting the needs of the mentee in real-time. Panopoulos and Sarri (2013) examined the variables with e-mentoring and found that the medium for which the mentor and mentee met did not matter. What mattered most was the frequency of the interactions. More engagement resulted in greater the career development and satisfaction whether in-person or via e-mentoring. Perhaps the use of e-mentoring can remove some of the barriers for the underrepresented with respect to obtaining engaged mentors. The mentee is no longer confined to finding mentors within his or her organization. The pool of mentors can be expanded globally using the technology. Leck and Wood (2013) suggest that e-mentoring is particularly beneficial to individuals of marginalized groups because the barriers associated with social status are less visible in the electronic exchange. Traditional mentoring relies on physical space. Stereotypes can surface and be applied both with and without conscious awareness. These biases can hamper the quality of the exchange between the mentor and mentee. Therefore, it may be reasonable to suggest that the dynamics that the authors discuss as *the old girls' network* may change in an e-mentoring relationship.

Today, health care exists within a complex microsystem. DNPs can have a profound impact on national and global health care. DNPs can serve as change agents and take the lead in addressing in health care delivery challenges by serving as interprofessional collaborators while simultaneously improving clinical practice and patient outcomes. Excellent mentorship should include cultural diversity and nurse empowerment to produce diverse, competent, and progressive health care leaders.

Mentorship can also cultivate successful role assimilation and professional identity; however, traditional, dyad, mentor–mentee relationships may not be sufficient. DNP students and graduates may need multiple mentors that form learning networks and linkages, which explore issues from multiple perspectives. Since developmental needs change over time, mentoring cannot not be a stagnant activity. A strong commitment by all parties is necessary for a doctoral role assimilation. E-mentoring may also provide a forum to close the gap associated with the lack of qualified mentors for the underrepresented. However, as the sole mentoring method, it is a short-term solution until we establish a larger pool of qualified culturally diverse nurse mentors. Seeking lifelong mentorship and menteeship for all in doctoral advanced nursing practice is a wise investment in *human capital,* which can ultimately improve the lives of the doctoral advanced nurse, as well as patients and families, globally.

■ REFERENCES

American Association of Colleges of Nursing. (2015). *New AACN data confirm enrollment surge in schools of nursing* [Press Release]. Washington, DC: Author.

Beech, B. M., Calles-Escandon, J., Hairston, K. G., Langdon, M. S. E., Latham-Sadler, B. A., & Bell, R. A. (2013). Mentoring programs for underrepresented minority faculty in academic medical centers: A systematic review of the literature. *Academic Medicine: Journal of the Association of American Medical Colleges, 88*(4), 541–549.

Brown, M. A., & Crabtree, K. (2013). The development of practice scholarship in DNP programs: A paradigm shift. *Journal of Professional Nursing, 29*(6), 330–337.

Cronenwett, L., Dracup, K., Grey, M., McCauley, L., Meleis, A., & Salmon, M. (2011). The doctor of nursing practice: A national workforce perspective. *Nursing Outlook, 59*(1), 9–17.

Leck, J. D., & Wood, P. M. (2013). Forming trust in e-mentoring: A research agenda. *American Journal of Industrial and Business Management, 3,* 101–109.

Panopoulos, A. P., & Sarri, K. (2013). E-mentoring: The adoption process and innovation challenge. *International Journal of Information Management, 33*(1), 217–226.

Interdisciplinary and Interprofessional Collaboration: Essential for the Doctoral Advanced Practice Nurse

Julie Cowan Novak

A series of Institute of Medicine (IOM) reports—*To Err Is Human: Building a Safer Health System* (IOM, 2000); *Crossing the Quality Chasm: A New Health System for the 21st Century* (IOM, 2001); *Health Professions Education: A Bridge to Quality* (IOM, 2003), and *The Future of Nursing: Leading Change, Advancing Health* (IOM, 2010)—were the tipping points in the discourse related to patient satisfaction, safety, quality, access, and cost-effective health care delivery; the *Triple Aim*, *"The Future of Nursing report*, had more Internet hits than any other IOM report" (Dr. Kenneth Shine, 2013, former vice chancellor of Health Sciences, University of Texas System and former IOM president, UT System, "Lessons Learned from a Lifetime of Quality Improvement"). The public reaction to these reports was significant. The reports catalyzed patient safety and quality research, improvement science, clinical translational science, evidence-based practice (EBP), and the critical role that nursing must play in the future of health care. These IOM reports were foundational to the development of the Doctor of Nursing Practice (DNP) degree. Health care summits across the United States resulted in common themes, including consumer-driven health care; basic universal health care for all; interoperability of electronic health records; new models of care for nurse-managed clinic systems; and interprofessional education (IPE), practice, and research to promote collaboration (Rapala & Novak, 2007). The reports were extremely helpful in developing early DNP programs from 2000 to 2005 before the American Association of Colleges of Nursing (AACN) DNP essentials (AACN, 2006). The Affordable Care Act (2010), the Centers for Medicare and Medicaid (CMS) Delivery System Reform Incentive Payment (DSRIP) program, and health care reform legislation at the regional, state, and federal levels further support this revolution in nursing education.

■ SCOPE

This chapter describes the development and sustainability of interprofessional partnerships for DNP program enrichment. Unique and traditional IPE and interdisciplinary partners and effects on curricular redesign are to be presented. Interdisciplinary practice inquiry projects that build the evidence base and lead to documented outcomes, supporting the critical need for interprofessional and interdisciplinary collaboration, are to be discussed. Finally, nurse-led clinics that provide a setting for DNP and IPE, practice, and research are to be described. Nurse-led clinics provide a learning collaboratory where students partner with communities design settings and systems where children, families, and adults learn, live, work, play, and pray (Novak, 2015). Over the past 50 years, academic nursing centers have been developing, implementing, and evaluating alternatives to the failing, mismanaged traditional U.S. health care delivery system. Most of these efforts have lasted only one to three years due to dependence on a single grant for funding support. To address this problem, a model of sustainability, or a "mosaic of support" was created providing a framework for the continued success of a replicable nurse-managed health home model. The model emphasizes effective communication, a business plan, and a broad portfolio of sources of support (see Figure 17.1). DNP students and their interprofessional partners learn how to develop and sustain an integrated model of learning, discovery, and engagement with key components related to communication, collaboration, business principles, and diversification of funding streams. Interprofessional students and faculty meet monthly to innovate and sustain what they have developed in partnership with communities who have clearly identified their needs. The model reflects the triple aim at one third the cost of traditional medical models of the last and current century. DNP and other interprofessional students must learn to collaborate and communicate effectively in practice

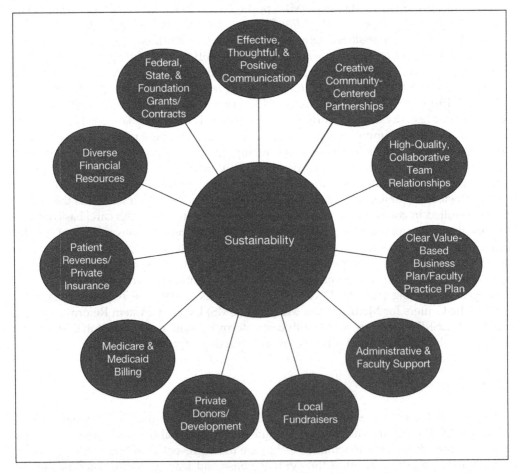

FIGURE 17.1   An integrated model of sustainability: Building a mosaic of support.
Source: Adapted from Novak (2004, 2016).

settings if health care's 17% gross national product is to be reduced, and significant improvements are to be made and sustained.

■ DEVELOPING INTERDISCIPLINARY PARTNERSHIPS FOR DNP PROGRAM ENRICHMENT

ACADEMIC

The academic patient safety's call-to-arms occurred in 2003 when the IOM published *Health Professions Education: A Bridge to Quality* (IOM, 2003). Initially, the education report did not benefit from the media exposure of the earlier reports; education is not as sensational as lost lives reported in *To Err Is Human: Building a Safer Health System* (IOM, 2000). The root cause to any problem or issue is complex. The revolution in health care must not lose momentum in solving fundamental education-related patient safety, quality, and systems issues. Education as a root cause of these issues is losing lives once-removed (Rapala & Novak, 2007). The lack of effective collaboration and communication leads to errors, added costs, patient dissatisfaction, unfulfilled community partnerships, and unsustainability.

In addition to a common patient safety language, the IOM multidisciplinary team suggested a group of five core competencies that should be incorporated into the curriculum of all health care education programs. The five competencies include the ability to: (a) provide patient-centered care; (b) work in interdisciplinary teams; (c) employ EBP; (d) apply quality improvement (QI); and (e) use informatics (IOM, 2003). The recommendations from this report have been further delineated in federal and foundation requests for proposals (RFPs), health care publications, and the popular press. The IOM Future of Nursing Report's (2010) recommendations further clarified the call to action including: (a) Nurses should practice to the full extent of their education and training; (b) achieve higher levels of education and training (remove APN practice barriers); (c) be full partners with physicians and others in redesigning health care in the United States; and (d) recognize that effective workforce planning and policy-making require better data collection and an improved information infrastructure.

If nurses are to be effective, transformative, innovative collaborators and team leaders, attention must also be paid to individual identity development as professionals (Charles, Bainbridge, & Gilbert, 2010). Professional identity development is dependent on interactions with the world around us. Student experiences across the curriculum must be designed with this in mind. Bookend leadership and IPE courses at the beginning and end of DNP programs are insufficient.

Just as it is difficult for health care providers to respond to and balance a myriad of patient safety issues from medication reconciliation to information systems implementation, it is difficult for nursing academe to balance patient safety with operations, research, and teaching (Rapala & Novak, 2007). All IOM reports serve as a blueprint for change. Removal of scope of practice barriers was the first and specific recommendation of the IOM future of nursing report (2010).

Competencies related to the DNP essentials (AACN, 2006), Quality, Safety, and Education of Nurses (Cronenwett et al., 2007) are teamwork, collaboration, EBP, QI, safety, and informatics, and Team Strategies and Tools to Enhance Performance and Patient Safety (TeamSTEPPS) (AHRQ, 2016) must be woven into the curriculum to address these core challenges. The TeamSTEPPS initiative is based on evidence derived from team performance, leveraging more than 30 years of research in military, aviation, nuclear power, business, and industry, to acquire team competencies. These team competencies affect knowledge (shared mental model), attitudes (mutual trust and team orientation), and performance (adaptability, accuracy, productivity, efficiency, and safety). Thus, a cadre of professionals who can participate in and lead team science (integrated multidisciplinary research teams), develop health homes, and integrate best current evidence with clinical expertise and patient/family preferences and values are to be created for the effective delivery of health care (Stevens, 2013). For effective health care team performance, nurses must come to the table with a clear professional identity and comprehensive leadership training and development.

To collaborate and mentor students effectively, nursing faculty must relinquish insular behaviors. Health care providers of the 21st century must function effectively within nursing and interprofessional teams, fostering open communication, mutual respect, and shared decision making to achieve a quality patient care. DNP programs must prepare the workforce for a complex health care environment, designing system-wide fixes. The siloed natures of professional schools and graduate programs with competing interests are barriers to collaboration. Joint curricular design replete with the opportunity for cross-walking core and cognate courses are essential. Interprofessional courses include genomics, systems, human factors influencing patient safety and quality, EBP, informatics, health economics, including value-based health care delivery (Elton & O'Riordan, 2016; Porter & Teisberg, 2006), health policy, and public-health/population-health principles and telehealth (Novak et al., 2016). Coordination and collaboration with other health care disciplines are difficult to achieve due to physical location, competing priorities, simple geography, profession program accreditation constraints, and asynchronous academic program calendars. Telehealth opportunities remove many barriers to interprofessional practice (IPP) and IPE.

Since the majority of educational and health care institutions were built before 1970, redesign of these facilities should promote opportunities for interdisciplinary collaboration, IPE, and student success. Interprofessional simulation centers and true interprofessional clinical settings in universities and health care agencies provide an opportunity for DNP practice inquiry projects related to patient safety and quality, simulation and device design, competency development, outcomes management, continuous learning, and systems improvement.

Nurses must think more broadly about potential collaborators in solving the problems of the health care delivery system. Disciplines such as industrial, biomedical, and mechanical engineering have much to offer as engineering principles are applied to DNP curricular development and hospital and clinic development, design, renovation, and sustainability. Nurse-led models emulate the triple aim to enhance the patient experience, improve quality, and reduce cost. The DNP was developed to reengineer health care (Novak, 2006) to achieve these goals through designing accessible, effective, efficient, safe, and high-quality health care delivery systems. The DNP addresses the complexity of the health care system head-on, including the information, knowledge, and technology explosion; spiraling costs; and the need for a systems approach to create new models of care and solve existing health care dilemmas (Wall, Novak, & Wilkerson, 2005).

The DNP student brings core capabilities of leadership development, health promotion, disease prevention, case management, patient safety and quality, and care of the individual, family, community, as well as a biopsychosocial, behavioral perspective, within a social justice and population systems context. The DNP graduate must understand resource utilization, and possess a strong service orientation. Engineering students bring expertise in root cause analysis, systems design, device design, simulation, and human factors. Melding these entities yields a dynamic, synergistic, and innovative environment, where each partner brings affiliations and skills to improve care that is evidence-based. This creates a horizontally and vertically integrated interprofessional learning environment where not only the students benefit, but also the nursing do, and other health science and engineering faculty learn and create new educational and practice models (Rapala & Novak, 2007).

These efficient and effective models have been shared with a variety of faculty and students from nursing, medicine, dentistry, nutrition/dietetics, and audiology in the UT Nursing Clinical Enterprise through the development of six nurse-led clinics (Novak, 2015). Each of these clinics has been guided by community invitation, and a community needs assessment, patient, parent and family focus groups and surveys, and the potential for long-term sustainability through a mosaic of support (see Figure 17.1). With this approach, interprofessional students at all levels learn that the community leads the process or "the dance." For community buy-in and long-term collaboration, the relationship with the community must be egalitarian and respectful. Conversely, hierarchical models of the past tied to a single grant may leave communities with disdain and mistrust and the inability or desire to sustain current or future partnerships or projects.

GOVERNMENTAL

Health policy didactic and residency courses are key elements of the DNP degree including in-depth policy design, implementation, and evaluation. Interprofessional health policy courses for nursing, other health sciences, engineering, business, communications, and political science students provide an optimal setting for curricular enrichment, systems change, and effective advocacy, and policy design. Residency experiences at the state and federal levels are invaluable. Enabling students to understand effective lobbying, cultivate relationships with key staff, work with professional organizations' legislative experts, share expertise through partnership development with legislators, gather data from community constituents and stakeholders, provide testimony, assist in drafting legislation, and enact and evaluate policy are essential components of professional development and the DNP degree. National nursing organizations, for example, Nurse in Washington Internships (NIWI), George Mason University, offer a week-long intensive policy experience on Capitol Hill.

Promoting worldwide health is mankind's greatest challenge. The DNPs and their interprofessional partners also have the potential to lead in the local-to-global health care policy arena. This requires an understanding of several global agencies, such as the World Health Organization (WHO), the Pan American Health Organization (PAHO), the United Nations, the United Nations International Children's Emergency Fund (UNICEF), the World Bank, and the Centers for Disease Control (CDC) (Novak, 2014). Currently, there are more than 180 PAHO/WHO collaborating centers in 15 countries in the Americas (PAHO, 2015). Ten WHO-collaborating centers are based in U.S. schools of nursing with areas of concentration in child health, nurse midwifery, gerontology, home health, and primary health care (PAHO, 2015).

All DNP practice inquiry projects should include health policy implications. For some projects, the relevant policy implications are to integrate policy with ethics, research, and education. Exemplars include care of vulnerable populations and the underserved, workforce and faculty shortages, funding for nursing education, employee and community wellness programs, and barrier removal to increased access to advanced practice nursing care. Recognizing the underutilization of DNPs knowledge and skills, the future of nursing report clearly recommends practice and licensure at the full extent of DNP knowledge and skill preparation and competency.

NONGOVERNMENTAL ORGANIZATIONS FOR GLOBAL SERVICE-LEARNING PROJECTS

Nongovernmental organizations such as the Carter Center, the Bill and Melinda Gates Foundation, Christel House International, and the Johnson & Johnson Foundation have supported global interprofessional service-learning projects for students in the health care disciplines (Richards & Novak, 2010). DNPs have the ability to establish new global models reflecting the future of nursing recommendations and evaluating their impact, all of which will lead to higher quality and more cost-effective care.

The Carter Center has three objectives: (a) to prevent and resolve conflicts, (b) to enhance freedom and democracy, and (c) to improve health (Carter Center, 2010). In the words of Carter Center co-founder and former U.S. President Jimmy Carter in his 2002 Nobel Peace Prize speech, "The bond of our common humanity is stronger than the divisiveness of our fears and prejudices. God gives us the capacity for choice. We can choose to alleviate suffering. We can choose to work together for peace. We can make these changes—we must" (Carter, 2002, para 39).

The Bill and Melinda Gates Foundation has local, national, and global objectives. Globally, the foundation focuses on reducing extreme poverty, improving health, and increasing the public library access. Within Africa, the foundation has had a profound effect on improving access to antiviral medications and the prevention and treatment for HIV/AIDS, tuberculosis (TB), and malaria.

The author has partnered with Christel House International and the Johnson & Johnson Foundation to enact an ongoing interprofessional service-learning project in Cape Town, South Africa. Christel House International is a public charity that operates learning centers (kindergarten through 12 [K-12] schools) in impoverished neighborhoods with the goal of creating sustainable social and educational impact. Between 1999 and 2002, Christel House opened five learning centers in Mexico, India, South Africa, Venezuela, and the United States. Christel House K-12 Academy in Cape Town helps children break the cycle of poverty, realize their hopes and dreams and become self-sufficient, contributing members of society through educational excellence. Teams of nursing and medical students have partnered with local community leaders to provide school and family health promotion, HIV/AIDS, TB, and malaria prevention and intervention, and educational programs. Direct care has been provided in the Themba Care Orphanage and the Tafelsig Community Health Center. Working with an interprofessional student team in caring for AIDS patients develops a depth of communication, and a deep sense of humanity and camaraderie. Students describe this service learning experience as deeply affecting their personal, moral, and ethical development and changing their professional goals. For example, after their service learning projects, nearly 50% of the 98 health-science student participants changed their professional goals to public health in global settings.

DNP practice inquiry projects with interprofessional partners in the health sciences and engineering are ongoing (Richards & Novak, 2010). As nursing's status in second- and third-world countries varies widely, these initiatives and their interprofessional and interdisciplinary frameworks will provide a foundation for global DNP program development. Student participants describe the experiences as "life-changing; promoting one's professional identity development while acknowledging health care as a team sport; new ways of knowing and doing; deep understanding that the community must lead the partnership for long-term sustainability, relevance, and rich student learning."

■ INTERPROFESSIONAL COLLABORATIVE RESEARCH

The focus of DNP Essential VII outcome (AACN, 2006) is the analysis of appropriate scientific data, the synthesis of concepts related to clinical prevention and population health to develop increased cultural awareness and proficiency, implement, and evaluate interventions to address health promotion/disease prevention, and to evaluate health care delivery models and/or strategies (AACN, 2006). The final practice inquiry project is a synthesis of theoretical concepts for program development combined with grounding in change and leadership theory, and concepts of program planning, implementation, and evaluation. It can take up to 17 years before the scientific findings become part of practice at the bedside or in the community setting (Charman, 2013; Morris, Wooding, & Grant, 2011). The DNP program emphasis on interdisciplinary, relevant, evidence-based projects is designed to significantly reduce that lag time. DNP graduates have the ability to translate bench research and apply improvement science across a wide range of health care settings.

This work is actualized in the DNP scholarly project. One exemplar is the community assessment, development of, and sustainability factors necessary for creation of nurse-managed clinics as a system of care. These "health homes" led by the pediatric nurse practitioner and family nurse practitioner/DNP students and faculty in our UT Nursing Clinical Enterprise promote enhanced collaboration with academic partners including community pediatrics, behavioral health, dentistry, and audiology; a new model of health care for 6,700 children enrolled in Head Start programs and the care of 14,000 patients across all UT Nursing Clinical Enterprise (UTNCE) clinics.

The DNP plays an important role in the evaluation of new, sustainable-care delivery models including clinic design, development, implementation, and evaluation and identification of strategies that lead to positive outcomes, a healthy operating margin, and long-term sustainability. The DNP integrates principles of QI, psychosocial, and cultural concepts and utilizes models and theoretical concepts to explain the observed phenomena. The DNP utilizes principles of EBP and health care economics to evaluate these models. An understanding of health economics and finance, including a cost analysis as a standard component of the final practice inquiry project, is critical. Practice inquiry exemplars might include an analysis of medicare and medicaid access and recommendations for system improvement and a gap analysis of county-level health departments for a national accreditation. These access and public health system improvements require effective interdisciplinary communication and collaboration.

The AACN (2006) criteria for the scholarly project describe a reflection of the breadth of education and synthesis of knowledge gained in the course of study. The projects demonstrate evidence of scholarship in other disciplines such as behavioral science, business, engineering, and pharmacology. The scholarly project is enriched through an interprofessional curriculum and interdisciplinary final project committees, ultimately resulting in collaborative peer-reviewed presentations, manuscript submissions, and other professional and lay publications. At this critical juncture, DNP projects must be relevant to patient populations and meaningful, sustainable systems of care. The DNP projects and development of new ways to deliver effective IPE have the potential to be transformative in nursing practice not only from health care system perspectives, but also in terms of the transformation of nurses themselves.

■ SUMMARY

DNP students and graduates face many exciting challenges in health care reform and in designing effective systems of health care delivery. These include being responsive to emerging needs and health issues for individual patients, their families, and local to global populations. Recognizing that traditional, hierarchical, models of the 20th century do not work, new interprofessional practice models must adhere to the triple aim principles of "reengineered" primary health care across diverse settings in the context of a reengineered health care system and attitude of health care professionals. Social justice, wellness, mutual respect, and value-based health care must replace insular silos of hierarchy, insecurity, competition, and spiraling costs. Students must be developed as leaders who truly collaborate with other disciplines and their communities, embracing the opportunity to work together in an equalitarian and sustainable model. Opportunities for interpersonal interactions and diverse educational experiences must be provided. Whether a simulation lab, a newborn and family assessment experience, sharing a caseload of patients with interprofessional students, developing and sustaining a refugee clinic or working with audiologists to deliver hearing health care through telepractice, students must have diverse IPE experiences each semester on an ongoing basis. One course or practice experience at the beginning or end of the program will not achieve interprofessional understanding, mutual respect, and the depth of collaboration that the complexities of health care require. DNPs have the potential to mobilize research translation and dissemination, and practice implementation strategies to ensure EBP as the norm rather than the exception (Novak, 2014).

Practice inquiry exemplars can emanate from Center for Medicaid (CMS; these projects do not pertain to Medicare). Delivery System Reform Incentive Payment (DSRIP) projects ranging from access to primary care, to chronic care management, to behavioral health, to public health infrastructure, and to readmission rates. These DNP initiatives promote team science and clinical translational research. DNP programs, now exceeding 250, are "just in time" in preparing nurses as clinical professionals who can make critical decisions, lead discourse and change, and write, implement, and evaluate health policies. In order for DNPs to be effective collaborators in their new roles, the individual DNP must be willing and prepared for personal change and growth concurrent with system level change and improvements. The ability to focus on social justice and the greater good is the essence of true leadership and collaboration.

■ CRITICAL THINKING QUESTIONS

1. *Consider your own clinical practice experience. How much interprofessional communication do you employ?*
2. *Discuss whether you think nursing operates too much within its "nursing silo" or not.*
3. *Identify any way in which your DNP education curricula are structured for interdisciplinary experiences.*
4. *Who do you perceive will be your primary non-nursing doctorally prepared collaborators when you complete your degree and enter the workforce as a DNP graduate? Discuss how you might enhance this collaboration.*
5. *Give some thought to who you might select as possible preceptors in your DNP program and identify at least one non-nurse doctorally prepared mentor with whom you might collaborate.*
6. *Debate whether you believe bachelor of science in nursing (BSN) education does an adequate job teaching interprofessional and interdisciplinary collaboration.*
7. *Discuss whether you believe master of science in nursing (MSN) education does an adequate job teaching interprofessional and interdisciplinary collaboration.*
8. *Identify one other health profession that you know the least about. Perform a Google search and discuss how you might collaborate with this health professional in a possible DNP-interprofessional role.*
9. *Go to the website of the* Journal of Research in Interprofessional Practice and Education, *www.jripe.org. Retrieve an article from one of the current issues from your library and discuss the article's relevance to your future DNP role.*
10. *Devise a clinical research question that would involve the expertise of nursing and at least one other discipline.*
11. *Describe Novak's Integrated Model of Sustainability and its usefulness for your practice.*

12. *Compare and contrast your current practice setting with* The Future of Nursing *recommendations regarding leadership, practice and interprofessional collaboration. What progress has been made?*

■ REFERENCES

Agency for Healthcare Research and Quality. (2016). TeamSTEPPS. Washington, DC: Author. Retrieved from www.AHRQ.gov\teamSTEPPS

American Association of Colleges of Nursing. (2006). *The essentials of doctoral education for advanced nursing practice.* Retrieved from http://www.aacn.nche.edu/DNP/pdf/Essentials.pdf

Carter Center. (2010). *About the center.* Retrieved from http://www.Cartercenter.org/about/index.html

Carter, J. (2002). Nobel lecture. Retrieved from http://nobelprize.org/nobel_prizes/peace/laureates/2002/carter-lecture.html

Charles, G., Bainbridge, L., & Gilbert, J. (2010). The University of British Columbia model of interprofessional education. *Journal of Interprofessional Care, 24*(1), 9–18.

Charman, E. (2013). Medical research council. Measuring time: Getting research from bench to bedside. Retrieved from Insight.mrc.ac.uk

Cronenwett, L., Sherwood, G., Barnsteiner, J., Disch, J., Johnson, J., Mitchell, P., . . . Warren, J. (2007). Quality and safety education for nurses. *Nursing Outlook, 55*(3), 122–131.

Elton, J., & O'Riordan, A. (2016). *Healthcare disrupted: New generation business models and strategies.* Hoboken, NJ: John Wiley.

Institute of Medicine. (2000). *To err is human: Building a safer health system.* Washington, DC: National Academies Press.

Institute of Medicine. (2001). *Crossing the quality chasm: A new health system for the 21st century.* Washington, DC: National Academies Press.

Institute of Medicine. (2003). *Health professions education: A bridge to quality.* Washington, DC: National Academies Press.

Institute of Medicine. (2010). *The future of nursing: Leading change, advancing health.* Retrieved from http://books.nap.edu/openbook.php?record_id=12956&page=R1

Morris, Z. S., Wooding, S., & Grant, J. (2011). The answer is 17 years; what is the question: Understanding time lags in translational research. Retrieved from jrs.sagepub.com

Novak, J. (2006). The doctor of nursing practice: Reengineering healthcare. New York, NY: The Helene Fuld Healthcare Trust.

Novak, J. (2014). Globalization and international health. In M. A. Nies & M. McEwen (Eds.), *Community health nursing: Promoting the health of populations.* St. Louis, MO: Elsevier.

Novak, J. (2015). Addressing RHP 6 community needs through the 1115 Waiver–2015. Retrieved from http://www.texasrhp6.com/addressing-rhp6-community-needs-through-the-1115-waiver

Novak, R. E., Cantu, A. G., Zappler, A., Coco, L., Champlin, C. A., & Novak, J. C. (2016). The future of healthcare delivery: IPE/IPP audiology and nursing student/faculty collaboration to deliver hearing aids to vulnerable adults via telehealth. *Journal of Nursing & Interprofessional Leadership in Quality & Safety, 1*(1). Retrieved from http://digitalcommons.library.stmc.edu/utoustonjqualsafe/vol%201/iss1/1

Pan American Health Organization. (2015). PAHO/WHO collaborating centers. Retrieved from http://www.paho.org/collaboratingcenters

Porter, M. E., & Teisberg, E. O. (2006). *Redefining healthcare.* Cambridge, UK: Harvard Business School Publishing.

Rapala, K., & Novak, J. (2007). Integrating patient safety into curriculum: The doctor of nursing practice. *Journal of Patient Safety and Quality Health Care,* 17–23. Retrieved from http://docs.lib.purdue.edu/cgi/viewcontent.cgi?article=1014&context=rche_pre

Richards, E., & Novak, J. (2010). From Biloxi to Cape Town: Curricular integration of service learning. *Journal of Community Health Nursing, 27*(1), 46–50.

Stevens, K. R. (2013). The impact of evidence-based practice in nursing and the next big ideas. *The Online Journal of Issues in Nursing, 18*(2), 4.

Wall, B., Novak, J., & Wilkerson, S. (2005). The doctor of nursing practice: Reengineering healthcare. *Journal of Nursing Education, 44*(9), 396–403.

CHAPTER SEVENTEEN

Reflective Response 1

Grant Charles

Whether we acknowledge it or not, we are intimately connected with members of other professions. We cannot fully function even in the most isolated of practice settings without the direct or indirect support of numerous other professionals. Yet despite this, we spend little time in our entry-level training or in our subsequent practice, thinking or learning about these other professions. If we think about them at all, it is often through the egocentric lens of our own profession and particular job roles. We often struggle to understand the worldviews of the other professions. We know our view is the correct one and become frustrated when others express other perspectives. There are, of course, people who work hard to understand other professions although not as many as are needed. As a result and as Novak rightfully identifies, there is a price patients pay when members of the various health professions do not relate well to each other. It has been well documented in a number of jurisdictions that when there is a lack of collaboration between the health professions, there is a corresponding increase in intervention errors and patient death (Kohn, Corrigan, & Donaldson, 2000; Romanow, 2002).

Novak correctly calls for increased attention to be paid to how relationships with other practitioners and with patients can be improved. She discusses the need for nurses to let go of traditional insular behaviors and to reach out and learn with and from other professions especially during their foundational training. I commend her statements on this issue. She has rightfully identified the beginning point for collaboration and for creating significant changes in the health care system.

It is unfortunate though that she gives the nurse-managed health home model as an example of how this collaboration could work. This is more of an interdisciplinary approach. The same is true of the service-learning project she describes later in the chapter. Both are interesting projects but I would respectfully suggest neither appear to me to be interprofessional. The difference between interprofessional and interdisciplinary is critical. Interprofessional education (IPE) is when two or more professions purposefully interact in order to learn with, from, and about each other (Charles & Alexander, 2014a). The goal is to learn to see the world through the perspective of the other. Interdisciplinary is more about using the knowledge of two or more professions to achieve a desired outcome (Charles & Alexander, 2014a). The goal is to take knowledge from a number of professions to provide the best service. There are obviously connected concepts and adhering to an interprofessional approach can increase the likelihood of incorporating the best approaches needed for any given service. However, they are not the same thing. Working side by side is not the same as trying to actively understand another profession.

At the core, IPE and practice helps us not only learn with, from, and about other professions, but also helps us to be able to actively express to members of other professions that their knowledge, skills, and worldviews matter to us. Mattering is the active process of expressing that we understand and accept others and that what they think and believe are important to us (Charles & Alexander, 2014b). This is a critical point that is rarely discussed with regard to our interactions with others. Feeling that "we matter to others" is key in decreasing interprofessional conflicts. In the absence of this sense of mattering, there is a high likelihood of territorial conflict between professions and personal conflict between individuals. Mattering is a way of validating other professions and, in turn, feeling validated by them.

Novak falls into the same trap that others do when writing in this area. She identifies where we should be going without really identifying why we struggle to get there. What is lacking from the chapter is a clear sense of how our professional training can hold us in place rather than helping us to develop new ways of being. Without a serious examination of our role in contributing to the current state of affairs, we risk changing only how we talk about collaboration and partnership rather than actually helping develop new ways of working with others. My response to Novak focuses on why we need to pay close attention to the points she raises regarding interprofessional practice and service learning, while, at the same time, calling for even further examination of not where we can go, but why we are not getting there.

Perhaps the best place to start in this response is to provide an overview of how we develop our identity as professionals. While a great deal has been written on the education of health care professionals, little attention has been paid to our individual identity development as professionals (Charles & Alexander 2014a; Charles, Bainbridge, & Gilbert, 2010). It is our sense of "who we are" rather than just "what we know" that dictates how we interact with each other and with service users within the health care environment. Humans change over time. This change is dependent on how we create meaning and form ideas about ourselves and our environment (Alexander, 2007; Valsiner, 2000). It is this process of determining meaning in interpersonal interactions that strongly influences who we become as individuals and professionals and, in turn, continues to influence how we relate to members of our own profession, other professionals, and the people for whom we provide services.

This development of "who we become" as a member of a profession begins with our earliest entry level training. While still under the influence of the broader context of society and personal relationships outside of their college or university, students are immersed in both academic and practice settings during the course of their professional training. Simply put, "who we become" in the course of our training is in part dictated by the environment in which we are trained and in part by the people with whom we interact. This is the foundation of most professional training. For example, if as nursing students we spend our time in our training primarily interacting with other nursing students, then as nurses we likely assume the general values, attitudes, and knowledge modeled for us daily. In fact, if we do not incorporate these values, attitudes, and knowledge, then there is a good chance that we will not complete our training.

As we progress through our entry-level training, we increasingly see the world from the viewpoint of our profession. This signals that we are becoming a member of our profession. It is easy to begin to think that the way our profession sees the world is the only "true" way to view it. This uniprofessional focus ensures the development of a worldview that has traditionally been seen as being appropriate to our profession. However, the lack of systematic exposure to other professions means that we do not have the opportunity to learn that there is more than one valid way of seeing the world. In fact, our training encourages loyalty to our own profession with the corresponding risk that we may reject, at least partially, the other ones.

It is this narrowing of perspectives that can create so many of the communication misunderstandings regularly seen between the various health professions (Charles et al., 2010). For example, how one interprets an interaction with a practitioner from another profession is dependent on one's own profession's world view, which is largely formed in each individual through professional training. If we have not had systematic exposure to other professions, then it is easy to assume that the way we see the world is "correct." Not only does one not automatically try to see the world from the other's perspective, but often we are not even aware that there is another perspective. It is easy to think that if a member of another profession does not agree with us, it is because they are wrong, misinformed, or maybe just not as well-trained. When two people from different professions take this position when interacting with each other, it is quite understandable that there could be serious disagreement and conflict.

Unfortunately, we tend to take this early way we see the world into our practice. Unless successfully challenged, these ways of interacting with others continue and can easily be entrenched throughout our practice careers and through the acquisition of advanced level degrees. Further education does not guarantee that we will become more open to the viewpoints of other professions. Indeed, there are powerful forces at play within the practice and academic communities that contribute to ongoing interprofessional difficulties.

There have been a number of barriers identified that inhibit the implementation of an interprofessional agenda within practice and academic sites (Charles, Bainbridge, Copeman-Stewart, Art, & Kassam, 2006; Charles, Bainbridge, Copeman-Stewart, Kassam, & Tiffin, 2008; Paul & Peterson, 2002; Salhani & Charles, 2007). These include, as mentioned, different philosophies of working and values of the various professions (Loxley, 1997; Miller, Freeman, & Ross, 2001). Also, there can be a fear of deskilling or deprofessionalization (Loxley, 1997; Miller et al., 2001). The push for closed role boundaries and the protection of our own professional knowledge also contributes to the creation of barriers (Miller et al., 2001). Other identified barriers include power differences between the professions, territoriality and fear of domain infringement (Geva, Barsky, & Westernoff, 2000; Hornby & Atkins, 2000), role insecurity (Hornby & Atkins, 2000), and the perceived need for clinical freedom or autonomy (Loxley, 1997). The power of these barriers to hold us in our old ways of doing things should not be underestimated. Most of the health professions have struggled long and hard to find their place in the system and are loath to take any actions that would put them at risk regardless of their stated commitment to collaborative practice. However, until we begin to address our part as individual practitioners and as members of a profession in contributing to the development and maintenance of these barriers, we cannot truly develop healthy interprofessional partnerships. Collaboration of this type means being willing to invite members of other professions into areas of our practice that we have traditionally claimed as our own. It also means that being willing to accept that other ways of doing things can be as effective as the way we have traditionally done them.

Novak also mentions in her chapter how service learning opportunities can contribute to the development of an improved health care delivery system. I strongly agree with her central message, although once again I would push the unspoken core concept of what she is saying to examine how these types of experience can help us find new ways of developing our sense of professional identity, thus changing how we interact with others. Service learning, similar to interprofessional collaboration, is an attempt to redefine how we interact with others. It is meant to break down the often rigid, one-way, top-down relationships that characterize traditional provider–patient interactions (Charles & Dharamsi, 2010; Charles, Dharamsi, & Alexander, 2011). Community service learning has been developed in part as a response to a growing realization that while professional education produces good technical practitioners, it does not necessarily contribute to the development of socially responsible citizens. Student involvement in service learning projects can help foster an applied rather than abstract sense of civic responsibility (Waterman, 1997). Benefits for students have been seen to include positive changes in moral development, civil responsibility, critical thinking, problem analysis, cultural awareness, and increased understanding of the connection between people and their social environments (Bordelon & Phillips, 2007; Lemieux & Allen, 2007; Ngai, 2006; Roos et al., 2005). Perhaps most importantly, service learning experiences teach students about the power of "patient voice." Community members are used as teachers and not solely recipients of services. This represents a significant shift in the relationship. The provider–patient partnership becomes reciprocal rather than unidirectional.

This shift in the relationship has tremendous potential for changing how we perceive ourselves as professionals and for how we interact with others. We are really only now also beginning to understand that we become who we are as professionals in part through our interactions with the people we serve (Alexander, 2008, Alexander & Charles, 2009; Garfat & Charles, 2007). Traditionally (and continuing to today), we have tended to see the provider-patient relationships as being one way. We give our skills and knowledge and they receive. Their role in this process is seen as being relatively passive. Our traditional way of interacting with patients has always ignored the true nature of relationships. Whether we want to acknowledge it or not, human relationships, even those of a professional nature, are bidirectional. There is always a two-way process in any human interaction (Valsiner, 2000). The motivation for trying to develop "professional" distance from those with whom we work is commendable. We have believed that this protects patients. However, what it can really do is dehumanize and invalidate them (and us) in the process. This is not healthy for anyone. Rather than denying the two-way nature of relationships, we need to challenge the underlying philosophy behind our interactions with patients and the reasons we provide service the way we do. The same holds true in our interactions with other professions.

There has to be room in our development of our professional identity to acknowledge the importance of mutuality in relationships. We need to begin to openly accept that if we want to work effectively with patients and other professions, then we need to develop a sense of shared relationship. This requires that we strive to ensure that there is room and opportunity for a joint investment in the relationship by each participant. This is not to say that we shift the focus from task to process, thus preventing a timely delivery of service. Rather, it is a call for an acceptance that a focus on reciprocity and mutuality can enrich the quality of the interaction and the outcome for both the patient and the provider.

All of this is to say that if we truly want to develop a healthier and more effective delivery system, we need to challenge the way in which we interact with members of other professions and with the people we serve. We need to seriously examine how we develop our professional identities in order to identify those aspects of it that are holding back the development of reciprocal and respectful relationships with colleagues and patients. We need to seriously ask ourselves what is it in our profession's worldview and way of doing things that reinforces barriers and boundaries. We also need to appreciate that the other professions can help us achieve the goals of our profession rather than seeing them as a potential threat.

In order to do any of this, we have to reconceptualize how we train entry-level students—in this case, new bachelors of science in nursing (BSN)-to-DNPs (particularly) and post-master's DNPs too. It is not enough to change any single aspect of how we develop as professions. We must examine the interplay between professional identity development, the reciprocity of relationships with patients and other service providers, and the boundaries we create that, however well-meant serve to distance ourselves from others. We cannot do this by simply calling for greater collaboration. We have to be willing to challenge our professional worldview. This is no easy task giving the context within which we have developed and maintained our worldview. There can be no denying that many people will find this a risky proposition. However, if we do not do it, then the likelihood that we effect significant change in our delivery systems and patient outcomes is minimal.

I fully agree with Novak's call for increased interdisciplinary and interprofessional collaboration although I would give the later the priority. Interprofessional understanding can lead to more effective interdisciplinary collaboration. This involves challenging how advanced practice nurses or doctoral advanced practice nurses become who they become. This requires seriously question how nursing cannot only contribute to an advancement of collaborative practice, but also how nursing also helps create the barriers that hinder or block these efforts. If change could be brought about simply by agreeing on where we should be going, then we would already all be working in healthy and collaborative delivery and academic settings. Change is difficult and can come about only through the efforts of people willing not just to try to change the system but also themselves. This is the essence of true leadership.

■ REFERENCES

Alexander, C. (2007). You are what you do. *Relational Child and Youth Care Practice, 20*(3), 17–21.

Alexander, C. (2008). Accepting gifts from youth: Reciprocity makes a difference. *Relational Child and Youth Care Practice, 21*(2), 27–35.

Alexander, C., & Charles, G. (2009). Caring, mutuality and reciprocity in social worker-client relationships. *Journal of Social Work, 9*(1), 5–22.

Charles, G., & Alexander, C. (2014a). An introduction to interprofessional practice in social and health care settings. *Relational Child and Youth Care Practice, 27*(3), 51–55.

Charles, G., & Alexander, C. (2014b). Beyond attachment: Mattering and the development of meaningful moments. *Relational Child and Youth Care Practice, 27*(3), 26–30.

Charles, G., Bainbridge, L., & Gilbert, J. (2010). The University of British Columbia model of interprofessional education. *Journal of Interprofessional Care, 24*(1), 9–18.

Charles, G., & Dharamsi, S. (2010). Service learning, interprofessional education and the social work placement: The case for combining the best of all worlds. In E. Ralph, K. Walker, & R. Wimmer (Eds.), *The practicum in professional education: Canadian perspectives* (pp. 69–88). Calgary, AL, Canada: Detselig Press.

Charles, G., Bainbridge, L., & Gilbert, J. (2010). The University of British Columbia model of interprofessional education. *Journal of Interprofessional Care, 24*(1), 9–18.

Charles, G., Bainbridge, L., Copeman-Stewart, K., Kassam, R., & Tiffin, S. (2008). Impact of an interprofessional rural health care practice education experience on students and communities. *Journal of Allied Health, 37*(3), 127–131.

Charles, G., Bainbridge, L., Copeman-Stewart, K., Art, S. T., & Kassam, R. (2006). The Interprofessional Rural Program of British Columbia (IRPbc). *Journal of Interprofessional Care, 20*(1), 40–50.

Charles, G., Dharamsi, S., & Alexander, C. (2011). Interprofessional field education: Reciprocal learning for collaborative practice. In J. Drolet, N. Clark, & H. Allen (Eds.), *Shifting sites of practice: Field experience in Canada* (pp. 253–263). Toronto, ON, Canada: Pearson.

Garfat, T., & Charles, G. (2007). How am I who I am? Self in child and youth care. *Relational Child and Youth Care Practice, 20*(6), 6–16.

Geva, E., Barsky, A., & Westernoff, F. (2000). Developing a framework for interprofessional and diversity informed practice. In E. Geva, A. Barsky, & F. Westernoff (Eds.), *Interprofessional practice with diverse populations: Cases in point* (pp. 1–28). Westport, CT: Auburn House.

Hornby, S., & Atkins, J. (2000). *Collaborative care: Interprofessional, interagency and interpersonal* (2nd ed.). Malden, MA: Blackwell Science.

Kohn, L. T., Corrigan, J. M., & Donaldson, M. S. (2000). *To err is human: Building a better health system.* Washington DC: National Academies Press.

Lemieux, C. M., & Allen, P. D. (2007). Service learning in social work education: The state of knowledge, pedagogical practicalities, and practice conundrums. *Journal of Social Work Education, 43*(2), 309–325.

Loxley, A. (1997). *Collaboration in health and welfare: Working with difference.* London, UK: Jessica Kingsley Publications.

Miller, C., Freeman, M., & Ross, N. (2001). *Interprofessional practice in health and social care: Challenging the shared learning agenda.* London, UK: Arno.

Ngai, S. S. (2006). Service-learning, personal development, and social commitment: a case study of university students in Hong Kong. *Adolescence, 41*(161), 165–176.

Paul, S., & Peterson, C. Q. (2002). Interprofessional collaboration: Issues for practice and research. *Occupational Therapy in Health Care, 15*(3-4), 1–12.

Romanow, R. J. (2002). *Building our values: the future of health care in Canada-final report.* Ottawa, ON, Canada: Commission on the Future of Health Care in Canada.

Roos, V., Temane, Q. M., Davis, L., Prinsloo, C. E., Kritzinger, A., Naude, E., & Wessels, J. C. (2005). Service learning in a community context: Learners' perceptions of a challenging training paradigm. *South African Journal of Psychology, 35*(4), 703–716.

Salhani, D., & Charles, G. (2007). The dynamics of an interprofessional team: The interplay of child and youth care with other professions within a residential treatment milieu. *Relational Child and Youth Care Practice, 20*(4), 12–20.

Valsiner, J. (2000). *Culture and human development.* London, UK: Sage.

Waterman, A. S. (1997). An overview of service-learning and the role of research and evaluation in service-learning programs. In A. S. Waterman (Ed.), *Service-learning: Applications from the research* (pp. 1–11). Mahwah, NJ: Erlbaum.

Reflective Response 2

Jihane Hajj

Novak accurately described the crucial role of doctorally prepared advanced practice nurses (APNs) in bringing to the table "a clear professional identity and comprehensive training and development." APNs surely need not pursue a doctoral degree if their sole responsibilities are in firm adherence to the core competencies set forth by their governing entities. It is true that the goal of a Doctor of Nursing Practice (DNP) degree is to prepare and equip the graduate with the skills to enhance the interdisciplinary and interprofessional collaboration potentials with the goal of overcoming the many challenges of our health care system. The following response serves to provide the reader with concrete examples that each one is invited to apply in his or her own area of specialty. Through reflection, I will be exercising the true meaning of this act that gives me the complete *freedom* as a thinking being to examine the end results of my actions and in this case my role as a doctorally prepared APN (Gasche, 1986). In this response, I will be strictly referring to concrete examples in the area of prevention and more specifically cardiovascular prevention. As it is very well known, challenges in the health care system encompasses various specialties and these concrete examples should be merely a guide to expand your thoughts in your future practice as doctorally prepared APNs.

There exist numerous roles of doctorally prepared APNs' contributions in the area of clinical research, evidence appraisal, and guidelines development, and health policy development. Each of these areas are discussed separately resorting to concrete examples from the field of cardiovascular prevention. As a preventive cardiology APN, I specialize in evaluating and managing individuals' cardiovascular risk. It is very well-documented that cardiovascular diseases (CVD) remain the leading cause of death in men and women, and more importantly traditional risk factors (i.e., smoking, lack of exercise, obesity, diabetes, hypertension, hyperlipidemia) do not fully explain the reason individuals get coronary artery disease (CAD). In fact, 60% of patients with CAD have 0 to 1 risk factor, which makes it more challenging to understand the process of atherosclerosis and a tremendous opportunity for research (Nasir et al., 2012). The interdisciplinary collaboration opportunities are unlimited in this field of study. While it is established that APNs possess the ability of understanding and applying the nationally accepted guidelines to decrease cardiovascular risk, the doctorally prepared APN should play additional roles in clinical research to unveil the many mysteries surrounding this nagging disease process. What factors keep CAD the leading cause of death among men and women? What is the role of biomarker of inflammation and how are the newly approved agents (i.e., proprotein convertase subtilisin/kexin type 9 or PCSK9 inhibitors) affect the inflammatory biomarkers, and what are their effects on progression of atherosclerosis? All these questions and many others should be addressed by doctorally prepared APNs in collaboration with other specialists in other disciplines.

The professional identity of the doctorally prepared APN should be flourished in the area of evidence appraisal and guidelines development. Doctorally prepared APNs will be equipped to appraise the evidence. In the area of cardiovascular prevention, there are numerous randomized controlled trials (RCTs) being performed. The American College of Cardiology (ACC) and the American Heart Association (AHA) released in 2013 a set of recommendations to reduce atherosclerotic cardiovascular risk in adults (Stone et al., 2013). These recommendations were set forth by an expert panel from the medical field who reviewed high-quality evidence such as RCTs. The DNP program will prepare the APNs not only to understand and apply the evidence behind our practice but to be part of the expert panel that sets forth the national guidelines pertaining to our practice in this field.

The doctoral prepared APN will also be expected to possess a set of skills in the area of health policy development pertaining to the APN's field of practice. It has been demonstrated through many state initiatives that policy change is a staggering way to enhance public health (Centers of Disease Control and Prevention [CDC], 2013, 2014). Therefore, unlike the counterargument that governing one's health is an individual's responsibility, doctorally prepared APNs are expected to induce policy changes that positively impact their specialty practices. Policy changes are greatly needed in the field of cardiovascular prevention. The soaring costs of CVD expected to reach $275 billion in 2030 are not reflective of preventive costs but purely short- and long-term costs of CVD (Heidenreich et al., 2011). Policy changes are needed in the area of insurance coverage for cardiovascular risk assessment testing. Numerous studies demonstrated that a substantial percentage of individuals diagnosed with CVD and heart attacks did not qualify (before the cardiovascular event) for long-term preventive treatments due to lack of major risk factors (Nasir et al., 2012; Ridker, Buring, Rifai, & Cook, 2007; Wilson et al., 2008). Therefore, individualizing one's risk by evaluating for subclinical atherosclerosis (presence of atherosclerosis in the absence of clinical symptoms) is predictive of CVD and cardiovascular events and is the recommended testing measure, which unfortunately comes with an out-of-pocket cost and not covered by private or governmental insurance agencies (Blaha et al., 2009; Budoff et al., 2007; Detrano et al., 2008; Sarwar et al., 2010). The only exception was with the Texas Heart Attack Prevention Bill that was passed in 2009 and mandated insurance companies to cover the costs of computer tomography (CT) scan for the heart that measures coronary artery calcification scores and/or ultrasonography for the neck vessels (carotid arteries) that measures vessel thickness and evaluate for the presence of atherosclerosis (Beller, 2009). Inducing policy change at this level is a function expected from doctorally prepared APN while collaborating at the interdisciplinary and interprofessional levels.

In summary, I described within this response a few concrete examples of the continuously growing role of the doctorally prepared APN. Through interdisciplinary and interprofessional collaboration, doctorally prepared APNs are capable of inducing many of the much-needed changes in our complex and expensive health care system. When reflecting on your role in your specialized area of practice, do that with complete *freedom*. As Aristotle described freedom being the cause of itself (Liberum est quod Causa sui est), or in other words, freedom calls for knowing self and the truth/value within self. It is imperative to use this freedom in order to envision and design your role in this profession and the unlimited potential that this role has to improve the health care system in general and public health in specific. As a DNP graduate, how would you impact our complex health care system?

■ REFERENCES

Beller, G. A. (2009). The Texas Heart Attack Prevention Bill mandating coverage for CAD Screening tests. *Journal of Nuclear Cardiology, 16*, 681–682. doi:10.1007/s12350-009-9130-0

Blaha, M., Budoff, M. J., Shaw, L. J., Khosa, F., Rumberger, J. A., Berman, D., . . . Nasir, K. (2009). *Journal of the American College of Cardiology Cardiovascular Imaging, 2*(6), 692–700. doi:10.1016/j.jcmg.2009.03.009.

Budoff, M. J., Shaw, L. J., Liu, S. T., Weinstein, S. R., Mosler, T. P., Tseng, P. H., . . . Berman, D. S. (2007). Long-term prognosis associated with coronary artery calcification: Observations from a registry of 25,253 patients. *Journal of the American College of Cardiology, 49*(18), 1860–1870. doi:10.1016/j.jacc.2006.10.079

Centers for Disease Control and Prevention. (2013). *State indicator report on fruits and vegetables*. Retrieved from http://www.cdc.gov/nutrition/downloads/State-Indicator-Report-Fruits-Vegetables-2013.pdf

Centers for Disease Control and Prevention. (2014). *2014 state indicator report on physical activity*. Retrieved from http://www.cdc.gov/physicalactivity/downloads/pa_state_indicator_report_2014.pdf

Detrano, R., Guerci, A. D., Carr, J. J., Bild, D. E., Burke, G., Folsom, A. R., . . . Kronmal, R. A. (2008). Coronary calcium as a predictor of coronary events in four racial and ethnic groups. *New England Journal of Medicine, 358*(13), 1336–1345. doi:10.1056/NEJMoa072100

Gasche, R. (1986). *The tain of the mirror: Derrida and the philosophy of reflection*. Cambridge, MA and London, UK: Harvard University Press.

Heidenreich, P. A., Trogdon, J. G., Khavjou, O. A., Butler, J., Dracup, K., Eze-Kowitz, M. D., . . . Woo Y. J. (2011). Forecasting the future of cardiovascular disease in the United States: A policy statement from the American Heart Association. *Circulation, 123*, 933–44.

Nasir, K., Rubin, J., Blaha, M. J., Shaw, L. J., Blankstein, R., Rivera, J. J., . . . Budoff, M. J. (2009). Interplay of coronary artery calcification and traditional risk factors for the prediction of all-cause mortality in asymptomatic individuals. *Circulation: Cardiovascular Imaging, 5*, 467–473.

Ridker, P. M., Buring, J. E., Rifai, N., & Cook, N. R. (2007). Development and validation of improved algorithms for the assessment of global cardiovascular risk in women: The Reynolds Risk Score. *Journal of the American Medical Association, 297*(13), 1433.

Sarwar, A., Shaw, L. J., Shapiro, M. D., Blankstein, R., Hoffmann, U., Cury, R. C., . . . Nasir, K. (2010). Diagnostic and prognostic value of absence of coronary artery calcification. *Journal of the American College of Cardiology Cardiovascular Imaging, 2*(6), 675–688. doi:10.1016/j.jcmg.2008.12.031

Stone, N. J., Robinson, J. G., Lichtenstein, A. H., Bairey Merz, C. N., Blum, C. B, Eckel, R. H., . . . Tomaselli, G. F; American College of Cardiology/American Heart Association Task Force on Practice Guidelines. (2013). 2013 ACC/AHA guideline on the treatment of blood cholesterol to reduce atherosclerotic cardiovascular risk in adults. *Circulation, 129*(25, Suppl. 2), S1–S45. doi:10.1161/01.cir.0000437738.63853.7a

Wilson, P. W., Pencina, M., Jacques, P., Selhub, J., D'Agostino, R. Sr., O'Donnell, C. J. (2008). C-reactive protein and reclassification of cardiovascular risk in the Framingham Heart Study. *Circulation: Cardiovascular Quality and Outcomes, 1*, 92–97.

The DNP-Prepared Nurse's Role in Health Policy and Advocacy

Sr. Rosemary Donley and Carmen Kiraly

This chapter discusses the value of *Essential V, Health Care Policy for Advocacy in Health Care*, in actualizing the role of the advanced practice nurse (APN). In order to place Essential V and the others from *The Essentials of Doctoral Education for Advanced Nursing Practice* (American Association of Colleges of Nursing [AACN], 2006) in context, the authors briefly examine the evolution of the AACN's Position Statement on the Practice Doctorate in Nursing (AACN, 2004).

■ THE EVOLUTION OF THE PRACTICE DOCTORATES

The 11 authors of the report, *The Essentials of Doctoral Education for Advanced Nursing Practice*, linked their proposal to the Doctor of Nursing (ND) program that was developed at Case Western Reserve in 1979. Briefly describing the trajectory of clinical doctorates, they noted that in the early 1960s some schools of nursing offered doctoral degrees focused on practice rather than research. Most readers are familiar with the Doctor of Nursing Science (DNS, DNSc, or the DSN) programs and degrees. Scheckel (2009) provides a time-oriented context about the emergence of the Doctor of Nursing Practice (DNP) degree describing four phases in the development of doctoral education in nursing: the doctor of education (EdD; 1900–1940), a PhD degree in the basic or social sciences (PhD: 1940–1960), a PhD in the basic or social sciences with a minor in nursing (PhD: 1960–1970), and the proliferation of two pathways (DNSc and PhD: 1970–present). Other authors have discussed the motivation behind these early efforts. Commenting on the EdD in nursing education first offered at Columbia University in 1924, Grace explains that education was an attractive field for nurses who envisioned academic careers because Schools of Education were receptive to students from other practice disciplines. Although PhD programs in education and in the basic or social sciences did not include nursing theory or science, pursuit of these degrees was stimulated by the federally financed Nurse Scientist Program (Edwardson, 2004; Grace, 1989). That talented men and women sought advanced research or education degrees outside of the discipline of nursing reflected not only the state of nursing science in the 1950s and

1960s, but also the norms and social climates of universities, academic medicine, and the health care establishment. Nursing was viewed as a practice rather than a scholarly discipline (Bullough & Bullough, 1984). One window into how nursing was perceived in this period is given by Meleis (1988) in her allusion to the obstacles that nursing faculty faced as they tried to advance a PhD degree in nursing. Graduate councils and provosts rejected their proposals because of the state of nursing science and the lack of qualified faculty with active programs of research. Although the purpose of this chapter is not to revisit nurses' struggles to become accepted within academia and health care circles, it is important to recognize that the DNP is the newest pathway in nurses' journey toward academic and professional recognition.

The AACN (2016a) document, *Advancing Health Care Transformation: A New Era for Academic Nursing,* reports that most leaders in academia and in practice do not hold influential positions in academic health centers. Absent from the policy tables, they are not positioned to inform or direct health care transformation. However, because about 63% of 2.8 million registered nurses (RNs) work in the nation's hospitals in-patient and out-patient settings, nursing is on the agenda of academic health centers, even when nurse leaders are not visible in academic health centers' circles of power (Health Resources and Services Administration [HRSA], 2013). *Essential V* speaks about the present and the future.

Ironically, the initiative to develop professional or practice degrees also comes at a time when traditional PhD programs are being challenged as irrelevant, time consuming, and too narrowly focused on scholarly research (Nyquist, 2002). In describing the Re-visioning PhD Education Project funded by the Pew Foundation and carried out at the University of Washington, Edwardson (2004) compares their findings to the state of doctoral education in nursing in the early years of the 21st century. The Re-visioning Project described: over-production of PhDs, ritualistic degree requirements, overuse of doctoral students in undergraduate education, low program completion rates, long periods of doctoral and postdoctoral training, limited job availability in universities and colleges, and lack of a diverse student body. In her thesis, Edwardson states that PhD programs in nursing lack diversity and that some students spend a long time completing degree requirements (Edwardson, 2004).

Although doctoral programs in nursing were not included in the Re-visioning Project, nurse educators are considering how this report and the loss of faith in traditional PhD education affect their discipline. Nurse leaders are very aware that less than 1% of the nursing workforce holds a PhD in nursing or a related field (Anderson, 2000; Hinshaw, 2001; Robert Wood Johnson Foundation [RWJF], 2013). There is attention to the diversity and the age of nurses who compose PhD student cohorts. The government, private foundations, and schools of nursing have had some success in recruiting, retaining, and graduating men and women of color. Some schools have accepted the challenge of the RWJF to shorten the length of their PhD programs. RWJF's Focus on Scholars program seeks to decrease the age of new PhD nursing graduates by offering significant grants to nurses who enroll in 3-year PhD programs (RWJF, 2013). Other schools have adopted the AACN's proposal to develop bachelor of science in nursing (BSN) to PhD programs as another way of shortening the time that nurses spend in post-baccalaureate studies (Loomis, Willard, & Cohen, 2006). Equally significant as the age of new PhD graduates and the small percentage of nurses with PhDs is the lack of a robust PhD pipeline, a factor frequently emphasized in policy statements about nurse faculty shortages and the rise of DNP education (AACN, 2015c; Berlin & Seachrist, 2002; Martsolf, Auerbach, Spetz, Pearson, & Muchow, 2015).

It is also interesting that more than 10 years after the AACN's proclamation on DNP education, nurses who evaluate DNS programs continue to compare practice-oriented doctorates to research doctorates (AACN, 2014; Fulton & Lyons, 2005; Loomis et al., 2006). Sometimes, the comparisons are critical (Meleis & Dracup, 2005); usually they are descriptive efforts to differentiate the purpose, the educational and/or clinical content, and the intended outcomes of each program (AACN, 2014, 2015b). The 2015 report from AACN's task force on the implementation of the DNP program is AACN's latest effort to restate the intent of the DNP degree; emphasize the incorporation of *The Essentials of Doctoral Education for Advanced Nursing Practice* into curriculum and outcome assessments; and re-state its position that the DNP degree is the educational pathway to advanced practice (AACN, 2015b).

Martsolf et al. (2015) note that although many schools have developed and value DNP education as the route to advanced practice, only about 30% of the schools offer the BSN to DNP program as the entry level into advanced practice. Their data also suggest that the master of science in nursing (MSN) remains a viable and perhaps preferred option for advanced practice education. As yet, there are no published studies that link patient outcomes to the educational pathway of the DNP-prepared APN. Outcome studies do support the quality of care provided by MSN-prepared APNs (Cronenwett et al., 2010; Stanik-Hutt et al., 2013).

Although the doctorate of nursing practice is relatively new, it is being embraced by the nursing community; its rapid growth also heightens concern about the PhD pipeline. Early objectors to the DNP program saw this new degree as adding another dimension to the confusing and unresolved debate about the educational preparation for entry into practice (Meleis & Dracup, 2005). Others acknowledge that nurses aspiring for clinical or administrative careers would select DNP programs because they are shorter and are more appropriate for their future roles (Loomis et al., 2006).

There is also strong support for DNP education from national organizations, notably the AACN, the American Association of Nurse Practitioners (AANP), the American Academy of Nurse Practitioners (AANP), the National Association of Pediatric Nurse Practitioners (NAPNAP), and the National Organization of Nurse Practitioner Faculties (NONPF, 2015). Their websites actively market the significance and the importance of the practice doctorate. The literature also presents opinion articles, survey data, and reports of interviews and studies of nursing schools' approaches to: the BSN to DNP or the post-master's DNP (Martsolf et al., 2015). Almost 30 years ago, Downs (1989) observed that educators have debated the differences surrounding doctoral education since it began in the United States. It seems that nursing has now found a way to continue the entry into practice debates at the doctoral level.

■ THE DNP DEGREE

What can be said about the state of the DNP? There has been an amazing response from schools of nursing to the AACN's 2004 statement on practice doctorates. In a recent review of the AACN's (2016) website, the month after the 2015 transition deadline for recognizing the DNP degree as the entry level into advanced nursing practice had passed, 271 schools of nursing offered DNP programs and another 100 programs were said to be in planning stages. In Figure 18.1, the AACN shows a comparison between the growth of DNP and PhD programs between 2006 and 2014 (AACN, 2015a).

The AACN (2015b) notes, however, that the variability among existing DNP programs transcends the different entry pathways: the BSN to DNP or post-master's DNP. Institutional, academic, regulatory, professional, and economic factors influence how each dean and faculty plan, implement, evaluate, and fund the DNP program of studies and establish admission standards (AACN, 2014).

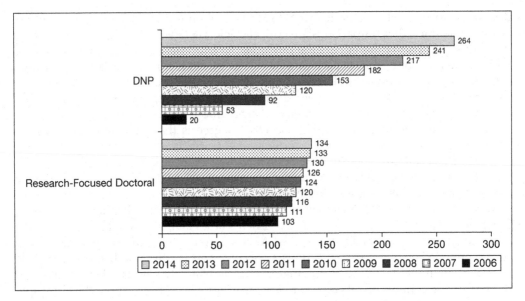

FIGURE 18.1   Comparison of growth between PhD and DNP programs from 2006 to 2014.

DNP, Doctor in Nursing Practice.

Source: American Association of Colleges of Nursing (2015a).

The drafters of the 2004 position statement envisioned that the competencies and scope of practice of DNP graduates would transcend the institutional walls of the Academy (AACN, 2015b). Citing the Institute of Medicine's (IOM) classic studies on medication errors and patient safety, *To Err Is Human* (1999) and *Crossing the Quality Chasm* (2001), the authors argued that a new type of APN was needed if this country were to improve quality of health care. Guided by the proposal, *Health Professions Education: A Bridge to Quality* (2003), the IOM spoke of a new care delivery system that was patient centered, evidence based, interdisciplinary, informed by informational technology, and oriented to improve quality of care.

In proposing practice doctorates in nursing, the AACN (2004) increased the educational competencies of master's-prepared APNs, slightly lengthened advanced practice programs to establish educational parity with other health professionals, sought to improve practice and patient care outcomes, and increased the supply of clinical faculty.

Essential V, Health Policy for Advocacy in Health Care is identified as a core concept in doctoral education for advanced nursing practice (AACN, 2004). Any nurse who aspires to a position of leadership in nursing or health care needs to be grounded in health policy.

■ HEALTH POLICY COMPETENCE AND THE ADVANCED PRACTICE NURSING

While there are many definitions of health policy, most authors purport that policies are decisions about the allocation of resources made by persons with authority (Longest, 2016; Mason, Gardner, Outlaw, & O'Grady, 2016). In the United States, health care decision making resides in both the public and private sectors. This public/private engagement is unique in developed countries because in other developed countries health care is a benefit of citizenship. The Department of Health and Human Services (DHHS, 2014) reported that 4 years after the Patient Protection and Affordable Care Act (PPACA) had been enacted the number of uninsured adults decreased by 10.3 million. However, 5 years after the passage of the PPACA of 2010, the employer-based commercial health plans remain the major source of health insurance for the majority of American workers and their families (Kaiser Family Foundation [KFF], 2014a). The aged, the poor, the totally and permanently disabled, and special populations such as active duty military and their dependents, and veterans participate in health insurance programs supported by the federal and state government insurance plans. At the time of the enactment of the PPACA, it was estimated that approximately 47 million Americans (18% of the population) were underinsured (KFF, 2014b). Despite its complexity and the engagement of the government and the private sector, American health care faces three persistent policy challenges: the iron-triangle of access, cost, and quality (McClellan & Rivlin, 2014).

ACCESS

Without health insurance there is limited access to health care services unless a person has the ability to pay his own health care bill. For the majority of Americans, health insurance is obtained through enrollment in: employer-supported health insurance plans; plans purchased from private sector insurance brokers; the ACA's health exchange; or government-sponsored health plans such as Medicare and Medicaid. Each option requires that enrollees and their dependents meet eligibility requirements, adhere to enrollment timelines, and pay required premiums and fees. As the major purpose of the PPACA (2010) is to reduce the number of uninsured Americans, the law includes mandates to enable all people to obtain affordable health insurance. These mandates affect: employees, insurance providers, employers that offer insurance plans, and all under- or uninsured citizens. Those who fail to comply with the mandates pay fines. These mandates are not popular; efforts to rescind them or challenge their constitutionality have been engaged at all levels of government. The PPACA is an issue in the 2016 Presidential election; members of Congress have introduced repeated bills to rescind the ACA and/or change some of its provisions; the Supreme Court has ruled on its constitutionality in *The National Federation of American Business (NIFIB) v. Sebelius, 2012* and *King v. Burwell, 2015* (Center for Health Law, 2012; Scotus Blog, 2015). Although anyone who works in, profits from, or cares about personal or population health care is a stakeholder, education in health policy is required to actualize this responsibility. *Essential V* urges nurses, especially APNs, to actively participate in health policy development and evaluation.

COST

Another important goal of the PPACA is the reduction in the growth of health care costs. Although America has the highest health care costs in the world and invests 17% of its gross domestic product (GDP) in health care (World Bank, 2011–2015), cost control is challenging. McClellan and Rivlin (2014) suggest three complementary strategies to slow cost escalation: avoid wasteful spending, especially waste linked to inefficiencies; increase market competition; and improve population health. Waste reduction is a popular political theme, because waste accounts for about 20%

of health care expenditures (Berwick & Hackbarth, 2012). These authors delineate six categories of wasteful behavior: overtreatment, lack of care coordination, failure in care delivery processes, administrative complexity, pricing failures, and fraud and abuse. Another common theme in post-ACA's discussions is the cost of medication errors in acute care settings. While most patients have not read the IOM's trilogy on patient safety, they know that medication errors are more than costly; they can cause death (IOM, 1999). Nationally, there are many efforts within the health care, medical, nursing, pharmacological, technological, and accreditation communities to improve medication practices and make hospitals safer places. At the governmental level, beginning in 2009, Medicare changed its hospital payment system and withheld additional payments to hospitals when patients were found to have acquired infections, pressure ulcers, or injuries from falls during their hospital stays (Watcher, Foster & Dudley, 2008).

Insurance plans compete on product design and price. Health care is a lucrative business; capitalism rewards the most successful health entrepreneurs. Market forces are influenced by supply and demand, not vulnerability, poor health status, need, or poverty. Cost plays an important role in the American health care establishment because health care affects all sectors of the economy. Berwick and Hackbarth (2012) are not alone in thinking that competition among health care providers will bring down costs. Yet, this assumption about the health care marketplace has yet to produce a health care delivery system that improves health status, enhances the quality of care, and lowers health care costs in America.

POPULATION HEALTH AND BUILDING A CULTURE OF HEALTH CARE

Although population health has been a mantra in public health circles for years, it is now identified as an *Essential VI* in the AACN's *Essentials of Doctoral Education for Advanced Nursing Practice* (AACN, 2004; Marmot, 2005). Interest in population health speaks about a global awareness that treatment of disease provides only a partial answer to improving health status of individuals and populations (Starfield & Shi, 2002). The social, environmental, and living situations that determine health are increasingly linked to improved health status, reduced health disparities, and cost control (Centers for Disease Control [CDC], 2015). The IOM (2016) recently published a high-level framework to educate future health providers about the importance of the *Social Determinants of Health*. In 2013, the RWJF working with the RAND Corporation embarked on an ambitious project, a Culture of Health Initiative (Acousta et al., 2016). Their vision was expressed as six priorities: bridging health and health care; building demand for healthy places and practices; eliminating health disparities; engaging business for health; strengthening vulnerable children and families; and leadership (RWJF, 2015). Plough (2015) describes this initiative as a challenge for the public health workforce. *Essential VI, Clinical Prevention and Population Health for Improving the Nation's Health*, identifies DNP-prepared APNs as leaders in population health (AACN, 2004). Although the DNPs' role in promoting and transforming health care into a culture of health is yet to be articulated in the nursing literature, the AACN's (2004) essentials document and the newly released AACN (2016a) report on *Escalating Academic Nursing's Impact on Transforming Health and Health Care* are compatible with this vision. Plough's related call to learn how to use big data sets is also very relevant to any nurse leader or researcher who aspires to analyze patterns of population health in real time.

QUALITY OF CARE

Quality of care is the most elusive and difficult concept to define and measure among the access, cost, and quality triad. Quality is increasingly linked to achieving successful outcomes rather than describing and measuring structures, processes, or patient satisfaction (Torgerson & Raftery, 1999). Since the implementation of PPACA, attention is focused on value-based incentives to improve outcomes by changing providers' practice patterns and reframing payment strategies (Centers for Medicare & Medicaid Services [CMS], 2016). If successful, these new payment systems will replace the old fee for service payment models. Moving away from familiar fee-for-service systems to value modifiers and meaningful use of payment systems creates management and political challenges (Miller, 2012). Yet, there is growing traction among policy makers around strategies that link value-based payments and care management practices to produce demonstrable patient outcomes (McClellan & Rivlin, 2014). Another popular fiscal strategy, designed to lower costs and enhance quality of care, is bundled payments. Bundling provides single payments for a defined treatment, compressing all the possible charges for an episode of care into a single payment. Because bundling is used for common and predictable procedures, as knee replacements, providers and insurers can estimate and manage the risks of accepting bundled payments rather than fees for service (Delbanco, 2014).

The American health care establishment also relies on technology to deliver and advance patient care. Initially, the technology was medically oriented. Now, high technology medicine competes with sophisticated informational technology, as the electronic medical record (EMR), in institutional and community-based centers and practices. There is a compelling need to access timely, accurate and secure data by patients, clinicians, insurance companies, and the government. Competing concerns about privacy and appropriate access to health data challenge the health care establishment to rethink where it spends its 3 trillion dollar health care budget. If one aspires leadership in nursing or health care, competence in health policy is a necessity. Advocacy must be balanced and informed.

HEALTH POLICY COMPETENCE

When Longest (2016) speaks of policy competence, he notes that anyone who wants to influence health policy must understand the policy process and comprehend how health policies are made. This knowledge gives leaders the skill in scanning policy and political environments, and identifying the threats and opportunities on the horizon. These insights help leaders shape the policy environment for the benefit of their group's interest. Longest is speaking of federal and state health policy, but his advice also applies to nongovernmental sectors, because U.S. health policy arises from the private as well as the public sector. Advocacy is ineffective if the person or group desiring change does not grasp the workings of extant systems and the powerful forces that sustain them.

Longest (2016) also proposes that successful policy advocates possess two skill sets: the ability to gain access to policy environments and the organizational acumen to build consensus around an agenda. In this context, access means that nurses know their elected representatives and can get their attention; they have the power to bring issues of importance to government. That nurses can have access to political power brokers is not surprising. American nurses (2.8 million RNs and 690,000 licensed practical nurses [LPNs]) are a large, geographically distributed group of health care providers. Approximately

55% of the 2.8 million RNs hold BSN degrees; approximately 11% have master's or doctoral degrees. While the majority of nurses live in urban areas, about 445,000 RNs and 166,000 LPNs live in rural communities where 52 million people also reside (HRSA, 2013). The number and the geographical locations of nurses give them natural access to members of Congress, especially members of the House of Representatives. Four large nursing organizations that represent practicing nurses, educators, researchers, accreditors, and administrators, the American Nurses Association (ANA), the National League for Nursing (NLN), the AACN, and the American Organization of Nurse Executives (AONE), form the Tri-Council for Nursing. This alliance of autonomous nursing organizations periodically issues policy and position papers that represent the view of its member organizations. The Tri-Council for Nursing (n.d.) also discusses and advocates for policies that cross and occasionally unite the special interests in nursing.

What constitutes the policy agenda of the Tri-Council? Given that it is an alliance and not another nursing organization, the best clue to its business is contained in the policy websites of its four constituent members. It can be said that securing and increasing funding for Title VIII, the Nursing Workforce Development Programs, and obtaining funding from the National Institute of Nursing Research is high on the agenda of the Tri-Council.

The ANA (2016), the official spokesperson for nursing, lists as its legislative issues: safe staffing, safe handling and mobility of patients, home health, nurse workforce development, health reform, advanced practice registered nurses (APRNs) and durable medical equipment, APRNs and veterans, and RN nursing home staffing. Their website also publishes information about the ANA-PAC (political action committee), the fundraising and political support arm of the ANA. The AACN's (2015d) ambitious federal policy agenda includes five familiar goals: advance policies to prepare a more highly educated and diverse nursing workforce, focusing on seamless academic progression, affordability, and interprofessional education; amplify nurses' role in transforming America's health care delivery system into one that is patient centered and team based; obtain federal investment in academic nursing's infrastructure; secure federal funds to support research; and elevate the role of nursing. The AONE identifies Title VIII re-authorization, elevation of nursing research and data, promotion of the value of nursing, and sustaining and growing funding for nursing. The NLN (2015–2016), the accreditor of all programs that lead to licensure and graduate programs at the master's and DNP levels, lists its 2015–2016 governmental affairs agenda as: access, education, diversity, and workforce. However, these four organizations alone or in alliance are joined by other voices that speak for nursing. These voices represent the interest of members of specialty nursing organizations, exemplified by the American Association of Critical-Care Nurses (AACN, 2016b). This group traces its four decade engagement in health policy on their website. Although most nursing associations are not registered as lobbyists, many hire Washington-based lobbying firms to advise them about bringing their issues to Congress or the Executive Branch of government. All these organizations and a large number of specialty nursing organizations employ policy experts on their staffs or contract with public policy staffs. These individuals frequently visit the Hill and bring their organizations' elected and appointed leaders to meet with members of Congress and their committee and office staffs. The ANA, the AACN and the NLN have offices based in Washington so that they can easily access policy makers.

ORGANIZATION

Then, there is the question of organization. Nurses do not agree or rally around a common agenda. Although there are many nursing organizations, no group speaks for all nurses. At the federal level, from the Tri-Council and many of the large specialty groups, there is support for nurse traineeships (Title VIII) and the education of APNs; deans, individually and through the AACN, join the research community to lobby for additional funds for research and evidence-based practice. In the states, issues revolve around licensing reform and efforts to assure a full scope of practice for nurse practitioners and other APNs. At the state level, nurses and their organizations engage in power battles with organized medicine and hospital and nursing home associations over access to care, cost, and quality.

Abood (2007) makes an important contribution when she observes that bedside nurses know that cost containment and lack of coordination can affect their patients' quality of care. She also insists that if nurses are to address access, cost, and quality of care in meaningful ways, they must move out of their comfort zones. Although Abood is examining policy or practice change at the micro level, she affirms that if nurses are to bring about changes in policy, they need the access to power, the will to carry their activities forward, the time, and the energy. Her observations about the level of commitment that policy change requires can be generalized to state and federal policy work.

■ SUMMARY

As has been stated frequently in this chapter, AACN's *Essential V* challenges DNP graduates to become engaged in health policy. Their engagement in the world of health policy at federal and state levels will not create a common voice for nursing in policy arenas or breakdown the silos that limit interdisciplinary collaboration. However, their direct engagement in the policy process will bring first-hand observations of patient care experiences to policy tables. It is well recognized that unidentified problems cannot be solved. Because APNs work in institutions, primary practices, urgent clinics, and in communities, they can inform systems thinking, decision making, and innovative, evidenced-based practice. In discussing what leadership means for DNP-educated APNs, Walker and Polancich (2015) posit that contemporary practice requires the application of specialized knowledge, clinical expertise, and the capacity to discern appropriate interventions and policy changes that will improve care. Leadership requires a mix of cognitive, clinical, and interpersonal skills.

Years ago, Hildegarde Peplau said that nurses can win the battle for quality of care at the bedside but lose it at the policy table. *Essential V* challenges DNP graduates to advocate for quality of care, not only at unit and service centers in institutions, but also in board rooms, in the literature, and in public forums. APNs must speak in the places where decisions that affect practice and patient care are made.

■ CRITICAL THINKING QUESTIONS

1. *Discuss the engagement of DNP-prepared APNs in creating health policy changes?*
2. *Be specific about steps that DNP-prepared APNs can take to actualize AACN's (2006) Essential V. How can these nurses influence policy change at federal and/or state levels?*
3. *How can DNP-prepared APNs provide leadership in improving the quality of community-based care?*
4. *Describe the differences between MSN and DNP-prepared nurses' engagement in health policy.*
5. *How can a DNP-prepared APN impact the health care policy challenges known as the iron-triangle: access, cost, and quality?*
6. *Describe how a DNP-prepared APN can reduce health care disparities at the population level?*

7. *To what do you attribute the increasing number of DNP-prepared graduates versus PhD-prepared graduates?*
8. *Emphazing impact, what health policy issues do you think have been properly emphasized by the authors of this chapter?*
9. *What issues would you additionally include as policy areas where the DNP-prepared APN can have a critical impact?*
10. *Describe how you might individually impact local, regional, national, or global health policy.*

■ REFERENCES

Abood, S. (2007). Influencing health care in the legislative area. *The Online Journal of Issues in Nursing, 12*(1). Retrieved from http://www.nursingworld.org/MainMenuCategories/ANAMarketplace/ANAPeriodicals/OJIN/TableofContents/Volume122007/No1Jan07/tpc32_216091.html

Acousta, J. D., Whitley, M. D., May, L. W., Dubowitz, T., Williams, M. V., & Chandra, A. (2016). *Perspectives on a culture of health.* Santa Monica, CA: RAND Corporation.

American Association of Colleges of Nursing. (2004). *Position statement on the doctor of nursing practice (DNP).* Retrieved from http://www.aacn.nche.edu/publications/position/DNPpositionstatement.pdf

American Association of Colleges of Nursing. (2006). *The essentials of doctoral education for advanced nursing practice.* Retrieved from http://www.aacn.nche.edu/publications/position/DNPEssentials.pdf

American Association of Colleges of Nursing. (2014). Key differences between DNP and PhD/DNS programs. Retrieved from http://www.aacn.nche.edu/dnp/ContrastGrid.pdf

American Association of Colleges of Nursing. (2015a). DNP fact sheet. Retrieved from http://www.aacn.nche.edu/media-relations/fact-sheets/dnp

American Association of Colleges of Nursing. (2015b). The doctor of nursing practice: Current issues and clarifying recommendations. Retrieved from http://www.aacn.nche.edu/aacn-publications/white-papers/DNP-Implementation-TF-Report-8–15.pdf,1-23

American Association of Colleges of Nursing. (2015c). Nursing faculty shortage. Retrieved from http://www.aacn.nche.edu/media-relations/fact-sheets/nursing-faculty-shortage

American Association of Colleges of Nursing. (2015d). 2015 federal policy agenda. Retrieved from http://www.aacn.nche.edu/government-affairs/legislative-goals

American Association of Colleges of Nursing. (2016a). *Advancing healthcare transformation: A new era for academic nursing.* Washington, DC: Author.

American Association of Critical Care Nurses. (2016b). History of health policy at AACN. Retrieved from http://www.aacn.org/wd/practice/content/publicpolicy/publicpolicyhistory.pcms?menu=practice

American Nurses Association. (2016). Take action America. Retrieved from http://www.rnaction.org/site/PageServer?pagename=nstat_issues

Anderson, C. A. (2000). Current strengths and limitations in doctoral education in nursing: Are we prepared for the future? *Journal of Professional Nursing, 16*(4), 191–200.

Berlin, L. E., & Sechrist, K. R. (2002). The shortage of doctorally prepared nursing faculty: A dire situation. *Nursing Outlook, 50*(2), 50–56.

Berwick, D. M., & Hackbarth, A. D. (2012). Eliminating waste in U.S. healthcare. *Journal of the American Medical Association, 307*(14), 1513–1516.

Bullough, V. L., & Bullough, B. (1984). *History, trends, and politics of nursing.* Norwalk, CT: Appleton-Century-Crofts.

Centers for Disease Control. (2015). Social determinants of health. Retrieved from http://www.cdc.gov/socialdeterminants

Center for Health Law and Policy Innovation, Harvard Law School. (2012). Summary of the decision by the U.S. Supreme Court on the Patient Protection and Affordable Care Act. Retrieved from http://www.chlpi.org/wp-content/uploads/2013/12/SCOTUS_ACA_Summary_6-29-12.pdf

Centers for Medicare & Medicaid Services. (2016). Value-based payment modifier. Retrieved from https://www.cms.gov/medicare/medicare-fee-for-service-payment/physicianfeedback program/valuebasedpaymentmodifier.html

Cronenwett, L., Dracup, K., Grey, M., McCauley, L., Meleis, A., & Salmon, M. (2010). The doctor of nursing practice: A national workforce perspective. *Nursing Outlook, 59,* 9–17.

Delbanco, S. (2014). The payment reform landscape: Bundled payment. Retrieved from http://health affairs.org/blog/2014/07/02/the-payment-reform-landscape-bundled-payment

Department of Health and Human Services FY 2014. (2014). *HHS Agency financial report.* Retrieved from http://www.hhs.gov/sites/default/files/afr/fy2014-agency-financial-report-final.pdf

Downs, F. S. (1989). Differences between the professional doctorate and the academic/research doctorate. *Journal of Professional Nursing, 5*(5), 261–265.

Edwardson, S. R. (2004). Matching standards and needs in doctoral education in nursing. *Journal of Professional Nursing, 20*(1), 40–46.

Fulton, J. S., & Lyon, B. L. (2005). The need for some sense making: Doctor of nursing practice. *The Online Journal of Issues in Nursing, 10*(3). Retrieved from http://www.nursingworld .org/MainMenuCategories/ANAMarketplace/ANAPeriodicals/OJIN/TableofContents/ Volume102005/No3Sept05/tpc28_316027.html

Grace, H. K. (1989). Issues in doctoral education in nursing. *Journal of Professional Nursing, 5*(5), 266–270.

Health Resources and Services Administration. (2013). The U.S. nursing workforce: Trends in supply and education. Retrieved from http://bhpr.hrsa.gov/healthworkforce/reports/nursingworkforce/ nursingworkforcefullreport.pdf

Hinshaw, A. S. (2001). A continuing challenge: The shortage of educationally prepared nursing faculty. *The Online Journal of Issues in Nursing.* Retrieved from http://www.nursingworld.org/ MainMenuCategories/ThePracticeofProfessionalNursing/workforce/NursingShortage/ Resources/ShortageofEducationalFaculty

Institute of Medicine. (1999). *To err is human.* Washington, DC: National Academies Press.

Institute of Medicine. (2001). *Crossing the quality chasm.* Washington, DC: National Academies Press.

Institute of Medicine. (2003). *Health profession education: A bridge to quality.* Washington, DC: National Academies Press.

Institute of Medicine. (2016). *A report brief: A framework for education health professionals to address the social determinants of health.* Washington, DC: The National Academies of Sciences, Engineering, Medicine.

Kaiser Family Foundation. (2014a). Health insurance coverage of the total population. Retrieved from http://kff.org/other/state-indicator/total-population

Kaiser Family Foundation. (2014b). The uninsured at the starting line: Findings from the 2013 Kaiser survey of low-income Americans and the ACA. Retrieved from http://kff.org/uninsured/report/the -uninsured-at-the-starting-line-findings-from-the-2013-kaiser-survey-of-low-income-americans -and-the-aca

Kohn, L. T., Corrigan, J. M., & Donaldson, M. S. (Eds.). (2000). *To error is human: Building a safer health system.* Washington, DC: National Academies Press.

Longest, B. B. (2016). *Health policymaking in the United States.* Chicago, IL: Health Administrative Press.

Loomis, J. A., Willard, B., & Cohen, J. (2006). Difficult professional choices: Deciding between the PhD and DNP in nursing. *The Online Journal of Issues in Nursing, 12*(1).

Marmot, M. (2005). Social determinants of health inequalities. *Lancet, 364*(9464), 1099–1104. Retrieved from http://www.thelancet.com/action/showAbstract?pii=S0140673605742343

Martsolf, G. R., Auerbach, D. I., Spetz, J., Pearson, M. L., & Muchow, A. N. (2015). Doctor of nursing practice by 2015: An examination of nursing schools' decisions to offer a doctor of nursing practice degree. *Nursing Outlook, 63*(2), 219–226.

Mason, D. J., Gardner, D. B., Outlaw, F. H., & O'Grady, E. T. (2016). *Policy and politics in nursing and health care.* St. Louis, MO: Elsevier.

McClellan, M., & Rivlin, A. (2014). *Health policy issue brief: Improving health while reducing growth: What is possible?* Washington, DC: The Brookings Institution.

Meleis, A., & Dracup, K. (2005). The case against the DNP: History, timing, substance, and marginalization. *Online Journal Issues in Nursing, 10*(3). Retrieved from Nursingworld.com

Meleis, A. I. (1988). Doctoral education in nursing: It present and future. *Journal of Professional Nursing, 4*(6), 436–446.

Miller, H. D. (2012). Ten barriers to healthcare payment reform and how to overcome them. Center for HealthCare Quality and Patient Reform. Retrieved from http://www.chqpr.org/downloads/overcomingbarrierstopaymentreform.pdf

National League for Nursing. (2014). Nursing student demographics. Retrieved from http://www.nln.org/newsroom/nursing-education-statistics/nursing-student-demographics

National League for Nursing. (2015–2016). Public policy agenda. Retrieved from http://www.nln.org/docs/default-source/advocacy-public-policy/public-policy-brochure2015-2016.pdf?sfvrsn=0

National Organization of Nurse Practitioner Faculties. (2015). The doctorate of nursing practice NP preparation: NONPF perspective. Retrieved from http://c.ymcdn.com/sites/www.nonpf.org/resource/resmgr/DNP/NONPFDNPStatementSept2015.pdf

Nyquist, J. (2002). The PhD: A tapestry of change for the 21st century. *Change, 34*(6), 12–20.

Patient Protection and Affordable Care Act, 42 U.S.C. § 18001 et seq. (2010).

Plough, A. L. (2015). Building a culture of health: A critical role for Public Health Services Research. *American Journal of Public Health, 105*(Suppl. 2), S150–S152.

Robert Wood Johnson Foundation. (2013). Focus on nursing scholars. Retrieved from http://futureofnursingscholars.org

Robert Wood Johnson Foundation. (2015). Our areas of focus. Retrieved from http://www.rwjf.org/en/our-focus-areas.html

Scheckel, M. (2009). Nursing education: Past, present, future. In G. Roux & J. Halstead (Eds.), *Issues and trends in nursing education: Knowledge for today and tomorrow* (pp. 27–55). Burlington, MA: Jones & Bartlett.

Scotus Blog. (2015). King v. Burwell. Retrieved from http://www.scotusblog.com/case-files/cases/king-v-burwell

Stanik-Hutt, J., Newhouse, R. P., White, K. M., Johantgen, M., Bass, E. B., Zangaro, G., . . . Weiner, J. P. (2013). The quality and effectiveness of care provided by nurse practitioners. *Journal of Nurse Practitioners, 9*(8), 492–500.

Starfield, B., & Shi, L. (2002). Policy relevant determinants of health: An international perspective. *Health Policy, 60*(3), 201–218.

The American Organization for Nurse Executives. (2016). Key issues. Retrieved from http://www.aacn.nche.edu/membership/awards/aone

Torgerson, D., & Raftery, J. (1999). Measuring outcomes in economics evaluations. Retrieved from https://www.researchgate.net/profile/David_Torgerson/publication/12963497_Economics_notes_measuring_outcomes_in_economic_evaluations/links/0deec51a4be91256c7000000.pdf

Tri-Council for Nursing. (n.d.). Joint statement from the Tri-Council for Nursing on recent registered nurse supply and demand projections. Retrieved from https://www.google.com/?gws_rd=ssl#q=what+is+the+Tri+Council+in+nursing

Walker, D. K., & Polancich, S. (2015). Doctor of nursing practice: The role of the advanced practice nurse. *Seminars in Oncology Nursing, 31*(4), 263–272.

Watcher, R. M., Foster, N. E., & Dudley, R. A. (2008). Medicare's decision to withhold payment for hospital errors: The devil is in the details. *The Joint Commission Journal on Quality and Patient Safety, 34*(2),116–123.

World Bank. (2011–2015). Health expenditure, total (%GDP). Retrieved from http://data.worldbank.org/indicator/SH.XPD.TOTL.ZS

CHAPTER EIGHTEEN

Reflective Response

Irene C. Felsman

Donley and Kiraly provide a compelling argument regarding the importance of solid preparation of the Doctor of Nursing Practice (DNP) level advanced practice registered nurse (APRN) to participate in policy development regarding advocacy for quality health care, based on *Essential V of Doctoral Education for Advanced Nursing Practice.* (American Association of Colleges of Nursing, 2006). The authors' analysis of the origin and history of doctorates in the field of nursing is thorough and engaging, beginning with development of the doctor of education (EdD) degree at the turn of the 20th century, and concluding with the current structure of two complementary doctoral level pathways, the PhD and the DNP. A foundation is laid for understanding the distinction between, as well as the interface of these two roles as a basis for discussion of the responsibility for all professional nurses in positions of leadership to engage in health and public policy development. A particularly important point that the authors make is that there appears to be variability in level of rigor among DNP programs as developed by different institutions since the inception of this degree in 2004. Clearly, regulation of program certification is essential if the DNP role is to be seen as credible, particularly in the leadership and health policy arena.

While in accordance with all the issues presented by the authors, I particularly resonate with the concept that the professional nurse in the DNP role is potentially most powerful in terms of representing patient/client experiences in the policy arena. DNPs, given their often intimate and sustained exposure to vulnerable and marginalized populations, are uniquely placed to advocate for policy changes in health care, with the ultimate aim of assuring access to quality, affordable services. Indeed, it may be argued that the expertise of a DNP-prepared nurse is invaluable in terms of representing the realities of underserved populations, those most affected by adverse social determinants of health (SDOH).

Given, as the authors quoted, that less than 1% of the nursing workforce holds PhD in nursing or related fields (Robert Wood Johnson Foundation, 2013), how effective are PhD-prepared nurses functioning alone as advocates for change in health policy that benefit the disenfranchised? Nursing professionals must begin to move beyond differences in educational preparation, complement the strengths of different educational and experiential preparation, and recall the true advocacy nature of our caring profession if there is to be movement toward a health policy agenda which addresses more equitable allocation of resources in our society, the basic premise of the PPACA (2010). Professional nurses at *all* levels of nursing, particularly those of us in leadership and advanced practice roles, must commit to becoming competent in health policy development and evaluation. "Advanced practice registered nurses (APRNs) have positioned themselves to serve an integral role in national health care reform. A successful transformation of the nation's health system will require utilization of all clinicians, particularly primary care providers, to the full extent of their education and scope of practice" (Stanley, Werner, & Apple, 2009).

Health policy competence, as described by Donley and Kiraly in this chapter, includes two primary areas of expertise: the ability to gain access to policy environments and the organizational acumen to build consensus around an agenda. Crucial to this process is the ability to articulate and communicate clearly both the agenda of nursing as a profession as well as the needs of the most vulnerable in ways that will be heard by policy makers. Donley and Kiraly state: "Advocacy is ineffective if the person or group desiring change does not grasp the workings of extant systems and the powerful forces that sustain them." This statement implies an obligation for health care providers to inform and educate clients regarding rights and privileges with regard to their voice in developing health policy, in order to encourage all to engage in action toward a "Culture of Health" (RAND Corporation, n.d.). An awareness of the need to elicit the strength and power of a community or population in addressing their own health care access needs is essential in order for policy to have meaning. For how will change occur if a great majority of the population remains disenfranchised and powerless to affect change? By providing mechanisms for community participation, professional nurses can ensure that voices of the vulnerable will be heard.

As the largest group of health professionals in the world, there is a great potential for nurses to create forward movement regarding a healthy society. I am in agreement with the authors of this chapter that we have fallen short as a profession thus far. Kostas-Polston, Thanavaro, Arvidson, and Taub (2015) articulate a clear mandate: "APNs must come to see political engagement as a professional obligation and health policy as something that they can shape rather than something that happens to them."

In conclusion, it is essential for DNPs to stay abreast of current population's health issues and to fully engage in health policy development. This engagement is inherently multilayered and complex, from the education and representation of clients at the individual and community level to the representation of nursing issues at the local, state, and national levels. The ultimate goal is a safe, equitable, and affordable health care system, ensuring an improved health and well-being of the population (RAND, n.d.).

■ REFERENCES

American Association of Colleges of Nursing. (2006). *The essentials of doctoral education for advanced nursing practice.* Retrieved from http://www.aacn.nche.edu/publications/position/DNPEssentials .pdf

Kostas-Polston, E. A., Thanavaro, J., Arvidson, C., & Taub, L. F. (2015). Advanced practice nursing: Shaping health through policy. *Journal of the American Association of Nurse Practitioners, 27*(1), 11–20. doi:10.1002/2327-6924.12192

Patient Protection and Affordable Care Act. (2010). PUB L 111–148, 124 Stat., March 23, 2010, 119–1024. Retrieved from https://www.gpo.gov/fdsys/pkg/PLAW-111publ148/pdf/PLAW-111publ148.pdf

RAND Corporation. (n.d.). Building a national culture of health. Retrieved from http://www.rand .org/pubs/research_reports/RR1199.html

Robert Wood Johnson Foundation. (2013). Focus on nursing scholars. Retrieved from: http://futureof nursingscholars.org

Stanley, J. M., Werner, K. E., & Apple, K. (2009). Positioning advanced practice registered nurses for health care reform: Consensus on APRN regulation. *Journal of Professional Nursing, 25*(6), 340–348. doi:10.1016/j.profnurs.2009.10.001

Enhancing the Doctoral Advanced Practice Nursing Role With Reflective Practice

Graham Stew

By three methods we may learn wisdom: first, by reflection, which is the noblest; second by imitation, which is the easiest; and third by experience, which is the bitterest.
—Confucius

This chapter is addressed to the advanced practice nurse (APN) studying at a doctoral level, and it explores the concept of reflective practice and its relevance for you and your work. This chapter examines definitions of reflective practice and how the art and science of nursing can be combined with reflection to produce praxis—advanced nursing practice based on scholarship, expertise, and critical thinking. The teaching of reflective practice appears to be more predominant in nursing curricula outside of the United States, and so some of these concepts may be new to you. However, this chapter hopefully reminds you that there is no end point to learning, and that reflection can support further exploration of your practice.

■ WHAT IS REFLECTION AND REFLECTIVE PRACTICE?

The challenge for most writers in this field is to agree on a satisfactory definition of reflection, and the literature is full of worthy attempts. Despite differences in these texts and the plethora of definitions, one dominant assumption among these writers is that reflection is worthwhile and can enhance practice. In the context of learning, reflection is a generic term for intellectual and affective activities in which individuals engage their experience to create and clarify meaning in terms of self, which results in a changed conceptual perspective (Boud, Keogh, & Walker, 1985). John Dewey (1938) summarized the process: "we learn by doing and realizing what came of what we did" (p. 12). Is it simply learning from experience?

Over the years, experienced nursing professionals like yourselves have developed practical knowledge and working intelligence as you made sense of your work in theoretical ways (Schön, 1983). Much of this learning has been subconscious, meaning that you may know more than you consciously realize. Through reflection, this tacit knowledge (or knowing-in-action) can be made conscious and explicit (Argyris & Schön, 1974). Taylor (2000) defined reflection as "the throwing back of thoughts and memories, in cognitive acts such as thinking, contemplation, meditation and any other form of attentive consideration, in order to make sense of them, and to make contextually appropriate changes if they are required" (p. 3). This definition allows for a wide variety of thinking as the basis for reflection, and it is similar to many other explanations by suggesting that reflective thinking is a rational process that produces positive change (Boud et al., 1985; Boyd & Fales, 1983; Mezirow, 1981).

In simple terms, reflection enables you to learn from experience through a systematic process of thinking. You are probably already familiar with Kolb's (1984) well-known learning cycle, which is helpful here (Figure 19.1).

Unless the individual moves through all four stages of this cycle:

1. The actual experience
2. Reflecting on it
3. Relating these reflections to existing knowledge and creating a new perspective on the experience
4. Returning to the practice setting ready to test new understandings then conscious learning in its fullest sense has not occurred

Kuiper and Pesut (2004) defined reflection as a metacognitive process that supports thinking about one's own thinking related to an experience and within a conceptual framework. Jarvis (1992) distinguishes reflective practice from thoughtful practice, and suggests reflective practitioner as one who is able to "problematise many situations of professional performance so they can become potential learning" (p. 180). How to *problematize* practice? The challenge for experienced practitioners like yourselves is to somehow make the familiar strange, and to become aware of (and question) many of your assumptions about practice. This process of unpacking existing knowledge can facilitate *unlearning* many aspects of previous practice, which then opens up possibilities for fresh learning. Unlearning can require a significant break with previous

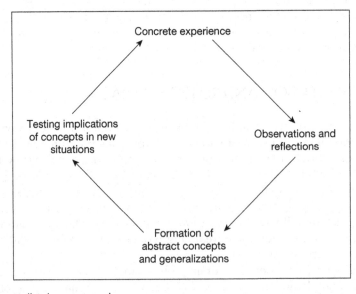

FIGURE 19.1 Kolb's learning cycle.
Source: Kolb (1984).

modes of understanding, doing, and being (Rushmer & Davies, 2004). This intellectual work of change can naturally create tensions between *outside-in* or research knowledge, and *inside-out* or practice knowledge (Hargreaves, Earl, Moore, & Manning, 2001). Nevertheless, changes in understanding that do not lead to changes in practice are meaningless, while changes in practice that are not associated with changes in understanding will not lead to meaningful or lasting improvement (MacDonald, 2002). As advanced practitioners, aspects of your practice can be so familiar that you may spend a good deal of time on *automatic pilot*, hardly aware of your responses to routine situations. Is this intuitive expertise at work, or is it simply unthinking ritual?

■ WHY BOTHER TO REFLECT?

So why, you may be asking, should you bother to reflect? After all, your skills and knowledge have been developed over many years, and your clinical practice has probably achieved a high standard. In my experience, APNs who undertake doctoral study face the unsettling tasks of examining their practice and of challenging many things they once took for granted. This unpacking of assumptions and questioning of the evidence base for your practice can be acutely uncomfortable, as customary ways of working over the years are exposed as perhaps having little justification or theoretical foundation. It is here that reflection can come to the rescue. Some comments from my United Kingdom students on the professional doctorate in nursing program may give you a sense of their experience of reflection:

> I question why we do things more in practice, and reflection has opened up a totally new concept of what nursing means to me.

> I cannot believe how many assumptions I held about my practice...stripping these away has been scary but enlightening and empowering!

> I ponder and question everything now; nothing is taken for granted, unless I can give myself a sound rationale for doing that. It's not comfortable, but I now see how necessary it is.

> I suggest that as a doctor of nursing practice graduate you will be expected to extend the boundaries of professional knowledge and practice, and that this contrasts with the role of the MSN graduate, whose role is to demonstrate mastery of the discipline. Because of this increased expectation of the *doctoral advanced practice nurse*, the skills of reflective practice become even more essential. (Dreher & Montgomery, 2009; Teekman, 2000)

In striving to develop and enhance your nursing practice, the function of critical reflective inquiry is to "correct and improve the practice through self-reflection and criticism and...[to] generate models of 'good practice'" (Kim, 1999, p. 1206). By bringing together head, hands, and heart (understanding, application, and emotion), you can develop practical wisdom, or *phronesis*. Originally used by Aristotle (trans. 1975), *phronesis* was one of three ways of knowing or "intellectual virtues," the other two being *episteme* and *techne*. *Episteme* is concerned with universal, scientific, and context-free knowledge, whereas *techne* is related to practical, context-dependent, and craft-based knowledge. *Phronesis*, however, involves ethical deliberation that is

> Based on values, concerned with practical judgement and informed by reflection. It is pragmatic, variable...and orientated toward action. (Kinsella and Pitman, 2012, p. 2)

It is the ability to decide what we should do in any given situation, and to consider one's actions in order to deliver change, especially to enhance the quality of one's practice. The key to unlocking this practitioner wisdom is reflection, and the key to reflection is self-awareness.

■ WHAT IS SELF-AWARENESS?

Reflection involves sensitive introspection, and thus, a vital aspect of reflective practice is self-awareness. Self-awareness is central to the process of reflection and can be defined as the

> Process [over time] of noticing and exploring aspects of the self, whether behavioural, psychological or physical with the intention of developing personal and interpersonal understanding.... To become more aware of and to have a deeper understanding of ourselves is to have a sharper and clearer picture of what is happening to others. (Burnard, 2002, pp. 30–31)

Thus, self-awareness is the foundation for reflective practice as the outcome from being self-aware underpin the whole process. When self-aware, you become conscious of your beliefs, values, qualities, strengths, and limitations. In other words, self-awareness involves an honest examination of who you think you are. It allows you to see yourself in a particular context, and identify how your presence and actions affect a situation. Through self-awareness, we are able to learn how to consciously use ourselves in interactions with others (Forbes, 2008). Burnard (2002) states that being self-aware enables us to

> Select therapeutic interventions from a range of options so that the patient or client benefits more completely. If we are blind to ourselves we are also blind to our choices. We are blind, then, to caring and therapeutic choices that we could make on behalf of our patients. (p. 36)

Associated with self-awareness is mindfulness, which can be deceptively simple. It is moment to moment awareness, being totally in the present. Experiences and sensations are observed as they are experienced, without being caught up in the mental events that usually follow sensations. Thoughts and feelings are noted and acknowledged as they arise, but judgment and analysis is avoided (Kabat-Zinn, 2005). If reflection is a necessary prerequisite for learning, then mindfulness is a prerequisite for experience. It represents a simple awareness of what is present from one moment to the next. By being totally present to whatever arises in your practice, you can respond appropriately and authentically to the needs of your patients and the situation. Mindfulness is increasingly recognized as being beneficial in nursing practice (White, 2014). As a Doctor of Nursing Practice (DNP) student, mindful self-awareness also assists you with identifying your own learning needs and the ways in which your learning needs can be met. It is then involved in your evaluation of whether those needs have been met.

■ HOW DO YOU REFLECT ON PRACTICE?

Donald Schön (1987) noted differences between *reflection-on-action* happening after practice, and *reflection-in-action* happening in the moment of practice. For example, as a clinical situation unfolds around you, you may be thinking on your feet and making apparently instant decisions (reflection-in-action), and then later, thinking over what happened in order to make sense of it (reflection-on-action). In this way, Schön (1983) argued that each practitioner builds a situational repertoire that is forever being expanded and modified to meet new situations. Often, the alternations from practice to theory and back to practice, and so on are so fast that it seems like one integrated process, and

> It is this entire process of reflection-in-action which is central to the 'art' by which practitioners sometimes deal well with situations of uncertainty, instability, uniqueness, and value conflict. (Schön, 1983, p. 50)

There is also the concept of "reflection-*for*-action," which refers to the process of anticipating, planning, and thinking about what is to come in the clinical situation (Thompson & Pascal, 2012). As a doctoral advanced nurse practitioner (NP)/clinician, you have accumulated a huge practice repertoire of knowledge, skills, and actions, most of which you may be largely unaware. In short, as an expert, you possess "a deep background understanding of clinical situations based upon many past paradigm cases" (Benner, 1984, p. 294), and "know more than you can tell" (Polanyi, 1983). In your clinical setting, you may practice *intuitively*, which probably involves a complex recognition of patterns within the situation, to which you can respond without conscious deliberation. You *just know* what needs to be done, and when called upon to explain your actions, you can be at a loss to provide a rational justification.

This is where structured reflection can help to *unpack* your tacit knowledge, bring it into awareness, and explicate it for others. There are many published models of reflection to use (e.g., Atkins & Murphy, 1993; Johns, 2004, 2007; Taylor, 2000), but three simple questions can be used to explore any event or experience: *What?, So What?, and Now what?* This sequence of questioning moves us through the processes of description, analysis, and synthesis. If you wish, please work through the critical questions at the end of this chapter, which will guide you through this process and are relevant for all levels of reflection. These simple questions are based on Johns's (2007) model of structured reflection shown in Exhibit 19.1.

Many nurses (in my experience) complain that their work situation allows very little space and time for reflection: "we're just too busy...patients can't wait for us to reflect!" My response would be that reflective practice does not demand extra time or energy, but an altered relationship to one's work. Although in many settings, groups of nurses reflect together on specific clinical incidents and may keep reflective journals to assist in making sense of their experience; however, these structured methods are not always necessary. I encourage all my doctoral nursing students in the United Kingdom to maintain a reflective research journal that helps to capture their changing thoughts and feelings as they progress through their program. The journal entries act as an excellent resource for student/supervisor meetings, a guide for the reflective elements of their final thesis, and also a way to reinforce the students' reflexivity throughout the research process. If you (as a doctoral APN) can make sense of your practice as you go about your daily work using systematic and thoughtful reflection, not only will this reflection increase your personal understanding, it will also likely result in your continued professional growth and self-empowerment.

EXHIBIT 19.1   **Johns's model of structured reflection, 15th edition.**

- Bring the mind home.
- Focus on a description that seems significant in some way.
- What particular issues seem significant to pay attention to?
- How were others feeling and what made them feel that way?
- How was I feeling and what made me feel that way?
- What was I trying to achieve and did I respond effectively?
- What were the consequences of my actions on the patient, others, and on myself?
- What factors influenced the way I was feeling, thinking, and responding?
- What knowledge did or might have informed me?
- To what extent did I act for the best and in tune with my values?
- How does this situation connect with previous experience?
- How might I respond more effectively given this situation occurs again?
- What would be the consequences of alternative actions for the patient, others, and on myself?
- What factors might constrain me from acting in new ways?
- How do I *now* feel about this experience?
- Am I more able to support myself and others better as a consequence?
- Am I more able to realize desirable practice?

Reprinted from Johns (2007) with permission from Sage Publications.

■ WHAT ABOUT NURSING KNOWLEDGE?

You may be asking yourself "It's all very nice being reflective, but what about the development of nursing knowledge?" The dominant paradigm for nursing knowledge over the past few decades has been one of *technical rationality*, supported by the rise in research-based practice. The term technical rationality originated with Habermas (1970) and was employed by Schön (1983) to refer to the dominance of theory over practice (and hence of theorists over practitioners).

The development of nursing science has been the result of a one-way flow of information from researchers through academic journals and textbooks, to nursing practitioners. Grounded in technical rationality (Aristotle's *episteme*), new developments in nursing practice have been driven by the findings of scientific (usually quantitative) research studies and the writing of theorists (Rolfe, 2006). Hypothetico-deductive positivist models of research, working from the general to the specific, generate *middle-range* or *grand* theories to be translated into everyday practice. In actual fact, they produce evidence *of* or *from* phenomena, and not evidence *for* practice, as is usually assumed. Such assumptions are an act of belief, and give evidence-based practice a spurious respectability. Nursing theory created by academics away from the clinical setting (on the *high, hard ground* of technical rationality) cannot be easily incorporated into practice (in the *swampy lowlands*), in the same way that oil and water cannot mix. The incommensurability between these two discourses or worldviews has led to the theory–practice gap, much discussed and lamented by educationalists and practitioners alike. Although some nursing theories are developed inductively from practice, the gap still exists because they are not returned for testing or implementation in their own original setting (the practice–theory–practice gap).

This problem, however, can be addressed through reflective inquiry, which turns technical rationality on its head by starting with the individual nurse's experience, and then *unpacking* it to discover what can be learned and applied in future situations. Reflection, therefore, offers an alternative, inductive approach to learning and knowledge generation. It challenges the usual hierarchy of evidence by shifting the emphasis from the findings of large-scale research studies to the knowledge generated by individual practitioners from their own practice, thereby promoting practitioners to the status of researchers and theorists in their own right (Rolfe, Freshwater, & Jasper, 2001).

Central to this process is a specific practice event experienced uniquely by individuals, from which a number of more abstract generalizations may be derived. It is consistent with the essence of nursing, where no two clinical situations are ever the same. Through exploring specific incidents in practice and generating new theoretical perspectives, other types of knowledge that are essential to you as a doctoral advanced NP can be utilized and valued. In addition to *propositional* knowledge (from published research and textbooks), you use *personal* knowledge (self-awareness and ethical values), and *practice* knowledge (the cumulative wealth of experience from previous clinical situations). All three types of knowing are embedded in the expert nurse's everyday practice in order to provide high-quality and holistic patient/client care, and this combination of different ways of knowing and their application to practice can be termed *praxis* (the action component of phronesis).

Praxis or *wise action* effectively dissolves the traditional theory–practice gap by making theory and practice mutually dependent upon one another. Nursing praxis is a bringing together of theory and practice that involves a continual process of hypothesizing and testing out new ideas, and of modifying practice according to the results. Therefore, I would argue that all practitioners are not only *theorists*, but also *researchers*, engaged in numerous pieces of action research and the generation of informal theory. In its everyday use, the phrase "research-based practice" limits the knowledge deemed acceptable for practice. However, reflective NPs can access other types of knowledge through the kind of critical inquiry that takes place within nursing praxis, producing "practice-based evidence." Practice knowledge created through reflection can be judged by its own criteria—its relevance and value to care—rather than any external criteria normally reserved for positivist research. Such research may have a sample of one, and might not be generalizable beyond that single person. Nevertheless, it is still a valid research and represents what Rolfe and Gardner (2005) called a nursing science of the unique, concerned with *persons* rather than *people*.

As a consequence, distinctions between research and practice, and between the generation and application of knowledge merge into one. Theory does not determine practice, but is generated from practice. In fact, the process is circular with practice-generating theory and theory-modifying practice, which generates new theory and so on. Nursing praxis is a fusion of knowing and doing, in which research is incorporated into everyday practice, and in which theory and practice become two sides of the same coin. The doctoral APN is thus not just a nurse with a lot of experience, but instead a practitioner who can freely move between different ways of knowing, and who is able to select and transform knowledge appropriate to the situation. Trusting your intuitive personal and practice knowledge requires courage and conviction, because it requires a shift from reliance on abstract, propositional thinking to thinking based on clinical reasoning related to concrete experiences. Do you have the ability to pay attention to and learn from everyday practice with the aim of realizing the optimal standard of care for your patients? This ethical artistry, in my opinion, is the hallmark of an advanced and expert practitioner, and also denotes doctoral level practice. The resulting science and art of nursing are then woven into a rich tapestry of practice, which honors the intuitive and holistic nature of experience.

■ PARADIGM WARS?

The dominant discourse or paradigm in nursing has been, and remains, the *natural science* approach of evidence-based practice and the randomized controlled trial. So long as this positivist worldview dominates contemporary science, it will probably continue to hold sway in nursing. Yet, the profession would be enriched if it could also accommodate the *human science* tradition. Mitchell and Cody (1992) summarized their overview of human science with the assertion that the

> Lived experience, the world as experience, meaning, and understanding are all aspects of a unitary process of human life and cannot be adequately described, explained, or analyzed through objectification, measurement, or reduction. (Mitchell and Cody, 1992, p. 55)

Watson (1999a) has identified similar philosophical and conceptual foundations for human science, adding that human science epistemology "allows not only for empirics, but for advancement of esthetics, ethical values, intuition, and process of discovery" (p. 16). Essentially, human science aims at knowledge development that enhances understanding of the multidimensional meanings inherent in human existence, rather than that which seeks to explain, predict, and control human phenomena, as in the natural science tradition.

Nurse scholars such as Newman (1986), Paterson and Zderad (1988), Parse (1981, 1998), and others have promoted human science perspectives in the interests of humanistic nursing. Can we combine nursing science with the artistry of nursing? Self-awareness and mindful reflection can be the way forward to producing thoughtful, innovative, and critical practice. It is when the nurse is in this place of personal wisdom, gaining new and deeper insights, that a caring moment becomes more possible (Watson, 1979, 1999b).

■ SUMMARY

Reflective practice is something more than thoughtful practice. It is that form of practice that seeks to problematize many situations of professional performance, so that they can become potential learning situations and you, as a doctoral advanced NP, can continue to learn, grow, and develop in and through your practice. As you journey through your doctoral program, you will be developing the qualities related to this level of study— critical thinking and reflexive self-awareness—in addition to extensive specialist knowledge, practical research skills, and scholarship. Doctoral study involves mastering procedures not only for generating knowledge, but also for becoming aware of different ways of knowing and of the limits of knowledge. It means tolerating uncertainty and realizing that all knowledge is provisional, and that we can be certain of nothing in science (Popper, 1969). It is this shift in the breadth and depth of intellectual perspective that distinguishes master's from doctoral-level study, from MSN-prepared APN to the doctoral DNP or DrNP graduate.

The reflective skill set of the doctorally prepared APN includes challenging assumptions about evidence, learning to think and write reflexively, developing your own characteristic voice, and producing practice-based knowledge. Your professional identity and self-awareness will be transformed through your doctoral journey, and both your practice and research will be underpinned by sensitive and insightful reflection. By developing both praxis (mindful action) and phronesis (practical wisdom), you can expand your concepts of what constitutes knowledge and reality. As doctorally pre-pared nurse scholars (whether in direct practice roles or not) you will have the skills of generating nursing knowledge from practice, and mindful, reflective awareness will enable you to achieve excellence in your own professional nursing performance. This approach honors your patients, yourself and your profession. Do you not owe it to your patients, yourselves, and your profession?

■ CRITICAL THINKING QUESTIONS

1. *Identify a situation or incident in your recent clinical experience that was significant, pow-erful, or memorable in some way* (either positively or negatively). *Tell the story briefly, either in writing or verbally within your group. What happened?* (What?)
2. *What were you thinking and feeling? Why did you act or not act as you did?*
3. *What was good and bad about the experience?*
4. *What factors influenced your decisions and actions?*
5. *What sense can you make of the situation?* (So what?)
6. *What else could you have done, and what would have been the result?*
7. *How has your practice changed as a result of this experience?*
8. *If a similar situation arises again, what will you do?* (Now what?)
9. *What have you learned from this experience?*
10. *How can you share this learning with others? Is it nursing knowledge?*

■ REFERENCES

Argyris, M., & Schön, D. (1974). *Theory in practice: Increasing professional effectiveness.* San Francisco, CA: Jossey-Bass.

Aristotle. (1975). *The Nicomachean ethics.* Boston, MA: D. Reidel.

Atkins, S., & Murphy, K. (1993). Reflection: A review of the literature. *Journal of Advanced Nursing, 18*(8), 1188–1192.

Benner, P. (1984). *From novice to expert: Excellence and power in clinical nursing practice.* Menlo Park, CA: Addison-Wesley.

Boud, D., Keogh, R., & Walker, D. (1985). *Reflection: Turning experience into learning.* London, UK: Kogan Page.

Boyd, E. M., & Fales, A. W. (1983). Reflective learning: Key to learning from experience. *Journal of Humanistic Psychology, 23*(2), 99–117.

Burnard, P. (2002). *Learning human skills: An experiential and reflective guide for nurses and health care profes-sionals* (4th ed.). Oxford, UK: Butterworth Heinemann.

Dewey, J. (1938). *Experience and education.* New York, NY: Macmillan.

Dreher, H. M., & Montgomery, K. E. (2009). Let's call it "doctoral" advanced practice nursing. *The Journal of Continuing Nursing Education, 40*(12), 530–531.

Forbes, J. (2008). Reflexivity in professional doctoral research. *Reflective Practice, 9*(4), 449–460.

Habermas, J. (1970). Technology and science as "ideology." In J. Shapiro (Trans.), *Toward a rational soci-ety.* Boston, MA: Beacon Press.

Hargreaves, A., Earl, L., Moore, S., & Manning, S. (2001). *Learning to change: Teaching beyond subjects and standards.* San Francisco, CA: Jossey-Bass.

Jarvis, P. (1992). Reflective practice and nursing. *Nurse Education Today, 12,* 174–181.

Johns, C. (2004). *Becoming a reflective practitioner,* (2nd ed.). Oxford, UK: Blackwell Publishing.

Johns, C. (2007). Toward easing suffering through reflection. *Journal of Holistic Nursing, 25*(3), 204–210.

Kabat-Zinn, J. (2005). *Coming to our senses: Healing ourselves and the world through mindfulness.* London, UK: Piatkus Books.

Kim, H. S. (1999). Critical reflective inquiry for knowledge development in nursing practice. *Journal of Advanced Nursing, 29*(5), 1205–1212.

Kinsella, E. A., & Pitman, A. (2012). *Phronesis as professional knowledge: Practical wisdom in the professions.* Dordrecht, Netherlands: Sense Publishers.

Kolb, D. A. (1984). *Experiential learning—Experience as the source of learning and development.* Upper Saddle River, NJ: Prentice-Hall.

Kuiper, R. A., & Pesut, D. J. (2004). Promoting cognitive and metacognitive reflective clinical reasoning skills in nursing practice: Self-regulated learning theory. *Journal of Advanced Nursing, 45*(4), 381–391.

MacDonald, G. (2002). Transformative unlearning: Safety, discernment and communities of learning. *Nursing Inquiry, 9*(3), 170–178.

Mezirow, J. (1981). A critical theory of adult learning and education. *Adult Education, 32*(1), 3–24.

Mitchell, G. J., & Cody, W. K. (1992). Nursing knowledge and human science: Ontological and epistemological considerations. *Nursing Science Quarterly, 5,* 54–61.

Newman, M. (1986). *Health as expanding consciousness.* St. Louis, MO: Mosby.

Parse, R. R. (1981). *Man-living-health: A theory of nursing.* New York, NY: Wiley.

Parse, R. R. (1998). *The human becoming school of thought: A perspective for nurses and other health professionals.* Thousand Oaks, CA: Sage.

Paterson, J. G., & Zderad, L. T. (1988). *Humanistic nursing.* New York, NY: National League for Nursing Press.

Polanyi, M. (1983). *The tacit dimension.* Gloucester, MA: Peter Smith.

Popper, K. (1969). *Conjectures and refutations.* London, UK: Routledge & Kegan Paul.

Rolfe, G. (2006). Nursing praxis and the science of the unique. *Nursing Science Quarterly, 19*(1), 39–43.

Rolfe, G., & Gardner, L. (2005). "Do not ask who I am...": Confession, emancipation and (self)-management through reflection. *Journal of Nursing Management, 14,* 593–600.

Rolfe, G., Freshwater, D., & Jasper, M. (2001). *Critical reflection for nursing and the helping professions: A user's guide.* New York, NY: Palgrave.

Rushmer, R., & Davies, H. T. O. (2004). Unlearning in health care. *Quality and Safety in Health Care, 13*(Suppl. II), ii10–ii15.

Schön, D. A. (1983). *The reflective practitioner.* London, UK: Temple Smith.

Schön, D. A. (1987). *Educating the reflective practitioner.* London, UK: Jossey-Bass.

Taylor, B. (2000). *Reflective practice: A guide for nurses and midwives.* Buckingham, UK: Open University Press.

Teekman, B. (2000). Exploring reflective thinking in nursing practice. *Journal of Advanced Nursing, 31*(5), 1125–1135.

Thompson, N., & Pascal, J. (2012). Developing critically reflective practice. *Reflective Practice 13*(2), 311–325.

Watson, J. (1979). *Nursing: The philosophy and science of caring.* Boston, MA: Little, Brown.

Watson, J. (1999a). *Nursing: Human science and human care.* Sudbury, MA: Jones & Bartlett.

Watson, J. (1999b). *Postmodern nursing and beyond.* New York, NY: Churchill Livingstone.

White, L. (2014). Mindfulness in nursing: An evolutionary concept analysis. *Journal of Advanced Nursing, 70*(2), 282–294.

Reflective Response

Rosalie O. Mainous

Reflection should be a component of nursing curricula at all levels of nursing practice, but it is also essential for doctorally prepared advanced practice nurses. As expert clinicians, consumers of research, and skilled in evidence-based practice, those with the professional practice doctorate must utilize reflection to bring together what is known, what is clinically relevant, and what can be improved on.

The author identifies several key components of reflective practice. First, the unlearning of old ways of doing to allow for a new paradigm to emerge is critical. Those who are pursuing a doctorate in nursing practice must examine the "old" practice and apply a new skill set, while reflecting upon progress towards improved patient outcomes. Self-awareness is also necessary; as we are self-aware, we are cognizant of our strengths and weaknesses in any given situation. Mindfulness, that is being in the moment and totally present to the clinical scenario faced, is taking on an increasingly important role. Johns's model of structured reflection (Exhibit 19.1) clearly demonstrates the connections among self-awareness, mindfulness, and the "unpacking" of knowledge understood.

The author describes the way most new knowledge reaches the bedside. It has been driven by the work of theorists and researchers, moving from the general to the specific with the generation of middle range theories. These theories are then tested clinically, and may be altered or give rise to new theoretical constructs. Generation of new knowledge has indeed been unidirectional. However, while many theories are developed in a practice vacuum, there is great support for a new model whereby new knowledge and translational work is performed by interprofessional teams that include clinical researchers, practicing clinicians, and a cadre of scientists from a variety of disciplines. The theory–practice gap, which continues to exist, is due in part to the underuse of new knowledge and the slow translation of science to the bedside. The author makes the point that much of the work generated by the PhD, or those with research doctorates (one step removed from the clinical setting), contributes to the gap as the knowledge generated is not easily used at the bedside. Reduction of this theory–practice gap is now a national priority. When teams are formulated with Doctors of Nursing Practice (DNPs) and PhDs, the researchers (PhDs) trained in specific research methodologies together with expert practitioners (DNPs) pose a clinical question for testing; practitioners test the theory utilizing a researcher formulated design in the clinical setting and then reflect on the findings; the findings are evaluated through the lens of an experienced clinician with in-depth analysis by the researcher, at which point the team makes sense of the findings and determines what can be translated back to the bedside as evidence for practice and further testing. This process is enhanced with reflective inquiry which allows for use of the clinician's knowledge from past experiences, critical to the development of useable patient-centered interventions.

This chapter highlights the importance of clinician knowledge, which should be recognized by theorists and researchers alike, as valuable and a unique contribution to science. I agree. Some clinical knowledge is created through reflective practice. The two primary academic methods of reflection include journaling and group discussion (Caldwell & Grobbel, 2013), but classroom, case conferences, and other methods are being utilized. Reflective case studies that focus on the needs of the patient and the values of the nurse have been shown to have a significant impact on the advanced practice nursing student's understanding of his or her role (ter Maten-Speksnijder, Grypdonock, Pool, & Streumer, 2012). The movement away from critical thinking and toward clinical reasoning is enhanced through critical reflection (Raterink, 2016).

The author points out the inevitable merging of traditional research as the generation of new knowledge with reflective practice, and its contribution to the body of evolving science for the discipline. This movement has been fully conceptualized in the newly emerging field of Synthesis Science, that of the language and methodology of evidence-based practice. In evidence-based practice models, while randomized controlled trials are seen as the gold standard, many other forms of knowledge are accepted including clinician expertise (which in best practice should derive in part from reflection) to qualitative findings. Schön (1987), the father of reflective practice, suggests that an epistemology of practice that traditionally has had a positivist slant, termed *technical rationality*, now incorporate the experience of the practitioner, which is evident in many different models of evidence-based practice. According to Kinsella (2007), Schön's position of adding reflective practice to the understanding of a clinical scenario does not denigrate traditional research knowledge, but instead is additive and has important ramifications for those applying it to practice. Reflective practice together with evidence-based practice has been suggested to be the two skills necessary to form a model of professional thinking (Bannigan & Moores, 2009).

As with any pedagogical strategy, it must be leveled appropriate to the student population. Just as pharmacology is taught one way and with a specific set of outcomes to be achieved at the baccalaureate level, it becomes more complex with different outcomes and different teaching strategies at the master's level. Reflection as a strategy for mastery differs from every level of nursing practice. Reflection for the doctoral advanced practice nurse will be at a high level and incorporate several ways of knowing.

■ REFERENCES

Bannigan, K., & Moores, A. (2009). A model of professional thinking: Integrating reflective practice and evidence based practice. *Canadian Journal of Occupational Therapy, 76*(5), 342–350.

Caldwell, L., & Grobbel, C. C. (2013). The importance of reflective practice in nursing. *International Journal of Caring Sciences, 6*(3), 319–326.

Kinsella, E. A. (2007). Technical rationality in Schon's reflective practice: Dichotomous of nondualistic epistemological position. *Nursing Philosophy, 8,* 102–113.

Raterink, G. (2016). Reflective journaling for critical thinking development in advanced practice registered nurse students. *Journal of Nursing Education, 55*(2), 101–104.

Schön, D. (1987). *Educating the reflective practitioner.* London, UK: Jossey-Bass.

ter Maten-Speksnijder, A. J., Grypdonock, M. H. F., Pool, A., & Streumer, J. N. (2012). Learning opportunities in case studies for becoming a reflective nurse practitioner. *Journal of Nursing Education, 51*(10), 563–569.

CHAPTER TWENTY

Enhancing the Doctor of Nursing Practice Degree With a Mandatory Study-Abroad Program

H. Michael Dreher, Mary Ellen Smith Glasgow, Vicki D. Lachman,
Rick Zoucha, Melanie T. Turk, Scott Oldfield,
Cynthia Gifford-Hollingsworth, and Margie Molloy

Although the study-abroad attendance at the undergraduate level is increasing in the United States (after decreasing post-9/11), still only an extremely small number of students ultimately study abroad, and there is no real data on the number of undergraduate nursing students who participate (Conant, 2010). In academic year 2013 to 2014, the number of U.S. students studying abroad for credit increased by 5.2% (to 304,467 students), but this growth still only represented 1.5% of all U.S. students enrolled at institutions of higher education in the United States (NAFSA, 2016). At the graduate level, there is an absence in the literature of study-abroad programs that focus exclusively on graduate nursing students. In 2006, Drexel University started what was perhaps the first mandatory study-abroad program for any nursing program in the United States. Drexel focused its 2-week study-abroad program on its Doctor of Nursing Practice (DrNP) program. Duquesne University initiated its own Doctor of Nursing Practice (DNP) study-abroad program in 2008 and it will become mandatory in 2016. As stated in a 2014 paper titled, *What Will it Take to Double Study Abroad: A "Green Paper" on the Big 11 Ideas From IIE's Generation Study Abroad Think Tank* "educators must do more to prepare today's students to succeed in the global economy. Study abroad enables today's students— future leaders from all backgrounds in all sectors—to gain access to international experiences that will better prepare them for the world they will enter after graduation" (Institute of International Education [IIE], 2015, p. 4). This chapter describes both programs and the experiences of the faculty and students who have participated in the programs in London, Dublin, and Rome.

■ WHY STUDY ABROAD FOR DOCTORAL NURSING STUDENTS?

In an increasingly geopolitical, global-oriented world, it is incumbent that that the most educated health professionals, including doctoral-prepared clinicians, scientists, and scholars, have the kinds of real-world experiences that will give them the best context for discussing the international implications of health issues and in making informed decisions about health policy and practice. Indeed, the rise of the severe acute respiratory syndrome (SARS) virus, the H1N1 flu virus, the deadly Ebola virus, and now the emergence of the Zika virus (Dreher et al., 2004; Gardner, 2009; Lupton, 2016; Robert Wood Johnson Foundation, 2014) are vivid recent examples of why nurses, now more than ever, know that the health of someone on one continent may have a direct impact on the health of citizens on another.

Increasingly, the international higher education is a big business. Foreign students contribute to more than $30 billion to the U.S. economy each year, with the United States currently by far the largest host country, with more than a quarter of the world's foreign students (Institute of International Education, 2015). Even with the global recession, the global education still grew (Redden, 2009a). However, the Institute of International Education annually tracks study-abroad numbers (both foreign students studying in the United States and the U.S. students going abroad), the previously reported 1.5% overall rate of participation by the U.S. students is still very low (NAFSA, 2016). The International Association of Universities (IAU, 2014) global survey, conducted in 2013 revealed, "More than twice as many U.S. respondents than all respondents indicated that internationalization was of low importance to institutional leaders (11 percent versus 5 percent)" (Green, 2014, p. 2). However, a current survey of employers found that nearly 40% reported that their organizations have missed out on international opportunities because they did not have trained personnel (Daniel, Xie, & Kedia, 2014). A 2006 to 2007 report found that only 5.1% of all the study-abroad students was among those in the health profession majors. At least since 1996, Zorn suggested that internationalizing the nursing curriculum was essential to prepare the nurses for the challenges of the 21st century (Zorn, 1996). One critique is that the current nursing curricula fail to properly acknowledge the global environment (Benton, 2012; Duffy, 2001), and that any significant movement to more formally globalize nursing curricula in the United States has been largely absent. A review of the literature identified several peer-reviewed articles describing U.S.-based study-abroad programs (Breitkreuz, 2010; Carpenter & Garcia, 2012; Christoffersen, 2008; Fennell, 2009; Folse, Jarvis, Swanlund, & Timan, 2015; Gilliland, Attridge, Attridge, Maize, & McNeill, 2016; Johanson, 2006; Levine, 2009; Parker, Locsin, & Longo, 2006; Saenz & Holcomb, 2009), but there were no study-abroad programs that focused on graduate nursing students exclusively, much less doctoral students.

Nevertheless, in 2006, the forward thinking doctoral nursing faculty at Drexel University were convinced that a short-term formal study-abroad experience would be an innovative enhancement to its DrNP program. It would ideally prepare the students to better face the contemporary global problems that highly educated nursing and other health professionals will increasingly be challenged to solve. Similarly, the Duquesne School of Nursing faculty thought about the importance of an international education component in their own Doctor of Nursing Program. This chapter provides practical information related to the approval and funding process necessary to implement these types of programs and, given the lack of graduate (or doctoral) nursing study-abroad programs described in the literature, highlight the perspectives of both faculty and students who have participated in both programs.

■ THE DREXEL DrNP PROGRAM'S INTERNATIONAL STUDY-ABROAD PROGRAM

WHY WAS IT CREATED?

The initial idea for the program began with the doctoral nursing department chair who became aware that the LeBow College of Business sent their master of business administration (MBA) students abroad for 1 week as part of the standard curriculum. With a new provost on campus seriously interested in promoting the Drexel brand more internationally, and with a renewed focus on encouraging international programs for both undergraduate and graduate students, it seemed plausible that the new doctoral program could also embed a study-abroad program in the curriculum. Further, if master's students were spending 1 week abroad, it seemed logical that doctoral students should stay longer.

The Drexel DrNP[1] program's international study-abroad program was thus first conceived in early 2006, and the first doctoral nursing students and faculty participated in the inaugural program in London in April 2007. The DrNP International Study Abroad Program is a 2-week intensive program that is offered in the second year of study. It takes place during the student's last quarter of study (spring quarter) before completing all the formal doctoral coursework and beginning with the clinical dissertation seminar in the subsequent summer quarter. Because the DrNP program was designed for the working adult, with classes 1 day a week, a 2-week program was deemed the most feasible. Although a 2-week study-abroad program may not seem like a long time, indeed short-term study-abroad programs (2–8 weeks in duration) predominate, attracting 57% of all study-abroad students in 2011 (Chow & Villarreal, 2011), and the standards for short-term study-abroad programs are now being published in the literature (Kurt, Olitsky, & Gels, 2013; Redden, 2009b). In retrospect, the new DrNP curriculum was well positioned to both integrate and accommodate a short-term study-abroad program. The first course in the 3-year part-time doctoral program was the Politics of Health: Implications for Nursing Practice, and there was a desire by the course chair and the doctoral faculty to include the content on how doctoral-prepared nurses should and could participate more fully in a dialogue and in the activism regarding international health issues (Dreher, Lachman, Smith Glasgow, & Ward, 2008). This idea of a 2-week program seemed ideal and feasible, and in consultation with the MBA program, the chair and teaching faculty had a precedent campus-based graduate program model that provided with the design guidance.

WHY IS THE PROGRAM "MANDATORY"?

One of the very first decisions the faculty made was that if it was decided to truly implement the program, it would be mandatory, not optional. This view was rooted in fairly egalitarian ideals. At the undergraduate level, too often study abroad becomes an "elite" activity for privileged students. This is widely recognized and has been perpetuated by the international standards for study abroad, which carry a high social prestige (Fry, 1984). The current data from NAFSA still indicate that "Although the diversity of study abroad participation has increased in recent years, minority students are still greatly underrepresented in study abroad" (NAFSA, 2016, p. 1). Though the first 11 doctoral students all worked full time; they certainly had financial obligations beyond the typical undergraduate, and some even had children in college (the mean age of the first class was 43 years). Yet, it was calculated that an affordable program could be created; however, the concern was that if the activity were optional, it likely would not have a full participation. Thus, the goals of making the DrNP program more innovative with an emphasis on global learning would not be complete. Further, the department chair did not see administratively how the DrNP program could be operated effectively with some students going abroad and others not. As this program was conceived after the first class matriculated in September 2005, the 11 enrolled students were approached in January 2006 about their willingness to participate. The program proposal would only move forward if all 11 students agreed to participate. Initially, only 10 of 11 students were willing, but with some coaxing the one recalcitrant student agreed. Thus began what turned into a full year of planning in order to get the graduate study-abroad program designed, approved, funded, and then scheduled.

HOW IS THE PROGRAM FUNDED?

The germination of this idea came at an opportune time for the DrNP program. The Drexel annual budget planning process for the following academic year usually begins each February and this allowed strategic time to create and submit a proposal to the associate dean for Doctoral Education and Research, to the college dean, and to the university provost using the standard budget procedures. There were two strategies taken that were critical for the rapid and ultimate approval in the first cycle submission. First, this new graduate study-abroad program closely matched the evolving mission of the university to enhance its international image and reputation; one way was by increasing study-abroad offerings to students. This program's particular emphasis on graduate students, specifically doctoral students, was deemed highly innovative in the approval process. Second, the department chair proposed of using a creative financing procedure that would make the offering more palatable to prospective students, who might initially think they could never afford to attend both a 3-year doctoral nursing program and participate in a 14-day study-abroad program which would certainly require them to take time off from work. The faculty believed the idea of a mandatory study program would be attractive to students who were looking for a distinctive DrNP doctoral program, but in the end, the idea had to become "real" to the prospective student. Since funding the doctoral study-abroad program involved funding both student and faculty travel, each will be discussed separately.

Funding Doctoral Students Studying Abroad

To make the program both attractive and "doable" for prospective students, the decision was made to take the full cost of the program (airfare, housing, events, health insurance, and administrative costs) and to divide the total cost of the program to each individual student into a DrNP international study fee paid in eight separate quarterly payments. Because Drexel is on quarters, this allowed the first-year students to make a payment of some $450 over four quarters in year 1 and 2, and thus attend the study-abroad program in their seventh quarter (spring quarter) in year 2. On their return, they did make one final payment in the summer quarter.[2] If the students are on financial aid (and many of them are), their international study fee is considered part of their financial aid package as the program is mandatory. This is a very critical point. If it were optional, financial aid would not cover it. This procedure had been followed for years, and has been very effective. Even students who are not on financial aid do not view the quarterly charge as excessive. Later, with new billing procedures, the program billed students over 12 quarters (the full 3-year program of study) but in an attempt to simplify billing, the intra-college budgetary implications were impacted, especially if a student later went to a one course per semester program of study.

Certainly, the international study fee is a creative way to provide for the financing of doctoral students (or any student in any degree) to attend the program. Their eight-quarter (or 12-quarter) fee went into a designated college account whereby the department chair could then annually fund the group airfares, the shared apartment accommodations abroad (two students share one apartment and single upgrades at the individual student's expense were usually available), the costs for all tours, the events, the additional local guest scholars for the two courses that were offered abroad each year, and the administrative fee charges by the study-abroad company partner, the London-based Foundation for International Education (FIE). Because Drexel University was one of the founding schools to participate in FIE's London program, they had experience with Drexel University and the quarter system. However, the Drexel DrNP program was not just FIE's first short-term study-abroad program they sponsored, but also the first graduate and first doctoral program they hosted.

Funding Accompanying Doctoral Faculty Abroad

Although the quarterly international study fee covers the expenses for the participating doctoral students, it does not cover the expenses of the participating faculty. Doctoral study-abroad programs are inherently different from undergraduate study-abroad programs, and may even be different from the most master's study-abroad programs. It would be inconceivable to simply place a full cohort of doctoral students in another institution abroad and have them taught completely by external faculty. However, this is the model for most undergraduate study-abroad programs (especially language study-abroad programs; Institute of International Education, 2007), these doctoral students follow a certain prescribed curriculum; and its departmental teaching faculty (by rotating which courses are scheduled to be taught abroad) rotate going abroad. Indeed, this study-abroad program was not exclusively designed for the students, but its mission was also designed to benefit the program's doctoral nursing faculty scholars as well. By also including a faculty objective for this program, traveling teaching faculty are then able to make international contacts that could lead to global collaborations, which in turn, could further enhance Drexel's international image and reputation. In preparation for each year's program, the selected teaching faculty secured local scholars to come into the classroom as guest speakers to enhance each course's content.

The Drexel program's emphasis on the international benefits to the doctoral teaching faculty is one real difference in undergraduate versus graduate study abroad. Second, securing guest scholars for rotating different doctoral level courses is an activity that cannot easily be outsourced to another host school or institution. Recruiting scholars with a very specific type of expertise or area of scholarship requires that the traveling faculty (who know a year in advance what courses are going to be offered abroad and who will be teaching them) make international connections, and through their network of referrals, approach the best local or regional university scholars, and invite them to speak. Because the 2-week program was structured with one course offered usually 9 a.m. to 12 noon Monday through Thursday, and the second class 1:30 p.m. to 4:30 p.m.[3] (Fridays were reserved for class field trips and the weekends were free for students and faculty), typically there were two guest speakers per class per week. Additionally, the program was successful at arranging a full day off campus at another host institution (Dublin Trinity College, Kingston University/St. George's of London, and the University of Brighton). As mentioned previously, since Drexel operates on a 10-week quarter system, students attend class on campus in weeks 1 and 10 only, and weeks 3 and 4 are typically entirely abroad. Thus, the students are not on campus in Philadelphia for the other 6 weeks and all 30-class hours in the quarter are met using this model.

As Drexel's DrNP program relies on its own doctoral faculty traveling abroad to teach, network, and act as semiformal guides for student activities (undergraduate students must be chaperoned and supervised to a larger degree than graduate students to avoid risks to the university), there must be a separate budget for faculty expenses (housing, food, and travel). The Drexel DrNP program typically sent two or three faculty abroad each year with each class of students. For the fourth annual program in London in 2010, there was a new day program at the University of Brighton with their professional doctoral students and faculty, and this was the program's first experience with Drexel DrNP students networking with other international students in professional nursing and other health-related doctoral programs.[4]

Courses taught abroad were selected by the department chair as part of the annual nursing teaching schedule procedures. Doctoral nursing courses were purposefully rotated so that a diverse set of faculty could take part in the experience. However, there was no standard procedure for faculty selection (e.g., by seniority), the philosophy of the department chair was mostly to use the experience to reward highly productive faculty who had been awarded tenure, received a major grant, or had exceptionally high teaching evaluations in the doctoral program. If the international mission of a university or college is important, then annual requests to fund this particular faculty activity can become part of the normal budget process.

■ THE DrNP-IN-LONDON PROGRAM: A FACULTY PERSPECTIVE

London is a cosmopolitan historical city rich in health care and public health history. Therefore, setting up meaningful extracurricular adventures with opportunities for learning with FIE was easy. The study-abroad experience in London began the first weekend upon arrival. Since this is a doctoral study-abroad program, a decision to eschew the typical dorm experience used for undergraduates was made, and the doctoral students were housed instead in an affordable hotel/apartment in Kensington within easy walking distance to all FIE facilities. After an overnight Friday transcontinental flight, a very light day-1 schedule was recommended. Students were given a brief late afternoon orientation to the FIE facilities and a quick overview of the neighborhood. On day 2, both students and faculty attended a guided walking tour of the Kensington neighborhood, including an intriguing view of the homes of John Stuart Mill and Robert Browning, as well as Kensington Palace and Hyde Park. A Sunday afternoon guided coach tour of London gave the group (students and faculty) an overview of greater London, including some of the beautiful historical sites such as Westminster Abby, Tower of London, and House of Parliament. London is the home of the Florence Nightingale Museum which holds a unique collection of artifacts clearly depicting the life of this notable woman, and students were provided tickets to attend this museum on their own. During a Medical Walking Tour (especially designed for us by a historian at FIE) later in the program, students and faculty covered the streets of London's medical quarter and beyond, giving us views of the old hospitals for sick children and poor immigrants. A day trip to Cambridge granted a view of an ancient university city with college buildings of all architectural styles and meadows leading down to the River Cam. Their King's College Chapel has some of the finest Gothic fan vaulting in England. The theater opportunities on London's West End rival New York City's Broadway, and the students and faculty attended dramatic performances of *Blood Brothers* at the Phoenix Theatre and *Billy Elliot* at Victoria Palace Theatre. In year 2, students and faculty were also given a tour of the Royal College of Surgeons, which included a view of the Hunterian Collection, an outstanding collection of over 3,500 natural history specimens assembled by the surgeon and anatomist John Hunter. One benefit of working with FIE is that they have traditionally provided complimentary admission to teaching faculty to all scheduled events and provided a private office, computer support, and cell phones to the faculty as well.

Coursework formally began on the first Monday after arrival. The speakers who visited our classrooms were selected to bring to students the "English view" on a variety of topics, just as the sites provided them with a flavor of England's architecture, arts, and history. The following was a sample year-1 itinerary and roster of speakers in our all-day visit to Kingston University and St. George's University of London:

- Dignity in Everyday Nursing Practice—Dr. Ann Gallagher, Senior Research Fellow
- Nursing Leadership in the Modern NHS—Ms. Jayne Quigley, Head of Nursing, Leadership Development, St. George's Healthcare NHS Trust
- Leading Nursing in a London Hospital—Dr. Geraldine Walters, Director of Nursing, St. George's Healthcare NHS Trust and Visiting Professor, Buckinghamshire Chilterns University College
- Leading and Researching Nursing in a Multi-Professional Faculty—Ms. Kath Start, Deputy Dean and Head of School of Nursing, Faculty of Health and Social Care Sciences
- The Nurse Consultant Role in Critical Care—Ms. Deborah Dawson, Nurse Consultant in Critical Care, St. George's Healthcare NHS Trust

The students and faculty were also privileged to have a lively discussion of educational differences in doctoral education with Professor Fiona Ross, dean of the Faculty of Health and Social Care Sciences.

Over the 2 years, speakers in one of the two courses taught abroad, Clinical and Applied Ethics in Nursing Practice (which had been taught twice), have included Dr. Verena Tschudin, then a reader and director of the International Centre for Nursing Ethics (ICNE), who spoke on "International Dimensions of Nursing Ethics," as well as "Human rights issues: Women and nurses," and Dr. Paul Wainwright, professor, Kingston University and St. George's University of London on "Research Ethics in the UK." In addition, there was the eminent international biomedical ethics scholar Professor Donna Dickenson, who won the Fourth International Spinoza Lens Award 2006 for Ethics (the first woman to win this award). She used a very dynamic reflective questioning style with the doctoral students. In the 2007 session, she selected assigned readings from her new book, *Property in the Body: Feminist Perspectives* (Dickenson, 2007), and in 2008 the program focused on her book *Body Shopping: The Economy Fueled by Flesh & Blood* (Dickenson, 2008). In 2008, the doctoral students also had the opportunity to take part in an interactive presentation with Dr. Christopher Johns. Dr. Johns (2006) is recognized internationally as a pioneer of reflective practice within nursing and health care. During this half-day session, students gained a thorough understanding of the true meaning of reflection, its application in health care practice settings, and how to incorporate reflective practice into their future roles as doctoral-prepared nurses and clinical scholars.

All of the educational sessions and extracurricular activities were designed to give students a deeper understanding of a different perspective on nursing and health related ethical, legal, and educational issues that the United Kingdom faces. Students typically get the course syllabi a couple of weeks before the quarter begins, so they might complete most of their readings before traveling abroad. What we have clearly gleaned is that *reading* about socialized medicine, nursing education, or reflective practice is not the same as hearing and experiencing the strengths and problems with these very different systems. The evaluations repeatedly have supported our decision to immerse our doctoral students, including some who have never been abroad, in this different world.

■ **CASE STUDY I: The DrNP-in-London Program: A Doctoral Student's Perspective**

As I boarded the Virgin Atlantic Boeing 747 in the spring of 2008, I was filled with anticipation. Weeks leading up to our departure, I poured over the itinerary and gathered as much travel information as I could about London and the surrounding countryside. Despite my best intentions to sleep during the flight, I diligently read the course material while we flew over the Atlantic. But my eyes periodically drifted from my articles on ethics and pedagogy sitting on my tray table to the clouds out of my window, as I daydreamed about the time yet to be spent 5,700 km across the ocean. With an hour remaining in the flight, some skeptical thoughts also interrupted my pleasant escape. Although the required experience abroad was one of the intriguing elements of the Drexel University DrNP degree, I harbored a small amount of doubt regarding the impact this experience was going to have in changing how I viewed the world around me. Our itinerary allowed for two full days of acclimation before the start of the class. I spent my first day familiarizing with the local surroundings. Nestled in west London, our accommodations off Gloucester Road in the Borough of Kensington were equal distance between Hyde Park and Kensington Palace, and the nearest tube stop and the building housing the classrooms. The neighborhood streets were lined with several foreign embassies and a variety of eclectic restaurants, including several "Gastro Pubs" which I frequented often during my 2-week stay. The next day, we took a walking tour of Kensington in the morning and a bus tour of London in the afternoon, which truly gave me the lay of the land. That evening, as I sat preparing for the following day's classes, I stared out my hotel window at the street lights below, once again daydreaming about the experiences yet to be had. I awoke the following morning to the start of a 2-week journey filled with discovery in and out of the classroom. In addition to the intellectual rigor fostered by the Drexel faculty and readily embraced by my peers, something I had grown to expect over the last year in the DrNP program, I was challenged by several guest lecturers specializing in the field of nursing ethics. Dr. Wainwright provided a perspective on research ethics, not entirely unfamiliar, but still unique to the United Kingdom. Dr. Gallagher lectured on virtue ethics, inviting a dialogue impossible not to

(continued)

■ CASE STUDY I: The DrNP-in-London Program: A Doctoral Student's Perspective *(continued)*

join. We also had the honor of having Dr. Dickenson, who spoke on reproductive ethics, and much of the concepts she presented that morning in late April were ideas shared from her soon-to-be-published book. Particularly memorable was a pleasant train ride to the University of Bedfordshire, north of London, to hear Professor Christopher Johns, author of several books including *Engaging Reflection in Practice: A Narrative Approach* (Jones, 2006), used the previous semester before our London experience. Dr. Johns lectured as if he was telling a story, a format many of the British lecturers seemed to follow. We were encouraged to discuss our own personal experiences, and by the end of our time together, a tapestry of our reflections had been woven together as a testament to the power of reflective practice. Hearing from, interacting with, and then being escorted through the reflective process was far more enriching than my previous attempt at reading his book and then attempting to synthesize reflective practice into my everyday life. A visit to the St. George's Healthcare National Health Service Trust main campus in Tooting, southwest London, one of the United Kingdom's largest teaching hospitals and associated with the renowned St. George's University of London, provided an opportunity to observe and compare a socialized health care system to our own capitalistic health care system in the United States. Perhaps the highlight of the visit for me was speaking with the nursing staff on their vascular unit. I was encouraged to find far more similarities than differences in the management of clients with vascular disease. It was also refreshing to see the importance placed on the nursing contribution to the care of the patient. By the completion of the visit I had a true appreciation for the National Health Services and the attempt to provide every citizen with availability and access to primary health care. The remainder of the time not taken up with academic and professional pursuits was spent with my classmates touring Cambridge, exploring the culture, people, and historical sites of London, including a fascinating medical walking tour and a visit to the Florence Nightingale Museum. On the last day of my London adventure, I took a walk into Hyde Park, a stroll I became quite fond of over the previous 2 weeks. As I slowly walked along the edge of Round Pond, my mind was no longer consumed with daydreams of anticipated future experiences or skepticism. Instead, it was filled with the knowledge, experiences, and memories obtained from the past 2 weeks. Knowledge gleaned from the exceptional guest lecturers who so willingly shared their expertise. Experiences fostering an international perspective of nursing, and a realization of the responsibility I bear to my profession that goes beyond the door of my institution and is not limited by borders. And memories of people and places that I will carry with me for the rest of my life.

Scott Oldfield, DrNP, CRNP, Vascular Surgery Clinic, Geisinger Medical Center, Danville, Pennsylvania, Drexel University, Class of 2006

■ THE DrNP-IN-DUBLIN PROGRAM: A FACULTY PERSPECTIVE

In London, students learned to love the city. In Dublin, students learned to love and appreciate the people of Ireland. Initially, many of the students were less than enthusiastic about having their study-abroad experience in Ireland. They wanted to go to a country that they perceived as culturally sophisticated and known for its theatre and museums. Instead, they were introduced to a country that had its own charm, unique culture, and rich history. The program's study tour guide in 2009, Colin Hogan, was an American graduate student from Chicago studying at the Dublin School of Business. Colin helped students and faculty navigate the city as well as shared his experiences as an international student.

Again after a short Saturday orientation, the second day in Ireland began with a medical walking tour conducted by Pat Liddy, a well-known Dublin historian, author, and artist who has developed a unique walking tour service for Dublin. Indeed, we were the first medical walking tour that Mr. Liddy ever conducted. On this tour alone students learned about the Irish Healthcare System, the potato famine, religious oppression, women's health care, and the political and religious landscape's effect on childbearing rights, as well as had a visit to the Rotunda Hospital which specializes in women's health and midwifery services. The hospital, founded in 1745, was the original Dublin Lying-In Hospital and maternity training hospital, the first of its kind in Europe. There the students had an opportunity to have a question and answer session with the nursing administrator on call, and began to get a glimpse of nursing education and nursing practice in Ireland.

Two doctoral courses were offered during the Dublin study-abroad experience: Legal Issues Confronting Nursing Faculty and Administrators and Qualitative Methods for Clinical Nursing Inquiry. Irish guest lecturers were invited to the classes to present the "Irish Perspective" on assigned topics and readings. The legal issues course used a case-based approach to examine the multitude of legal and ethical issues that confront the contemporary nursing faculty member in the classroom, in clinical settings, or in situations in their professional role as a faculty member. A lecturer from the University of Limerick discussed basic Irish nursing education from both a historical and current perspective. Students and faculty learned that Ireland moved swiftly to the bachelor of science in nursing (BSN) entry only in the 1990s, and unlike the United States, undergraduate nursing students specialize early on in their education in one of five specialties: general population, intellectual disabilities, psychiatric mental health, midwifery, and child nursing.

The program also consisted of a day at Trinity College School of Nursing and Midwifery, which provided an opportunity to interact with their doctoral students and faculty, and also to hear a lecture on our host country's health system, always an integral part of our program. Drexel students attended a presentation on the PhD Program in nursing and midwifery outlining the school's research resources, and they attended a PhD proposal defense. Trinity students heard a similar Drexel DrNP program presentation. All students were then able to compare and contrast institutional research infrastructure, including release time, research support, and incentives, as well as the differences related to research start-up packages and salary incentives, which were greater for Drexel. Although doctoral nursing education was relatively new to Trinity College, the institution had a wide and historic international legacy, educating both Oscar Wilde and James Joyce, among others.

Trinity College provided a wealth of guest scholars for our qualitative methods course and a wider discussion of graduate nursing education in Ireland. Guest lecture topics included:

- *Ethical considerations in qualitative research*—using a study on women's experiences of carrying a fetus with an abnormality as an exemplar

- *Qualitative research data collection strategies*—using a study on women's experiences of myocardial infarction as an exemplar
- *Mixing data, design and analysis: Triangulation as a qualitative research strategy*—using examples from studies on student midwives' views of their education and quality of life at end-of-life care
- *Qualitative sampling issues*—using field notes, memoing, and interviewing, focusing on a grounded theory approach and using a study on sexuality in mental health nursing as an exemplar

Unlike the prevailing paradigm in the United States, Trinity College of Nursing and Midwifery faculty are trying to hone their quantitative research program, while American nursing faculty are still grappling with balancing qualitative and quantitative research as equal partners. These presentations provided valuable opportunities for discussion, as the Drexel DrNP program is a hybrid nursing doctorate, and all doctoral candidates complete a clinical dissertation. Thus, the PhD students at Trinity and the DrNP students from Drexel appreciated and benefited from exploration of each other's research projects during our day visit.

In the context of their multicultural study-abroad education, students and faculty experienced such activities as the Unmanageable Revolutionaries: Women in Irish History Walking Tour, a Dublin Literary Pub Crawl, and an incredible night of tragic drama attending Arthur Miller's *All My Sons* at the famed Gate Theater in Dublin. During the Irish women's history tour, it was startlingly apparent to us that the accomplishments of Irish women were sadly missing as a major aspect of Irish history. Foreign domination, a historically patriarchal society, religious oppression, and lack of childbearing rights appear to have largely contributed to Irish women's invisibility in Irish history. This walking tour alone led to a great discussion about the Irish role of women and of women's right globally that permeated the classroom. Having attended the London program once and now the Dublin program, each was uniquely different, and both were incredibly rewarding for students and faculty.

■ CASE STUDY II: The DrNP-in-Dublin Program: A Doctoral Student's Perspective

As an adult doctoral student with multiple responsibilities, including a full-time career and family, the thought of adding an international study-abroad program seemed daunting. As the time neared, however, with all the planning and packing upon us, the excitement grew. Spending 2 weeks in Ireland with my 11 peers, learning about health care and health care education, as well as taking two courses would soon be a reality, and not just a paragraph on paper, or as a small blurb describing the DrNP program. The courses selected to be taken in Ireland were oriented to qualitative research methods and legal issues in nursing academia, both very appropriate for study abroad. I do not think we could have experienced and learned more about qualitative research in any better way than with the opportunities we were given in Ireland. We had multiple qualitative researchers, all well established in their fields, coming to the Dublin School of Business and give us lectures about their own research, as well as various

(continued)

■ CASE STUDY II: The DrNP-in-Dublin Program: A Doctoral
Student's Perspective *(continued)*

methods used in their research. Each lecturer was well prepared and willing to
entertain questions from each of us. Also, after the lectures, our professor from
Drexel would summarize and clarify any questions raised during the morning's
session and prepare us for the next day. I think we were each impressed how
each lecturer brought to us a living classroom from which we were able to ab-
sorb much more than if we had just read their articles and discussed them in
class in Philadelphia. We also spent a day at Trinity College with the doctoral
nursing students in the morning and in the afternoon learned about their educational system, types of research being pursued by the students, and strengths
of their program. During lunch, there were informal opportunities to share personal experiences of doctoral education and our own research interests with the
Trinity students and faculty. We discussed the differences between the United
States and Ireland, as well as the differences between Drexel University and
Trinity College. Many of us also visited the *Book of Kells* and Trinity Library that
same day. In our time off, we enjoyed taking in the sights and tastes of Ireland.
Each of us wandered in our own directions, some of us taking in Howth, Belfast,
Galway, the Cliffs of Moher, and Cork, to name a few. We enjoyed watching
football and rugby from the local taverns, and of course had to spend some time
in the Temple Bar Area listening to Irish music and enjoying the Guinness (we
were doctoral students!). As a group, we visited Glendalough and the Wicklow
mountains on our last day in Ireland. We even got used to the rainy damp weather and appreciated the beautiful days we had, as well. The country of Ireland
is beautiful, and the people could not have been more welcoming. The camaraderie among many of us was enhanced significantly, and was a bonus to everything else we experienced and learned on this short, but expansive learning experience. Many other programs *encourage* their students to study abroad, but we
were privileged that this was a mandatory part of our curriculum. I know some
of my classmates clearly underestimated the impact this trip would have on our
lives. I am sure if it were only optional, our chief nursing officer colleague, for
example, would have said she could not afford to leave her high-powered position for 2 weeks. Instead, she had to go and, indeed, had a ball. For any doctoral
students studying abroad, it will most likely be an unforgettable, life-altering
experience, well worth the inconveniences it may have caused in the life of a
doctoral student.

Cynthia Gifford-Hollingsworth, DrNP, CRNP, CPNP, Surgical Research Nurse Supervisor,
Department of Surgery, College of Medicine, Drexel University, Class of 2007

■ WHAT WE LEARNED FROM BOTH EXPERIENCES

When Drexel planned and implemented the mandatory 2-week study-abroad experience, the faculty was not clear on the direct impact that such an experience would have
on the overall student's global and doctoral educational experience. In year 1, faculty
were immediately and pleasantly surprised how deep an impression the study-abroad
experience had on the students, both personally and professionally. Simply based on

assessments from first-year faculty, students, and FIE partners in London, the study program became a standard part of the DrNP curriculum, and it was advertised as "mandatory" for the second class of 2006.

During the first 4 years of this program, it was evident that many of the students had never ever been abroad, and others who had traveled abroad had not visited London or Dublin. This is actually not surprising when one recognizes that the most typical doctoral nursing student (even today) is a woman in her forties often managing families, education, and a full-time career. Although some students were reticent about going abroad due to family responsibilities, most adapted quite well and enjoyed the experience immensely. Students not only learned course content, but were able to experience a different culture for a 2-week period and be exposed to a different health care system, educational system, research viewpoint, and perspective. In Ireland, students were quite interested to learn about the religious oppression of the Irish people and its effects even today. Many modern Irish who themselves had not experienced oppression still spoke about the psychological pain of oppression in their normal dialogue with the students. Many of the students identified with these feelings and their pain resonated with them. In London, students were able to experience an incredibly massive, cosmopolitan city that probably provided a more diverse cultural experience, but certainly less intimate and personal, than Dublin. The faculty were particularly observant of the impact Ireland had on many of our students who were of Irish descent and in the country for the first time.

Overall, the DrNP study-abroad experience provided students with an opportunity to experience another country and learning another culture while maintaining full-time or part-time employment in the States. These doctoral students, all studying part-time, had an opportunity to immerse themselves in their studies for a 2-week period and also bond as a group, becoming familiar with each other as individuals, students, and professionals. Students also learned about London or Dublin in the classroom and out in the field without the immediate pressures of family and work. They learned that largely Anglophilic London and Dublin are indeed very different from their own American culture, and that despite having an accent, or having a different educational system or health care system, we are still at the core more alike than different.

■ SUMMARY

From 2007 to 2010 and the fifth, sixth, and seventh study-abroad programs (which added a 4-day experience in Edinburgh, Scotland, when DrNP students attended the Second International Conference on the Professional Doctorate in 2011 as part of their London program; in 2012, the program returned to Dublin; and in 2013, the students split time with 1 week in London and then to Rome for the Third International Conference on the Professional Doctorate), it became clear that this innovation had become an integral part of the curriculum. Even with the downturn in the economy with the global recession in 2007, the program was sustainable and able to only modestly increase the quarterly fee each year (e.g., 1 year due to increased fuel charges and another due to fluctuating currency exchange rates). The initial intention was never to be based solely in London, although partnering with the London-based FIE made the job of planning such a short-term study-abroad program much easier. It should be noted that despite the trend toward globalism and outreach to new international locations like China and India, almost 40% of current U.S. students complete their study-abroad experience in just four countries, the United Kingdom, Italy, Spain, and France (NAFSA, 2016).

Still, it takes an incredible amount of planning to put a high-level, scholarly program together. The Drexel faculty were adamant to communicate that this program was not a "vacation" but truly a study-abroad experience. Families were not even permitted (of course as far as that could be enforced), until week 2 of the program, so students could at least have 1 week where they could concentrate on themselves and this formative experience without the distractions of family obligations. A doctoral study-abroad program requires meticulous planning to secure scholars to come to a new, foreign-based doctoral seminar classroom. It requires months of networking and, indeed, the program compensated the visiting classroom scholars with modest honoraria. The faculty continuously debated to what extent this should be a "cultural immersion" experience. The department chair tried to take the program to Madrid 1 year, but unfortunately there was a scarcity of scholars fluent in English who could guest lecture on the focused topics. A faculty scout (who was traveling nearby in Spain at the early planning stages of the program for the following year) found the accommodations and suburban location of the host school unacceptable. Indeed, graduate students, and particularly doctoral students, will not want to be treated as undergraduates or thrown in with them in the same type of accommodations. The majority of the Drexel students worked full time, so they did typically have discretionary income that would allow them to pay a little more for more upscale accommodations and amenities. The department chair actually flew to Dublin to inspect the facilities (again, he was traveling nearby) and having satisfactory accommodations for graduate students, even more so than "Spartan" accommodations that undergraduates may not flinch at, became critically important when returning students discussed their study-abroad program with students who had just begun their program.

Finally, it was discerned that the amount of time necessary to plan such a program required more time for graduate students than undergraduates. The Drexel MBA colleagues have also confirmed this. Therefore, one of the doctoral nursing faculty serves as a study-abroad facilitator and works in concert with the chair each year to plan the micro details of the program. The department chair has typically gone in the first year of a new venue so the second-year experience can be highly fine tuned, but this is not necessarily a permanent practice. But when a department chair is walking in Dublin with a fellow faculty member who says, "Wow, I am so privileged to be here," then the expectations that these faculty will use their new international experiences to network, collaborate, and ultimately increase their global scholarly reputations (and hence to the college and university) become realized (and well worth the investment).

After many successful program years, the overall evaluation has been that this mandatory international experience is an important and distinctive part of the DNP program. If this model was used for PhD in nursing programs, PhD students could perhaps be matched up with an international faculty mentor in the host city and have DNP and PhD students share one course and take another separately. London and Dublin have become excellent alternating sites, but in 2014 and 2015, students were sent to Ontario, Canada with mixed success as the Canadian site was not deemed "an international destination" by the students. However, this overall experience suggests that a short-term model could be easily replicated by international doctoral nursing students coming to the United States and certainly for other U.S.-based doctoral nursing programs. With the rise of globalization, it is critical that nursing students, particularly doctoral-educated clinical nursing scholars, have an enhanced understanding of international health issues. Participation in a mandatory study-abroad program for doctoral nursing students is one way to accomplish this. So when the article "So What Did You Learn in London" was republished on the Internet (Redden, 2007), it caught both the students' and faculty's eyes, and the answer is, "a lot."

■ THE DUQUESNE DNP-IN-ROME STUDY-ABROAD OPPORTUNITY: A FACULTY PERSPECTIVE

Students enrolled in the Duquesne University DNP program have the opportunity to participate in a 10-day study-abroad experience as part of a required course they take during the summer, "Transcultural and Global Health Perspectives." The School of Nursing has a rich history of being involved in international initiatives with primarily undergraduate students. When the DNP program was developed in 2008, the faculty felt strongly that including a cultural immersion experience outside of the United States for graduate students would assist students in thinking about health and illness from a perspective different from that of the U.S. health care system. The study-abroad component has not been a requirement of the course, but was strongly encouraged; in 2016, it will become mandatory. However, since the inception, an overwhelming majority of students chose to study abroad. With the inclusion of this course and study-abroad experience, DNP students learn to become advanced practitioners who can design systems of care that are culturally competent and congruent for diverse clients, families and communities within the context of their professional settings.

The DNP study-abroad experience has been available to students since the summer 2009, and the Rome experience has been taking place since 2011. Because the university has an Italian campus in Rome that is used by undergraduate students during the fall and spring terms, going to Rome with the DNP students in the summer seemed to be a natural fit. Two faculty members accompany the students to Rome and work closely with the assistant director of the Italian campus to plan the 10-day experience. All graduate courses at the school of nursing are online, and the course is structured as a 12-week summer course; this allows the students to complete some course requirements before and after the study-abroad period. Thus, the city of Rome becomes the classroom during the 10 days abroad. Planned activities are designed to immerse students in the Roman culture and engage them in fieldwork, which facilitates observation of the cultural influences on health and the health care system. For example, students use a metro pass to travel throughout the city via public transportation including the bus system and underground metro system. The campus itself is located just outside the main confines of the city, requiring students to take a bus and then the metro to get to the city-center area of Rome. This is an intentional element of the experience because students then travel throughout the city as Romans do. Students must also consider and plan for common occurrences on public transportation, such as pickpocketing, that Roman citizens encounter every day.

Students have the opportunity to engage in a variety of experiences that highlight the influences of historical and contemporary culture as well as religion and faith on individuals and the health care system. Through 2 to 3 hours dinners and the camaraderie students witness and experience, students learn the value and importance placed on food and the experience of coming together for a meal. Three to four group meals are planned with the students and faculty at well-established restaurants in Rome. Other activities include a special Ancient Rome walking tour with a professor of ancient history through the Colosseum and Roman Forum, including St. Cosmus and Damian Church, the most important church for the history of medicine in Ancient Rome, the Pantheon, and Piazza Navona. The excursion emphasizes the rich and extensive history of Rome and the influence on its citizens. Students participate in an expedition of the Vatican Museums and Sistine Chapel with a Vatican art historian who is also a professor of art history. Students listen to and have the opportunity to ask questions of these knowledgeable and experienced professors during the experiences. As a group, we attend the Papal Audience at St. Peter's Square, held on Wednesday mornings during the summer, where students hear short readings and prayers, and receive a blessing in several languages including Spanish, German, Italian, French, Arabic, and English, to name a few. Certain visiting groups from various countries are announced as attendees of the Papal Audience, and our group is announced as "pilgrims from Duquesne University in Pennsylvania." This is one of the many experiences that call attention to the impact of religion on the Italian culture.

Because one of the objectives of the course is for students to learn and write about health care environments outside of their usual frame of reference, many of the planned activities focus on health and health care contexts within the Roman culture. Examples of such activities include a private tour of the National Museum of Medical Art at the Santo Spirito Hospital with the former Director of the Red Cross in Italy, tours of private hospitals and public hospitals, such as the Salvator Mundi International Hospital and the San Giovanni Calibita Hospital on Tiber Island. During these experiences, students meet with physicians, nurses and other hospital personnel to learn about each hospital's specialty areas and common practices relative to whether the facility is part of the private or public hospital system. Students conduct observational fieldwork and have the opportunity to ask questions based on their individual area of interest. In 2015, students visited the Lazzaro Spallenzani Hospital, specializing in infectious disease. This facility was a public hospital until 1996 when the Ministry of Health declared it an autonomous institution of recovery and research. Lazzaro Spallenzani Hospital was the facility that took care of the two patients with Ebola in Italy, both of whom were cured there in 2015.

An activity that has become a particularly meaningful tradition each year is a group dinner at the Trattoria degli Amici (Trattoria of Friends). This restaurant, which collaborates with the Comunità di Sant'Egidio, employs individuals with disabilities who are accompanied by medical professionals and adult volunteers. The restaurant owners and managers believe that friendships are made this way, through understanding and working together side by side. Because of this idea, they have created classes for individuals with disabilities on how to work in restaurants and have sponsored conventions with theme areas about successful employment of workers with mental and physical disabilities. After the dinner, students have the option of participating in a prayer service conducted each night by the Comunità di Sant'Egidio (Community of Sant'Egidio). This service is led by lay people and often focuses on praying about current global issues such as peace in war-torn countries like Syria. Following the service, students meet with a leader in the lay community to discuss the community-service initiatives of the Sant' Egidio community.

Student learning outcomes of this study-abroad experience have been incredibly meaningful from both a personal and scholarly perspective. One hundred and fifteen students have participated in the Rome study-abroad component of the course, and numerous students have described how the trip impacted, and even changed, their lives. Many students have described the study-abroad experience as life changing and transformational. They have described how the experience has assisted in helping them feel part of the global nature of nursing. Many have described a new-found empathy for working with immigrant and refugees in the United States. From a scholarly perspective, the major writing assignment for the course has been completed as a publishable manuscript by several groups of students, and three groups have published papers about their experience in peer-reviewed journals (Easterby et al., 2012; Gregg et al., 2013; Montenery, Jones, Perry, Ross, & Zoucha, 2013). Additional groups of students are planning to submit their manuscripts for publication. The study-abroad experience in Rome helps students to transfer these unique experiences to patients of diverse cultures when organizing and providing care within the U.S. health care system. Students who have engaged in this experiential learning in Rome reported that they were clearly able to recognize the importance of one's culture on health and well-being.

■ CASE STUDY III: A DNP Student's Perspective of a Global Immersion Experience in Italy

Many factors influenced my decision to attend Duquesne University School of Nursing's DNP program. Hearing about taking part in a global experience to explore a different health care system had a great appeal to me when introduced during the on-campus orientation week. Our cohort was given an overview of the various countries visited by the past groups of DNP students. Italy was mentioned as a possibility and I secretly hoped that we would be enjoying wine and pasta in the summer semester of June 2014. Once announced that Italy was the choice, the excitement was palpable on the class's discussion board. Flights were booked, work schedules cleared for 10 days, and lives in the United States put on hold to immerse in a new land where many of us had never ventured.

Drs. Turk and Zoucha were assigned to be our course faculty. They supported us with not only writing our learning objectives but also ignited excitement about taking in the sights and sounds of Rome and Florence. Despite suffering from jet lag when we arrived in Rome, we readied ourselves to attend a Papal Audience at St. Peter's Square. Whether or not you are a Catholic, this was an impactful experience. The message of love from Pope Francis filled the hot, steamy square. Especially memorable was the verbal announcement of special visitors from the podium. Our group of DNP students cheered like concert goers when Duquesne University School of Nursing was announced. I was impressed with my fellow cohorts' enthusiasm and lungs. This day set the tone for a great study abroad with a group of fellow students that we had previously known exclusively through our interaction on an e-learning management system. How special it was to finally get to know each other face to face and build personal and professional bonds that will extend well past our May 2015 graduation date.

Our home base for the trip was the Duquesne's Italian Campus (Sede Italiano) located on the Generalate grounds of the Sisters of the Holy Family of Nazareth in Rome. The beautiful campus is located west of downtown Rome, just beyond Vatican City and St. Peter's Basilica. The nuns' kind, spiritual, and simple way of life was demonstrated by a lovely presentation of yogurt and fruit for breakfast, and included sliced deli meat that was very European indeed. Highlights of our itinerary included tours of the Vatican, Sistine Chapel, the Coliseum and the Duomo. Since Duquesne has a strong faculty presence in Italy, these tours were led by Duquesne faculty who are based in Italy and have inside knowledge and access to many things that made our group feel like VIPs.

Importance of family and food in Italy are engrained in the Italian culture. It was evident to our group as we strolled through the squares and saw these customs unfold in front of us. Many of our meals were shared together and dinner conversations were filled with interesting topics, ranging from various aspects of the Italian health care system, sights seen on our tours, and of course shopping. Our cohort became infamous for making friends with the vendors at the Florence leather market. Many of our suitcases weighed significantly more on the way back home.

In the global world in which we now live, it is imperative that as DNP students we have a working knowledge of the health care needs/utilization of

(continued)

■ CASE STUDY III: A DNP Student's Perspective of a Global Immersion Experience in Italy *(continued)*

our global neighbors. The National Health System of Italy was highlighted with a tour of San Giovanni Calibita Hospital on Tiber Island. Our group was greeted by nurse leaders and given an insight of health care delivery in Italy and the role of the nurse. Perhaps the best photo opportunities of the trip occurred at the shrine to Florence Nightingale in the famous Santa Croce (Holy Cross). If only Florence knew what a powerful impact she would have on the future of nursing.

I, for one, am glad that I cleared my work schedule for 10 days to go on this memorable study abroad. Looking back, my life was not put on hold but rather given the opportunity to immerse in the culture of a new land. Through the lens of a DNP student, I was able investigate a different health care system and compare it with the U.S. health care system. I will forever cherish these memories and will think about how I enjoyed many gelatos with my fellow DNP students!

Margie Molloy, DNP, RN, CNE, CHSE, Director, Center for Nursing Discovery, Duke University School of Nursing, Duquesne University School of Nursing, Class of 2015

■ ACKNOWLEDGMENTS

This chapter is dedicated to the memory of Dr. Kathy P. Falkenstein (December 7, 1952 to June 4, 2010), who accompanied traveling Drexel students and faculty to London in 2007 and Dublin in 2009.

■ CRITICAL THINKING QUESTIONS

1. *How important is it for you to be educated with a "global nursing scholar framework?"*
2. *Describe a couple of international nursing/health-related issues of which you believe you would have a better comprehension if only you had more live experience/experiential exposure to them.*
3. *How has international travel helped your global IQ, or have you had limited or no international travel experiences?*
4. *Undergraduate study-abroad models have proliferated. Should graduate study abroad be as prevalent? Why or why not?*
5. *Our research indicates there is a shortage of nursing study-abroad opportunities. Why is this so and what could be done about it?*
6. *If you had to design an international clinical practicum in your DNP degree, what would it entail?*
7. *Americans, even educated ones, are notoriously monolingual. Do you speak a second language, and what value to international health in the context of your career trajectory would being proficient in a second language be?*
8. *Describe how a lack of study-abroad opportunities for nurses, particularly doctoral graduate nursing students, impacts the health of the average global citizen. Or does it?*
9. *What did you learn from the three narrative experiences of the two Drexel and Duquesne DNP students who described their study-abroad program in London, Dublin, and Rome?*
10. *How would you go about helping to implement a similar study-abroad program in your own DNP program?*

■ NOTES

1. The Drexel DrNP was a hybrid professional doctorate combining advanced nursing practice with the conduct of clinical research, and all students completed a clinical dissertation. The DrNP changed to a DNP with very minor curriculum changes in 2015 (Dreher, Donnelly, & Naremore, 2005).
2. For the first class, the students were simply required to make eight quarterly payments which began the subsequent quarter after the program was approved. Starting with the second class in 2006, students began making quarterly payments immediately on matriculation.
3. The students were given a lunch break of 1.5 hours between classes to better reflect on the UK/European culture, which takes a more leisurely attitude toward gastronomy. Predictably, the first class asked to decrease the mealtime to get out of the class early and the faculty refused. In the end, the longer lunch mealtimes were evaluated favorably.
4. Much to our dismay, the active volcanoes in Iceland in April 2010 delayed the study-abroad program by a week, and so the decision was made to Skype in most of all the planned speakers as the students completed week 1 on campus. Students did attend week 2 in London and many stayed abroad longer after the formal program ended.

■ REFERENCES

Benton, D. (2012). Advocating globally to shape policy and strengthen nursing's influence. *The Online Journal of Issues in Nursing, 17*(1), 5.

Breitkreuz, K. (2010). In support of global health in the nursing curriculum: A nurse educator's view from the road less traveled. *DEAN's Notes, 31*(3), 1–4.

Carpenter, L. J., & Garcia, A. A. (2012). Assessing outcomes of a study abroad course for nursing students. *Nursing Education Perspectives, 33*(2), 85–89.

Chow, P., & Villarreal, A. (2011). *Open doors: Report on international educational exchange.* Institute of International Education. Retrieved from http://www.iie.org/en/Research-and-Publications/Publications-and-Reports/IIEBookstore/Open-Doors-2011

Christoffersen, J. E. (2008). Leading a study-abroad group of nursing students in Nicaragua: A first-timer's account. *Nursing Forum, 43*(4), 238–246.

Conant, E. (2010). Students without borders: Why more college kids are choosing to travel—alone—to far flung locales. Newsweek.com. Retrieved from http://education.newsweek.com/2010/09/12/students-find-study-abroad-adventure.html

Daniel, S. J., Xie, F., & Kedia, B. L. (2014). *2014 U.S. business needs for employees with international expertise.* Paper presented at the Internationalization of U.S. Education in the 21st Century. The Future of International and Foreign Language Studies: A Research Conference on National Needs and Policy Implications, April 11–13, Williamsburg, VA. Retrieved from http://globalsupport.tamu.edu/Footer-Links/Resources-Center/Global-Publication/2014-US-Business-Needs-for-Employees-with-Internat.aspx

Dickenson, D. (2007). *Property in the body: Feminist perspectives.* Cambridge, UK: Cambridge University Press.

Dickenson, D. (2008). *Body shopping: The economy fueled by flesh & blood.* Oxford, UK: Oneworld.

Dreher, H. M., Dean, J. L., Moriarty, D. M., Kaiser, R., Willard, R., O'Donnell, S., . . . Phung, L. (2004). What you need to know about SARS now. *Nursing, 34*(1), 58–63; quiz, 63.

Dreher, H. M., Donnelly, G., & Naremore, R. (2005). Reflections on the DNP and an alternate practice doctorate model: The Drexel DrNP. *The Online Journal of Issues in Nursing, 11*, 1. Retrieved from http://www.nursingworld.org/MainMenuCategories/ANAMarketplace/ANAPeriodicals/OJIN/TableofContents/Volume112006/No1Jan06/ArticlePreviousTopic/tpc28_716031.aspx

Dreher, H. M., Lachman, V. D., Smith Glasgow, M. E., & Ward, L. S. (2008). *Educating the global clinical scholar: The first doctoral nursing program to institute a mandatory study abroad program.* AACN Doctoral Education Conference, Captiva Island, FL, January 2008.

Duffy, M. E. (2001). A critique of cultural education in nursing. *Journal of Advanced Nursing, 36*(4), 487–495.

Easterby, L. M., Siebert, B., Woodfield, C. J., Holloway, K., Gilbert, P., Zoucha, R., & Turk, M. W. (2012). A transcultural immersion experience: Implications for nursing education. *The ABNF Journal, 23*(4), 81–84.

Fennell, R. (2009). The impact of an international health study abroad program on university students from the United States. *Global Health Promotion, 16*(3), 17–23.

Folse, V. N., Jarvis, C. M., Swanlund, S. L., & Timan, M. R. (2015). The creation of a synchronous learning environment to support a study abroad program for nursing majors at a traditional liberal arts university. *Journal of Professional Nursing, 31*(3), 233–241.

Fry, G. (1984). The economic and political impact of study abroad. *Comparative Education Review, 28,* 203–220.

Gardner, A. (2009). Pandemic (H1N1) update—The role of nurses. *Australian Nursing Journal, 17*(5), 7.

Gilliland, I., Attridge, R. T., Attridge, R. L., Maize, D. F., & McNeill, J. (2016). Building cultural sensitivity and interprofessional collaboration through a study abroad experience. *The Journal of Nursing Education, 55*(1), 45–48.

Green, M. (2014). *The best in the world? Not in internationalization.* Trends and Insights for International Education Leaders, NAFSA and International Association of Universities—Institute of International Educators (pp. 1–5). Retrieved from http://www.nafsa.org/Professional_Resources/ Research_and_Trends/Trends_and_Insights/The_Best_in_the_World__Not_in_Internationalization

Gregg, K., Houck, N., Irwin, R., Kattan, M. B., Kramer, N., Stayer, D., . . . Turk, M. (2013). Fieldwork as a way of knowing: An Italian immersion experience. *Online Journal of Cultural Competence in Nursing and Healthcare, 3*(3), 1–15.

Institute of International Education. (2007). *Current trends in U.S. study abroad and the impact of strategic diversity initiatives.* IIE Study Abroad White Paper, Meeting America's Global Education Challenge. Retrieved from http://www.iienetwork.org/file_depot/0-10000000/0-10000/1710/ folder/62450/IIE+Study+Abroad+White+Paper+I.pdf

Institute of International Education. (2014). What will it take to double study abroad: A "green paper" on the big 11 ideas from IIE's generation study abroad think tank. Retrieved from file:///C:/Users/ Micheal/Downloads/Green-Paper-What-Will-It-Take-To-Study-Abroad-November-2014 .pdf

Institute of International Education. (2015). *Special reports: Economic impact of international students.* Retrieved from http://www.iie.org/Research-and-Publications/Open-Doors/Data/ Economic-Impact-of-International-Students#.V_Ksbb83K9Y

Johanson, L. (2006). The implementation of a study abroad course for nursing. *Nurse Educator, 31*(3), 129–131.

Johns, C. (2006). *Engaging reflection in practice: A narrative approach.* Hoboken, NJ: Wiley-Blackwell.

Kurt, M., Olitsky, N. H., & Gels, P. (2013). Assessing global awareness over short-term study abroad sequence: A factor analysis. *Frontiers: The Interdisciplinary Journal of Study Abroad, 23,* 22–41.

Levine, M. (2009). Transforming experiences: Nursing education and international immersion programs. *Journal of Professional Nursing, 25*(3), 156–169.

Lupton, K. (2016). Zika virus disease: A public health emergency of international concern. *British Journal of Nursing, 25*(4), 198, 200–202.

Montenery, S. M., Jones, A. D., Perry, N., Ross, D., & Zoucha, R. (2013). Cultural competence in nursing faculty: A journey, not a destination. *Journal of Professional Nursing, 29*(6), e51–e57.

NAFSA. (2016). Trends in U.S. study abroad. Association of International Educators. Retrieved from http://www.nafsa.org/Explore_International_Education/Advocacy_And_Public_Policy/ Study_Abroad/Trends_in_U_S__Study_Abroad

Parker, M., Locsin, R., & Longo, J. (2006). Global communities and healthcare transition: Analysis of a study-abroad course to Thailand. *International Journal for Human Caring, 10,* 86–87.

Redden, E. (2007). So what did you learn in London? Retrieved from http://insidehighered.com/ news/2007/06/01/research

Redden, E. (2009a). In global recession, global ed still growing. Retrieved from http://insidehighered .com/layout/set/print/news/2009/29/international

Redden, E. (2009b). Standards for short-term study abroad. Retrieved from http://www.insidehighered .com/news/2009/01/30/standards

Robert Wood Johnson Foundation. (2014). Ebola care is nursing care. Retrieved from http://www.rwjf .org/en/library/articles-and-news/2014/11/_ebola-care-is-nursing-care.html

Saenz, K., & Holcomb, L. (2009). Essential tools for a study abroad nursing course. *Nurse Educator, 34*(4), 172–175.

Zorn, C. R. (1996). The long-term impact on nursing students of participating in international education. *Journal of Professional Nursing, 12*(2), 106–110.

CHAPTER TWENTY

Reflective Response

Joyce J. Fitzpatrick

The authors, faculty, and students at Drexel University and Duquesne University, are to be commended for the success in implementing a study abroad experience in their respective Doctor of Nursing Practice (DNP) programs. The Drexel program stands out for the mandatory requirement of a study-abroad experience. This is a unique and innovative curriculum requirement, and one that will not only attract students to the program, but also benefit all the participants.

Most importantly, it will change the students' view of the world, and orient them to the challenges in global health, from the perspective of other countries. As the student participants report the short 2-week experience changes one's perception of the world. I have always believed that one learns as much about oneself as about others through travel. And the learning that has occurred for the students in the Drexel and Duquesne programs is noteworthy. They will be better global citizens in our professional world of nursing for having participated in the study-abroad program. And as the authors note, nursing is now global. We can no longer isolate ourselves from the diseases, and particularly from the viruses that can travel just as easily, and perhaps faster, than we can. We can no longer ignore the conflicts of war and famine, and poverty that afflicts those in our country and throughout the globe. My colleagues and I have argued for a more knowledgeable nursing workforce, attuned to the health disparities that result from the lack of resources, both material and professional (Lee et al., 2015). This perspective is the result of my global work, and that of professional nursing colleagues.

One enhancement of the current program would be to extend the experience to counties in Africa, Asia, Australia, Latin America, and the Middle East, so as to introduce students to a broader perspective on health ethics, population health, and health disparities. Although this would present several additional challenges, it would also provide a rich and broadening experience. Perhaps this could be offered as an elective experience to begin, and then evaluated for its value as the program dimensions are formalized. Of course, the time frame might also need to be extended, but even in 2 weeks, one can travel to most countries and have a rich introductory experience. There are special opportunities to connect with colleagues in Hong Kong as there is a similar professional doctorate currently offered at Hong Kong University (HKU). Several U.S. professors and I have consulted with HKU colleagues, and many of the U.S. professors have served as visiting faculty at HKU. In particular, there are opportunities for collaborative global health projects that can be initiated by DNP students and faculty.

My own experience with international and global partnerships through the DNP program at Case Western Reserve University (CWRU) are many and varied. The primary partnership has been with colleagues at University College Cork in Cork (UCC), Ireland where I served as a Fulbright Scholar from 2007 to 2008. During that year and the following 2 years, Professor Geraldine McCarthy and I designed the first Doctor of Nursing (DN) program and modeled the course work after the DNP program at CWRU. There have been three cohorts of student enrolled thus far, and Professor McCarthy and I have continued to teach in the program and mentor students toward publication and global work. The students in each of the three cohorts were expected to be knowledgeable about, and connected to, global nursing. In formal classes, students were introduced to nurse leaders via Skype, during both the nursing theory and nursing leadership classes. One of the most significant outcomes of the leadership classes from cohorts one and two was the publication of books on nurse leaders, with doctoral students interviewing the nurse leaders and contributing chapters based on these interviews (McCarthy & Fitzpatrick, 2012, 2013). For many of the doctoral students this was their first professional publication, and one that has the potential for replication in other countries. It is our strong belief that no one should exit a doctoral program without publishing their scholarly work, and it is the responsibility of faculty to mentor students toward success in this endeavor. There are several additional publications that provide evidence of success among UCC DN students and UCC and CWRU faculty (Day, McCarthy, & Fitzpatrick, 2016; Day, Wills, McCarthy, & Fitzpatrick, 2010).

Another dimension of the collaboration, particularly relevant to the chapter by Dreher and colleagues, is the study-abroad component of the CWRU DNP program in which students are encouraged to build global experiences into their DNP practicum objectives. Two U.S. experts in emergency nursing took advantage of this opportunity and spent part of their practicum time at UCC, connecting to a leading nurse expert in emergency care in Ireland, who at the time was a DN student at UCC. One of the CWRU students and the UCC student (both of whom have now graduated) continue to collaborate on research and professional practice specific to emergency nursing. Six other CWRU DNP students have participated in course work at UCC as part of the practicum requirements in their own doctoral program. All CWRU student participants are expected to share their expertise with UCC students, delivering at least one formal presentation. Most of the study-abroad experience, however, comes from the informal networking that occurs between UCC and CWRU students.

Another dimension of the CWRU and UCC collaboration has been the conferences held at UCC. CWRU DNP students have participated in research and theory conferences. This provides another opportunity to connect those with similar professional interests and has sparked additional collaborative ongoing research. Two prior collaborative research projects have been published (Coffey et al., 2013, 2016; Weathers et al., 2015).

CWRU DNP students also have connected with colleagues in Hong Kong as part of their DNP practicum. Two students traveled to a Hong Kong nursing conference and presented their work to not only HKU DNP students but also nurse leaders from a range of Hong Kong health care facilities. These two DNP students then traveled on to the International Council of Nurses (ICN) Congress that was being held in Melbourne, Australia, and had the opportunity to connect with global nurse leaders. These students would describe this as the highlight of their DNP education, and continue their commitment to working with colleagues from other countries.

An important recent outcome of the CWRU UCC collaboration has been the publication of two nursing theory books, with CWRU DNP and UCC DN students as chapter authors (Fitzpatrick & McCarthy, 2014, 2016). Faculty from both institutions and PhD students from UCC also have participated, those expanding the collegial relationships across doctoral programs. These collaborations in theory development have led to plans for future research projects, coupling the ideas shared in the books with extension and replication studies.

I introduce global nursing leadership in the introductory nursing leadership course in the CWRU DNP program. Though many of the students have not initially considered themselves leaders beyond their current positions, they express a commitment to embark on leadership paths at a national and global level, through opportunities presented at ICN and the United Nations. There are currently plans underway to formalize global nursing leadership opportunities as part of the doctoral program.

In contrast to the Drexel University process for supporting the study-abroad programs, all CWRU students who select to go abroad fund their own experiences directly. However, it is acknowledged that this limits the opportunities to only those who have resources readily available because it is an elective experience, this mirrors the model that is used at CWRU for the undergraduate nursing students who choose to do their community health experience abroad.

There is no better experience than learning about a country or culture than that of experiencing it firsthand. Although all of the study-abroad experiences described here and in Chapter 20 are short term, even the small periods of exposure can change perceptions and perspectives. The Chinese proverb is indeed relevant: "A journey of a thousand miles begins with the first step." Through global educational experiences, we are taking the first steps toward an understanding of the global health among the future nurse leaders.

■ REFERENCES

Coffey, A., McCarthy, G., Weathers, E., Freidman, M. I., Gallo, K., Ehrenfeld, M., . . . Fitzpatrick, J. J. (2013). Nurses' preferred end-of-life treatment choices in five countries. *International Nursing Review, 60*(3), 313–319.

Coffey, A., McCarthy, G., Weathers, E., Freidman, M. I., Gallo, K., Ehrenfeld, M., . . . Fitzpatrick, J. J. (2016). Nurses' knowledge of advance directives and perceived confidence in end-of-life care: A cross-sectional study in five countries. *International Journal of Nursing Practice, 22*(3), 247–257.

Day, M. R., Wills, T., McCarthy, G., & Fitzpatrick, J. J. (2010). The power of life story books. In M. L. Wykle & S. H. Gueldner (Eds.), *Aging well: Gerontological education for nurses and other health professionals*. Sudbury, MA: Jones & Bartlett.

Day, M. R., McCarthy, G., & Fitzpatrick, J. J. (2016). *Self-neglect*. New York, NY: Springer Publishing.

Fitzpatrick, J. J., & McCarthy, G. (Eds.). (2014). *Theory in nursing: Application to research and practice*. New York, NY: Springer Publishing.

Fitzpatrick, J. J., & McCarthy, G. (2016). *Nursing concept analysis: Application to research and practice*. New York, NY: Springer Publishing.

Lee, H., Kim, S., DeMarco, R., Aronowitz, T., Mtengezo, J., Kang, Y., . . . Fitzpatrick, J. J. (2015). Recognizing global disparities in health and in health transitions in the 21st century: What can nurses do? *Applied Nursing Research, 28*(1), 60–65.

McCarthy, G., & Fitzpatrick, J. J. (Eds.). (2012). *Leadership in action: Influential Irish women nurses' contributions to society*. Cork, Ireland: Oak Tree Press.

McCarthy, G., & Fitzpatrick, J. J. (Eds.). (2013). *Leadership in action: Influential Irish men nurses' contributions to society*. Cork, Ireland: Oak Tree Press.

Weathers, E., McCarthy, G., Landers, M., Porter, C., Cortese, M., & Fitzpatrick, J. J. (2015). Nurses' caring behaviors: A comparative study in Ireland and the United States. *International Journal for Human Caring, 19*(3), 30–35.

The DNP Certification Examination: Yes? No? You Decide

Bobbie Posmontier and Sandra N. Cayo

In August 2000, Mary Mundinger, who was both president of the Council for the Advancement of Comprehensive Care (CACC) and dean of Columbia University School of Nursing invited educational leaders in nursing and medicine to discuss the future role and preparation of advanced practice registered nurses (APRNs; National Board of Medical Examiners [NBME], 2009). The work of this first conference resulted in suggesting the Doctor of Nursing Practice (DNP) degree as the entry-level degree for the APRN and set the stage for the eventual development of a DNP certification examination by the joint efforts of the NBME and the CACC (Mundinger, 2008a). Since the administration of the first DNP certification examination in 2008, however, a storm of controversy has ensued regarding its value (Mundinger, 2008b). In order to understand the controversy, this chapter reviews its major components and explore the arguments for and against the DNP certification examination.

■ WHAT IS THE DNP EXAMINATION?

The NBME and CACC proposed a voluntary two-tiered examination to assess clinical knowledge, diagnostic skills, and independent clinical management of patients across the lifespan in a variety of health care settings in order to validate advanced DNP clinical competencies (American Board of Comprehensive Care [ABCC], 2009). The purpose of this voluntary examination was to provide an extra level of standardized assurance of safety and competency to the public and other medical professions (NBME, 2009). Once the examination was passed, the ABCC would then designate the DNP as a diplomate in comprehensive care (DCC) by the ABCC and permit use of the title "doctor" in clinical practice (Landro, 2008; Mundinger, 2009).

   The examination consists of questions that evaluate the diplomate candidate's ability to assess the severity of disease, make clinical judgments, and manage patient-centered mainstream high-impact diseases (ABCC, 2009). Although the examination was mainly designed to test the advanced clinical skills of adult and family nurse practitioners with a DNP, other APRNs with a clinically focused DNP degree were also invited to sit for the examination if they believed they have mastered the examination's content. To help clearly understand who falls under the category of APRN, the American Nurses Association (ANA) and American Nurse Credentialing Center (ANCC) categorize APRN under four domains: certified nurse-midwife (CNM), certified registered nurse anesthetist (CRNA), clinical nurse specialist (CNS), and certified nurse practitioners (CNP).

The actual 2-day examination is based in part on Step 3 of the United States Medical Licensing Examination (USMLE). It consists of two 5-hour tests administered in 60-minute blocks allowing 90 seconds per question (ABCC, 2009). The examination is comprised of two dimensions including: (a) 336 multiple-choice questions that require action-oriented clinical decisions and judgment for normal development and disease, and (b) a series of dynamic interactive patient vignettes that evaluate the diplomate candidate's ability to apply knowledge and to manage a variety of patient problems across various health care settings along a simulated-time format. Acting as primary health care providers, diplomate candidates manipulate simulated time in a variety of acute or chronic patient cases by advancing the computer clock to find out results of diagnostic tests, procedures, and patient conditions so that additional assessments, treatment orders, consultations, and interventions can be formulated. Diplomate candidates are allotted 25 minutes to complete each patient vignette, and scoring is based on algorithms derived from codified policies of experienced health care providers.

Diplomate candidates are expected to possess advanced-level knowledge in normal development, mechanisms of disease, and general principles of patient-care management (ABCC, 2009). In addition, they are expected to provide evidence of an in-depth understanding of disorders of the blood and of the central nervous, mental, skin, musculoskeletal, respiratory, cardiovascular, gastrointestinal, renal and urinary, male and female reproductive, endocrine, and immunologic systems. The diplomate candidate is also expected to demonstrate expertise across a variety of clinical tasks including the ability to perform history and physical assessments, order appropriate diagnostic tests, formulate diagnoses and prognoses, order appropriate medications, perform health maintenance, understand disease prevention, provide clinical interventions, communicate with multidisciplinary health care team members, demonstrate an understanding of legal and ethical issues, and demonstrate an understanding of patient-care management across a variety of health care settings.

Three eligibility criteria are required to sit for the examination: national certification as an APRN, graduation from an accredited DNP program, and recognition or licensure by a state board of nursing as an APRN (ABCC, 2010). Although the DNP examination was not designed to replace national certification or guide curriculum development, the NBME and CACC consider it an additional assurance to the public of a high level of clinical competency and safety of the DNP graduate. A controversial issue that has not been fully addressed is whether future non-DNP-educated doctoral APRNs with a different doctorate degree (e.g., PhD) may be eligible to sit for the examination, because at present they are not eligible.

■ ARGUMENTS FOR THE DNP EXAMINATION

Proponents of the DNP certification examination argue that it was never designed to evaluate clinical expertise among nonclinical DNP graduates (administrative and education tracks; NBME, 2009). According to the NBME and CACC, the DNP examination was designed to assure the public that clinical DNP graduates function within the boundaries of their practice as well as meet the standards of their profession. They further assert that evaluation reflecting national standards of practice is the only mechanism that can ensure safe and high-quality patient care.

According to proponents of the DNP examination, the line between physician and DNP practice is very clear, because the context and scope of the examination are different from those of the three-step USMLE examination for physician certification (NBME, 2009). Unlike the physician USMLE examination, the DNP certification examination is a shorter examination, which does not require prior formal clinical skills assessment and prior fundamental scientific knowledge, as required by physician certification candidates. Because the DNP certification examination should reflect the same level of clinical acumen as primary care physicians, proponents also defend the choice of the NBME as the developer of the examination (Kane, 2009; Mundinger, 2007).

In contrast to physician certification, proponents also argue that the DNP examination more comprehensively evaluates the training of DNPs in patient care coordination to facilitate access to care and meet health care disparities (NBME, 2009). Unlike physicians, DNPs represent a new generation of primary care providers who not only manage complex illnesses in hospitals, emergency departments, and outpatient offices, but also coordinate care among various health care providers and health care settings, and provide preventive services that encompass contextual components such as social and family support and cost-effective health care (Kane, 2009; Landro, 2008). Rather than replicating the physician USMLE examination, the DNP examination contains different dimensions of the USMLE Step 3 that reflect advanced nursing practice. Mundinger (2009) argues that opposition to the examination may be fueled in part from physicians who worry that competition from DNP diplomates may lower their income and prestige.

Proponents of the DNP examination assert that concerns about physician regulation of APRN practice are unfounded (Mundinger, 2008a, 2008b; NBME, 2009). Justification for this position is based on the fact that the DNP examination is only one component of the certification process. In order to receive a diplomate status, DNPs must also possess national certification as an APRN, graduate from an accredited DNP program, and be recognized or licensed by a state board of nursing as an APRN, all of which are governed almost exclusively by nursing associations (with the exception of the CNM, which is governed by the American College of Nurse-Midwives [ACNM]). In addition, the DNP examination may actually assist in better defining the boundaries between doctoral advanced practice nursing and medicine.

The DNP examination represents expert input from both nursing and medicine professionals; these both support a multidisciplinary health care team approach that better serves the needs of primary care patients. According to the NBME and the CACC, future health care will require the collaboration of multidisciplinary health care teams whose individual members possess a variety of educational backgrounds and clinical expertise to meet the health care gaps created by an increasing shortage of primary care providers (Mundinger, Starck, Hathaway, Shaver, & Woods, 2009). Nonphysician primary care providers such as DNPs are vital to reduce the fragmentation and inefficiency of patient care, especially among the medically underserved. Without a sufficient pool of primary care providers, proponents of the DNP examination assert that there will be increased cost, decreased quality of care, and decreased patient satisfaction. They further argue that the increased use of DNPs will require additional assurance that DNPs have met national standards of care expected of all primary care disciplines. Each primary care discipline, however, will need to define its boundaries and standards in patient-care management. With the ultimate goals of patient safety and excellent health care, the NBME and CACC promoted the development of the DNP examination to provide evidence of high-quality standardized assessment of DNPs who practice within the boundaries of their profession and provide care that is complementary to other primary health care professions. The NBME and CACC also view the DNP examination as complementary to the goals of uniform regulation of APRN practice via LACE (licensing, accreditation, certification, education), which emphasizes the achievement of competency-based standards of practice (American Psychiatric Nurses Association [APNA], 2010).

Proponents of the DNP examination also assert that the DNP examination reflects more in-depth knowledge, training, and skills than master's-prepared APRNs, and that this distinction is necessary to assure the public of safe and high-quality care (Landro, 2008). In contrast to opponents' negative views regarding the broadness of the examination, the ABCC asserts that the DNP certification examination was designed to be broad in scope to reflect the DNP diplomates' complex advanced practice knowledge, skills, and decision making (ABCC, 2009). Finally, according to proponents, the DNP examination, which is based on standards endorsed by medicine, assures the public that the DNP diplomate is not a second-tier professional (Landro, 2008).

Although some opponents argue that there is no distinct difference between master's-prepared and doctorally prepared APRNs, proponents argue that DNPs invest more time in education beyond the master's level to prepare them to act as leaders in translating research into practice and to address the faculty shortage (McGrath & Piques, 2009). According to proponents, each represents a distinct level of practice reflected in their essential components (Table 21.1). Although master's-prepared APRNs are more focused on a specific populations such as pediatric or women's health care in limited health care settings, the DNP is more focused on complex diagnosis, coordination of care, and management of individuals across a variety of health care settings (Landro, 2008). In addition, their extended training in medical practice and management is more similar to primary care physicians than to master's-prepared APRNs (Mundinger, 2009).

Compared to master's-prepared APRNs, who focus mainly on *understanding* theories of practice and health care policies, DNPs are expected to take *leadership* in translating theoretical knowledge into clinical practice, changing health care policy, organizing and facilitating financing of health care to eliminate health care disparities, and improving the overall quality of care to benefit patients (American Association of Colleges of Nursing [AACN], 1996, 2006). In contrast to master's-prepared APRNs who are expected to *utilize* evidence-based nursing in practice, DNPs are expected to *synthesize, translate, disseminate*, and *integrate* new evidence-based knowledge into practice. Although master's-prepared APRNs are educated to *deliver culturally sensitive care, promote health*, and *prevent disease* for specific patient populations, DNPs focus on improving the nation's health by *integrating* and *institutionalizing evidence-based nursing knowledge* for disease prevention and health promotion for individuals and populations. The DNP also takes health care management one step further by not only managing complex illnesses and conducting individual and systemic assessments, but by evaluating links between individuals, populations, and health care financing and policy.

According to ANCC, a majority of nurses have varying opinions and find it difficult to agree for or against the DNP certification examination (ANCC, 2010). In an ANCC survey of 4,284 nurses, where 71% were currently practicing as an APRN, respondents were asked, "What do you envision as the desired future for certification of nurses holding the DNP degree in the year 2015?" While 60% expressed the desire for a single endpoint examination, 40% expressed the desire for staged examinations where testing would occur at one or more midpoints during master's preparation with a final endpoint DNP examination.

TABLE 21.1   **Essentials of DNP Versus MSN Preparation for APRNs**

DNP Preparation[a]	MSN Preparation[b]
I. Theoretical Foundations for Practice—act as leaders to use the conceptual scientific foundation of nursing to translate knowledge into clinical practice to benefit patients in all practice environments	I. Theoretical Foundations of Nursing Practice—critiques, utilizes, and evaluates theory within practice
II. Organizational and Systems Leadership for Quality Improvement and Systems Thinking—taking the lead in changing policy, organization, and financing of health care to eliminate health disparities, improve quality and safety, and evaluate cost-effectiveness of care	II. Understanding policy, organization, and financing of health care
III. Clinical Scholarship and Analytical Methods for Evidence-Based Practice—synthesizes knowledge, translates research into practice, disseminates knowledge, and integrates new knowledge into practice	III. Initiate change and improve nursing practice
IV. Information Systems/Technology and Patient Care Technology for the Improvement and Transformation of Health Care	IV. Ethics—understand principles, personal values, and beliefs to frame nursing practice
V. Health Care Policy for Advocacy in Health Care—involves influencing policy design and development, analysis of policy, and political activism to decrease health care disparities, improve quality of care, and influence health care financing in all levels of government	V. Understanding how health care policy is organized and delivered
VI. Interprofessional Collaboration for Improving Patient and Population Health Outcomes—facilitates interdisciplinary collaboration	VI. Professional role development to operationalize theoretical principles and norms of specialty
VII. Clinical Prevention and Population Health for Improving the Nation's Health—leaders in integrating and institutionalizing evidence-based prevention for individuals and populations	VII. Human diversity and social issues to deliver culturally sensitive care to patients; health promotion and disease prevention for specific patient population
VIII. Advanced Nursing Practice—addresses complex medical management across a variety of health care settings; is able to manage more complex illness, conducts individual and systemic assessments, evaluates links between individual, population, health care financing and policy	VIII. Advanced health/physical assessment, physiology, pathophysiology, and pharmacology

APRN, advanced practice registered nurses; DNP, Doctor of Nursing Practice; MSN, master of science in nursing.
[a]Adapted from American Association of Colleges of Nursing (2006).
[b]Adapted from American Association of Colleges of Nursing (1996, 2011).

H. Michael Dreher, founding chair of the Doctoral Nursing Department at Drexel University, which has had a Doctor of Nursing Practice program since 2005, stated support for the examination, reporting:

While there is a great deal of opposition to this DNP exam, I am for it. I do not think it was prudent for the AACN to include the executive role in the

DNP degree construction and exclude the educator role. Therefore, the DNP exam emphasizes the clinical practitioner role and any credible credential that Doctor of Nursing Practice graduates can obtain that can differentiate their practice beyond the MSN, is worthy of at least further trial and study. (Dr. H. Michael Dreher, personal communication, May 10, 2010)

Dreher and Montgomery (2009) also suggest that the new term "doctoral advanced practice nursing" be used to differentiate "master's-level advanced practice nursing," and one could infer that this DNP examination may perhaps validate clinical practice beyond current master's APRN competencies.

In summary, proponents refute the criticisms of the DNP examination by asserting:

- It was never designed for nonclinical DNPs
- The boundaries between physician practice and even doctoral advanced practice nursing are quite clear
- Concerns of physician regulation of NP practice are unfounded
- Multidisciplinary health care teams with clear professional boundaries represent the future of primary care to meet the needs of the underserved
- The DNP certification is necessary to assure the public of high standards of care
- The DNP examination is worthy of further trial and study

In addition, proponents assert that the DNP certification examination supports the uniform regulation of APRN practice via LACE. Finally, proponents assert that there is a distinct difference between the practice of master's- and DNP-prepared APRNs.

■ ARGUMENTS AGAINST THE DNP EXAMINATION

The most salient arguments against the DNP certification examination question the validity of the examination for nonclinically based DNPs such as administrators and educators. In addition, nonclinically based APRN administrators and educators earning a DNP are only required to be actively certified by the ANCC in their respective roles. Those who oppose the examination cite the 50% pass rate achieved by 45 examinees in 2008, 57% pass rate among 19 examinees in 2009, 45% pass rate among 31 examiners in 2010, 70% pass rate among 22 examiners in 2011, and a 33% pass rate among 18 examiners in 2012 to bolster the argument against its validity (ABCC, 2015). The American Association of Nurse Practitioners (AANP), American College of Nurse Practitioners (ACNP), and some specialty groups of the American Medical Association (AMA) have publicly expressed their opposition to the DNP examination (Guadagnino & Mundinger, 2008; Hoyt & Proehl, 2009). Because those DNPs who pass the examination will use the title "doctor," some argue that the boundaries between medicine and nursing have been blurred to an extent that will cause public confusion. In addition, the use of the USMLE as the template for the DNP examination has raised some concerns that the public will be misled to think that DNP certification is equivalent to physician certification. Some opponents also express concern that NBME credentialing will ultimately result in physician regulation of APRN practice, because the NBME is viewed as a medical credentialing agency (National Organization of Nurse Practitioner Faculties [NONPF], 2008).

Opponents also argue that there are already psychometrically sound national certifying examinations for APRNs and question the utility of an additional certification examination (Counts & Dempster, 2008; Stanik-Hutt, 2008). They further argue that the

DNP certification examination is based on the practice of medicine and does not measure APRN expertise. Unlike current national certifying examinations for APRNs, opponents believe that the DNP examination is extraneous and unrelated to advanced practice nursing. NONPF (2008), which designed a population-based academic curriculum for the DNP, issued a statement that the individual-based DNP certification examination from the NBME is too broad to assess competency among DNP graduates with differing roles and specialties. This statement was also endorsed by six other organizations representing nurse practitioners including the AANP, ACNP, Association of Faculties of Pediatric Nurse Practitioners (AFPNP), National Association of Nurse Practitioners in Women's Health (NPWH), National Association of Pediatric Nurse Practitioners (NAPNAP), and National Conference of Gerontological Nurse Practitioners (NCGNP) (Johnson, 2008).

Several physicians have expressed concern regarding the ability of the DNP to practice independently (Guadagnino & Mundinger, 2008). In addition, some physicians have raised concerns that unsupervised DNP diplomates will ultimately decrease patient safety and quality of care. Some opponents also argue that there is no research to substantiate that DNP certification improves patient care (Michalski, Sagan, Moore, Bednash, & Rosseter, 2006). Finally, opponents argue that adding another layer of certification will dissuade nurses from becoming APRNs and further decrease the pool of available primary care providers (NONPF, 2008).

In summary, opponents argue that the DNP certification examination is irrelevant to nonclinical DNP graduates and DNP graduates who do not have expertise in family and adult advanced nursing practice. Furthermore, opponents believe that it:

- Blurs the lines between physician and doctoral advanced nursing practice (Guadagnino & Mundinger, 2008; Hoyt & Proehl, 2009)
- May result in physician regulation of advanced nursing practice (NONPF, 2008)
- Is unnecessary as a plethora of psychometrically sound national certifying examinations already exist (Counts & Dempster, 2008; NONPF, 2008)
- Is too broad to assess competency among DNP graduates with differing roles and specialties (NONPF, 2008)
- Could result in decreased safety and quality of care (Guadagnino & Mundinger, 2008)
- May dissuade nurses from becoming APRNs (NONPF, 2008)
- May add an extraneous certification examination that may increase barriers to practice (NONPF, 2008)

■ WHERE DO WE GO FROM HERE?

We are currently sitting at another crossroads in nursing history where proponents and opponents of the DNP competency examination are currently unable to find a middle ground between their two divergent positions. The nursing profession has continually experienced "growing pains" since the days of Florence Nightingale. While some innovations have flourished, others have failed, and yet others have undergone metamorphosis through lively dialogue. For example, when the National League for Nursing (NLN) refused to give nurse-midwives a special niche during their 1954 convention, a group of nurse-midwives formed the ACNM (Rooks, 1997). Despite the alienation that nurse-midwives felt from the nursing profession in the 1950s, today State Boards of Nursing, the Advanced Practice Registered Nurse Consensus Group, and the

ACNM are working side-by-side with other professional nursing organizations on *The Consensus Model for Advanced Practice Registered Nurses* (APRN Consensus Work Group & the National Council of State Boards of Nursing APRN Advisory Committee, 2008).

Representatives from both groups will need to come to the negotiating table to decide on the values they hold in common and work to achieve high standards of quality and safety from a common vision. Do they both agree that they need to meet the growing needs for primary care, remove barriers to practice, and better define practice as separate yet complementary to medicine? Do they agree with the majority of nurses in the ANCC survey who support a DNP certification examination? Both groups will need to discuss their differences and find a path that meets their diverse needs. Representatives from both groups will need to better define and determine the difference in competencies between the DNP and the master's-prepared APRN so that the purpose of a national DNP certification examination is clearer. They will need to address whether a competency examination endorsed by medicine is necessary for public confidence in DNP practice.

If both groups can agree on the value of the DNP certification examination, they will need to address the reasons for its low pass rate. Because the DNP certification examination is currently designed to evaluate the competence of DNPs from adult and family practice, representatives from both groups may need to discuss the possibility of revising or developing other specialty versions of examination so that it is a more valid measure of other clinical APRN specialties. In addition, both groups will also need to discuss the possibility of revising the DNP competency examination to better reflect the population-based focus of the DNP curriculum.

■ SUMMARY

As the doctoral APRN moves into the future, the nursing profession and individual APRN specialties will need to define the competencies that result in the highest-quality care for patients and their families, as well as set them apart from the practice of medicine. Both opponents and proponents of the DNP competency examination are needed at the negotiating table to explore what is ultimately best for patient care. As properly managed interpersonal conflict can result in opportunities for new learning and growth, the opinions of both sides may be needed to drive the growth of doctoral APRN practice to its fullest potential. So now, after having read this chapter, are you prepared for the new DNP certification examination? Yes? No? Perhaps you want to think about it more, and then decide.

■ CRITICAL THINKING QUESTIONS

1. *What are the major differences between master's- and doctoral-level certifications?*
2. *What do you think are pros and cons of the NBME's designing the DNP certification examination? Would another certifying body be more appropriate and why?*
3. *What are the major factors that differentiate the DNP practice from physician-based primary care practice?*
4. *Does the DNP certification examination promote or obstruct multidisciplinary collaboration? Why?*
5. *Does the DNP certification examination enhance public confidence? Why or why not? What is your rationale?*

6.   *Can a 50% pass rate support the arguments of both opponents and proponents of the DNP certification examination?*
7.   *Would another layer of certification dissuade or encourage nurses from becoming APRNs? What is your rationale?*
8.   *How could you argue that DNP certification improves patient care?*
9.   *How would you answer the criticism that there are already enough psychometrically sound APRN certification examinations?*
10. *What are your thoughts about the appropriateness of the DNP certification examination for APRN specialties other than family and adult advanced nursing practice? How would you answer the criticism that the examination is not appropriate for specialty APRNs such as pediatric and women's health care APRNs?*

■ REFERENCES

American Association of Colleges of Nursing. (1996). *The essentials of masters education for advanced practice nursing*. Retrieved from http://www.aacn.nche.edu/education-resources/MasEssentials96.pdf

American Association of Colleges of Nursing. (2006). *The essentials of doctoral education for advanced nursing practice*. Retrieved from http://www.aacn.nche.edu/dnp/Essentials.pdf

American Association of College of Nursing. (2011). The essentials of master's education in nursing, Retrieved from http://www.aacn.nche.edu/education-resources/MastersEssentials11.pdf

American Board of Comprehensive Care. (2009). Examination content for DNP certification examination. Retrieved from http://abcc.dnpcert.org

American Board of Comprehensive Care. (2010). Eligibility requirements. Retrieved from http://abcc.dnpcert.org

American Board of Comprehensive Care. (2015). About the ABCC and the CACC. Retrieved from http://www.abcc.dnpcert.org

American Psychiatric Nurses Association. (2010). An introduction to LACE. Retrieved from http://www.apna.org/i4a/pages/index.cfm?pageid=3498

APRN Consensus Work Group & the National Council of State Boards of Nursing APRN Advisory Committee. (2008). Consensus model for APRN regulation: Licensure, accreditation, certification & education. Retrieved from http://www.aacn.nche.edu/education-resources/APRNReport.pdf

Counts, M., & Dempster, J. (2008, April 4). Letter to the editor sent to the *Wall Street Journal*. *American Academy of Nurse Practitioners*. Retrieved from www.aanp.org/NR/rdonlyres/9A676C85-022C-460B-9FCD-63361829DF8A/0/wsjletter0408.pdf

Dreher, H. M., & Montgomery, K. E. (2009). Let's call it "doctoral" advanced practice nursing. *The Journal of Continuing Nursing Education*, 40(12), 530–531.

Guadagnino, C., & Mundinger, M. (2008). Growing role of nurse practitioners. *Physician News Digest*. Retrieved from https://physiciansnews.com/cover/508.html

Hoyt, S., & Proehl, J. (2009). Weighing in on the DNP examination. *Advanced Emergency Nursing Journal*, 31(4), 261–263.

Johnson, P. J. (2008). The DNP storm. *Neonatal Network*, 27(5), 297–298.

Kane, R. (2009). The advanced practice nurse: An answer to the primary care challenge. *Clinical Scholars Review*, 1(1), 37–38.

Landro, L. (2008). Making room for Dr. Nurse. *Wall Street Journal*. Retrieved from http://www.wsj.com/articles/SB120710036831882059

McGrath, J. M., & Piques, A. (2009). The past, the present, and the prospective student: Is there a recipe for the DNP? *Journal of Perinatal and Neonatal Nursing*, 23(3), 207–212.

Michalski, K., Sagan, C., Moore, K., Bednash, G., & Rosseter, R. (2006). Readers and authors respond to "Introducing the Doctor of Nursing Practice." Retrieved from http://www.medscape.com/viewarticle/543596

Mundinger, M. (2007). Who will be your doctor? *Forbes.com*. Retrieved from http://www.forbes.com/2007/11/27/nurses-doctors-practice-oped-cx_mom_1128nurses.html

Mundinger, M. (2008a). Certification is the answer: What is the question? *Clinical Scholars Review*, 1(1), 3–4.

Mundinger, M. (2008b). American Board of Comprehensive Care Certification (ABCC): Too close to medicine? *Clinical Scholars Review, 1*(2), 67.

Mundinger, M. (2009). The clinical doctorate 15 years hence. *Clinical Scholars Review, 2*(2), 35–36.

Mundinger, M. O., Starck, P., Hathaway, D., Shaver, J., & Woods, N. F. (2009). The ABCs of the doctor of nursing practice: Assessing resources, building a culture of clinical scholarship, curricular models. *Journal of Professional Nursing, 25*(2), 69–74.

National Board of Medical Examiners. (2009). Development of a certifying examination for doctors of nursing practice. Retrieved from http://www.nbme.org/PDF/NBME-Development-of-DNP -Cert-Exam.PDF

National Organization of Nurse Practitioner Faculties. (2008). Nurse practitioner DNP education, certification and titling: A unified statement. Retrieved from https://www.pncb.org/ptistore/ resource/content/forms/DNP_Unified_Statement.pdf

Rooks, J. (1997). *Midwifery and childbirth in America*. Philadelphia, PA: Temple University Press.

Stanik-Hutt, J. (2008). Debunking the need to certify the DNP degree. *The Journal for Nurse Practitioners, 4*(10), 739.

Reflective Response 1

Michael Clark

In my current role, I teach both master of science in nursing (MSN) and Doctor of Nursing Practice (DNP) nurse practitioner students. The MSN students frequently ask me if they "need the DNP." I tell them that "the market will dictate the answer." The only argument that makes sense to me about the validity of the American Board of Comprehensive Care (ABCC) is whether it is predictive of competence and success in the marketplace. Certification examinations should address both fiduciary and predictive concerns.

External market forces are driving an increase in the number of bachelor of science in nursing (BSN) graduates. Employers recognize that nurses need more sophisticated skill sets in order to meet quality standards and add value to their organization. Similar forces will drive DNP education.

Currently, there is an explosion of new DNP programs. There are quality concerns about rigor and variance among programs. I do think that more demanding measures of competence might have a positive impact on the quality of DNP programs. This has been seen in BSN education where Commission on Collegiate Nursing Education (CCNE) requires minimum pass rates for the National Council Licensure Examination (NCLEX). Currently, the only claim that can be substantiated regarding DNP graduates is that they take more courses.

There are, however, deeper issues. The ABCC primarily targets DNP essential eight (advanced nursing practice). Measurement of competence for this essential is necessary but not sufficient. We need to grapple with how we measure the other seven competencies.

DNP programs may make the case that the scholarly project or capstone is designed to evaluate multiple DNP essentials. However, there is no practical way to verify the scope and depth of capstone projects across programs. A test or series of tests that measure competencies across all eight essentials may serve to ensure minimum competence in all eight essentials.

It would take time and a good deal of money to develop quality psychometrics for certification examinations that measure DNP competence in multiple domains. Many of the constructs need to be developed within the paradigm of improvement science. These constructs must incorporate many sources of expertise including those of medicine, business and policy. Having a PhD in nursing does not ensure competence within the paradigm of improvement science. We would need DNP's and other experts in improvement science to design these tests.

We will not move forward unless we move beyond binary narratives such as PhD–DNP and nursing-medicine. The new narratives center on health care economics and quality metrics such as those found in the "Triple Aim." The identification and measurement of competencies must be informed by a consideration of these broader narratives.

■ CONCLUSION

In conclusion, the construction of the ABCC is an important first step in initiating a dialogue about the unique competencies that a DNP graduate must possess. We must continue to grapple with ways to identify and measure these competencies. Testing would need to accomplish two objectives. It must measure competence by utilizing valid constructs developed within the paradigm of improvement science. It must also be predictive of a selective advantage in the marketplace for the DNP graduate.

Reflective Response 2

Geraldine M. Budd

The American Board of Comprehensive Care's (ABCC) Doctor of Nursing Practice (DNP) generalist certification examination has existed for 8 years and was accredited by the National Commission of Certifying Agencies in 2011 (Carter and Moore, 2015). In the time the examination has been available, the trend is that less graduates take the examination each year (American Board of Comprehensive Care, 2016). It is likely that this will continue and the DNP generalist examination will not gain acceptance or prominence for nurse practitioners (NPs). Several factors contribute to this perspective including that the DNP examination (a) neglects the nursing leadership consensus of the advanced practice registered Nurses (APRN population specialties, (b) negates the core nursing beliefs, and (c) is not accepted by either individual state board of nursing or the national council of state boards of nursing. Each is discussed subsequently.

Shortly after the development of the DNP generalist certification examination, the NP profession transitioned to a paradigm that precludes the inclusion of a generalist comprehensive NP certification. Driven by the 2008 *Consensus Model for Advanced Practice Registered Nurses (APRN): Licensure, Accreditation, Certification and Education* (American Nurses Association [ANA], 2008), NP licensure, education, and certification now encompass the population foci of family (across the life span); adult-gerontology; women's health; and pediatric, neonatal, or psychiatric population focus. Adult-gerontology or pediatrics NPs are further clarified as acute care or primary care. Although all types of NPs are needed, educational preparation has been divided depending on the role, population, and specialization.

The motivation for the Consensus Model for APRNs (2008) was inconsistencies in NP education, certification, and regulation. The Consensus Model was developed with input from more than 60 nursing organizations and on publication it was immediately endorsed by 48 nursing organizations (Stanley, 2012). As this book nears publication, the NP state boards, accreditors, certifiers, and professional organizations are closing in on integrating all the major elements of the Consensus Model (Cahill, Alexander, & Gross, 2014). Thus, state boards are requiring education and certification to be aligned with the role and population foci of the Consensus Model. Furthermore, the state board–approved NP certifying bodies (American Academy of Nurse Practitioners [AANP] Certification Program [AANPCP], 2016; American College of Cardiovascular Nursing [AACN] Certification Corporation, 2016; American Nurses Credentialing Center

[ANCC], 2016; Pediatrics Nursing Certification Board [PNCB], 2016) have all adopted the Consensus Model tenets. Role and population education consistent with the model is required to register for certification examinations. All the NP certification examinations direct testing toward the role and population foci. And, in the case of pediatrics and adult-gerontology, education and certification must be attained either as an acute or primary care NP (AANPCP, ACCN Certification Corporation, ANCC, and PNCB).

The ABCC DNP certification website lists the benefit of the ABCC certified diplomate certification as providing comprehensive care to complex patients across the life span (ABCC, 2016). ABCC applicants must be eligible for NP licensure, but no role of NP is specified. No population focus is indicated, although it is required that the applicant be educated in the area of "across the life span," and have completed a DNP program. Furthermore, Carter and Moore (2015) describe the examination as verifying that the ABCC-certified NP diplomate is prepared to deliver direct comprehensive care to complex individuals of all ages across the continuum of settings. A review of the website does not reveal any mention of the examination's congruence with the Consensus Model nor is this discussed in the two recent publications about the examination (Carter, 2013; Carter and Moore, 2015).

The core nursing beliefs are represented in the American Association of Colleges of Nursing (AACN, 2006) competencies. These competencies relate to the integration of science, leadership, quality care, technological literacy, inquiry, health policy, ethics, and independent practice. For NPs, the DNP competencies are intended to be complemented by the National Organization of Nurse Practitioner Faculties (NONPF) specialty competencies (NONPF, 2016). In contrast, the established DNP competencies do not suggest a single clinical proficiency pathway for either family across the life-span NPs, other specialty NPs, or for other APRN roles. Yet, the ABCC certification examination eligibility singles out the generalist or "across the lifespan" NP practice competencies as the defining characteristic of a qualified DNP. This incongruence negates the potential that different NP specialty competencies offer toward advancing the U.S. health agenda.

The likelihood of wide adoption of a generalist DNP certification examination is also unlikely because of the increased market demand for APRNs in various specialties. Some authorities have reasoned that the need for specialty health care is what drove the development of the licensing, accreditation, certification, education (LACE) Consensus document (ANA, 2008; Rounds, Zych, & Mallory, 2013). The aging of the American population and a shortfall of physicians in specialty care by 2025 (Dall, West, Chakrabarti, & Iacobucci, 2015) will undoubtedly increase the need for NPs to provide specialty care (Coombs, 2015). Furthermore, NPs often desire and seek specialty care employment because of prior hospital experience in a similar specialty area (Budd, Wolf, & Hass, 2015).

The huge need for specialty care has extended beyond the original specialties recommended in the Consensus Model and has spawned a number of secondary specialty NP certifications for those already certified. New specialty examinations in oncology, cardiology, dermatology, and emergency medicine have been developed (Tegler, 2016). These secondary certifications will likely continue to expand as the need to hire more specialty NP providers expands. The specialty certification examinations are aligned with the Consensus Model (2011) and can help to ensure the NP is operating within particular scope of practice. This enhances public safety and promotes the profession.

In 2011, the Institute of Medicine (IOM, 2011) published *The Future of Nursing Report: Leading Change, Advancing Health.* The publication's goal of removing practice barriers has promoted nursing organizations to work to change state legislative and regulatory language so that NPs will have full practice authority and be able to move their license to all 50 states. The *Future of Nursing* outlined suggestions to enhance the ability of nurses to promote health.

State boards dictate NP licensing requirements and these typically include the type of education and certification required (Blackwell & Neff, 2015). According to Blackwell and Neff, numerous state boards of nursing have ambiguous scope of practice regulations resulting in the NP education and certification being the determinants for scope of practice. Education requirements are a graduate degree in all but two states (Indiana and South Dakota; AANP, 2016). At this writing, all but three states require certification for NP licensure (California, Kansas, and New York; AANP). State boards of nursing must approve the NP certification examinations (Blackwell & Neff, 2015). The ABCC certification examination is not approved for NP licensure and no information suggests that any state plans to do so. States have either adopted or are moving toward full adoption of the approved NP roles as defined in the Consensus Model. The ABCC certification is not consistent with the Consensus Model NP roles. This is likely to pose a barrier to getting state approval for the examination.

The aforementioned reasons provide a strong argument as to why the consensus of multiple NP stakeholders and organizations should prevail and the ABCC's DNP examination should not be adopted as a certification.

■ REFERENCES

AACN Certification Board. (2016). ACNPC-AG—Certification for adult-gerontology acute care nurse practitioners. Retrieved from http://www.aacn.org/wd/certifications/content/acnpc-ag -landing.pcms?menu=certification

American Association of Colleges of Nursing. (2006). *The essentials of doctoral education for advanced nursing practice.* Retrieved from http://www.aacn.nche.edu/publications/position/DNPEssentials.pdf

American Association of Colleges of Nursing. (2011). *The essentials of master's education in nursing.* Retrieved from http://www.aacn.nche.edu/education-resources/MastersEssentials11.pdf

American Association of Nurses Credentialing Center. (2016). APRN consensus model. Retrieved fromhttp://nursecredentialing.org/Certification/APRNCorner

American Association of Nurse Practitioner Certification Board. (2016). FAQs: Contact information. Retrieved from https://www.aanpcert.org/faq-certification

American Association of Nurse Practitioners. (2016). State practice environment. Retrieved from https://www.aanp.org/legislation-regulation/state-legislation/state-practice-environment

American Board of Comprehensive Care. (2016). 2009 pass rates. Retrieved from http://abcc.dnpcert .org/exam-pass-rates

American Nurses Association. (2008). ANA issue brief: Consensus model for APRN education. Retrieved from http://www.nursingworld.org/cmissuebrief

Blackwell, C. W., & Neff, D. F. (2015). Certification and education as determinants of nurse practitioner scope of practice: An investigation of the rules and regulations defining NP scope of practice in the United States. *Journal of the American Association of Nurse Practitioners, 27*(10), 552–557.

Budd, G. M., Wolf, A., & Haas, R. E. (2015). Addressing the primary care workforce: A study of nurse practitioner students' plans after graduation. *Journal of Nursing Education 54*(3), 130–136.

Cahill, M., Alexander, M., & Gross, L. (2014). The 2014 NCSBN consensus report on APRN regulation. *Journal of Nursing Regulation, 4*(4), 5–12.

Carter, M. (2013). Certifying competency in comprehensive care. *Clinical Scholars Review, 6*(2), 87–88.

Carter, M. A., & Moore, P. J. (2015). The necessity of the Doctor of Nursing Practice in comprehensive care for future health care. *Clinical Scholars Review, 8*(1), 13–17.

Coombs, L. A. (2015). The growing nurse practitioner workforce in specialty care. *The Journal for Nurse Practitioners, 11*(9), 907–909.

Dall, T., West, T., Chakrabarti, R., & Iacobucci, W. (2015). *The complexities of physician supply and demand: Projections from 2013 to 2025.* Washington, DC: Association of American Medical Colleges.

Institute of Medicine (US); Committee on the Robert Wood Johnson Foundation Initiative on the Future of Nursing. (2011). *The future of nursing: Leading change, advancing health.* Washington, DC: National Academies Press.

National Organization of Nurse Practitioner Faculties. (2016). Competencies for nurse practitioners: Core competencies for nurse practitioners. Retrieved from: http://www.nonpf.org/?page=14

Pediatric Nursing Certification Boards. (2016). The acute care PCNP. Retrieved from http://www.pncb .org/ptistore/control/exams/ac/ac_role

Rounds, L. R., Zych, J. J., & Mallary, L. L. (2013). The consensus model for regulation of APRNs: Implications for nurse practitioners. *Journal of the American Academy of Nurse Practitioners, 25,* 180–185.

Stanley, J. M. (2012). Impact of new regulatory standards on advanced practice registered nursing: The APRN Consensus Model and LACE. *Nursing Clinics of North America, 47,* 241–250.

Tegler, E. (2016). Nurse practitioner subspecialties. In American Academy of Nurse Practitioners (Ed.), *Celebrating 50 years of nurse practitioners* (p. 79). Austin, TX: American Academy of Nurse Practitioners.

Advising Doctor of Nursing Practice "Clinicians" and How Their Role Will Evolve With a Practice Doctorate: Perspectives From a 35-Year Nurse Practitioner

Joan Rosen Bloch

How similar or different are advanced practice nurses who are Doctor of Nursing Practice (DNP) graduates from master of science in nursing (MSN) graduates? Since the inception of the DNP academic degree, the debate about the right academic degree for entry into nurse practitioner (NP) practice continues. Will roles be different for any of the four groups of advanced practice registered nurses (APRNs[1]) who first obtained MSN degrees and built up on that with their nursing practice-focused doctorate degrees? How will they differ? How will they differ from APRNs who obtain research-focused doctorate, PhD degrees? Will the roles evolve by inductive or deductive development—or perhaps a combination of both? What determining factors will shape the roles of APRNs with different "levels" of education preparation? Must we be prescriptive and restrictive about roles for clinicians with DNP degrees during a time when many changes are underway in health care and health care systems? We must not jeopardize the flexibility and creativity of professional nursing roles that continue to evolve. Perhaps, with knowledge and skills acquired from doctoral studies, empowered doctorally prepared nurses can build up on their prior education and practice experiences, and grow their professional journey in flexible ways that best serve three main stakeholders: the profession of nursing, health care systems, and, of course, the people served by both the profession of nursing and systems of health care.

Considering the unprecedented number of APRNs who have sought doctoral education since the introduction of the practice doctorate in 2004, this is an exciting time for nursing (Auerbach et al., 2015). It is exhilarating for students and professors to participate together in doctoral journeys as there is much passion to learn more to better serve society's needs for caring and healing. Working together to build bridges and solutions to the *big* health problems that threaten all people is an important shared goal. Together, through nursing doctoral education, we have great opportunities to create important think tanks where innovative solutions may be born.

If you are a clinician embarking on this DNP journey, which requires a tremendous investment in time, money, and professional energy, there are important questions to ponder. As a profession and for each individual contemplating their degree—the impact of the DNP degree on the individual professional nurse and the larger health care context is quite relevant. We now enter the second decade of having this practice-based nursing doctorate academic degree. DNP graduates have entered the nursing market place—both in the academic and practice settings to fill positions that are meeting workplace needs (Auerbach et al., 2015).

■ MUST *YOUR* ROLE BE DEFINED AT THIS TIME? WHAT IS *YOUR* VISION?

Reading this chapter for a clear vision of how either your role will be shaped differently, or how, as an educator, you can facilitate shaping the role of your DNP students differently from MSN students may be problematic. By now, you may be wondering if the preceding paragraph has created "double talk" with no clear vision. You are probably right. If you think you will find a clear role description that separately delineates APRN roles based on the MSN and DNP degrees, pause right now . . . because . . . the vision is being shaped *now* by all of us. We are the next generation of what Dunphy, Youngkin, and Smith (2004) coined as the "rebels, renegades, and trailblazers" (p. 25) of nursing's future. The rebels, renegades, and trailblazers of yesteryear shaped the current myriad of APRN roles as we know them today. Yet, as you read in previous chapters of this book, formalization of the APRN role into the construct as we now know it took multiple decades. Remember, Loretta Ford, EdD, RN, PNP, FAAN, the pioneer of the NP movement, met tremendous resistance from the discipline of nursing as she forged forward with her visionary model of nursing practice with the NP role (Ford, 1997; Ford & Gardenier, 2015). (See earlier chapters to learn more about the history of the APRN role as we know it today. Carefully consider the barriers that those bold and brave nurses confronted. Are there parallels today?)

Shaping the future role possibilities of a nursing workforce with practice doctorates occurring today and in years to come rests with all of us. Not only is this a time of creativity, but a time for critical evaluation of why one is considering the DNP degree and not the traditional PhD. Deep, honest reflection of this basic question should yield great insights to guide a myriad of possibilities that should enhance the nursing profession's tripartite contributions (practice, research, and education) for the greater good of society.

History has shown us that the boundaries of practice are pliable and flexible enough to change with time and context to meet the needs of all stakeholders (Aiken & Fagin, 1992; Fairman, 2008, 2010; Stanley, 2005). Passage into this millennium with the nursing practice doctorate presents new opportunities for the profession of nursing to empower those most passionate about nursing, who have the perseverance to pursue and accomplish a terminal degree in the discipline of nursing. The practice doctorate *must* differ from the traditional PhD to take the nurse on a trajectory beyond the "research walls" of academia in which the PhD is expected to advance nursing science as a full-time research scholar (Bloch, 2005; McGrath & Piques, 2009). Though the degree is separate, but equal, nursing doctorate graduates *must* work together for the greater good of nursing and health care.

Nursing is central to the key policy issues and has the ability to shape health care reform (Fairman, 2010). Nursing made great strides in the last half of the 20th century, with profound role successes in practice as APRNs and in academia as PhD scholars. The fight for the development and acceptance of nursing PhD programs and the APRN role did not happen overnight, but took more than a quarter century (McGrath & Piques, 2009). The work of the past century emphasized getting our foothold into academia and into independent practice arenas where we are now more visible to other "players" (i.e., beyond those of our patients who were cared for by nurses). The profession is now well positioned to participate in shaping and *improving* the health and health care system of our nation. Yet, much improvement is needed. There is a significant health disadvantage of the American people compared to those in countries of comparable wealth (Institute of Medicine [IOM], 2013). Despite the fact that the United States is the wealthiest country in the world and spends the most money on health care, health indicators such as infant mortality rates are the worst compared to all other nations of comparable wealth (IOM, 2013). It is quite apparent that our health care system is broken and desperately needs help. As we forge ahead, we must allow our insights from our nursing disciplinary lens to be shared and heard at interdisciplinary forums.

With the success of nursing roles (the independent role of APRNs in practice and PhD scholars in academia), it is exciting that the evolving practice doctorate has been embraced nationally, and in record speed. This is evidenced by the rapid growth in the number of DNP programs. Nearly half of all nursing schools with any graduate-level nursing education ($N = 564$ schools) offer a DNP program ($N = 251$ DNP programs) (Auerbach et al., 2015). The need exists for another level of expertise that builds on MSN education in practice, despite a clear prescription for the role in the marketplace for the DNP graduate. As McGrath and Piques (2009) explain, nursing's commitment to this practice doctorate reveals our commitment to advancing health care by educating a generation of very motivated nurses to create unprecedented opportunities within a multilayered, complex health care environment. Unity and coalitions between all those in nursing, regardless of all degrees and the "alphabet soup of credentials" within the nursing profession are necessary. Thus, the future roles will be shaped by the expertise the DNP brings to health care practice and policy.

■ MSN VERSUS DNP: WHICH IS BETTER ENTRY INTO APRN CLINICAL PRACTICE?

Should the DNP degree be required for entry into APRN practice? As many are aware, this was proposed by key nursing stakeholders and then endorsed by the American Association of Colleges of Nursing's (AACN's) proclamation that all master's programs that educate APRNs to enter practice should transition to the DNP by 2015 (AACN, 2004). Well, the year 2015 has come and gone, and this did not happen. Though some schools transitioned their APRN master's degree programs into DNP programs, most have not. The MSN remains the predominant entry-level academic degree for APRN practice (Auerbach et al., 2015). The introduction of the DNP degree can be viewed as a catalyst of major changes introduced in the last decade. However, nonetheless, NPs still acquire their critical clinical skills in diagnosis and management of patients in preparation for practicing independently in the master's degree programs (Roush, 2014). APRN MSN education has been revamped and is described subsequently.

During the last decade, concurrent with developing the academic practice doctorate degree, debates ensued among nursing leadership about restructuring APRN educational curriculum, certification, and licensure related to APRN practice. With much confusion and uncertainty that led to rumors, concerns, and dissension, the leaders of key nursing organizations, who were stakeholders in current and future roles for APRNs, formed a task force to reach a consensus (APRN Consensus Work Group, 2008). Although during the period from mid-1990s to 2003, the organizations made individual and collaborative efforts to address the myriad of regulatory APRN issues, it was not until 2003 that they all came together. After a 6-year period, they reached an agreement on a consensus model for APRN regulation and education. The model established guidelines for titling, education, certification, accreditation, and licensing for the four clinical APRN roles—(a) certified registered nurse anesthetists (CRNAs), (b) certified nurse-midwives (CNMs), (c) clinical nurse specialists (CNSs), and (d) certified nurse practitioners (CNPs). This model, endorsed by 44 national nursing organizations, was a great feat for nursing; for in addition to developing nationally recognized standards for APRN regulation, the consensus model clarified the role and scope of APRNs, which assists policy makers and the lay public with the understanding of the key roles of APRNs (Stanley, Werner, & Apple, 2009).

The consensus model, referred to by the acronym LACE (licensure, accreditation, certification, and education) was released years after the AACN announced their position that the DNP degree should be the academic degree for entry into APRN practice. It is imperative to understand that the LACE model *does not repute the value of MSN as entry into APRN clinical practice.* Though AACN and other organizations recommend the practice doctorate for clinical APRN roles, there is currently no movement to actually restrict APRN licensure and certification only to DNP graduates. Dr. Anne O'Sullivan, a member of the consensus group and former president of the National Organization of Nurse Practitioner Faculties (NONPF), in her report on April 18, 2010 at NONPF's annual conference held in Washington, DC, clarified, on behalf of the consensus group, that there is no current plan to dissolve the MSN degree requirement as the entry degree for APRN practice. She emphasized that there is absolutely no evidence that the public would be better served by changing the MSN-required degree to a DNP degree as entry into clinical APRN practice. On the contrary, it was emphasized that there is a plethora of evidence documenting the positive impact that the master's-prepared APRNs have had on improving health outcomes among diverse populations with various health conditions throughout the United States (Joel, 2004; Stanley, 2005). So, why should entry into APRN practice be changed from requiring an MSN degree to a DNP degree?

The two officially recognized accreditation agencies for nursing by the U.S. Secretary of Education, The National League for Nursing Accrediting Commission (NLNAC) and Commission on Collegiate Nursing Education (CCNE), have clarified that they will continue to accredit master's-level educational programs, and their standards have not changed to require doctoral preparation for NP programs. Although the AACN's (2006) document, *The Essentials of Doctoral Education for Advanced Nursing Practice*, recommended 2015 as a date for transition from master's to DNP degree programs for APRN education; they have clarified that this date was only a recommendation (NONPF, 2010). Furthermore, the recent RAND Report commissioned by the AACN confirms that, as of 2015, there is insufficient evidence of any added value in terms of outcomes of direct patient care provided by DNP-prepared APRNs over MSN-prepared APRNs (Auerbach et al., 2015). However, the number of schools that offer DNP programs continues to expand. Moreover, there is quite a robust demand for the DNP by APRNs for many are seeking DNP degrees (Auerbach et al., 2015).

■ WILL THE PRACTICE DOCTORATE EDUCATIONAL JOURNEY PROVIDE ADDITIONAL KNOWLEDGE AND SKILLS TO CHANGE THE CLINICIAN ROLE?

The DNP is an academic degree, not a specific prescribed clinical role. At the current time, it is designed to build on former academic nursing degrees to enhance and provide knowledge above and beyond that provided at the MSN and bachelor of science in nursing (BSN) levels. With a practice doctorate, however, it is anticipated that current advanced practice clinical nursing roles will be enhanced so that doctoral advanced practice nurses can apply new knowledge and skills to improve health outcomes and health care systems. The AACN's (2006) aforementioned key document, *The Essentials of Doctoral Education for Advanced Nursing Practice*, outlines and defines eight foundational outcome competencies for graduates of practice doctorate programs. These eight foundational competencies were previously cited in Chapter 4 and throughout this text. Educators consider these competencies as the key roadmap to creating innovative and integrated curricula to meet these competencies.

With critical evaluation of these competencies, one should be able to identify that there are developmental components that are woven throughout nursing curricula from undergraduate to doctoral levels. For example, at the undergraduate level, the required basic science courses introduce BSN students to scientific underpinnings of practice, and clinical rotations based in hospitals introduce BSN students to complex systems. Yet, professional roles differ developmentally. At the baccalaureate level, professional role development requires understanding the role of the nurse. Upon graduating with a MSN degree, the professional role is developmentally focused on their "new" advanced nursing practice role, a role different from their BSN nursing role.

The problem for nursing leadership and advancement in today's complex health care systems is that the current curricula for master's educational programs are filled to capacity with little room for additional courses or content (Newland, 2010). Therefore, the practice doctorate is a natural next step for clinicians who want more from their professional role. Thus, DNP curricula, by design, include higher level and expanded content. Dr. Jamesetta Newland, the editor-in-chief of *The Nurse Practitioner: The American Journal of Primary Healthcare* and a Fellow of the American Academy of Nurse Practitioners (FAANP), justified the need for additional education with the formation of a practice doctorate. She argued that leadership skills must be part of the curriculum, and not dependent on acquisition of these skills as "on the job training" often "under fire." To meet the extensive learning objectives for today's practice as an APRN, the typical length of an MSN nursing program is insufficient to provide the requisite knowledge for NPs to grow into leadership positions that can really maximally impact improvements in health care systems. In addition, the need for professional parity was at the forefront of all DNP discussions. Newland (2010, p. 5) summed this up in her following statement:

> Why should nursing not have a practice doctorate as do other major health care professions? . . . The DNP is a practice doctorate conceived to prepare advanced clinical leaders in developing the skills necessary to bring about

change within the health care organization to improve quality of care and health outcomes.

■ AN ECOLOGIC EDUCATIONAL FRAMEWORK APPROACH TO THE PRACTICE DOCTORATE

Initially, the goal held by many educators is that future roles for DNP graduates would be in practice (Bloch, 2005; Boland, Treston, & O'Sullivan, 2010; Newland, 2010). This is not necessarily where most NPs end up once completing their DNP degree due to the dire market need of NP faculty with doctorate degrees. Nonetheless, curricula are designed to allow the doctoral educational journey to be one of professional growth and empowerment that builds on clinical experience and expertise shaped by prior MSN preparation. The educational journey for APRNs can be viewed as an advanced version of the "novice to expert" progression from entry into APRN practice with a MSN degree to a more expert role with a DNP degree. With this novice to expert construct applied to APRN roles, the goal for the DNP role is that DNP graduates are well positioned (with their new doctoral level knowledge) to seize new opportunities. They can leverage their academic credential (DNP) to open doors, be creative, and help transform their workplace or the health care system where they seek employment. This theme can be seen in the published literature on DNP outcomes, such as the descriptive longitudinal study of 22 DNP graduates from the University of Washington (Brown & Kaplan, 2010). The graduates emphasized that their doctoral work enhanced their practice roles in multiple ways, including that it increased their parity with physician colleagues with better clinical skills and opportunities to translate research to practice and policy (Brown & Kaplan, 2010). Students who are deciding between a practice doctorate (DNP) or a research doctorate (PhD) should decipher where they really would like to see themselves. Do they envision a role that is (a) entrenched in the real world of health care practice and clinical teaching or (b) behind the "ivy towers" entrenched in building and sustaining a program of research?

A PhD is a research degree and can prepare one to lead research teams to advance nursing knowledge through competing for the fiercely competitive research grants. The old adage of "publish or perish" still prevails in the work environment for PhD-prepared nursing faculty. Yet, these two worlds are intersecting in academia. Those with DNPs are demonstrating an important academic role educating future APRNs. Likewise, DNPs are contributing significant scholarship to the nursing profession. Therefore, the dichotomy between PhD and DNP is not so clear and the nursing discipline should look at other disciplines (e.g., medicine, dentistry, law) where practitioners and researchers often move between both worlds. Merged communities of researchers and practitioners are essential for effective feedback loops of knowledge dissemination and translation necessary for evidence-based practice and practice-based evidence (Bloch, 2015; Lyons, 2009).

Conceptualizing the possibilities of DNP roles and their subsequent impact on health and health care can be understood by an ecological education framework emphasizing how the DNP academic degree is built on the BSN and MSN academic degrees. Within an ecologic framework, a systems perspective is viewed, consisting of the health care system and various but distinct nursing systems, integrating within this larger system with complex microlevels and macrolevels. This synergy of systems demands multidisciplinary participants having educational competencies that allow progression from entry to expert levels, preparing the practitioner with developmental knowledge and skill sets transferable to practicing within complex health care systems. The BSN degree provides core competencies for entry into practice. The MSN degree builds up on this and allows the professional nurse to focus in a particular specialty area of nursing. In general terms, the specialization can be within the systems of nursing education, administration, or clinical practice. For APRN clinical specialties, there are regulatory licensures and professional certifications required for the specific APRN clinical practice (see Chapter 3). Though the historical evolution of APRN roles and resulting regulatory requirements dependent on first obtaining professional certification occurred over several decades, MSN education today is more prescriptive and shorter than those in the 1970s that produced the "rebels, renegades, and trailblazers" of yesteryear. Specific MSN programs differ depending on the knowledge and skills needed. For example, MSN nurse-anesthetist programs are quite different from pediatric NP and nurse-midwifery programs. At the completion of a master's degree, advanced practice nurses have a concrete idea of what their clinical role will be as an MSN-prepared APRN; they choose their specialty area. Their studies are focused on their specific specialty role and socialization to that specialty APRN role. Their classroom and clinical practicum experiences are therefore tailored to meet learning goals for their clinical specialty APRN role.

■ PATHWAYS TO POTENTIAL DNP ROLES

With a leap of faith, a love of clinical nursing, and a passion for learning, DNP students are ripe for an empowering journey in academia during their doctoral studies. Acquisition of a terminal degree, which allows an individualized approach to self-direct clinical experiential learning during doctoral studies, is an amazing post-master's nursing experience. Intensive advisement from doctoral nursing faculty facilitates this process and simultaneously creates a synergistic relationship between doctoral faculty and doctoral students. Thus, doctoral education differs dramatically from master's APRN-prescriptive education. Prepare to disrupt yourself and your thinking, as innovative change is needed (Samit, 2015). Grow how you think, broaden your perspectives and be part of the change that will happen to our challenged health care systems.

Glowing as it sounds, what about the practicalities? What exactly will the graduate do? Will employers want to hire, and even pay more for a practice doctorate? This line of reasoning has never interfered with the attainment of higher academic degrees. Do students pursue PhDs in the humanities because of potential salaries? A PhD in early American Victorian romance literature surely was not a ticket to becoming a millionaire. However, it may have provided the particular individual with an irreplaceable intellectual satisfaction above and beyond any other. Should clinical nurses not have advanced educational opportunities that permit them to build up on what they already know, and occupy professional roles that can advance practice, perhaps in ways in which the PhD graduate cannot? The evidence confirms that nurses, staff nurses, and APRNs often take a salary reduction after obtaining a PhD and transitioning to faculty positions (Yucca & Witt, 2009). Imagine, practice-based APRNs can advance their academic degree and remain in practice. Perhaps their income will change—maybe for a higher rate, but not necessarily; however, their opportunities will expand. If a position requires independent thinking, creativity, innovation, and leadership, it is only natural that the applicant with the best credentials is most likely to get it. It may be the academic degree that differentiates the applicants. Thus, having a DNP degree should trump an MSN degree if all other qualifications are equal. Graduates of practice doctorate programs are in the marketplace across the nation.

AN IMPORTANT EVOLVING ROLE OF NPs WITH DNP DEGREES: ACADEME

During the 20th century, the NP role transformed nursing practice and education, thus leading to increasing numbers of NPs assuming faculty positions and engaging in full tripartite activities in teaching, practice, and scholarship (Buchholz, Bloch, Westrin, & Fogg, 2015). The evidence is clear that NPs who have DNP academic degrees are filling an important professional role as clinical educators (Auerbach et al., 2015). Despite the fact that the DNP degree was never explicitly designed to prepare NP educators, it is a documented reality that DNP graduates are actively being hired into NP faculty positions. The market demand is strong.

AACN's (2006) eight essentials for DNP education guide curriculum that prepares advanced practice nurses to practice at the highest level. But, DNP curricula are purposely designed *not* to prepare nurse-educators, despite the fact that many NPs are eligible to teach in collegiate nursing programs after obtaining a terminal degree in the discipline of nursing (AACN, 2015). Considering that there is a strong need for NP Nurse Educators, it behooves the NP-DNP student to garner some educational experiences during their DNP program, if possible. Remember, opportunities to self-direct clinical experiential learning experiences exist, so clever ways to incorporate such should be possible. The NP-DNP student can carve out ways to incorporate clinical hours that can bridge practice and academia in innovative ways. Just think out of the box!

ROLE OF DNP AS SCHOLAR

DNPs, like PhDs, have professional responsibilities as scholars. One intense debate is whether the DNP degree prepares the scholars to generate new knowledge. AACN (2015) clearly states that it does, and furthermore, provides some guidance to distinguish between research-focused and practice-focused scholarship:

> Graduates of both research- and practice-focused doctoral programs are prepared to generate new knowledge. However, research-focused graduates are prepared to generate knowledge through rigorous research and statistical methodologies that may be broadly applicable or generalizable; practice-focused graduates are prepared to generate new knowledge through innovation of practice change, the translation of evidence, and the implementation of quality improvement processes in specific practice settings, systems, or with specific populations to improve health or health outcomes. New knowledge generated through practice innovation, for example, could be of value to other practice settings. This new knowledge is considered transferrable but is not considered generalizable.

What does the preceding statement by AACN (2015) really mean? In reality, dwelling too much on interpreting what the statement means and how to differentiate DNPs from PhDs may be missing the mark by distracting from the real work needed by DNPs and PhDs. Nonetheless, it is an important question that many are asking. Key messages are needed to our intradisciplinary and interdisciplinary colleagues in academia and practice who may be confused about the new practice doctorate in nursing? One way is to differentiate the DNP from the PhD is by the types of "gold-standard" federally funded grants that PhDs and DNPs could strive to achieve as principal investigators. A quick differentiation that seems to resonate with many is that PhDs should strive for writing *research* grants that hopefully could be funded, one day, by the National Institutes of Health (NIH). In contrast, DNPs should strive for writing *program* grants that could be funded, one day, by the Health Resources and Service Administration (HRSA). This distinction seems to resonate well when used.

Writing program grants to implement evidence-based programs, which are aimed to improve health outcomes is logical for practice-based DNP scholars. Writing a program grant such as a HRSA grant is different from writing a research grant. DNP students should seek insight into developing this skill during their doctoral journey. Seek faculty who understand this, for few PhD and DNP nursing faculty have been schooled in such. But, some have been extremely successful, such as those who write program grants for nurse-managed centers and other specialized funded health service programs. An example can be found in the article that describes a funded breast health services program in two nurse-managed centers (Tsai, Peterman, Baisch, Ji, & Zwiers, 2014).

Dissemination and Implementation Science

Roles exist for DNP and PhD scholars in the evolving *transdisciplinary* field of dissemination and implementation science. The discipline of nursing has much to contribute to advance broader and deeper understandings of this science (Bloch, Clark, & Faust, 2016). This is a ripe frontier for innovative nursing opportunities. The NIH and Academy Health jointly sponsor an annual conference on dissemination and implementation science. The focus of the conference is relevant to nursing science, practice, and policy. This is evident by reviewing the topics that were listed in the call for abstracts for the Eighth Annual Conference on the Science of Dissemination and Implementation in Health (see Table 22.1; http://diconference.academyhealth.org/callforabstracts/aof). From this list, it is evident that there is much overlap with nursing science and practice. Dissemination and implementation science incorporates key principles of methods related to quality improvement, community-based participatory research, evidence-based practice, and health program planning and evaluation. More about all these practice-based scholarly methods, not traditionally taught in nursing research courses, can be found in Bloch, Courtland, and Clark's (2016) textbook. More focus on these nontraditional research methods are needed. For example, APRNs who focus their practice in community settings versus hospitals, need to learn more about conducting community needs assessments, which are often required for submitting program planning grants. Also, logic models are also often required. Many DNP documents mention quality improvement methods (AACN, 2015), but additional methods are also critically needed in DNP education.

■ SUMMARY: EMBARKING ON PRACTICE DOCTORAL STUDIES— ADVICE FOR YOUR FUTURE ROLES

As a 35-year veteran NP who embarked on returning to academia for advanced nursing degrees in 1981 (MSN) and 1997 (PhD), I offer some advice. Keep an open mind and take the educational opportunity to learn about ways in which your contribution

TABLE 22.1 **Areas of Focus for the Eighth Annual Conference on the Science of Dissemination and Implementation in Health**

Focus Area	Specific Topics for Presentations
Behavioral health	• Studies that develop transformative research strategies to promote implementation, adoption, accessibility, and sustainability of evidence-based practices in behavioral health • Studies that optimize the reach of hybrid effectiveness-implementation research designs • Innovative implementation studies designed to improve behavioral health outcomes among diverse, vulnerable, and underserved populations around the globe • Studies that improve implementation strategies for behavioral health that ensure engagement of patients, decision makers, health care organizations, and other key stakeholders • Studies that advance implementation designs that address the complexities in behavioral health, from multifaceted interventions, to patient comorbidities, and contextual factors
Big data and technology for dissemination and implementation research	• Best practices and innovations in research methods and designs using big data for evaluating implementation • Integrating and effectively using big data technology to improve health care delivery, care quality, and population health • The role of various technology platforms in promoting the implementation of evidence • Using big data to address complexity in implementation science (e.g., complex and multilevel interventions, multiple conditions, variations in implementation processes, and contextual factors) • Scale-up and sustainability considerations for big data-based implementation research
Clinical (i.e., primary, specialty, hospital, etc.) care settings	• Dissemination and implementation of transitional care models (emergency room to outpatient, inpatient to outpatient, or between acute care and other residential facilities) • Rigorous observational studies of practice-led dissemination and implementation processes • Economic evaluation in dissemination and implementation research in clinical settings • Implementation science to improve health outcomes in underserved groups across highly variable primary care practice settings
Global dissemination and implementation	• Designs, implementation strategies, and outcomes for complex, combination multilevel interventions in international settings • Integrating new and expanding technologies (including low-tech) and methodologies to reach high risk, difficult to reach populations to improve health care delivery and population health • Opportunities to learn from scale-up and sustainability studies in low and middle income countries and other resource poor settings • Use of dissemination and implementation research methods from the field of international development • Building capacity for dissemination and implementation research in low- and middle-income countries

(continued)

TABLE 22.1   **Areas of Focus for the Eighth Annual Conference on the Science of Dissemination and Implementation in Health**   *(continued)*

Focus Area	Specific Topics for Presentations
Health policy dissemination and implementation	• Scientific study of implementation of state, local, regional, or national policies, including but not limited to major changes in health care delivery systems (e.g., bundled payments, population health, care coordination). These changes may be fostered by federal/state/private decision makers and/or regulations. • Evaluations of initiatives to promote the use of evidence in policymaking in various domains of health policies, including cross sector policies (e.g., in juvenile justice, education, etc.) • Methods/designs for evaluations of policy implementation, for example, randomized program evaluation, stepped-wedge, in-depth analyses • Rigorous evaluations of implementation outcomes of policies, including unintended consequences and economic dimensions, such as return on investment (ROI) • Studies testing optimal strategies to implement or enhance uptake of policies
Models, measures, and methods	• Measures and methods to capture the dynamic evolution of interventions and the contexts in which they are implemented • Studies demonstrating the application of simulation and statistical modeling techniques to implementation research questions • Research designs to maximize the value of observational studies for design and implementation (D&I; including but not limited to natural experiments such as the impact of major policy rollouts) • Research developing theories/methods/measures to study de-implementation • Research that focuses on the development and testing of theoretical and evaluation models for D&I processes
Prevention and public health	• Applications of prevention science methods within dissemination and implementation research studies • Studies of the implementation of hospitals and health care systems collaboration with community organizations and/or governmental public health to promote disease prevention • Studies of evidence-based multifaceted and multilevel interventions to disseminate and implement prevention programs • Use of community-based participatory research in disease prevention and health promotion

(continued)

TABLE 22.1 **Areas of Focus for the Eighth Annual Conference on the Science of Dissemination and Implementation in Health** *(continued)*

Focus Area	Specific Topics for Presentations
Promoting health equity and eliminating disparities	• Culturally based approaches to dissemination and implementation research • Understanding key barriers to implementation in diverse communities and underserved populations and effective strategies to overcome those barriers • Scaling up evidence-based interventions to address health disparities at the population level • Sustainability within settings and systems that address health disparities and health inequalities • Building capacity to address health disparities in dissemination and implementation research • Studies addressing health disparities in low-income settings through policy implementation

This table was created from information that was posted on the following website. Retrieved from http://diconference.academyhealth.org/callforabstracts/aof

to the greater good of society can grow through your potential role as a nurse. The beauty of returning to academic studies is that you are exposed not only to new knowledge from the courses you are enrolled in, but you are also exposed to others within nursing and outside of nursing. This can expand your network for future opportunities directly and indirectly. Perhaps directly by being offered an employment opportunity by someone you have met along this journey, or indirectly by exposing you to new types of employment opportunities that you would have never considered before.

As shown in Table 22.2, I have created "tips for success" that are developed from my 35 years of integrated experiences as a practicing NP and educator.

Embarking on journeys for new academic degrees that resulted in new roles has always further strengthened my love and devotion to the discipline of nursing. Little did I know about the actual roles I would eventually assume at the completion of my first academic degree; however, I successfully found roles I did not imagine before. These new roles, enabled by my newly acquired academic degrees, provided me with immensely satisfying professional opportunities and growth. Remember that what is good for the people is good for nursing. Thus, my advice to those considering embarking on a journey for a practice doctorate is to take a leap of faith with an open mind and enjoy the doctoral journey.

TABLE 22.2   **Student Tips for Success in Creating Your New and Expanded DNP Role**

Tips	Examples
1. Use your educational journey to build on your prior professional experiences. Critically evaluate your knowledge deficits and how your prior professional settings may have limited your exposures and experiences.	• Knowledge is power. Empower your future opportunities by gaining more knowledge. Put yourself in settings that you may not have had access to before. • Take courses not exposed to before (e.g., finances, basic science, advanced informatics); something that will give you an advantage in the area in which you seek your role development.
2. Take this educational journey as an opportunity to expand your horizons. Explore different role options as NPs have much to offer as key stakeholders in public, population, and community health. Use the opportunity of your "student" status to shadow experts in those roles.	• Reach out to a Centers for Disease Control and Prevention (CDC) official working in your area of interest. Perhaps you can visit the CDC and schedule a focused visit that meets your individually created objectives. You can "test out" such a position to see if that is what you may want to work toward. • Go to community policy meetings or shadow top "administrators or policy makers" to broaden your perspectives of the micro- and macro-environments. • If your NP practice is community-based, try to partner with an agency or health department conducting a formal needs assessment. This is a crucial step in program planning, implementation, and evaluation. Unless your NP practice is hospital based, much of the language and processes of "quality-improvement" are not used in community and population health. acute care.
3. Peer-mentor your classmates and let yourself be peer-mentored by your classmates.	• Strong bonds are created during doctoral studies, especially when you are the ones shaping the future roles of nurses with practice doctorates. Learn the strengths that each of you has and how you may collaborate in a way that builds on what each of you can "bring to the table."
4. Intradisciplinary and interdisciplinary collaboration will be essential for the success of your new role. Remember that professional relationships are built on trust, honest communication, and integrity. Professional behavior built on these qualities will enhance your ability to serve as a positive role model of the practice doctorate (Chism, 2009). This may be your best asset after your title of *doctor* opens new doors.	• As the first generation with practice doctorates, you serve as a role model. Your professionalism and ethical nursing practice must prevail at the highest standards. Others will be testing you; if you pass, opportunities will be presented. If you use your doctoral degree unwisely to wield power and control, you will meet much resistance (Houdin, Naylor, & Haller, 2004; McGrath & Piques, 2009).

(continued)

TABLE 22.2 **Student Tips for Success in Creating Your New and Expanded DNP Role** *(continued)*

Tips	Examples
5. Lastly, never complain about the costs of your doctoral degree. When you negotiate your role and compensation, do your homework. Know your market worth and do not expect your future employer to pay more just for the *doctor* title unless you can *articulate* the returns on their investment will be above and beyond what is being offered. Seeking a practice doctorate was your choice!	• "Attitude, attitude, attitude" is critical in the workplace environment. Attitudes reflecting gratitude for the opportunities your employer has provided will win support when you propose your award winning ideas. Attitudes of resentment that you are undervalued and underpaid contaminate workplace morale. If you truly believe that is your situation, it is time to "move on" and, equipped with your practice doctorate, find a different role for you.

DNP, Doctor of Nursing Practice; NP, nurse practitioner.

■ CRITICAL THINKING QUESTIONS

1. *Reflect deeply within yourself and identify at least three reasons you are considering a doctoral degree in nursing.*
2. *Identify how you hope your professional role would change as a DNP graduate.*
3. *Consider the barriers that those bold and brave nurse practitioners of yesteryear confronted as the role evolved. Discuss the parallels today with the new DNP academic degree.*
4. *Discuss the leadership knowledge and skills you feel you need as you translate your insights from practice during this time of national health reform.*
5. *Explain the roles and responsibilities of DNP graduate APRNs in evidence-based practice and practice-based evidence.*
6. *In what ways would your skills need to be enhanced to meet the AACN's essential outcome competency "Information Systems/Technology and Patient Care Technology for the Improvement and Transformation of Health Care?"*
7. *Describe your position, with its rationale, in the debate of which academic degree should be entry into APRN practice: the MSN versus the DNP.*
8. *Identify strategies (at least two) to ensure the development of another academic degree in nursing, the DNP, helps to unify and strengthen the worlds of nursing research and practice.*
9. *Develop a sample of a formal memorandum of understanding between you, in your role as a DNP with a colleague, a research nurse with a PhD, for knowledge dissemination, translation, and implementation collaboration.*
10. *Using the AACN's eight outcome competencies for DNP education, write a new job description in your clinical setting for yourself with the enhanced knowledge and skills you will gain with a DNP.*

■ NOTE

1. APRN is defined as a nurse who has met the education, certification, and licensure requirements to practice in one of four direct patient care roles: (a) certified nurse-midwife (CNM), (b) CRNA, (c) CNS, and (d) nurse practitioner (NP; AACN, 2015). In this chapter, APRN is not used

synonymously with a more general term, advanced nursing practice (APN). APN is a more general term used for all MSN roles, not these specific four APRN direct care roles.

■ REFERENCES

Aiken, L., & Fagin, C. (1992). *Charting nursing's future: Agenda for the 1990s*. Philadelphia, PA: J. B. Lippincott.

American Association of Colleges of Nursing. (2004). *AACN position statement on the practice doctorate in nursing*. Retrieved from http://www.aacn.nche.edu/dnp/dnp-position-statement

American Association of Colleges of Nursing. (2006). *The essentials of doctoral education for advanced nursing practice*. Retrieved from http://www.aacn.nche.edu/DNP/pdf/Essentials.pdf

American Association of Colleges of Nursing. (2015). The doctor of nursing practice: Current issues and clarifying recommendations. Retrieved from http://www.aacn.nche.edu/aacn-publications/white-papers/DNP-Implementation-TF-Report-8-15.pdf

APRN Consensus Work Group & National Council of State Boards of Nursing APRN Advisory Committee. (2008). Consensus model for APRN regulation: Licensure, accreditation, certification & education. Retrieved from http://aacn.nche.edu/education/pdf/APRNReport.pdf

Auerbach, D. I., Martsoff, G., Pearson, M. L., Taylor, E., Zaydman, M., Spetz, J., & Dower, C. (2015). The DNP by 2015: A study of the institutional, political, and professional issues that facilitate or impede establishing a post-baccalaureate doctor of nursing practice program. Retrieved from http://www.aacn.nche.edu/dnp/DNP-Study.pdf

Bloch, J. (2005). The doctor of nursing practice (DNP): Need for more dialogue. [Letter to the Editor]. *Online Journal of Nursing Issues, 10*(3). Retrieved from http://www.nursingworld.org/MainMenuCategories/ANAMarketplace/ANAPeriodicals/OJIN/LetterstotheEditor/Letter-to-the-Editor-from-Joan-Rosen-Bloch.html

Bloch, J. R. (2015). Will nursing faculty hinder or facilitate innovation in nurse executive DNP students? In A. Rundio & V. Wilson (Eds.), *The doctor of nursing practice and the nurse executive role* (pp. 17–37). Philadelphia, PA: Wolters Kluwer Health.

Bloch, J. R., Clark, M., & Faust, J. (2016). Implementation research. In J. R. Bloch, M. Courtney, & M. Clark (Eds.), *Practice-based clinical inquiry in nursing for PhD-DNP research: Looking beyond traditional methods* (pp. 157–185). New York, NY: Springer Publishing.

Bloch, J. R., Courtney, M., & Clark, M. (2016). *Practice-based clinical inquiry in nursing for PhD-DNP research: Looking beyond traditional methods*. New York, NY: Springer Publishing.

Boland, B. A., Treston, J., & O'Sullivan, A. L. (2010). Whether you seek a DNP program that offers online, full-time, or part-time options, prospective students should know what to look for when pursuing this esteemed degree. *The Nurse Practitioner, 35*(4), 37–41.

Brown, M. A., & Kaplan, L. (2010). *Opening doors: The practice degree that changes practice*. Poster session presented at the 36th Annual Meeting of the National Organization of Nurse Practitioner Faculties, Washington, DC.

Buchholz, S. W., Bloch, J. R., Westrin, D., & Fogg, L. (2015). Nurse practitioner faculty research: Results from the 2012 National Organization of Nurse Practitioner Faculties Survey. *Journal of the American Association of Nurse Practitioners, 27*(12), 664–670. doi:10.1002/2327-6924.12250

Chism, L. A. (2009). *The doctor of nursing practice: A guidebook for role development and professional issues*. Sudbury, MA: Jones & Bartlett.

Dunphy, L. M., Youngkin, E. Q., & Smith, N. K. (2004). Advanced practice nursing: Doing what had to be done—Radicals, renegades, and rebels. In L. A. Joel (Ed.), *Advanced practice nursing: Essentials for role development* (pp. 3–30). Philadelphia, PA: F. A. Davis.

Fairman, J. (2008). *Making room in the clinic: Nurse practitioners and the evolution of modern health care*. New Brunswick, NJ: Rutgers University Press.

Fairman, J. A. (2010). Historic and historical opportunities: Nurse practitioners and the opportunities of health reform. In E. M. Sullivan-Marx, D. O. McGivern, J. A. Fairman, & S. A. Greenberg (Eds.), *Nurse practitioners: The evolution and future of advanced practice* (pp. 3–14). New York, NY: Springer Publishing.

Ford, L. (1997). A voice from the past: 30 Fascinating years as a nurse practitioner. *Clinical Excellence for Nurse Practitioners, 1*(1), 3–6.

Ford, L., & Gardenier, D. (2015). Fasten your seat belts—It's going to be a bumpy ride. *The Journal for Nurse Practitioners, 11*(6), 575–577.

Houdin, A. D., Naylor, M. D., & Haller, D. G. (2004). Physician–nurse collaboration in research in the 21st century. *Journal of Clinical Oncology, 22*(5), 774–776.

Institute of Medicine. (2013). Health in international perspective: Shorter lives, poorer health. National Academy of Sciences. Retrieved from http://iom.nationalacademies.org/Reports/2013/US-Health-in-International-Perspective-Shorter-Lives-Poorer-Health/Report-Brief010913.aspx

Joel, L. A. (2004). *Advanced practice nursing: Essentials for role development*. Philadelphia, PA: F. A. Davis.

Lyons, J. S. (2009). Knowledge creation through total clinical outcomes management: A practice-based evidence solution to address some of the challenges of knowledge translation. *Journal of Canadian Child and Adolescent Psychiatry, 18*(1), 38–45.

McGrath, J. M., & Piques, A. (2009). The past, the present, and the prospective student. *Journal of Perinatal and Neonatal Nursing, 23*(3), 207–212.

Newland, J. A. (2010). In defense of the DNP. *The Nurse Practitioner: The American Journal of Primary Healthcare, 35*(4), 5.

National Organization of Nurse Practitioner Faculties. (2010). APRN consensus model frequently asked questions. Retrieved from http://www.nonpf.com/associations/10789/files/FAQsfinal2010.pdf

Roush, K. (2014). Whatever happened to the clinical DNP? Are current doctor of nursing practice programs a good fit for NPs in direct patient care? *American Journal of Nursing, 114*(6), 11.

Samit, J. (2015). *Disrupt you!* New York, NY: Flatiron Books.

Stanley, J. M. (2005). *Advanced practice nursing* (2nd ed.). Philadelphia, PA: F. A. Davis.

Stanley, J. M., Werner, K. E., & Apple, K. (2009). Positioning advanced practice registered nurses for health care reform: Consensus on APRN regulation. *Journal of Professional Nursing, 25*(6), 340–348.

Tsai, P. Y., Peterman, B., Baisch, M. J., Ji, E. S., & Zwiers, K. (2014). Providing and funding breast health services in urban nurse-managed health centers. *Nursing Outlook, 62*(3), 204–211.

Yucca, C. B., & Witt, R. (2009). Leveraging higher salaries for nursing faculty. *Journal of Professional Nursing, 25*(3), 151–155.

Reflective Response 1

Carol Savrin

Dr. Bloch begins her chapter by asking who "we" are. I think that at this juncture, that is a reasonable question that needs to be addressed. She clearly states that the individual with a Doctor of Nursing Practice (DNP) degree is just that, a person with a degree, and that does not necessarily confer a new role. How will we all as advanced practice registered nurse's (APRN) change with the increase in the number DNPs? The future lies in all of us as we move forward.

If one looks at the history of the nurse practitioner (NP) role, one will see that the role has been evolving and changing ever since it was envisioned by Loretta Ford in the 1960s. The advanced practice roles developed out of a need that was identified and nurses were the ones who stepped in to fill the need. In the case of the nurse anesthetist, the job was being done by the surgeons, but since they had a greater interest in the surgery than in the anesthesia, the job was not being done well (Diers, 1991). The midwife role was initially brought here from England and filled a need in rural and underserved areas where people could not afford a doctor to assist with delivery. With the advent of the World War I, there were not enough English midwives who either came to or stayed in the United States, and so the Frontier Nursing Service (FNS) under Mary Breckinridge began to train nurse midwives to fill the need (FNS, 2000). In the second reflective response in Chapter 3, Dr. Zuzelo writes that Dr. Hildegard Peplau is credited with first coining of the term "clinical nurse specialist" in 1938 to describe "an advanced practice nurse with expertise in nursing practice in the care of complex patients." The final advanced practice role to develop was the NP role, which began in the 1960s and 1970s in direct response to a shortage of primary care physicians in the underserved areas, especially the rural areas of the country. Traditionally, the role is agreed to have begun with the continuing education program developed by Loretta Ford and Henry Silver in Colorado during the period from 1965 to 1966 (Ford, 1967).

All of the advanced practice roles have been fluid. They have changed over the years, and have evolved as the society changed and as the need changed. The latest development in the advanced practice nursing (APN) role is that it is evolving globally (Savrin, 2009). The individual culture of the local entity clearly shapes the role, so that the APN role in Botswana is different from the APN role in Singapore, which is different from the APN role in South Korea. Although students might find it comforting to be told by current educators exactly what the role will be in the future, it is not how nursing has evolved, nor is it how the APN role has evolved. There was a point in time when nurses were not allowed to take blood pressures, and clearly that has changed over time. To paraphrase the overly quoted Gandhi (b. 1869, d. 1948), we have to "be the change that you want to see in the world,"[1] or in our case, the change we want to see in the NP world.

Interestingly, to some extent, the DNP or practice doctorate role has to wait for society to catch up with the responsibilities and embrace the role. When Rozella Schlotfeldt first envisioned the practice doctorate in the 1970s (Schlotfeldt, 1973), society was not ready for nurses to be educated at a doctoral level and people did not understand the role. It took many years for people to understand and embrace the role and the concept of a practice doctorate. Dr. Schlotfeldt envisioned that the ND (nursing doctorate) would affirm nursing's place as a profession and with recognition within the health care profession and as an important discipline. She envisioned the practice doctorate as very different from the PhD or research doctorate.

Whether APRNs entry to practice should be at the master of science in nursing (MSN) or DNP level is currently highly controversial. However, whether they continue to be educated at the MSN or DNP level, they will continue to evolve and will continue to meet the needs within society. We have thousands of APNs who are desirous of further education and have embraced the DNP with enthusiasm. Additionally, many schools have found it easier to establish a post-master's DNP prior to the establishment of a post-baccalaureate DNP. It remains to be seen if in the future the DNP becomes a post-baccalaureate program only, as the American Association of Colleges of Nursing (AACN) has suggested, or if the MSN will continue to be offered for the basic APN education and the DNP offered for a more extensive advanced education.

Dr. Bloch rightfully identifies the DNP as a degree and not a role. The role is the certified nurse practitioners (CNM), certified registered nurse anesthetists (CRNA), NP, or clinical nurse specialists (CNS) all of which are very different from the basic RN role. The degree makes the recipient think differently and therefore create innovative change. To argue for education at the DNP level, all APRNs should learn about culture and behavior of organizations, the role of policy in the provision of health care, and the business of health care. It is possible that the APRN in the initial stages must spend so much time learning about the pathophysiology, diagnosis, and treatment of diseases, and the pharmacological and non-pharmacological treatment of diseases that they are not ready to incorporate the organizational systems, the policy issues, and the business aspects into their practice settings. At this time, the post-MSN DNP is therefore transformational in changing the thinking patterns and enhancing the approach to APRN practice for those folks who choose to pursue it. The post-MSN DNP students have: (a) mastered the diagnosis and treatment of the patients they see; (b) are ready to incorporate research into practice as a way of thinking; (c) to enhance practice through creating coalitions with other health care providers; and (d) working together to change the policies that govern the health care environment. The DNP can be a clinician, a scholar and innovator, and an educator, although the educational role is somewhat controversial due to the stance of AACN. At this time, a significant number of DNP graduates are in fact educators, so that stance will likely change over time. As with the NP degree, it is a constantly changing environment. I agree with Dr. Bloch that we are embarking on a journey with the practice doctorate, and that we all need to embrace the journey and see where it takes us.

Dr Bloch provides a very salient and informative table at the end of the chapter with important points for the DNP student to think about as they embark on their journey in the DNP world. These points are very well thought out and will be extremely helpful to the DNP student as they are trying to maneuver this new degree. She rightly states, what is good for the people, is good for nursing.

■ NOTE

1. Quote widely cited.

■ REFERENCES

Diers, D. (1991). Nurse midwives and nurse anesthetists: The cutting edge in specialist practice. In L. Aiken, H. Aiken, & C. M. Fagan (Eds.), *Charting nursing's future: Agenda for the 1990's* (pp. 159–180). New York, NY: Lippincott.

Ford, L., & Silver, H. (1967). The expanded role of the nurse in child care. *Nursing Outlook, 15,* 43–45. *Care, 19,* 38A–39A.

Frontier Nursing Service. (2000). *The frontier nursing service: A history.* Wendover, KY: Frontier Nursing Service.

Savrin, C. (2009). Growth and development of the nurse practitioner role around the globe. *Journal of Pediatric Health Care, 23*(5), 310–314.

Schlotfeldt, R. (1973). Planning for progress. *Nursing Outlook, 21,* 766–769.

Reflective Response 2

Ann B. Townsend

In Chapter 22, Dr. Bloch highlights key issues and challenges that have emerged both within the profession of nursing and on an individual practitioner level since the American Association of Colleges of Nursing's (AACN's) recommendation in 2004 that the Doctor of Nursing Practice (DNP) be the entry requirement for advanced practice nurses (AACN, 2004). The DNP, a clinical practice doctorate, prepares expert practitioners to function as organizational catalysts in practice, leadership, and education. The basis for the AACN's recommendation in 2004 was in response to an identified need to re-conceptualize the educational preparation of health care professionals to confront the present and emerging complexities of the health care delivery system (AACN, 2015). Subsequently, the AACN's decision has sparked concerns, dialogues, and debates regarding the DNP as a terminal degree for the advanced practice registered nurse (APRN). Generally, identified issues include title confusion, the DNP or PhD as a terminal nursing degree, role and scope of practice, faculty resources, and professional parity (Brar, Boschma, & McCuaig, 2010).

Despite these overarching controversies that have surrounded the DNP clinical practice doctorate as reiterated in Dr. Bloch's discussion, nurses have enrolled in DNP programs in exponential numbers. From 2013 to 2014, the enrollment in DNP programs increased from 14,688 to 18,352 with the number of DNP graduates rising from 2,443 to 3,065 (AACN, 2015). Now, as in the past, nurses in clinical practice have positioned themselves to accept new roles and responsibilities to meet society's need for accessible, affordable, quality health care.

Nursing professionals embarking on the DNP journey, should keep two important points made by Dr. Bloch in mind: (a) the DNP is an academic degree, not a prescribed clinical role; and (b) the responsibility to envision and actualize the DNP role rests with us. The construction of that vision has definitely progressed over the past decade and the APRN-DNP role seems to be emerging with clarity. As Dr. Bloch highlights, APRN-DNP are finding new opportunities for scholarship in clinical, leadership, and educator roles. Despite limited outcome data to date on the influence and impact of the DNP role on the profession and the health care system (Pritham & White, 2016), APRN-DNP graduates reported that throughout their DNP program they acquired evidence-based practice, leadership, and teaching skills (Graff, Russell, & Stegbaur, 2007). DNP graduates described an enhanced perspective in clinical practice (Hlabse, Dowling, Lindell, Underwood, & Barsman, 2016) and identified a wider range of opportunities to change practice at the system level, rather than on an individual client basis (Brown & Kaplan, 2016). With an intrinsic drive towards leadership, vision, and knowledge, along with an persistent extrinsic need for health care reformation, the APRN-DNP seeks to effect change where clinical practice occurs through the translation of research into evidence-based practices, enhanced clinical knowledge, and evaluation of quality outcomes. This approach to improving care and quality at the point of practice shares a central premise with positive deviance, a powerful strategy that postulates problems within a community are best solved within that community (Bradley et al., 2009). Positive deviators, such as the those in the emerging APRN-DNP role, are innovators whose perspectives and behaviors allow them to obtain better results than others using the same resources within the system (Jaramillo et al., 2008) The positive deviance approach, which has improved complex health problems in various public health settings, identifies positive deviants with best practices and through qualitative study, generates and tests hypotheses to disseminate their quality strategies (Bradley et al., 2009). This approach supports the necessary collaboration between the researcher (PhD) and the practitioner (APRN-DNP) to bridge the research–practice gaps that affects quality in health care (Buchholz, Yingling, Jones, & Tenfelde, 2015). The APRN-DNP's focus is as an expert in clinical practice, evidence-based practice, quality improvement, translational research, and in the evaluation of the outcomes of these applications in clinical settings (Vincent, Johnson, Velasquez, & Rigney, 2010). Thus, using a positive deviance approach, APRN-DNPs are establishing their roles as vital to link research, practice, and quality outcomes at the point of care, ultimately impacting overall health system quality.

So, as we continue to actualize the DNP role, consider Dr. Bloch's cautionary message "that we must not jeopardize flexibility and creativity of professional nursing roles," particularly during this time of unprecedented health care system changes. As APRNs, it is our vision, our journey, and our responsibility to shape the future of nursing.

■ REFERENCES

American Association of Colleges of Nursing. (2004). *AACN position statement on the practice doctorate in nursing.* Retrieved from http://www.aacn.niche.edu./DNP/pdf/DNP.pdf

American Association of Colleges of Nursing. (2015). The doctor of nursing practice (DNP) fact sheet. Retrieved from http://www.aacn.nche.edu/media-relations/fact-sheets/dnp

Bradley, E. H., Curry, L. A., Ramanadhan, S., Rowe, L., Nembhard, I. M., & Krumholz, H. M. (2009). Research in action: Using positive deviance to improve quality of healthcare. *Implementation Science, 4*(25). Retrieved from http://implementationscience.biomedcentral.com/articles/10.1186/1748-5908-4-25

Brar, K., Boschma, G., & McCuaig, F. (2010). The development of the nurse practitioner preparation beyond the master's level: What is the debate about? *International Journal of Nursing Education Scholarship, 7*(1), 1–15.

Brown, M. A., & Kaplan, L. (2016). Opening doors: The practice degree that changes practice. *The Nurse Practitioner, 41*(4), 35–42.

Buchholz, S. W., Yingling, C., Jones, K., & Tenfelde, S. (2015). DNP and PhD collaboration: Bringing together practice and research expertise as predegree and postdegree scholars. *Nurse Educator, 40*(4), 203–206.

Graff, J. C., Russell, C. K., & Stegbauer, C. C. (2007). Formative and summative evaluation of a practice doctorate program. *Nurse Educator, 32*(4), 173–177.

Hlabse, M. L., Dowling, D. A., Lindell, D., Underwood, P., & Barsman, S. G. (2016). Supports and barriers to successful progression in a DNP program students' and graduates' perspectives. *Nurse Educator, 41*(5), 256–261.

Jaramillo, B., Jenkins, C., Kermes, F., Wilson, L., Mazzocco, J., & Longo, T. (2008, April). Positive deviance: Innovation from the inside out. *Nurse Leader,* 30–34.

Pritham, U., & White, P. (2016). Assessing DNP impact: Using program evaluations to capture healthcare system change. *The Nurse Practitioner, 41*(4), 44–53.

Vincent, D., Johnson, C., Velasquez, D., & Rigney, T. (2010). DNP-prepared nurses as practitioner-researchers: Closing the gap between research and practice. *The American Journal for Nurse Practitioners, 14*(11/12), 28–34.

When the DNP Chair Is a DNP Graduate: The DNP in the Academic Role

Susan DeNisco and Sandra Bellini

In the past decade, there has been an explosion of post-baccalaureate and post-master's-prepared nurses entering and completing Doctor of Nursing Practice (DNP) programs. These graduates leave armed with a wealth of new knowledge, including leadership, policy, informatics, systems analysis, evidence-based practice methodology, and clinical skills that make them uniquely prepared to enter academic settings as nursing faculty members. More than 50% of new DNP graduates are interested in obtaining a nursing faculty appointment on graduation (Loomis, Willard, & Cohen, 2007). DNP-prepared nurses are contributing considerably to nursing education in academic leadership roles, such as dean, associate dean, chair, director, or chief administrator of nursing programs and schools. Their effective leadership and strong influence can be witnessed at small nursing programs at liberal arts colleges and schools of nursing at large research-intensive universities (Danzey et al., 2011). However, there is much controversy in academic circles, which revolves around the discussion that DNP-prepared nurses may have an inadequate foundation to teach nursing students, let alone lead academic programs compared with their research-prepared colleagues. In the faculty hiring section of a National League for Nursing (NLN, 2012) annual survey (2011–2012) the data showed that research-prepared faculty scored slightly higher on curriculum development and assessment but ranked notably lower than both DNP and master's-prepared faculty on clinical skills. Still there is a paucity of literature regarding DNP graduates as effective faculty members, let alone their potentiality to lead academic units. This chapter offers insight on the way DNP graduates are positioned to be contemporary and clinically competent educators at both graduate and undergraduate levels and also possess the capacity to lead academic programs at their institutions.

■ ROLE AND PREPARATION OF NURSE EDUCATORS

The role and preparation of nurse educators may be one of the most contentious issues in nursing education (DeNisco & Barker, 2016). In the landmark report, *The Future of Nursing: Leading Change, Advancing Health* the Institute of Medicine calls to double nurses holding a doctoral degree in an effort to expand the pool of diverse nurse faculty and researchers (IOM, 2011). The report's other recommendations are in direct alignment with the American Association of Colleges of Nursing's (AACN's) *Essentials of Doctoral Education for Advanced Nursing Practice* (AACN, 2006) and has revolutionized the nursing education by recommending a curriculum to prepare a future workforce, which will lead change and implement reform in our fragmented health care delivery system. According to the NLN (2016), the nurse educator role requires specialized preparation and every nursing faculty member engaged in academia must be prepared to implement that role successfully. Nurse educators remain the key resource in preparing a nursing workforce that will provide quality care to respond to the health care needs of demographically aging and ever increasing diverse population. As nursing is a practice discipline it makes sense that whether employed in an academic or clinical setting the nurse educator must be a competent clinician. However, while being a good clinician is essential, some would say it is not sufficient for the faculty role. According to the AACN (2006), a DNP degree is not necessarily adequate preparation for the role of a nurse educator yet neither is a nursing research doctorate. Both the NLN and the AACN have suggested that advanced practice nursing faculty should have didactic course work in curriculum design and evaluation and teaching methodologies. Although the original intent of the DNP degree was not meant to prepare a nursing education workforce it is clear they are filling that void and will continue to do so. DNPs are serving as nursing faculty in associate, baccalaureate, master's, and DNP programs and are moving into administrative academic roles at a rapid pace. One of the main questions relates to how academic institutions accommodate new DNP-prepared faculty members as didactic nurse educators when they have only received clinical preparation. In a cross-sectional descriptive study of 137 DNP program characteristics it was found that only 11.7% of the programs offered nursing education electives (Udlis & Mancuso, 2012). However, DNP programs that do offer education elective courses or educational leadership options provide experienced master's-prepared nurses with formal preparation in educational theory, testing, evaluation, curriculum development, and an educational practicum (Danzey et al., 2011). The DNP degree with a focus on education embodies all aspects of the NLN Core Competencies for Nurse Educators (NLN, 2005). DNP programs that accept post-master's students with or without an advanced practice nursing degree are frequently employed in a faculty or staff development role or serve as clinical preceptors or mentors in their organizations. Another causative factor to the confusion in clearly defining DNP curriculum and roles is that many nursing faculty members designing and teaching in DNP programs have limited understanding of evidence-based practice and educational pedagogy as they are often rigorous researchers (Melynck, 2013).

■ SUPPLY AND DEMAND FOR NURSING FACULTY AND ACADEMIC ADMINISTRATORS IN NURSING

Health Resources and Services Administration (HRSA) has projected a large increase in demand for nurses, from about 2.8 million full-time equivalents in 2012 to about

3.5 million in 2025 (Table 23.1). Meeting this projected demand will require a significant increase in nursing graduates, perhaps by as much as 50%, to fill new nursing positions as well as to account for attrition from an aging workforce. This corresponds to an increase in the demand for nursing faculty. According to the AACN, U.S. nursing schools turned away 68,938 qualified applicants from baccalaureate and graduate nursing programs due to an insufficient number of faculty, clinical sites, classroom space, clinical preceptors, and budget constraints (AACN, 2014). In a survey of 714 baccalaureate and/or graduate nursing programs a total of 1,236 faculty vacancies were identified across the country. In addition, those surveyed reported the need to generate an additional 124 faculty positions to accommodate student demand (AACN, 2014). The survey also reported the critical issues related to faculty recruitment and were noted to be the limited pool of doctorally prepared faculty, finding faculty with the right specialty mix, faculty willing/able to conduct research, and faculty willing/able to teach clinical courses. Consequently, increased supply will require a major expansion of nursing faculty and other educational resources. With the "graying" of the current pool of nursing faculty and academic nursing administrators and a large number of expected retirements over the next decade, efforts must be made to convince more nurses and nursing students to pursue academic careers, and to do so earlier in their career trajectory. Careers in nursing education are typically marked by long periods of clinical practice or administration before entering a faculty role (DeNisco & Barker, 2016). The idea of advanced practice nurses with clinical doctorates versus research doctorates working in academia is supported by the National Organization of Nurse Practitioner Faculties (NONPF), the NLN and the AACN. The DNP degree is the answer to getting our most

TABLE 23.1 **Supply, Demand, Shortage of Nurses**

	Registered Nurses
Supply	
Estimated supply, 2012	2,897,000
Estimated supply growth, 2012–2025	952,000
New entrants	*1,950,000*
Attrition[a]	*(998,800)*
Change in average work hours[b]	*800*
Projected supply, 2025	3,849,000
Demand[c]	
Estimated demand, 2012	2,897,000
Estimated demand growth, 2012–2025	612,000
Changing demographics	*584,000*
ACA-related increase in the number of insured	*28,000*
Projected demand, 2025	3,509,000
Supply in excess of demand, 2025	**340,000**

ACA, Affordable Care Act.
[a]Includes RNs who exit to become APNs.
[b]This represents the change in nurse full-time equivalents resulting from a change in the demographic composition of the future workforce and the associated effect on average number of hours worked.
[c]The model assumes that demand and supply are equal in 2012.

Source: Data from U.S. Department of Health and Human Service (2014).

talented clinicians, executive leaders, managers, and educators the advanced practice experiences, which will deepen their critical thinking and analytic skills and widen their network of colleagues in leadership roles. This in turn will create a ready workforce not only on the service side but also on the academic side of nursing. With a terminal DNP degree the nurse educator will have the essential skill set to prepare a future nursing workforce who will be better able to respond to a changing patient population, lead interprofessional teams, and understand organizational systems.

SHORTAGE OF ACADEMIC LEADERS

One of the four key messages in the leading-edge document the *Future of Nursing: Leading Change, Advancing Health* (IOM, 2011) is the recommendation for strong leadership development in nursing and infusing this content into nursing curriculum. Although many academic leaders have had a 5- to 10-year plan of careful stepwise career planning many "fall into their roles" and are ill prepared to take the leap from faculty to "chair." In a recent search on the "Higher Education" employment website, there were 1,232 vacant full-time nursing faculty positions at 4-year institutions. In a related search for administrative academic positions in nursing, there were 408 postings for deans and associate deans across the country. The Indeed job search engine entering the key search term "nursing dean" came up with 1,161 administrator positions in the United States and 459 were deans or associate dean positions.

Role Preparation

According to Glasgow, Weinstock, Lachman, Suplee, and Dreher (2009) newly promoted academic administrators in higher education had little or no previous leadership experience. Very often junior faculty are promoted to the chair role as they are still working on their scholarship timeline and have may find it difficult to "do it all." According to Greene and Ridenour (2004) academic institutions have promoted their most senior faculty to the deanship role with more than 60% having been department chairs with little preparation for the transition. Compounding matters, new administrators may be faced with a lack of familiarity with the academic hierarchy in their institutions while at the same time trying to secure and mentor new nursing faculty, balancing a budget, and fund-raising at the time this country is facing faculty vacancies and clinical site shortages at an alarming rate. Undoubtedly, it takes knowledge, skills, and personal awareness to be a successful academic leader. It is safe to say that the best leaders are those who have knowledge of clinical nursing practice and as well as experience acquired in a nursing faculty role. There is little written about the DNP-prepared faculty members assuming leadership roles in academia. Many DNP faculty members come to their roles with established records as nurse educators, clinical specialists, nurse administrators, and expert practitioners. It seems that the "ideal" academic administrator would possess all of these traits and if not all a way to acquire skills that are inherent in each role. Wolverton, Gmelch, Montez, and Nies (2001) identified analytical competence, interpersonal competence, and emotional intelligence as the primary skills needed to assume a role such as an academic dean. One can argue that analytical competence can be gained from advancing one's education whether prepared as a PhD or DNP. In the clinical setting the DNP-prepared administrator is faced with a barrage of complex patient and systems issues that have honed their analytical skills and problem-solving ability. Interpersonal competence and emotional intelligence are skills that can be acquired through leadership development programs and mentoring; however, they are often innate traits found in individuals who enjoy working with and have the capacity to build partnerships, sustain relationships, and weather the emotional demands of an administrative role. The DNP program curricula provides an opportunity for the future academic "chair" to explore leadership theories, project management and evaluation techniques, business planning, policy, evidence-based practices, and change theories. This coupled with their real-life work experiences in the health care service industry provides the foundation to be a successful academic administrator.

PREPARATION FOR ACADEMIC ADMINISTRATION: CLINICAL VERSUS RESEARCH EDUCATIONAL PATHWAYS

As DNP-educated faculty is a relatively new phenomenon, there is naturally much discussion regarding what kinds of roles they may be prepared for in the academic setting. This is an important topic because DNP graduates are assuming faculty roles and are becoming integral to filling the nursing faculty. In the traditional triad of faculty roles and responsibilities, specifically *teaching, scholarship,* and *service,* it may be beneficial to explore the educational components of graduate nursing education for both practice-focused and research-focused doctorates to ascertain what kind of faculty graduates from such a program might be qualified to occupy.

A review of the DNP curricula across programs (AACN, 2016b) generally reflects incorporation of the DNP *Essentials* (AACN, 2006), although variation and further specialization are evident. Succinctly, DNP education focuses on preparing expert practice clinicians, or as aligned with Boyer's Model of Scholarship, scholarship of both *application* and *integration* (Boyer, 1990). Areas of emphasis in DNP programs include organizational systems, collaborative practice, policy, informatics, quality improvement, and populations-based health care for advanced practice nurses: both advanced practice registered nurses (APRNs) and nurse executives. Although students are groomed to assume leadership roles on graduation, including writing and disseminating for the profession, these activities are generally focused around outcomes studies or other form of scholarship; the main focus of a DNP program is not on traditional *discovery* scholarship. Additionally, some DNP programs feature specialization in nursing education (Danzey et al., 2011). These content areas would suggest solid preparation of future DNP-prepared faculty in teaching, practice-focused scholarship, and service. According to the literature, the majority of DNP-prepared faculty today is primarily engaged in teaching (Agger, Oermann, & Lynn, 2014), but also can include practice, scholarship, and administration (Bellini, McCauley, & Cusson, 2012).

Conversely, the main foci of research-focused doctoral programs in nursing is to prepare nurse scientists who will serve as stewards of the discipline and educate the next generation of nurse academicians and scientists (AACN, 2004); indeed the main focus is on developing future *discovery* scholars (AACN, 2010). Examination of general curricula for PhD programs is congruent with outcomes expectations, with coursework in: grantsmanship, theory, methods, and advanced statistics. Additionally, some programs offer additional optional preparation in education to optimize future success in the realm of nursing education (University of Connecticut Certificate in Health Professions Education, 2016). Together, these areas of focus in research-focused programs should prepare future graduates as faculty for teaching, research-focused scholarship, and service.

■ THE PREPARATION OF FUTURE NURSE LEADERS: THE GAP IN GRADUATE NURSING EDUCATION

Although both types of doctoral education prepare graduates as future faculty for *scholarship* and *service* minimally, and make available preparation for *teaching*, perhaps the true missing element in terms of preparing future academic administrators, is education specific to *leadership*.

An underlying theme of the DNP essentials (AACN, 2006) seems to emphasize leadership as an inherent part of DNP education, but is it enough? Similar to difference in the proportion of attention paid to various components of PhD versus DNP curricula surrounding policy, for example, leadership content may be "present," but substantively different between programs.

In DNP programs, emphasis on leadership content tends to rise from the DNP essentials (AACN, 2006) and focuses on systems leadership intended for the *practice* side of the academic practice environment. The goal is to educate both advanced practice nurses and nurse executives for upper level administrative roles. Interestingly, this move to advocating for doctoral-level preparation for nurse executives in the practice setting is relatively new and arguably has lagged behind previous advancements in educational requirements for advanced practice nurses. Yoder-Wise (2014) argues that preparation for upper level nursing leadership positions needs to be at the graduate level for both the academic *and* practice settings. At present however, it appears that the academic credentials for leadership in academia are generally higher than in health care settings.

Leadership content in PhD programs traditionally focuses on leading scientific research, either as a group or solo endeavor. Additionally, there is emphasis placed on mentoring for both students and faculty. According to Morin (2004) the goal of an academic administrator is really to reward faculty and create balance in a school in terms of faculty talents and diversity of scholarship making sure both are consistent with the overarching mission of the setting. Obviously, past experience as a successful researcher is very important in this role for research-extensive universities.

Perhaps a well-founded argument can be made that a new path in graduate nursing education needs to be established, which specifically focuses on leadership development (Aduddell & Dorman, 2010; Morton, 2014; Waite, McKinney, Smith-Glasgow, & Meloy, 2014). Such a program could include all of the necessary basic preparation for future faculty (teaching, scholarship, and service), yet would also include the breadth and depth of content necessary to prepare future administrators for both the practice and academic settings.

Future academic administrators will need skills that are different in many ways from those of the past. Perhaps going forward, qualities such as innovation, risk taking, and entrepreneurialism (Greene & Ridenour, 2004; Morton, 2014) may take precedence over past achievements in research or clinical practice, for example. To create programs to foster these skills however, nurse leadership positions in the practice setting will likely need to increase their minimal academic credentials for eligibility. Additionally, requiring certification as a nurse executive at the advanced level might be required for these positions, consistent with education and certification requirement for advanced nursing practice. Elevating the credentials and educational preparation of nurse administrators, be they in the academic or practice setting, would reflect positively on the discipline and assist in moving nurse leadership, similar to APRN education, beyond the apprenticeship model.

■ PERSPECTIVES FROM DNP CHAIRS: THE LIVED EXPERIENCE OF DNP-PREPARED ACADEMIC ADMINISTRATORS

As advanced practice nurses with nearly 60 years of collective experience in clinical practice, teaching, management, and academic administration the authors of this chapter share their lived experiences related to their career trajectories that prepared them for their administrative roles in academia in both a medium-sized private Catholic university and large research-intensive public university. A model case study of a DNP-prepared colleague who is serving as an associate dean in a medium-sized private Jesuit university was eager to share her expertise and successes in service, teaching, and leadership roles. The authors hope to demonstrate that DNP-prepared academic leaders possess distinctive abilities and skills that make for well-rounded and consistent leaders.

SANDRA BELLINI

The University of Connecticut is a research-extensive institution with a strong focus on scholarship. Common in many similar institutions, faculty engagement and productivity surrounding research activities have historically been considered more "valued" than other forms of scholarship, practice included. Early faculty opinions on whether the school of nursing (SON) should open a doctoral program with a non-research focus ranged from strong enthusiasm to strong opposition, typical of many schools over the past decade. Yet, the decision was made in 2007 by faculty vote that the school would develop and open a DNP program the following year.

The curriculum for the DNP program was created by a committee and approved across levels as required by both the state and the university. Given the strong emphasis on scholarship within the school, approval from the graduate school was sought and obtained for the program: the DNP degree would be conferred by the graduate school on par with PhD graduates from the SON and many other doctoral degrees across disciplines. In retrospect, the importance of securing this distinction was prescient for the future respect of the program within the research-extensive environment.

To serve as program administrator, the faculty felt it important that the candidate should be DNP prepared, with a strong background in advanced practice, and ideally experienced in teaching at the university level. Similar to the early decision to seek graduate school approval for the program, this second decision that the faculty made, specifically the desired qualifications for program leadership, was and remains a significant departure from the norm. It is certainly true that the availability of DNP-prepared graduates with the potential to develop into strong academic administrators was rare in the early days of DNP graduates, hence the majority of early DNP program administrators were PhD prepared. However, in the years that have elapsed, only a small number of schools have chosen DNP-prepared graduates as program directors (AACN, 2016b). Certainly, there are deans, associate deans, chairs, and program directors with the DNP credential, but the numbers remain proportionally small.

This phenomenon gives one pause for consideration given that DNP-prepared graduates would be unlikely viewed as qualified academically or experientially to guide the curriculum for a PhD program (Minnick, Norman, Donaghey, Fisher, & McKirgan, 2010). Why then, is a PhD graduate considered academically and experientially qualified to lead a practice-focused degree program when they do not possess that kind of educational background themselves? To some, the fact that the majority of DNP programs continue to be guided by faculty without DNP credentials seems incongruous when the number of available DNP graduates has soared in recent years (AACN, 2016a).

Accomplishments

Since the opening of the DNP program in 2008, the SON has refined the philosophical underpinnings for the program within the context of a research-extensive environment. Graduates of the program have demonstrated strong scholarship outcomes, including posters, podium presentations, and published manuscripts. It remains a point of pride that the DNP and PhD degrees are both conferred from the graduate school, as opposed to the DNP being conferred from the SON and therefore perceived as not quite "on par" with the PhD graduates. It is the philosophy of the school that preparing DNP graduates to be productive practice scholars may better prepare them as future faculty; important given the anticipated need for increased nurse educators in the future (Smeltzer et al., 2015; Smith-Glasgow, 2012). Over time, there has been more faculty investment in developing DNP students as practice scholars consistent with Boyer's Model of Scholarship (Boyer, 1990), which guides the SON. Concurrent with the more inclusive definition of scholarship, faculty practice and practice scholarship, have become more prominent within the school through the establishment of joint appointments. Creating appointments of this type can be beneficial to both the academic and practice settings (Walsh et al., 2012), as well as to individual faculty, creating a "win-win-win" opportunity.

Challenges

Although there has been significant progress toward faculty acceptance for the DNP over time, some resistance remains, as is likely commonplace in other research-extensive schools that have recently opened practice-focused doctoral programs (Agger et al., 2014). With the evolution and acceptance of DNP education, philosophy, and the more inclusive view of scholarship to include practice however, there remains a "glass ceiling" within the school and university for DNP (and PhD)-prepared clinical faculty. As is similar in many research-extensive universities, the infrastructure and criteria for tenure is not an option for clinical faculty at this time. To be sure, tenure is being offered as an option at many comprehensive schools and universities, but not at research-extensive universities (Agger et al., 2014). For some, this is an ongoing frustration that begs the question: If Boyer's Model is the framework that guides the school, then why is only discovery scholarship recognized as appropriate for tenure criteria? This is especially puzzling because nursing is, at its core, a *practice discipline*. If the rationale for this is related to the ability of faculty to establish revenue streams to support their salaries, then it is difficult to understand given the fact that clinical faculty in joint appointments are contracted to bring in revenue to support their salaries as a matter of course. In time, it will be interesting to see whether research-extensive universities will expand their tenure criteria to recognize practice scholarship. Failure to do so may result in great difficulty in recruiting and retaining clinical faculty who would have eligibility for tenure in other universities (Nicholes & Dyer, 2012).

SUSAN DeNISCO

Sacred Heart University (SHU) in Fairfield, Connecticut, is a relatively young (52 years old) private comprehensive institution of higher education. Embracing the Catholic intellectual tradition, the university's primary objective is to prepare students to live in and make contributions to the human community. Given this philosophy, the focus for faculty engagement is on teaching, scholarship, and service. The university has embraced the Boyer's Model of Scholarship; however, the scholarship of discovery is still the preferred and the most understood method of scholarship among faculty especially those colleagues in the college of arts and sciences. In 2008, a proposal to put forth a DNP program was supported by the nursing faculty and executive administration as the second practice doctoral program in the university with the physical therapy program offering the doctor of physical therapy (DPT) degree first. The DNP program admitted its first cohort in 2010 and has graduated approximately 50 post-master's prepared candidates. SHU has now added a practice doctorate in business administration (DBA) and has plans to begin a practice doctorate in education (EdD) in the near future. Given institutional support for providing programs that will help prepare students for careers in health care, finance, and education there has been a cultural shift to support faculty teaching in these programs to engage in the scholarship of application and integration and be supported for both clinical and tenure positions. As a family nurse practitioner, I was in the unique position to be on a clinical track appointment where I was promoted from clinical assistant to clinical associate professor based on very specific criteria. Following completion of my DNP degree, I received the dean's full support to transfer me as an associate professor to the tenure track where I applied 1 year of service toward my tenure timeline. I was the first faculty member in the history of SHU to be granted tenure and received a promotion to full professor, which is not typical for research faculty, let alone a DNP-prepared faculty member. To date there are four tenured professors in the college of nursing (CON), two with DNP degrees and the other two EdD prepared. There are currently four faculty eligible for tenure in the next several years and one of those is a DNP-prepared nurse new to academia but with years of progressive leadership experience in hospital administration. Unlike data presented by Dreher et al. there is a blend of nursing faculty terminal degree preparation at SHU and newly hired PhD-prepared faculty rely on their seasoned DNP-prepared colleagues as mentors as they transition into their roles at SHU. Although faculty enjoy scholarly discourse and bring unique perspectives based on their own nursing backgrounds and doctoral course, work there is not the tension of being a "second-class citizen" if DNP prepared. In the College of Nursing at SHU, DNP faculty chair curriculum and academic standards committees, participate in global initiatives, and are encouraged to attend AACN faculty development conferences. DNP faculty are high contributors to the life of the university.

Accomplishments

Since 2007, I have held several different academic leadership positions at SHU, including graduate nursing program director, DNP program director, and interim director of the SON. I have had administrative responsibility for four master's tracks, the development of the online master's programs and the development, implementation, and evaluation of the DNP program. During my year as interim director of the SON I was challenged to lead an increasing complex school with more than 1,100 students, 40 full-time faculty and staff, and a curriculum with strict national accreditation standards and guidelines. All of these roles involved having a skill set that one can argue DNP graduates attain in their curriculum and course work. The ability to lead, collaborate, work in systems, use data, make policy changes, and influence health outcomes are all skills that I obtained in my DNP course work and is in direct accordance with the AACN DNP *Essentials*. The ability to conduct a needs assessment, develop, obtain and manage grants, use research, understand clinical systems, and have business acumen makes the

DNP faculty member poised to lead academic programs and units. The post-master's DNP graduates from SHU are quite accomplished having peer-reviewed publications and presentations applying and extending their research in real time. They have gained confidence and increased competence and many have been selected for new positions in nursing administration, academia, and clinical practice.

Challenges

The DNP expert clinician who is in a program director, chair, associate dean or dean role has unique challenges to overcome. Juggling teaching, administration, scholarship, and practice are not easy. Having an organizational structure that builds clinical practice into the faculty workload may be one solution to the retention of talented help and reduction of burnout. SHU CON currently does not have a model that supports faculty practice so that advanced practice faculty who are in administrative roles have to add clinical practice on top of an already heavy workload. The individual trying to maintain clinical proficiency and develop as an academic administrator can be put in a precarious position and can be forced to choose one over the other. Keeping abreast of AACN, NONPF, American Association of Nurse Executives (AONE) as well as other national organization's position statements, curriculum, and accreditation guidelines is essential in being able to lead academic units and nursing faculty. Developing strategic relationships, fund-raising, creating a vision for a contemporary nursing curriculum, and producing revenue for the university are within the purview of the academic administrator. However, when that academician is nationally certified in an area of clinical expertise it can become difficult to maintain rigorous continuing education, licensure, and board certification requirements and minimum clinical practice hours. Although the scholarship of teaching, practice, and integration is what the DNP-prepared nurse educator is poised to accomplish, they often find themselves having to mature into and sustain the same scholarship agenda as their research-prepared colleagues.

■ CASE STUDY: DNP Graduate as an Associate Dean of Nursing

Dr. Audrey Beauvais BSN, MSN, MBA, DNP joined Fairfield University as the associate dean for undergraduate programs in the SON in 2014. She has more than 25 years of experience in academic and hospital settings as well as in the insurance industry. She earned her DNP degree from Case Western Reserve University in 2009. Although her formal educational preparation in the DNP program was invaluable, she had many work–life experiences that prepared her for her current administrative role. As she states all of those experiences have been "transferable" to her new position. Immediately before taking her current associate dean position, Dr. Beauvais began her career in academia as an assistant professor of the undergraduate nursing program at SHU. While she was a teaching faculty member she pursued her DNP degree and took both nursing education and leadership electives that enhanced her teaching methods and further developed her leadership skills. Her transition into an academic leadership role was challenging yet energizing. Her first academic leadership position was the

(continued)

■ CASE STUDY: DNP Graduate as an Associate
Dean of Nursing *(continued)*

assignment to the coordinator of the Patient Care Services Administrative Track where she led curriculum revision and implementation of this program into an online learning format. She was later promoted to director of the Undergraduate Nursing Program. For the 11 years before her employment at SHU, Dr. Beauvais worked in various leadership positions at Stamford Hospital, including nurse manager of the pediatric and psychiatric units, case manager, and performance improvement coordinator. Dr. Beauvais was the Magnet® coordinator that successfully led Stamford Hospital to be recognized as a Magnet hospital. These experiences, her graduate degree in business, her currency with literature and surrounding herself with excellent mentors in and outside of nursing equipped her with the skills necessary to lead an academic program.

ACCOMPLISHMENTS

Dr. Beauvais has been able to share her expertise, passion, and commitment to nursing to inspire the new generation of health care providers and nurse leaders. Besides her wealth of expertise in nursing leadership, education, and curriculum design, Dr. Beauvais has numerous scholarly activities, which are a credit to her philosophy that disseminating information to others is the way to make changes. Dr. Beauvais has earned a range of formal certifications in the areas of psychiatric and mental health nursing, nurse case management, clinical nurse leader, emotional intelligence, and trauma nursing. At both Sacred Heart and Fairfield Universities she has been charged with leading new programs, such as the clinical nurse leader and DNP programs. Her familiarity with NCLEX (National Council Licensure Examination) has made her an effective leader in helping programs improve their curriculum and testing methods to improve pass rates.

As a self-reported lifelong learner, Dr. Beauvais successfully studied for and passed the national examination as a clinical nurse leader so that she could have the same skill set that she was expecting of her master's students; this is another sign of her solid commitment to the nursing profession and academic excellence.

Dr. Beauvais has over 15 peer-reviewed presentations and articles and several book chapters, which speak to her contributions to the nursing profession and health care field. She is a peer reviewer for several referred nursing journals and is a sought after consultant by health care organizations applying for Magnet recognitions because of her expertise in this area. Her DNP education and work experiences have enabled her to obtain several grants to support her research on emotional, develop innovative teaching pedagogy, and establish community-based geriatric wellness programs.

Dr. Beauvais reports she has had numerous mentors who have helped her on her journey. As transformational leaders they created an atmosphere that supported her development as a faculty member and both as a service and

(continued)

■ CASE STUDY: DNP Graduate as an Associate
  Dean of Nursing *(continued)*

academic leader. She is now able to do the same with nursing faculty, students, and other colleagues. She helps individuals identify their strengths and inspires them to reach new heights in their nursing careers. She is receptive to new and innovative ideas whether it be curriculum development, increased use of simulation, adding new technology, supporting student remediation, service-learning projects, study abroad programs and mission trips.

CHALLENGES

Of course, clinical practice, nursing education, and administration are filled with challenges but as Dr. Beauvais has discovered practicing critical self-reflection has assisted her in capitalizing on her strengths and develop areas of perceived weakness so she can effectively lead. Her knowledge and expertise in emotional intelligence, which is the ability to recognize one's own and other people's emotions makes her an effective leader and able to handle frustrations that occur. At times, she feels the change process can be slow and learning to find effective ways of communicating to keep all stakeholders informed is essential. She identifies the challenges as the following: resources, nursing curriculum, and faculty.

RESOURCES

As in other business models, academic institutions also have limited resources and leaders must develop innovative models to create new revenue sources. This can be supported by fostering linkages among the university, other educational institutions, and clinical practice settings. Student clinical placements are limited, which makes the process of finding adequate training sites an incredible task. The ability to attract and retain qualified nursing faculty with lower salary bases than the service industry also contributes to the faculty shortage.

NURSING CURRICULUM

Providing a nursing curriculum to prepare future nurses for the complexity of today's health care environment is of paramount importance. Nursing curriculum has to keep pace with practice innovation and integration of change and be as nimble as their practice partners in this area. Creating a curriculum to bridge the gap between clinical practice and education is needed to improve the quality and safety of care. Another challenge is to increase funding to prepare a culturally diverse workforce and prepare the next generation of nursing faculty.

(continued)

■ CASE STUDY: DNP Graduate as an Associate
Dean of Nursing *(continued)*

FACULTY

Recruiting qualified faculty who is comfortable working in the culture of an academic institution can be challenging. Setting up a peer-mentoring program can be a solution to developing faculty new to nursing education. Salaries for clinicians and nurse administrators are traditionally higher than nursing faculty so it can be hard to sell to make this career shift. Faculty who hold advanced practice licenses find it challenging to maintain clinical practice and teach full time; promoting innovative practice models may help with faculty retention as well as provide clinical opportunities for students. In addition, it can be difficult to harness the collective knowledge and the experience of faculty colleagues to both honor and preserve nursing's unique heritage while at the same time drive innovative flexible and affordable curriculums.

■ ADVANCED EDUCATION FOR DNP CHAIRS: MINDING THE GAP

In the absence of formal educational pathways at the graduate level to prepare future academic administrators, we must make do with what we have for the time being. Set against the backdrop of the DNP essentials (AACN, 2006) and the experiential backgrounds of DNP graduates, it may be that we are off to a good start. True, a DNP-prepared graduate is probably not the best qualified to mentor research-track faculty or doctoral students exclusively, however, perhaps a general background in broader principles, such as mentoring, may be more valuable and more broadly applicable in most instances. In schools of nursing that are not research extensive, a DNP-prepared chair or dean might be well qualified for success having had formal preparation in finance, organizational systems leadership, collaborative practice, evidence-based care, and health policy for populations (AACN, 2006). These broader skills, which have been identified as important for the future success of the health care system, may fare just as well, or even improve on the traditional system of hiring administrators with backgrounds in research and methodology. In research-extensive schools, there is often a separate dean or associate dean whose charge is to shepherd the research mission of the school. In these circumstances, perhaps a team of DNP- and PhD-prepared administrators could bring the kind of collaboration and synergy between the two terminal degrees in nursing as has been advocated in recent literature (AACN, 2004; Murphy, Warshawsky, & Mills, 2014).

Until such time that formal graduate education programs are created to prepare academic administrators, consideration may be given to the current range of options available for this purpose at the post-graduate level. A number of professional organizations and funding sources sponsor such programs including AACN (AACN Leadership for Academic Nursing Program; AACN, 2016c), NLN (National League for Nursing Leadership Programs, 2016; www.nln.org/professional-development-programs/leadership-programs), Sigma Theta Tau International Leadership Institute (2013; www.nursingsociety.org/leadershipinstitute/nursefaculty/Pages/default.aspx), and the

Robert Wood Johnson Foundation Executive Nurse Fellows Program (www.rwjfleaders .org/programs/robert-wood-johnson-foundation-executive-nurse-fellows-program), among others. Perhaps the most desirable set of qualifications for a future DNP-program academic administrator would be equal academic preparation in areas of: education, leadership and practice, and scholarship. In the meantime, further educational preparation and professional development for new academic administrators appear to be dependent on a mix of mentoring programs, specific coursework available that best augments an administrator's current repertoire, and on-the-job training.

■ SUMMARY

It is an exciting time in nursing education. In the past 5 years the DNP degree is proving to be the most sought after terminal degree in nursing, which will undoubtedly meet societal needs for preparing a highly educated workforce, including more nurse educators and academic administrators. Nursing is the original practice discipline and for the nurse who wants to maintain relevance in the clinical arena, attain leadership skills to drive change in our health care delivery system, and develop business savvy, there is no question that this degree has much to offer. Of course, it would be desirable for the DNP graduate to have additional course work in nursing education but in reality most nursing educators including our colleagues prepared as researchers have not had these courses and have "learned on the job." Moreover, master of science in nursing (MSN)-prepared nurse practitioners have been teaching didactic and clinical content for years without curriculum development courses and have prepared thousands of competent clinicians. One can argue that who is a better role model for the student—the research-oriented faculty member who does not practice or the expert clinician who maintains an active clinical practice? Universities, schools of nursing, and academic administrators must consider formal and transparent succession planning models to retain their most talented and skilled faculty and promote them to leadership positions. Both the "graying" of the workforce and skill mismatches continue to be of great concern for schools of nursing across the country. Over the next decade, nursing education faces severe talent deficits due to what will be the demographic tidal wave of nursing faculty and deans. The nurse with a terminal clinical doctoral degree who is clinically expert, has a keen grasp of systems, understands translational research and data mining, and is grounded in the "practice discipline of nursing" are the nurse educators of today and the future.

■ CRITICAL THINKING QUESTIONS

1. *What competencies listed in the* The Essentials of Doctoral Education for Advanced Nursing Practice *prepare the doctor of nursing graduate for a career in academia? Give specific examples.*
2. *As a staff development nurse or a clinical preceptor you are faced with educating nurses for a variety of clinical roles. How were you prepared for those roles as an MSN graduate? How do you think your course work will prepare you in the DNP program?*
3. *How can a nursing faculty member with a DNP degree influence curriculum development? Give examples.*
4. *When applying for a faculty position how will you answer the following question: "Give an example of how you would handle a nursing student who was not meeting his or her clinical objectives."*

5. *What clinical, leadership, and research skills are essential to lead an academic unit? Does the DNP curriculum prepare the graduate to chair committees, lead curricular changes, and move faculty toward a shared vision for the future?*
6. *What traits make a strong leader in nursing? How does the DNP faculty member develop leadership skills?*
7. *Identify a nursing faculty member who has been your mentor. What skills does this individual possess that has inspired your nursing career?*

■ REFERENCES

Aduddell, K. A., & Dorman, G. E. (2010). The development of the next generation of nurse leaders. *The Journal of Nursing Education, 49*(3), 168–171.

Agger, C. A., Oermann, M. H., & Lynn, M. R. (2014). Hiring and incorporating doctor of nursing practice-prepared nurse faculty into academic nursing programs. *The Journal of Nursing Education, 53*(8), 439–446.

American Association of Colleges of Nursing. (2004). *AACN position statement on the practice doctorate in nursing.* Washington, DC: Author.

American Association of Colleges of Nursing. (2006). *The essentials of doctoral education for advanced nursing practice.* Washington, DC: Author.

American Association of Colleges of Nursing. (2010). PhD position statement. Retrieved from http://www.aacn.nche.edu/education-resources/phdposition.pdf

American Association of Colleges of Nursing. (2014). *Special survey of vacant faculty positions for academic year 2014–2015.* Retrieved from http://www.aacn.nche.edu/leading-initiatives/research-data/vacancy14.pdf

American Association of Colleges of Nursing. (2016a). DNP fact sheet. Retrieved from http://www.aacn.nche.edu/media-relations/fact-sheets/dnp

American Association of Colleges of Nursing. (2016b). DNP program directory. Retrieved from http://www.aacn.nche.edu/dnp/program-directory

American Association of Colleges of Nursing. (2016c). Leadership for academic nursing program. Retrieved from http://www.aacn.nche.edu/lanp

Bellini, S., McCauley, P., & Cusson, R. M. (2012). The doctor of nursing practice graduate as faculty member. *The Nursing Clinics of North America, 47*(4), 547–556.

Boyer, E. L. (1990). *Scholarship reconsidered: Priorities of the professoriate.* Princeton, NJ: Carnegie Foundation for the Advancement of Teaching.

Danzey, I. M., Ea, E., Fitzpatrick, J. J., Garbutt, S. J., Rafferty, M., & Zychowicz, M. E. (2011). The doctor of nursing practice and nursing education: Highlights, potential, and promise. *Journal of Professional Nursing, 27*(5), 311–314.

DeNisco, S., & Barker, A. (2016). *Advanced practice nursing: Essential knowledge for the profession.* Burlington, MA: Jones & Bartlett.

Glasgow, M. E., Weinstock, B., Lachman, V., Suplee, P. D., & Dreher, H. M. (2009). The benefits of a leadership program and executive coaching for new nursing academic administrators: One college's experience. *Journal of Professional Nursing, 25*(4), 204–210.

Greene, A., & Ridenour, N. (2004). Shaping a career trajectory in academic administration: Leadership development for the deanship. *Journal of Nursing Education, 43*(11), 489–495.

Higher Ed Jobs. (2015). Nursing faculty and nursing dean search. Retrieved from https://www.higheredjobs.com/search/advanced_action.cfm?PosType=1&InstType=1&Keyword=nursing+faculty&Remote=1&Remote=2&Region=&Submit=Search+Jobs

Institute of Medicine. (2011). *The future of nursing: Leading change, advancing health.* Washington, DC: National Academies Press. Retrieved from https://www.nationalacademies.org/hmd/~/media/Files/Report%20Files/2010/The-Future-of-Nursing/Future%20of%20Nursing%202010%20Recommendations.pdf

Loomis, J. A., Willard, B., & Cohen, J. (2007). Difficult professional choices: Deciding between the PhD and the DNP in nursing. *The Online Journal of Issues in Nursing, 12*, 16.

Melynck, B. M. (2013). Distinguishing the roles and preparation between doctor of philosophy and doctor of nursing practice graduates: National implications for academic curricula and health care systems. *Journal of Nursing Education, 52*(8), 442–448.

Minnick, A. F., Norman, L. D., Donaghey, B., Fisher, L. W., & McKirgan, I. M. (2010). Leadership in doctoral nursing research programs. *The Journal of Nursing Education, 49*(9), 504–510.

Morin, K. H. (2004). A conversation with Rheba de Tornyay, EdD, RN, FAAN. *Journal of Nursing Education, 43*(11), 486–488.

Morton, P. G. (2014). Preparing the next generation of academic chief nurse administrators. *Journal of Professional Nursing, 30*(4), 279–280.

Murphy, L. S., Warshawsky, N. E., & Mills, M. E. (2014). An assessment of the alignment between graduate nursing leadership education and established standards. *The Journal of Nursing Administration, 44*(10), 502–506. doi:10.1097/NNA.0000000000000108

National League for Nursing. (2005). Core competencies of nurse educators with task statements. Retrieved from http://www.nln.org/professional-development-programs/competencies-for-nursing-education/nurse-educator-core-competency

National League for Nursing. (2013). Annual survey of schools of nursing, Fall 2012. Retrieved from http://www.nln.org/newsroom/nursing-education-statistics/annual-survey-of-schools-of-nursing-academic-year-2011-2012

National League for Nursing Leadership Programs. (2016). Retrieved from http://www.nln.org/professional-development-programs/leadership-programs

Nicholes, R. H., & Dyer, J. (2012). Is eligibility for tenure possible for the doctor of nursing practice-prepared faculty? *Journal of Professional Nursing, 28*(1), 13–17.

Robert Wood Johnson Foundation Executive Nurse Fellows Program. (2013). Retrieved from http://www.rwjfleaders.org/programs/robert-wood-johnson-foundation-executive-nurse-fellows-program

Sigma Theta Tau International Leadership Institute. (2013). Retrieved from http://www.nursingsociety.org/learn-grow/leadership-new/international-leadership-institute

Smeltzer, S. C., Sharts-Hopko, N. C., Cantrell, M. A., Heverly, M. A., Nthenge, S., & Jenkinson, A. (2015). A profile of U.S. nursing faculty in research- and practice-focused doctoral education. *Journal of Nursing Scholarship, 47*(2), 178–185.

Smith-Glasgow, M. E. (2012). New developments in nursing education: A focus on contemporary content, pedagogies, deans, and trends. *Nursing Clinics of North America, 47*(4), xiii–xv. Retrieved from http://www.sciencedirect.com.ezproxy.lib.uconn.edu/science/article/pii/S0029646512000746

Udlis, K. A., & Mancuso, J. M. (2012). Doctor of nursing practice programs across the United States: A benchmark of information: Part I: Program characteristics. *Journal of Professional Nursing, 28*(5), 265–273.

University of Connecticut Certificate in Health Professions Education. (2016). Retrieved from http://health-professions-education-certificate.uconn.edu

U.S. Department of Health and Human Services; Health Resources and Services Administration; Bureau of Health Workforce; National Center for Health Workforce Analysis. (2014). The future of nursing workforce: National and state level projections 2012–2005. Retrieved from http://bhpr.hrsa.gov/healthworkforce/supplydemand/nursing/workforceprojections/nursingprojections.pdf

Waite, R., McKinney, N., Smith-Glasgow, M. E., & Meloy, F. A. (2014). The embodiment of authentic leadership. *Journal of Professional Nursing, 30*(4), 282–291.

Walsh, K., Kitson, A., Cross, W., Thoms, D., Thornton, A., Moss, C., . . . Graham, I. (2012). A conversation about practice development and knowledge translation as mechanisms to align the academic and clinical contexts for the advancement of nursing practice. *Collegian, 19*(2), 67–75.

Wolverton, M., Gmelch, W., Montez, J., & Nies, C. (2001). *The changing nature of the academic deanship.* San Francisco, CA: Jossey-Bass.

Yoder-Wise, P. S. (2014). The future of leadership. *The Journal of Nursing Administration, 44*(6), 318–320.

Reflective Response 1

Anne Marie Hranchook

Nurses who have earned a Doctor of Nursing Practice (DNP) degree are not only expert clinicians capable of assuming faculty roles, but are also uniquely prepared to fulfill administrative positions and lead academic programs in their respective schools and universities. The American Association of Colleges of Nursing (AACN) *Essentials of Doctoral Education for Advanced Nursing Practice* (AACN, 2006a), particularly *Essential II (Organizational and Systems Leadership for Quality Improvement and Systems Thinking)* is especially pertinent for the leader in an academic setting. This Essential assures that the DNP graduate has requisite knowledge in essential skills, such as advanced communication, leading quality improvement initiatives, business, finance, economic, and health policy principles. In addition, the DNP curriculum prepares graduates with administrative and leadership skills that are critical, such as understanding organizational culture, analysis of initiatives, and budgetary development.

The AACN takes the position in addition to leadership roles in a variety of settings, DNP graduates are eligible to teach at the collegiate level because they have a terminal degree in the discipline of nursing (AACN, 2015). Despite the AACN's endorsement, faculty possessing a practice degree may be surprised to find that there are barriers to advancing a career in academia (Roberts & Glod, 2013). Frequently, DNP-prepared faculty are advanced practice nurses who have been appointed to clinical track positions and they may not have the option to be tenured or in a tenure-track position. It is not uncommon that requirements for advancement into a chair or dean position in many colleges and universities includes a PhD and earned rank of professor. Faculty with a DNP degree may not be eligible for promotion and tenure and thus are never able to achieve the rank of professor. The primary focus of clinical track faculty is teaching, which includes clinical instruction, lecture, clinical practice, and participation in instructional committees. Although expert faculty clinicians are essential for guiding the clinical learning of undergraduate and graduate students, clinical expertise often remains unrewarded in the traditional academic evaluation required for promotion and advancement in academia (Paskiewicz, 2003).

To understand this better, one needs to know that academic progression builds on the basic tenets of what is commonly referred to as the standard triad: excellence in teaching, service, and scholarship. Whether primarily committed to program administration, research, or practice, teaching is a core responsibility for all faculty. Service is frequently classified in three areas: service to the university, to the profession, and to clinical practice (Finke, 2012). Within the triad, scholarship is frequently valued more highly than teaching or service. The classical interpretation of scholarship is the generation of new knowledge. When defined this way, it is frequently seen as the domain of PhD-prepared faculty. The priority an institution places on scholarship in its tenure and promotion decisions relies heavily on its Carnegie classification, the emphasis placed on research grants funded by the National Institutes of Health (NIH), as well as the institution's culture, values, and beliefs (Clark, Houten, & Percea-Ryan, 2010; Roberts & Glod, 2013). Traditional models of defining scholarship can pose barriers for DNP-prepared faculty in qualifying for tenure and promotion in some institutions.

Recognizing that the traditional boundaries of scholarship have not always fit the scholarly work of the discipline of nursing, the AACN (1999) developed a position statement defining scholarship based on the work of Boyer (1990). The AACN's model is an adaption of four areas proposed by Boyer (1990) and encompasses the scholarship of teaching, practice/application, integration, and discovery. This model supports the values of a discipline that brings together both scientific inquiry and application through professional practice and service (AACN, 1999). DNP-prepared faculty are clearly engaged in advancing the scholarship of nursing using this expanded definition.

In the document *DNP Roadmap Task Force Report*, the AACN (2006b) recommends that institutions offering a DNP should review their policies for promotion and tenure and, if the institution tenures faculty with other practice professional degrees (such as education, medicine, pharmacy, law, and audiology), then faculty with a DNP-practice doctorate should also be eligible for tenure. The AACN notes that in such cases, the standard for tenure should include a broad definition of scholarship consistent with Boyer's model (1990).

Although DNP-prepared faculty may face potential barriers to academic progression and appointment, the national nursing faculty shortage serves as a robust catalyst for change (Li, Stauffer, & Fang, 2016; Roberts & Glod, 2013). A special survey on vacant faculty positions completed by the AACN for academic year 2015 to 2016 revealed that there is a vacancy rate of 7.1% across the nation for full-time faculty positions (Li et al., 2016). Factors contributing to turnover include higher compensation in clinical and private sector settings, long hours, the desire to remain clinically active, and the perceived constraints of academia (Fitzpatrick, 2008; Lupien & Rosenkoetter, 2006; Potempa, Redman, & Landstrom, 2009). Although faculty roles can be highly complex, most regard the opportunity to lead in colleges and schools of nursing as extremely rewarding. Some of the most influential factors nursing faculty cite for accepting academic positions are academic freedom and the ability to use one's knowledge to teach and have an impact on the profession (Lupien & Rosenkoetter, 2006).

An increasing number of college and university nursing programs acknowledge that recruiting DNP-prepared faculty is not only an answer to the shortage of qualified doctoral faculty but also a much needed solution to meeting the educational needs of the next generation of nurses (Roberts & Glod, 2013). There are many factors that have profoundly influenced how schools of nursing conceptualize their curriculum. These factors include the growing complexity of our nation's health care system, the rampant growth in scientific knowledge and the increasing sophistication of technology. Benner, Sutphen, and Leonard (2010), the authors of a book titled *Educating Nurses: A Call for Radical Transformation*, strongly advocate for innovative teaching and learning approaches that bring nursing education and practice together. A viable solution to bridging the gap between education and practice is for schools of nursing to recruit DNP-prepared faculty. After all, nursing is a practice discipline and the purpose of the clinical doctorate is to provide affirmation for the highest level of preparation for advanced clinical practice.

The experience of certified registered nurse anesthetists (CRNAs) is not unlike that of other advanced practice nursing faculty. In 2007, the American Association of Nurse Anesthetists in collaboration with the Council on Accreditation of Nurse Anesthesia Educational Programs (COA) mandated that all nurse anesthesia educational programs transition to a doctoral framework. As part of this larger mandate, the COA also took the position that doctoral degrees are required for CRNA program administrators (program administrator and assistant program administrator) in all doctoral programs (COA, 2014). Although the COA did not mandate the type of doctorate, many program administrators have gone on to complete a practice doctorate to meet this requirement. Although I am personally in a tenure-track position and have earned a DNP as my highest degree, I am aware that the ability to be in a tenure-track position or attain tenure is not an option for many nurse anesthesia program directors across the country. I believe it is possible for DNP-prepared faculty to be successful as academic chairs, associate deans, and deans if given the opportunity and providing that the requirements for scholarship needed to advance a career in academia are reimagined.

■ REFERENCES

American Association of Colleges of Nursing. (1999). Defining scholarship for the discipline of nursing. Retrieved from http://www.aacn.nche.edu/publications/position/defining-scholarship

American Association of Colleges of Nursing. (2006a). *The essentials of doctoral education for advanced nursing practice*. Retrieved from http://www.aacn.nche.edu/dnp/Essentials.pdf

American Association of Colleges of Nursing. (2006b). *DNP roadmap task force report*. Retrieved from http://www.aacn.nche.edu/dnp/roadmapreport.pdf

American Association of Colleges of Nursing. (2015). The doctor of nursing practice: Current issues and clarifying recommendations. Retrieved from http://www.aacn.nche.edu/aacn-publications/white-papers/DNP-Implementation-TF-Report-8-15.pdf

American Association of Nurse Anesthetists. (2007). AANA position on doctoral preparation of nurse anesthetists. Retrieved from https://www.aana.com/ceandeducation/educationalresources/Documents/AANA_Position_DTF_June_2007.pdf

Benner, P., Sutphen, M., Leonard, V., & Day, L. (2010). *Educating nurses: A call for radical transformation*. San Francisco, CA: Jossey-Bass.

Boyer, E. (1990). *Scholarship reconsidered: Priorities for the professoriate*. Princeton, NJ: The Carnegie Foundation for the Advancement of Teaching.

Clark, N. J., Houten, L. A., & Percea-Ryan, M. (2010). Transitioning from clinical practice to academia. *Nurse Educator, 35*(3), 105–109.

Council on Accreditation of Nurse Anesthesia Educational Programs. (2014). Standards for accreditation of nurse anesthesia educational programs. Retrieved from http://home.coa.us.com/accreditation/Documents/Standards%20for%20Accreditation%20of%20Nurse%20Anesthesia%20Education%20Programs_January%202014.pdf

Finke, L. M. (2012). *Teaching in nursing: The faculty role*. In D. M. Billings & J. A. Halstead (Eds.), *Teaching for nursing: A guide for faculty* (pp. 1–14). St. Louis, MO: Elsevier.

Fitzpatrick, J. (2008). The #1 cause of the faculty shortage? It's the money! *Nursing Education Perspectives, 29*, 253.

Li, Y., Stauffer, D., & Fang, D. (2016). Special survey on vacant faculty positions for academic year 2015–2016. Washington, DC: American Association of Colleges of Nursing. Retrieved from http://www.aacn.nche.edu/leading-initiatives/research-data/vacancy15.pdf

Lupien, A. E., & Rosenkoetter, M. M. (2006). Nurse anesthetists as university faculty. *AANA Journal, 74*(5), 366–372.

Paskiewicz, L. S. (2003). Clinical practice: An emphasis strategy for promotion and tenure. *Nursing Forum, 38*(4), 21–26.

Potempa, K. M., Redman, R. W., & Landstrom, G. (2009). Human resources in nursing education: A worldwide crisis. *Collegian, 16*, 19–22.

Roberts, S. J., & Glod, C. (2013). Faculty roles: Dilemmas for the future of nursing education. *Nursing Forum, 48*(2), 99–105.

Reflective Response 2

Lisa A. Johnson

When asked to reflect on the preceding chapter, I was immediately impressed with the breadth and profundity of Drs. DeNisco and Bellini's effort and equally challenged by what was being requested of me. Why should this be such an arduous undertaking when I myself have completed a doctoral degree and chair students through the doctoral process? Perhaps my mêlée should be precisely what I write about and to do so I will lend the reader insight into my worldview as it pertains to doctoral nursing practice.

My career has gone from the traditional bachelor of science in nursing (BSN) student to the ranks of the tertiary care hospitals of various intensive and specialty care units, onward through my master of science in nursing (MSN) as an acute care nurse practitioner (NP). With a few years of NP practice under my belt, I made the decision to progress through a doctoral program. In 2007, I entered into a DrNP program with the intention of moving into the faculty role by the time I reached my mid-30s. During my doctoral work, I had education, research, and leadership courses; passed my comprehensive examinations; gave a proposal defense, completed a dissertation; and felt prepared to use the hybrid research degree in my academic endeavors. My DrNP, with an education track focus, provided me the knowledge to evolve as an educator of MSN Adult-Gerontology Acute Care Nurse Practitioner (A-GACNP) and DNP students.

With all the success and opportunities that have come my way since 2007, there has also been equal frustration and disappointment with the nursing profession. From the belief that a DrNP could not be considered for many tenured positions or research intensive opportunities, to the realization that, to some, my degree was viewed exactly as a DNP (yet it was not) was frustrating and likely equal to the thwarting of several DNP's I have interacted with. In addition to being the director of two acute care NP programs at very distinct universities, I still maintain a clinical practice in a local hospital system. Sadly, many practicing NP faculty would state the relevant clinical expertise that I bring to my students is not viewed as being as significant as the non-practicing registered nurse (RN) or NP who brings in research grants to their respective universities.

Not understanding me or my degrees, whether they be doctoral or master's level degrees, is not the issue. The issue is the profession itself, the profession I have embraced for the past 20 years, not taking pause to understand each other and what is best for our students. For me, the DNP was optimal. It may have fallen out of vogue, we have seen this with the nursing profession over the course of time, but I cannot help but think it might need to be reassessed from a curriculum standpoint. Simply stated, the authors who so eloquently wrote of the need for educational electives in DNP programs would have found the DNP had just that and were taught by doctorate in education (EdD)-prepared faculty. Formal preparation in curriculum development, educational theory, testing evaluation, and educational practicums were all part of the DNP educational track preparation. Yet, the research courses were taught by the PhD research-intense faculty, lending me their expertise in the gamut of qualitative of quantitative approaches.

I have often felt in the nursing profession that we complicate matters that really are quite simple at the core of their being. Who should teach in a DNP program is one such example. As a doctorally prepared NP that does not quite fit the mold of the PhD or DNP, I find myself almost an outsider looking in despite being in the blend of it all. Perhaps, what we need to concentrate on is not the degree one was conferred but rather the expertise of the faculty member on the particular subject matter being asked to teach. I agree with Dr. Bellini's question: "Why then, is a PhD graduate considered academically and experientially qualified to lead a practice-focused degree program when they do not possess that kind of educational background themselves?"

The majority of DNP programs continue to be guided by faculty without DNP credentials as we see a surge in the number of DNP offerings throughout the United States. What appears to be archaic in many schools is the infrastructure of the university rank and tenure constraints. There are also many institutions that are heavily survived by PhD-prepared faculty. Quite frankly, this seems to have become a "turf war" in a time when we have the largest numbers of doctorally prepared nurses entering the workforce and a nation in crisis over health care options. The majority of advanced practice nurse would say this is our time to make gains in the health care arena. Sadly, for those of us in academe we are also endeavoring to forge ahead in our own academic institutions, immobilized often by our own colleagues.

It was disheartening to learn that the university that granted me a DNP did not value me to be more than the equivalent of a middle manager. I was deemed qualified to educate MSN students, direct an NP program, maintain a clinical practice, but discouraged from any clinically based research and flatly informed that DNPs were not tenure worthy at my alma mater. To suggest that a non-PhD-prepared nurse is not a candidate for tenure, or for that matter to be considered into promotion for leadership and administrative roles at the same pace as a PhD, is troubling. For if that logic holds true then countless EdD-prepared colleagues should be some of the first to hold tenured positions as frequently they are the most prepared to perform the academic calling of professor.

As faculty and advanced practice nurses, we must be clear about what is and what is not a DNP. We have several organizations, such as the National Organization of Nurse Practitioner Faculties (NONPF), who have helped define the DNP yet, we still struggle when implementing DNP curriculum and pedagogy. NONPF has been a key driver in the practice doctorate movement since its inception (American Association of Colleges of Nursing, 2015; NONPF, 2002a; NONPF, 2002b; NONPF, 2005; NONPF, 2014; O'Sullivan, & Carter, Marion, Pohl, & Werner, 2005) and is currently working diligently to transition to a seamless, integrated curriculum for BSN-DNP programs throughout the country. We tussle with what DNP scholarly work should consist of, what committee member involvement entails, and what course content should be in the DNP curriculum, especially as we transition to the BSN-to-DNP structure. A DNP is not a PhD: It embraces its own tenets matching the advanced practice nurses' (APNs') necessities. A DNP-prepared nurse serves an important role in an ever-changing health care environment. Who better to appreciate the significance of the degree than the faculty who still practice as APNs? As described by the AACN's Task Force on the Implementation of the DNP "the Doctor of Nursing Practice (DNP) is widely recognized as one of the discipline's two terminal degrees and the preferred pathway for those seeking preparation at the highest level of nursing practice" (2015). The AACN's white paper also asks us to remember that the DNP is an academic degree, not a role, and that graduates of both research- and practice-focused doctoral programs are prepared to generate new knowledge (2015).

So while we preserve our ideals we have a calling in this country to be clinicians, scholars, and researchers; either we can embrace the uniqueness of our doctoral degrees, clinical backgrounds, and research interests or we can squabble like children on a playground. I would caution that while we deliberate, the sick are getting sicker, the learners are growing weary, and the realities remain the same. This is a period in history where we can be viewed as a unified nursing profession or a fragmented, highly educated assemblage who hold their particular ideals ahead of the greater good of the nursing profession.

■ REFERENCES

American Association of Colleges of Nursing Task Force on the Implementation of the DNP. (2015, August). The doctor of nursing practice: Current issues and clarifying recommendations. Retrieved from http://www.aacn.nche.edu/news/articles/2015/dnp-white-paper

National Organization of Nurse Practitioner Faculties. (2002a). Clinical doctorate initiative. Retrieved from http://www.nonpf.org/?page=83

National Organization of Nurse Practitioner Faculties. (2002b). Statement from the NONPF board of directors. Retrieved from http://www.nonpf.org/?page=83

National Organization of Nurse Practitioner Faculties. (2005). NONPF recommendations for the nursing practice doctorate and nurse practitioner preparation. Retrieved from http://c.ymcdn.com/sites/www.nonpf.org/resource/resmgr/imported/recommendationsstatement1105.pdf

National Organization of Nurse Practitioner Faculties. (2014). Nurse practitioner core competencies content. Retrieved from http://c.ymcdn.com/sites/nonpf.site-ym.com/resource/resmgr/Competencies/NPCoreCompsContentFinalNov20.pdf

O'Sullivan, A., Carter, M., Marion, L., Pohl, J., & Werner, K. (2005). Moving forward together: The practice doctorate in nursing. *The Online Journal of Issues in Nursing, 10*(3), Manuscript 4. Retrieved from http://www.nursingworld.org/MainMenuCategories/ANAMarketplace/ANAPeriodicals/OJIN/TableofContents/Volume102005/No3Sept05/tpc28_416028.html

A Critique of the 2006 Essentials of Doctoral Education for Advanced Nursing Practice: *Do They Guide Practice?*

David G. Campbell-O'Dell and H. Michael Dreher

It has been 10 years since the American Association of Colleges of Nursing (AACN) published *The Essentials of Doctoral Education for Advanced Nursing Practice*. In addition, while their call (it was never a mandate) to have advanced practice nurses begin to be prepared with the doctorate instead of the master's by 2015, nothing regulatory happened when 2015 came and passed. Nonetheless, the surge in nurses who have obtained and who seek the Doctor of Nursing Practice (DNP) degree is impressive. This chapter explores those 2006 essentials from two perspectives: a DNP-prepared, practicing clinician and an academic nursing dean who has helped launch two Doctor of Nursing Practice programs. These two authors offer their perspectives to the discussion of the relevancy of the essentials document to contemporary practice.

■ AN ADVANCED PRACTICE/CLINICIAN PERSPECTIVE

The eight *Essentials of Doctoral Education for Advanced Nursing Practice* published in 2006 by the AACN provide a foundation for curriculum development in order to advance education for this professional group of nursing students. These eight essentials are referenced and integrated into the course development of DNP programs. There is some controversy as to the level of consistency of how each program addresses each Essential, but that is a matter for those in academia to address. The intent of this discussion is to explore the idea of how these essentials may affect practice. The foundation question is: Is DNP-prepared practice based on the eight essentials?

As we evolve into this discussion, let us agree that this is not an attack on the 2006 *Essentials of Doctoral Education*. These essentials, discussed in great detail in other chapters, are not being questioned on their value when designing and delivering curriculum for the practice doctorate degree in nursing. These doctoral education essentials viewed in the context of all nursing education expectations provide continuity to the real foundations of how our discipline is educated. These essentials influence how our profession matures. However, is practice based on the essentials, and more specifically, is practice guided by the essentials? This approach opens several possibilities of exploration that includes a question of how competencies are determined in the academic setting that will confirm and propel the doctorally prepared nurse into practice. A broader question of the benefit and detractors of a structure that may (or may not) influence practice is worth exploring. Is the bureaucracy of academia complementing the bureaucracy of practice?

■ WHY EXPLORE PRACTICE AFTER GRADUATION?

An approach to consider before venturing forward is to ask why we consider this exploration in the first place. After graduation, is the doctorally prepared professional nurse beholden to the educational model comprised of these eight essentials to help structure processes that improve health care outcomes? This point can be debated in all disciplines and the value of considering this for the nursing profession cannot be discounted. Questions to be asked of all practice professionals that may address the value of our respective educational preparation is to challenge the application of our education as a mechanism of directing our actions. Does our cumulative education dictate what we do and why we do it? This is not an easy question to address.

Anecdotally, does the reader believe that those who practice as doctorates of pharmacology reflect back on the *structure* of their educational preparation when practicing their profession? Similarly, does a physician rely on the curricular structure in order to practice medicine, or does he or she rely on thinking processes gained as a result of the education when providing services? Similarly, we must reflect in our own discipline with the question of how curriculum delivery impacts practice. Do the eight essentials of doctoral education direct practice, or does the structure of the overall curriculum based on these essentials allow for independent and responsible thinking as a result of the overall education? The question of how the eight essentials address practice could be convoluted. Yet when brought down to the basic question of how is practice supported, the value of the eight essentials as an educational or curricular construct does not dictate the decisions made by the doctorally prepared nurse demonstrating the highest level of practice.

The following content explores practice and how it is manifested in comparison to the eight essentials of doctoral education. The conjecture is that these essentials do not guide practice, nor do they dictate thinking processes. Instead, they are conceptual structures that build the overall delivery of content for the purposes of building consistency in curriculum.

■ IS PRACTICE BASED ON THE *ESSENTIALS*?

Doctoral students' final work products may reflect how the essentials are incorporated into a cumulative project. However, not all final work products (capstones, scholarly projects, etc.), include all of the eight essentials of doctoral education. This may be acceptable to some DNP program leaders. From the perspective of the graduate in practice, the lack of inclusion of all essentials may not impact practice. Colleges and universities guide the inclusion of the essentials in an effort to assure that all elements of the educational process are achieved. This is not a bad expectation by the educators that are tasked to demonstrate a culmination of an academic process. Many DNP projects reflect great work that can be expanded in practice after graduation. However, for many, the final project is an artificial expectation driven by academia in anticipation that it will influence practice. Is this a successful approach? Most will agree that it is; not all projects on the doctoral level reflect practice as much as they reflect satisfaction of academic expectations. The work product completed in a DNP program reflects an understanding of the content of the program. As a result, the student hopefully gains a broader understanding of concepts and elements that can favorably affect practice outcomes, but this process does not necessarily reflect an improvement in practice. The onus of responsibility to improve outcomes is on the student as they synthesize knowledge gained and experiences demonstrated while a student.

Does doctorally prepared advanced practice nursing after graduation rely on the AACN's *Essentials* to guide practice? This question requires us to highlight the complexities of practice in an ever-changing delivery system in the context of an evolving society. When in practice, do DNP-prepared graduates reflect on the essentials after graduation in order to approach the challenges of patient services? This author believes that doctorally prepared nurses in practice are prepared to address the complexities of health care delivery systems and structures that impact patient outcomes. However, when working through identified challenges the doctorally prepared graduate is making decisions in the context of the environment to include the culture, economics, and personality dynamics of the system. Is the graduate thinking to himself or herself, "I am making a choice as I consider my clinical scholarship" or asking "How can I assure that this decision is addressing population health?" or even more specifically, "Is this decision before me reflective of advanced practice?" These and other essentials of doctoral education have been integrated into the thinking processes of the graduate. These essentials have built a foundation for thought, but are these essentials that spur exploration the basis for current practice? This may seem to be a fine line of distinction yet as an advanced practice nurse, I suggest that more often than not, practice decisions are made based on guidelines, system limitations, and human dynamics that mandate a response, and that the subtleties of the culture and context of the systems being negotiated. Did *The Essentials* help to prepare me for these issues? I believe so. Are *The Essentials* in my armamentarium to address needed decisions? I do not believe this to be true as practice is an ever-changing process. With a salute to *The Essentials*, a well-prepared doctorally educated nursing professional supports practice in order to improve outcomes, but these same essentials are not the basis for practice. Issues and dynamics outside the educational process influence practice. Do we owe a debt of gratitude to *The Essentials* to help us in this thinking process? I believe that we do, but in the same display of gratitude let us acknowledge that practice is not dependent on *The Essentials*.

■ DO *THE ESSENTIALS OF DOCTORAL EDUCATION* TRULY GUIDE PRACTICE?

As discussed earlier, this author believes that practice is guided by multiple dynamics that must be addressed and maneuvered by the doctorally prepared graduate. Can we state with confidence that this same educational preparation including the eight essentials truly guides practice? In order to explore this concept, a look at competencies is needed. A better question to consider is, are the eight essentials competencies of doctorally prepared practice? There are pros and cons to this argument, as the determination of competencies is an evolving process. Doctorally prepared practice can be grouped in one or more of the following categories: administration, practice, informatics, and policy. Absent from these categories of DNP practice is research and education. It is curious to think that a nursing scholar with master's preparation in research and education are not easily funneled into definitions of DNP-prepared practice. On the flip side of the concept that research and education are practice, consider that these actions do not directly impact patient outcomes, which is the mission of the DNP-prepared graduate. Are these roles nursing practice or the practice of academia? That is a topic for exploration outside of the discussions in this chapter. We keep our focus on examples of widely accepted DNP practice areas by exploring administration and clinical practice.

One example of DNP-prepared practice is nursing administration. Consider the competencies of the nurse executive as articulated by the American Organization of Nurse Executives (AONE, 2015). The main headings include: (a) communication and relationship building; (b) knowledge of the health care environment; (c) leadership; (d) professionalism; and (e) business skills. Each of these categories are expanded to include elements that address these headings. All activities address components that can be seen as competencies of practice. Though there are similarities and some could argue overlap with the eight essentials of doctoral education, can we state that the essentials on their own reflect competencies? These AONE criteria articulate expectations of practice in the context of the environment where practice takes place, not in an academic setting. Are these criterion competencies of practice? Most will agree that they are. If they do reflect practice, can we identify the essentials as reflection of competencies also?

Another example to consider is the competencies articulated by the National Organization of Nurse Practitioner Faculties (NONPF, 2012). The nurse practitioner (NP) core competencies are grouped into competency areas that include: scientific foundation, leadership, quality, practice inquiry, technology and information literacy, policy, health delivery system, ethics, and independent practice. Each of these areas expand to include NP core competencies and curriculum content to support competencies. How to actually measure these competencies to assure safe practice on graduation is a challenge that is being addressed by NONPF. One important caveat is the fact that no state is mandating the doctorate degree to perform as an advanced practice nurse. The master of science in nursing (MSN) degree is the required degree for all states to practice as an advanced practice registered nurse (APRN). The DNP degree has not yet become the minimum degree for APRN practice. Efforts are being made by the AACN to enhance the caliber of advanced practice education. In 2013, an APRN Clinical Training Task Force was formed. Consultation with multiple disciplines was incorporated into processes that included webinars and feedback sessions. Key stakeholders were invited to help gain consensus. Recommendations that were made as a result of this task force include the following:

1. Enhance APRN clinical education through simulation
2. APRN programs should adapt AACN-AONE principles for academic-practice partnerships
3. APRN clinical education and assessment should be competency based
4. Support the development of innovative APRN clinical education models

This task force and the recommendations that came from it are welcomed to help build and further develop the capabilities of advanced practice nursing. Though the eight essentials of doctoral education support these motives and to a large degree provide a foundation for these recommendations, they are not driving practice as is suggested by the evaluation of competencies. These essentials do not drive practice yet, as has been suggested earlier, but provide a foundation for thought that can lead to improved practice. As participants in the practice of nursing, we work to support education and practice in order to improve outcomes. As a discipline, we appreciate the distinction between the foundational support of the eight essentials and the elements that drive practice. It is necessary that we aim our focus on improving outcomes. As a discipline, the eight essentials of doctoral education are a good start in building a stronger nurse to contribute and enhance outcomes, but these same essentials are not competencies as written and adapted by the practice professional in nursing. Similarly, practice is not based on the implementation of the essentials. I suspect that some who read this last statement can offer an opposing argument against it. To further expand, please consider the following data.

■ ARE DNP-PREPARED PROFESSIONALS DEMONSTRATING IMPROVED OUTCOMES AS A RESULT OF THE EIGHT ESSENTIALS?

One organization that collects and disseminates data reflecting the perceived outcomes of DNP-prepared nurses is Doctors of Nursing Practice, Inc. (DNP, Inc., 2015). The mission of DNP Inc. is to improve health care outcomes by promoting and enhancing the doctorally prepared nursing professional. The organization is dedicated to (a) providing accurate and timely information; (b) supporting, developing, and disseminating professional practice innovation; (c) collaborating in a professional manner that demonstrates universal respect for others, honesty and integrity in communications and; (d) responding with open discussions and dialogues that promote the evolution of advanced nursing practice and the growth of the DNP degree. In an effort to address this mission and vision, several National DNP Outcome Surveys have been completed. Following are excerpts of results from the 2015 survey designed to determine characteristics of practice type, location, and satisfaction with practice of DNP-prepared graduates. The author is the president of this organization and has worked collaboratively with members of the organization to collect this information. The data in the following tables are approved for publication by DNP, Inc. (2015).

The information provided in Table 24.1 reflects the diversity of the respondent and the variety of tracks completed by these graduates. It is important to note that approximately 75% of the respondents identified themselves as working in academia. The survey did not determine the extent of this work compared with the percentage of colleagues in the clinical practice setting.

TABLE 24.1 **Characteristics of DNP Outcomes Survey Respondents (N = 697)**

Gender	88% Female (N = 603)
	10% Male (N = 68)
	2% Preferred not to respond (N = 12)
Degree program	94% MSN–DNP (N = 639)
	6% BSN–DNP (N = 44)
DNP educational track	70% APRN track (N = 478)
	17% Health systems leadership/admin (N = 120)
	11% Education in academia (N = 74)
	3% Public health (N = 19)
	2% Education in a health care system (N = 14)
	2% Informatics (N = 14)
	2% Health policy (N = 14)
	7% Other not identified (N = 45)

APRN, advanced practice registered nurse; BSN, bachelor of science in nursing; DNP, Doctor of Nursing Practice; MSN, master of science in nursing.

Table 24.2, describing the incorporation of the DNP essentials, may appear to be a compelling argument that the eight essentials can be considered as the basis for practice or perhaps that these directives guide practice. Though the majority of respondents acknowledge that each of these essentials are integrated or used in practice, the questions misses the mark in soliciting *how* these essentials are addressing practice. The responses here support the notion that practice is supported by the knowledge gleaned from an education based on the eight essentials, but again it fails to identify what aspects of practice are addressed through these academic guidelines. This information points to the perceptions of value of the eight essentials, yet does not capture how these essentials were applied to any given practice situation.

The national survey completed by the DNP Inc. organization in 2015 included questions designed to solicit information about activities of the DNP-prepared graduate after graduation. Fourteen questions were asked to reflect the level of participation or activities in work that is described in the eight essentials. Findings show that 11 of the 14 questions demonstrated that more than one fourth of respondents report no change in their professional activities after earning the DNP degree. Table 24.3 lists the questions and responses for each of these 14 questions. This is valuable information to both reflect the type of practice that may be seen in the DNP-prepared graduate, and also how the essentials may or may not have supported roles after graduation.

For example, 52.6% of respondents had either no change or a slight change in practice regarding their involvement in health policy as it related to their practice.

TABLE 24.2 **Incorporation of the DNP *Essentials* (*N* = 697)**

Question asked: Please indicate your level of agreement to the following statements.

	Disagree Strongly Disagree	Agree and Strongly Agree
I integrate scientific underpinnings into my practice. (Essential I)	2.3% (*N* = 16)	97.7% (*N* = 681)
I use organizational and systems leadership skills for quality improvement and systems thinking into my practice. (Essential II)	5.2% (*N* = 36)	94.8% (*N* = 659)
I apply clinical scholarship and analytical methods for evidence-based practice into my practice. (Essential III)	3% (*N* = 21)	97.0% (*N* = 674)
I use knowledge of information systems and technology and patient care technology for improvement and transformation of health care into my practice. (Essential IV)	6.5% (*N* = 45)	93.5% (*N* = 651)
I use health care policy for advocacy in health care in my practice. (Essential V)	8.9% (*N* = 62)	91.1 (*N* = 633)
I integrate inter professional collaboration to improve patient and population health outcomes in my practice. (Essential VI)	4.7% (*N* = 33)	95.3% (*N* = 663)
I apply clinical prevention and concepts of population health in my practice. (Essential VII)	6.3% (*N* = 44)	93.7% (*N* = 653)
I incorporate advanced nursing functions in my practice. (Essential VIII)	5.5% (*N* = 38)	94.5% (*N* = 658)

DNP, Doctor of Nursing Practice.

Just more than 52% of respondents reported a slight or no change in function as an administrator within their practice; 58.2% report no or minimal change in developing, implementing and/or evaluating information systems; 55.7% report no or minimal change in initiating a program to address disparities within a practice setting; and 50.3% report no or minimal change after graduation in initiating an organizational level change initiative. These and other characteristics of practice reflect the expectations of the eight essentials. This collection of information does not mean that the respondent is not doing good work, but does suggest that the efforts of their respective roles after graduation do not reflect the eight essentials that were the foundation of the DNP educational process.

Let us circle back to the question of whether or not DNP-prepared professional are demonstrating improved outcomes as a result of the eight essentials? To date, outcome data from DNP, Inc.-sponsored surveys reflect perceptions and self-reported examples of commitment to improving outcomes. Presentations typically take place in the context of an academic presentation, seminar, symposium, or conference that is reliant on the educational process for structure. Colleagues in academia strongly support this type of dissemination (and rightfully so). Scientific presentations of practice have indeed been made in practice-focused conferences for advanced practice nurses. These presentations use the eight essentials as a justification of the components and processes of the practice change the project reflecting the efforts of the student who completes the projects. Are practice conferences, symposia, and publications as responsive to the structure of practice or are these types of presentations reflective of the presenter's academic indoctrination?

■ SUMMARY

The question that has not been adequately addressed from the point of view of this author is if the DNP educational process that includes the eight essentials is influencing practice, or are practice issues being addressed outside of this academic structure? Surveys and presentations alone do not capture this information. Identifying and then evaluating the psychometrics of competencies to determine how they impact practice is the next step needed to support the growth of practice. The eight essentials play a role in this evaluation of competencies, but from the perspective of this practitioner, they are not competencies that guide practice. As discussed earlier, these essentials support the education of DNP students, but are not the basis for practice.

Quantifying the impact of DNP-influenced initiatives reflects outcomes and practice. This is accomplished within the context of the practice setting reflecting how the actions of the professional nurse successfully reflect practice change. This approach of measuring outcomes in the context of the setting steps outside of the eight essentials. The goal of improving outcomes is the responsibility of all in the health care delivery system and is supported by our individual and collective educational efforts that are later translated into practice. Building on the foundation of the essentials, the graduate influences systems and hopefully, successfully reflects the best kind of practice. This is the highest honor we can acknowledge for our education, recognizing that the academic process prepares us for practice, but this academic process does not mandate or guide practice. We are all rowing this boat together. Recognizing the strength of our respective oars is valuable in helping to move this ship forward.

TABLE 24.3 Changes in DNP Practice

Question: Since earning your DNP degree, please indicate how often you engage in the following compared with before earning your DNP degree.

	No Change	Slightly More Often	More Often	Considerably More Often	Not Applicable
...am involved in health policy issues related to my practice.	28.6% (N = 211)[a]	24.0% (N = 177)	22.6% (N = 167)	21.4% (N = 158)	3.4% (N = 25)
...function as an administrator within my practice.	39.9% (N = 295)	12.2% (N = 90)	13.1% (N = 97)	22.4% (N = 166)	12.4% (N = 92)
...develop, implement and/or evaluate information systems.	40.0% (N = 294)	18.2% (N = 134)	18.9% (N = 139)	14.6% (N = 107)	8.3% (N = 61)
...develop, implement and/or evaluate practice initiatives.	23.6% (N = 175)	19.3% (N = 143)	25.1% (N = 186)	27.2% (N = 201)	4.7% (N = 35)
...develop, implement and/or evaluate business plans related to practice.	39.5% (N = 291)	17.1% (N = 126)	16.7% (N = 123)	16.3% (N = 120)	10.4% (N = 77)
...incorporate health promotion and disease prevention.	27.3% (N = 201)	16.2% (N = 119)	23.1% (N = 170)	30.2% (N = 222)	3.3% (N = 24)
...actively incorporate evidence in your practice.	12.4% (N = 92)	12.7% (N = 94)	25.4% (N = 188)	46.6% (N = 345)	2.8% (N = 21)
...translate evidence into new practice initiatives.	15.9% (N = 118)	15.8% (N = 117)	24.9% (N = 184)	40.4% (N = 299)	3.0% (N = 22)
...participate in interdisciplinary teams.	27.1% (N = 201)	14.7% (N = 109)	21.3% (N = 158)	33.5% (N = 248)	3.4% (N = 25)
...lead interdisciplinary teams.	36.6% (N = 270)	14.8% (N = 109)	14.8% (N = 109)	28.7% (N = 212)	5.1% (N = 38)
...develop practice guidelines.	34.8% (N = 254)	19.2% (N = 140)	16.3% (N = 119)	22.6% (N = 165)	7.1% (N = 52)
...have initiated a program to address disparities within a practice setting.	41.4% (N = 304)	14.3% (N = 105)	15.2% (N = 112)	17.3% (N = 127)	11.8% (N = 87)
...used available technology to promote a change in practice.	29.5% (N = 218)	18.7% (N = 138)	22.2% (N = 164)	23.3% (N = 172)	6.2% (N = 46)
...have initiated an organizational level change initiative.	35.8% (N = 265)	14.5% (N = 107)	19.7% (N = 146)	24.1% (N = 178)	5.9% (N = 44)

DNP, Doctor of Nursing Practice.

[a] Information is provided by DNP, Inc.

AN ACADEMIC DEAN'S PERSPECTIVE

Many of the actual confluencing factors (e.g., expanding credit loads in master's of nursing programs and discussion of doctoral preparation in graduate-entry degrees across various health professions) and details surrounding the preliminary work on the DNP degree in the years preceding (chiefly 2004–2006) the announcement that the DNP degree should broadly replace the master's, have been identified and discussed in Chapter 1 of this book and in the previous edition. In the decade since publication of the 2006 *The Essentials of Doctoral Education for Advanced Nursing Practice* by the AACN, a lot of water has crossed under *and* over the bridge. Much of the opposition to the degree at the time is now supportive, but there are stakeholders and certainly individual practitioners and academics who retain their skepticism whether this was the right move at the time. This chapter is less about the politics and more about the relevance of the 2006 document to contemporary doctoral advanced nursing practice. As a DNP clinician and practitioner, Dr. David Campbell-O'Dell has presented a very internal perspective on the document and its meaning for actual DNP practitioners (inclusive of all traditional APRNs). This second perspective is from an academic dean's point of view and as an administrator who has now launched two very different DNP degrees in his career. First a DrNP at Drexel University, which focused on scalable clinical research with sample sizes that could advance practice knowledge generation, and now a DNP forthcoming at The College of New Rochelle, which will focus on advanced clinical care and is specifically designed to give the doctoral advanced practice graduate more advanced skills beyond the master's degree. And while the advancement of practice evidence is still essential, time has added some wisdom to this administrator and scholar, and more of the details surrounding "what is practice evidence?" have been filled in by the profession and the AACN in its recent white paper on the DNP (AACN, 2015). This second critique focuses chiefly on whether the eight 2006 DNP essentials are relevant a decade later. This critique ends with a summary conclusion whether there are curriculum elements that need to be added, deleted, modified, or whether more substantive change is required and a new updated, document is needed.

Essential I: Scientific Underpinnings for Practice

From the essentials document, this domain of knowledge for DNP practice includes:

1. The principles and laws that govern the life process, well-being, and optimal function of human beings, sick or well
2. The patterning of human behavior in interaction with the environment in normal life events and critical life situations
3. The nursing actions or processes by which positive changes in health status are affected
4. The wholeness or health of human beings recognizing that they are in continuous interaction with their environments (AACN, 2006, p. 8)

The understanding of most thought leaders in DNP education is that this essential encompasses the traditional scientific coursework for advanced nursing clinicians:[1] advanced pathophysiology, advanced pharmacology, and advanced health assessment. The NONPF, in their 2014 document *Nurse Practitioner Core Competencies Content*, also includes advanced content in genetics and communication skills in this domain (NONPF, 2014). It is an assumption that the accrediting and regulatory agencies of the other advanced nursing clinician or other APRN organizations would concur with this content. The disconnect, however, becomes apparent when one is considering whether the curriculum is focused on the bachelor of science in nursing

(BSN)-to-DNP or post-master's student. The BSN-to-DNP student does not have this basic advanced science background; the post-master's DNP student does, having had this content in required courses in their previous master's degree. Therefore, the predominant post-master's DNP programs do not build on this science content with rare exceptions. The Columbia University School of Nursing program has a course on incorporating genetics and genomics in advanced practice nursing (N9290), as does the University of Utah post-master's DNP (NURS 6240, Clinical Genetics) (Columbia University School of Nursing, 2016; University of Utah, 2016). However, this author could not find any other post-master's DNP program that required a doctoral level course in genetics/genomics. Certainly, it is not unusual that programs are uniquely different or have different requirements, even if they have common nursing accreditors that want to ensure that specific content is included in some format in a respective curriculum or degree. However, it is still widely not recognized that post-master's DNP programs are not required to be accredited, but is required of BSN-to-DNP programs that lead to certification and licensure (i.e., a BSN-to-DNP student that is preparing a new family NP or nurse anesthetist).[2]

The question raised here is why is there no specific additional science-specific content included in the DNP curricula? At Drexel, a focus group of newly graduated family nurse practitioner (FNP) students (from the MSN program) years ago indicated they thought they could have benefited from more advanced anatomy and new FNPs reported that during medical rounds, medical residents were far more proficient at identifying anatomical landmarks and at integrating this content in discussions with interdisciplinary colleagues than they were. In addition, while there were initial discussions about including an advanced human cadaver anatomy course/lab in the DrNP program, it never materialized. Why are there not additional pharmacology courses even available in post-master's DNP curricula? For whatever reason, advanced science-specific content is largely absent in post-master's DNP programs and this needs more discussion, particularly for DNP programs that are clinically focused.

The second area of this domain appears to more specifically related to scientific underpinnings in the discipline of nursing itself. In *Philosophy of Science for Nursing Practice: Concepts and Applications* (Dahnke & Dreher, 2016), the authors present a strong case for the inclusion of basic philosophy of science content for not just PhD in nursing/nursing science programs, but DNP programs as well. For a degree with such an emphasis on evidence-based practice, it is unclear whether there is enough content in DNP programs that includes substantive coursework on the nature of science, evidence, observation, explanation, and even the historical basis for the evolution of nursing thought and science. Dahnke and Dreher identify some of the DNP programs where there is an explicit inclusion of this content, and Vanderbilt's (NUR N410: Evidence-Based Practice I: The Nature of Evidence; 2016) and Oklahoma City University's (2016) DNP programs are examples of this implicit focus (NURS 7103 Philosophy of Science). The author recalls a DNP plenary speaker at an annual AACN Doctoral Education Conference being asked once why they included a philosophy of science course in their DNP curriculum (it was in there PhD program too—students took the course together)? She clearly understood the hidden context, which with the question was posed, being, "why do DNPs need this?" In a very explanatory way, she replied that no such course (with its emphasis on scientific concepts that often explored abstract, developmental theoretical philosophic content that supported practice inquiry too), created such an obvious shift in the student to "doctoral thinking," and beyond the kind of thinking required in very didactic, concrete-oriented master's courses. It was a reassuring concept, rightly addressed, and confirmed my own belief that this content was more than critical to any discussions of evidence-based or practice-based evidence, and essential to DNP student practice inquiry. Nevertheless, it is probably inappropriate to have discussion of nursing theory and nursing science at the doctoral level without a proper philosophical foundation in the philosophy of science. However, its omission in many DNP programs (or its cursory treatment) remains problematic, especially as the AACN has now acknowledged in its new white paper (2015) that indeed the DNP graduate should (and can) create *new* evidence for the discipline, specifically practice evidence.

Essential II: Organizational and Systems Leadership for Quality Improvement and Systems Thinking

In this essential, the AACN emphasizes that the DNP graduate should:

1. Develop and evaluate care delivery approaches, which meet current and future needs of patient populations based on scientific findings in nursing and other clinical sciences, as well as organizational, political, and economic sciences
2. Ensure accountability for quality of health care and patient safety for populations with whom they work
3. Develop and/or evaluate effective strategies for managing the ethical dilemmas inherent in patient care, the health care organization, and research (AACN, 2006, p. 9)

In many ways, this essential is strongly represented in most DNP curricula, with the exception of degree of emphasis on ethics at the doctoral level. First, however, quality and safety are paramount issues across all levels of nursing, from professional to advanced practice, and to doctoral advanced nursing levels (Dolansky & Moore, 2013). The newly renamed *Journal of Doctoral Nursing Practice* (2016; previously *Clinical Scholars Review*) publishes many studies authored or coauthored by DNP graduates whose focus is in the area of patient safety and quality. The Joint Commission (2016) core measure sets provides an enormous area of data areas where DNP student inquiry could be more focused, and where an emphasis on measures of quality and safety measures can be employed (see Table 24.4).

Although content and coursework on health care quality and safety is explicit in most DNP programs, such explicit emphasizes on ethics, whether clinical ethics or organizational ethics (for students in organizational/leadership-focused DNP programs), is uneven. This author believes that graduate content in ethics ought to be taught by faculty with specific training and education in ethics at the graduate level. This issue of the proper educational preparation to teach ethics has had some notice in the literature (Dreher, 2016a; Kalb & O'Conner-Von, 2007; Morse, 1999; Rizzuti, 1983). The Johns Hopkins Berman Institute of Bioethics has had a very purposeful focus on encouraging more ethics education in nursing. In a likely recent but undated statement, they state that in the area of ethics in nursing education there is "little or no faculty training" and seek to make "faculty ethics education and training a priority" (Johns Hopkins Berman Institute of Bioethics, n.d.). It is still a curious transition that in the revised 2011 AACN *Essentials of Master's Education in Nursing* ethics education was rewritten as one of the nine essentials to an area of emphasis within five of the nine essentials (AACN, 2011). Some could interpret that as progress, with ethics content integrated throughout most of the new essentials. Others could view an integration of content as a way that it can easily be de-emphasized, even nonpurposively. From my own practical curriculum experience, when an individual course loses its identity as a stand-alone course and the content is instead integrated across the curriculum, that is often the beginning of the

TABLE 24.4 **The Joint Commission Core Measure Sets**

Perinatal care

Stroke

Venous thromboembolism

Substance use

Tobacco treatment

Hospital outpatient department

Pneumonia measures

Heart failure

Acute myocardial infarction

Surgical care improvement project

Hospital-based inpatient psychiatric services

Emergency department

Immunizations

respective marginalization of that content. The issues of ethics in health care and nursing are complex and have become even more paramount. Nurses and nursing students generally have great interest in all aspects of ethics in nursing. Having more specialists (nurses and non-nurses) with clinical ethics training, not simply an interest in ethics, would likely be welcomed in the modern interdisciplinary and interprofessional health care environment.

Essential III: Clinical Scholarship and Analytical Methods for Evidence-Based Practice

There has probably been no more controversial essential than *Essential III*. From the very beginning there has been immense debate over what a scholarly end product should constitute, the culminating written document for a recipient of the DNP degree. One of my dean colleagues suggested in a conversation several years ago that the DNP actually should *not require* any such scholarly end product (like the dissertation that is expected and required of the PhD graduate). She explained that because the medical doctorate (MD) was a similar professional doctorate (just like the DNP) and does not require a scholarly project of any form, then neither should the DNP. She admitted it was a bold idea, but that her faculty would never vote to do such a radical thing. I actually gave her idea some considerable thought and began to revisit my own notions of what the DNP degree should require. With my colleague, Mary Ellen Smith Glasgow, now dean of the Duquesne University School of Nursing, we published "Global Perspectives on the Professional Doctorate" in the *International Journal of Nursing Studies* in 2011 (Dreher & Smith Glasgow, 2011). We noted that in the international community, there really is no such thing as a doctorate that does not include the conduct of "research" to a greater or lesser extent. The idea that a new practice doctorate (or professional doctorate) in nursing would not involve the generation of some kind of empirical (new) knowledge was characterized as an "idea that should not cross the ocean" (from the shores of the continental U.S. across the Atlantic of course). Over the course of a decade, we have now rightfully moved from the 2006 *Essentials* document with an admonition that "Research-focused doctoral programs in nursing are designed to prepare graduates with the research skills necessary for discovering new knowledge in the discipline. In contrast, DNP graduates engage in advanced nursing practice and provide leadership for evidence-based practice" (p. 11) to the new white paper which instead now states "Graduates of both research- and practice-focused doctoral programs are prepared to generate new knowledge" (p. 2). It actually is a proper evolution because nursing has always, beginning with the days of Nightingale who collected and analyzed data religiously, relied on its ability to create new knowledge derived from observation (and data) in practice. It is this data (transformed and interpreted into evidence) that over time advanced the health of patients, thus advancing the profession, and ultimately help nursing become a full-fledged discipline (Dreher, 2016b).

The DNP graduate is no longer restricted to a "capstone," and while the AACN now recommends the term "DNP Project," each nursing faculty does have the right to determine the content and title of what their DNP graduates will have to complete as a scholarly end product to the awarding of a doctoral degree at their institution. Whether it is a DNP thesis, doctoral practice dissertation, or a DNP project, it really only matters in the halls of the academy. But the global world of science (specifically the academy where many DNPs are employed) does not understand what a DNP project is, I assure you (remember, this degree is only about 10 years old). They do understand, however, what a doctoral thesis (or doctoral practice thesis) is. A simple review of what individual DNP programs call this end product is endless and some standardization will evolve with time. There is also significant diversity in PhD in nursing/nursing science programs and their quality, and in time DNP programs will likely normalize in comparison too. The DNP at research-intensive and research-oriented universities will likely highly emphasize practice knowledge development. To other DNP programs, this emphasis will vary. Physician practice, in comparison, really is not much different. In urban and suburban teaching universities where many physicians and members of the interdisciplinary health care teach, DNP practitioners are involved in the research enterprise and many hospitals (and networks) are absolutely dependent on federal research dollars. Physicians (and nurses) in more rural areas, are mostly fully engaged in just practice and may rarely have the need or demand to publish. These are the realities of modern health care and the expectations of knowledge production across disciplines. This author's chief concern is that if the DNP graduate does not publish his or her work and generate new evidence from his or her new practice environments, then the nursing discipline will suffer. As the largest health care profession, we have an enormous need for more evidence from which to base our practice. Our discipline and our contribution to improve the global health of all can only grow with the synergy of a community of doctorally prepared primary nursing clinicians, scholars, and clinician–scholars, who are uniquely qualified and extraordinarily prepared to bridge the gap between practice and the academy.

Essential IV: Information Systems/Technology and Patient Care Technology for the Improvement and Transformation of Health Care

In this essential, the following is expected of the DNP graduate:

1. Design, select, use, and evaluate programs that evaluate and monitor outcomes of care, care systems, and quality improvement, including consumer use of health care information systems.
2. Analyze and communicate critical elements necessary to the selection, use, and evaluation of health care information systems and patient care technology.

3. Demonstrate the conceptual ability and technical skills to develop and execute an evaluation plan involving data extraction from practice information systems and databases.
4. Provide leadership in the evaluation and resolution of ethical and legal issues within health care systems relating to the use of information, information technology, communication networks, and patient care technology.
5. Evaluate consumer health information sources for accuracy, timeliness, and appropriateness (AACN. 2006, p. 13).

Advancing the technology and informatics skills of all nursing students, not just DNP students, has been aggressively promoted since 2004 by the TIGER initiative—Technology Informatics Guiding Education Reform, and supported by many nursing and corporate organizations, including the AACN (Cheeseman, 2012; Hebda & Calderone, 2010). The 3-year and 10-year goals for the TIGER initiative are outlined in a white paper published by the Executive Steering Committee, led at the time by Marion Ball, EdD, of Johns Hopkins University School of Nursing and Diane J. Skiba, PhD, FAAN, FACMI, University of Colorado at Denver and Health Sciences Center, School of Nursing (co-chairs) (Tigersummit.com, 2007). Almost 10 years later, we can revisit whether the TIGER goals have been accomplished, and examine what role the DNP graduate is having in this area of knowledge management, data/evidence-driven health care, and the contribution health and nursing informatics is making to the efficient, safe, and effective delivery of health care (see Table 24.5)

In 2009, the Healthcare Information and Management Systems Society (HIMSS) published the latest report available on the TIGER initiative (it covered data through 2008) (thetigerinitiative.org, 2009). Part of the report focused on progress made by collaborative teams, which was charged with asking: Why does the nurse today need to know? (see Table 24.6).

Progress toward full TIGER implementation has been observed in the earmarking of some $19 billion to develop an interoperable medical record as part of the American Recovery and Reinvestment Act in 2008/2009. But this remains a continuing goal, perhaps even a "wicked problem" as movement to a full electronic record has increased time burden to health professionals according to some studies, has not increased efficiency simply by being automated, may take more time away from patients, nor improve health outcomes (Accenture, 2015; Freudenheim, 2012; Periyakoil, 2007). These findings only indicate that movement to a full electronic medical record can have some negative consequences.

TABLE 24.5 **Seven Pillars of the TIGER Vision**

1. Management and leadership
2. Education
3. Communication and collaboration
4. Informatics design
5. Information technology
6. Policy
7. Culture

TABLE 24.6   **Collaborative Teams**

1. Standards and interoperability
2. National Health Information Technology (IT) agenda
3. Informatics competencies
4. Education and faculty development
5. Staff development
6. Usability and clinical application design
7. Virtual demonstration center
8. Leadership development
9. Consumer empowerment and personal health record

Source: Thetigerinitiative.org (2009).

The second outcome on TIGER implementation is in mobilizing more nurses to be part of the national health care informatics infrastructure. However, the report states:

> Nurses are often at the center of care coordination for the patient and are well versed on the workflow and information flow critical to minimizing shortfalls with communication handoffs in the delivery of healthcare. Some practice specialty areas in nursing have been historically underrepresented in the development of use cases, technical infrastructure, and development of standards. This leaves a gap in creating interoperable electronic health records that cover the continuum of healthcare delivery through different practice environments. (tigerinitiative.org, 2009, p. 4)

Finally, there has been a goal to accelerate smart, standards-based, interoperable technology that will make advanced health care delivery by improving safety, quality, and outcomes, and making "health care" indeed more patient centered. The Planetree Model of Care is one organizational and institutional way to accomplish this, particularly its emphasis on advancing patient-centered care (Planetree.org, 2014).

The central question here is whether DNP education itself is moving health care and nursing IT forward? Some DNP programs have a specific course in the curriculum that focuses on many of the TIGER initiatives, while others take a "skill-based approach." This author favors the latter approach, with informatics education embedded (but prominently) throughout the curriculum. Developing these competencies, particularly at the beginning of the curriculum, is critical when students need to learn specifically how to navigate knowledge management. Simply, having one's smart phone programmed to trigger Medscape articles (germane to the student's specialty and clinical interests) weekly to the DNP student's email is a start. Using DNP orientations and residencies for quality time specifically devoted to an informatics update (an annual workshop perhaps) forces students to confront their own technology proficiency. Placing all this content in a stand-alone course often seems to backfire, with some students already off the curve (and ahead of the professor!) with their very honed technology skills and others left to languish sometimes just reorienting to a very technology-driven health care world.

The summary point for this essential is that the DNP clinician must be proficient in the kinds of technology support that others members of the interprofessional health care team use, and be adept at evaluating and then embracing new technologies. The clinical executive must be adept at knowing how to data mine for critical data points that might improve outcomes, revenues, or both. This DNP leader/manager must also be able to speak comfortably to the health care analytics team about how the compilation of big data can point to data trends, and again drive their own or the institution's evidence-based decision making.

Essential V: Health Care Policy for Advocacy in Health Care; Essential VI: Interprofessional Collaboration for Improving Patient and Population Health Outcomes; and Essential VII: Clinical Prevention and Population Health for Improving the Nation's Health

On reflection on the 2006 document, "advocacy" is very difficult to separate from the advocational communication and activities that promote patient safety and better health quality. Health care policy and health care politics are more easily differentiated, and so these two essentials are discussed together. *The Essentials* document indicates that, "Political activism and a commitment to policy development are central elements of professional nursing practice, and the DNP graduate . . . " (AACN, 2006, p. 13). The use of the words "political activism" seem particularly important today if we remember that the AACN's development and subsequent proclamations on the DNP all preceded both the global recession and the implementation of the Affordable Care Act (ACA). It is interesting, but nonetheless futile, to wonder whether had either of these events taken place earlier, would the path to the DNP have occurred at all or perhaps evolved differently? Nevertheless, "activism" has never been associated with the PhD degree. But its inclusion in the essentials document is a clear indication that the DNP graduate is charged to be a bigger leader at the grassroots practice arenas of the profession, not the traditional academic. This discussion is very similar to the medical profession's desire to always be the de facto leader of the modern Medical Home, again marginalizing APRNs and now doctorally prepared APRNs (i.e., DAPRNs). As part of current health reform, the Medical Home (first established in 1967 to coordinate complex pediatric care), is designed to comprehensively emphasize coordinated care, accountable care, preventive care, and an integrated payment system. A statement on the Joint Principles established by the American Academy of Pediatrics, American Academy of Family Physicians, American College of Physicians and American Osteopathic Association includes the following first three-bullet points:

- **Personal physician:** Each patient has an ongoing relationship with a personal physician who is focused on continuous and comprehensive care as part of a care team.
- **Physician leadership:** Practices are physician-directed and have a team approach to care delivery. All members of the team, including physician assistants and NPs are critical to the Primary Care Medical Home (PCMH) mission.
- **Whole person orientation:** The PCMH provides for all of the patient's healthcare needs or takes responsibility for appropriately arranging care with other specialists, clinicians and professionals (Bertka, 2011, p. 1).

Maybe the DNP student, who has "practice" at the core of their doctoral degree, should focus on the politics of health care and policy, rather than be educated in very traditional PhD-oriented health policy courses. Health policy is not the same thing as health activism, but health activism has to include health policy. Why cannot APRNs be the primary care provider in a Medical Home? Many of the barriers to comprehensive APRN practice, particularly of NPs, are multifactorial and not related to acquisition of the DNP (Hain & Fleck, 2014). However, the DAPRN has an even stronger argument for this role and for this seat at the table. It is likely the activism of the practitioner, particularly the doctorally prepared practitioner (or clinician who has similar credentials to medicine and other advanced health care providers), may provide the necessary leverage to expand the domains of nursing practice, particularly the domains of doctoral APRN.

Advocacy as a role function has a long history in nursing (Tomajan, 2012). One author describes the role of advocacy as "seeing a need and finding a way to address it" (Almidei, 2010, p. 4). However, this author does cringe when he hears nurses indicate they are the primary advocate for the patient, or the only advocate. The reality is an individual nurse *can be a very good advocate* for an individual patient, and can possibly be the primary advocate. But there are lots of interprofessional members of the health care team today who take their role of advocacy very seriously and may take offense to nursing viewing patient advocacy as chiefly in their domain of practice. This is where interprofessional education (IPE), particularly between NP students and medical students and residents (or similar comparative cohorts), may be very helpful. An excellent study ($N = 306$) has been reported in the *British Medical Journal of Quality and Safety*, which included nursing students, pharmacy students, physician assistant students, and residents focusing on IPE and safety (Brock et al., 2013). The field of "health care safety" is a very purposeful area where it can be easier to promote expert practice across various health care disciplines. This content, particularly in *Essentials V* and *VI* remains a strength since its inclusion in 2006. With the implementation and progress with quality and safety education for nurses (QSEN), TeamSTEPPS, Just Culture, and other quality, safety, and continuous improvement processes, there still needs to be an increasing permeation of this content directly and explicitly into nursing education not just in the DNP, but across all nursing educational degree levels (Lyle-Edrosolo, & Waxman, 2016; Penn, 2014; Sweigart et al., 2016).

The final piece to these two essentials (V–VI) and VII are comments on population health. Without a doubt, this is a popular buzzword in health care and nursing. In my own conversations with one of the leading health care executives in New York City recently, I was informed he thought the word *population health* was "overused" and queried "what does it really mean?" If one is talking about a capitated versus fee-for-service health care system (or network), then easily the capitated model of health care reimbursement is directly population focused and the most predominant (but slowly fading) fee-for service is technically, not. Another colleague has said "hasn't nursing always been doing population focused health?" Devore and Champion (2011) in *Health Affairs* write about accountable care organizations (ACOs) and their centrality to contemporary health care delivery, especially with the advent of the ACA:

> . . . the goals of an ACO are to empower people to take charge of their health and engage in shared decision making with providers; eliminate waste and unnecessary spending while also meeting patients' preferences for care; increase preventive care and other strategies that could help keep people well; and increase overall satisfaction with care. (pp. 41–42)

They also outline how ACOs could provide incentive, reimbursable dollars, when certain benchmark clinical health outcomes or metrics are made. This is capitated, population health, where a hospital network has control (or let us say accountability) for "covered lives"—the number of enrollees that any health care network has responsibility for from birth to death. Recently, there has been discussion whether short-term health promotion will actually save health care dollars (Levine, 2016). It is intuitive that it does, but when individuals seek costly preventive care (it is not free of course), the return on investment or savings from the slower progression of chronic or acute illnesses is not quickly seen. Whether the progression from a traditional fee-for-service model will disappear is unlikely, but market forces are suddenly focused more on value and outcomes, rather than net provider profitability. Writing in the *Harvard Business Review* Porter and Lee (2013) write of a values-driven health care model:

> We must move away from a supply-driven health care system organized around what physicians do and toward a patient-centered system organized around what patients need. We must shift the focus from the volume and profitability of services provided—physician visits, hospitalizations, procedures, and tests—to the patient outcomes achieved. (p. 50)

Certainly, health networks that choose capitation models of health care delivery are not the only networks of care that are focused on population health. But in traditional models of health care delivery that were at the nexus of why we needed health care reform, it does beg the question "what really is population-based health care and who is delivering it?"

Essential VIII: Advanced Nursing Practice

The domain of *Essential VIII* includes:

1. Conduct a comprehensive and systematic assessment of health and illness parameters in complex situations, incorporating diverse and culturally sensitive approaches
2. Design, implement, and evaluate therapeutic interventions based on nursing science and other sciences
3. Develop and sustain therapeutic relationships and partnerships with patients (individual, family, or group) and other professionals to facilitate optimal care and patient outcomes
4. Demonstrate advanced levels of clinical judgment, systems thinking, and accountability in designing, delivering, and evaluating evidence-based care to improve patient outcomes
5. Guide, mentor, and support other nurses to achieve excellence in nursing practice
6. Educate and guide individuals and groups through complex health and situational transitions, and
7. Use conceptual and analytical skills in evaluating the links among practice, organizational, population, fiscal, and policy issues (AACN, 2006, pp. 16–17)

Over the past 10 years this has been one of the two essentials (including *Essential III: Clinical Scholarship and Analytical Methods for Evidence-Based Practice*) that this author believes has been underdeveloped. With the BSN-to-DNP student this *Essential* is robust in most DNP curricula, as students in entry-level DNP programs have the usual required clinical content that is still required in master's advanced nursing practice programs (which still overwhelmingly predominate). It is in the post-master's DNP programs where this content is minimized.

As previously mentioned, the Columbia University DNP (again, formed as a DrNP initially) probably has the greatest emphasis on *Essential VIII* than any DNP program in the country. I have written about this program and its historical contribution to doctoral nursing in this text and in *Philosophy of Science for Nursing Practice: Concepts and Applications* (Dahnke & Dreher, 2010, 2016). A recent review of their curriculum indicates their emphasis on comprehensive care across the lifespan is even more explicit. But why do programs de-emphasize giving DNP students more advanced direct clinical care skills? Is it a curricular issue, whereas BSN-to-DNP students and post-master's DNP graduates need to be at the same eventual endpoint? We do not expect RN/BSNs (especially experienced RNs) to be at the same level of practice as generic BSN graduates, so why is this equivalency needed at the DNP level? Is this why NONPF abandoned their separate educational outcomes for DNP versus master's-prepared NPs? Was it too difficult to maneuver, to establish separate educational outcomes especially when it is not likely that any state Nurse Practice Act in the future is likely to abandon master's degrees in favor of doctoral degrees for entry into practice? Nevertheless, despite Columbia's innovation, it has yet to be copied and thus its critical impact on the profession is historical more than influential. Even the diplomate in comprehensive care (DCC credential; begun at Columbia), which this author highly supports, is given little attention today in the doctoral advanced practice arena. The chief critique of this *Essential* by this author is that the abandonment of separate competencies for doctoral practice has limited the expansion of the APRN role at the doctoral level.

Fairman, Rowe, Hassmiller, and Shalala (2011) explore some of the barriers and state restrictions on the scope of practice for NPs. Hain and Fleck (2014) estimate that only one third of states permit the full practice of APRNs. There is significant NP migration to states with expanded practice opportunities, but concurrent movement from general to specialty practice even among NPs is the result. Fairman et al. further state, "We believe that if we are to bridge the gap in primary care and establish *new approaches* (my italics] to care delivery, all health care providers must be permitted to practice to the fullest extent of their knowledge and competence" (p. 193). These authors may very well not be referring to DNP practice, but new approaches to care delivery would mostly be expected from practitioners with expanded credentials and additional education. It is an inference that is not unfounded.

Finally, many individuals also mistakenly think the Institute of Medicine (Institute of Medicine, 2011) report on nursing, *The Future of Nursing: Leading Change, Advancing Health*, included the DNP in their recommendation to double the number of nurses with a doctorate by 2020. Instead, they were specifically referring to the PhD. As in all IOM reports, there is an immense emphasis on data, and at the time of the report, there just was not sufficient evidence on the outcomes of the DNP degree versus the master's degree for APRNs. What is needed is not just a directive that future APRNs switch to doctoral rather than traditional master's practice, but also ongoing outcome data that analyzes this decision. The early arguments were made, but doctoral education is not just expensive to the student, but expensive to the health care consumer as extra education should mean "higher salaries" to most individuals who make that investment. As an employer, I would ask the DNP "what additional skills do you have that I could not get with a master's-prepared advanced practice nurse?" If I were that DNP-prepared job applicant, I think I would know exactly how to answer that and I would have practiced my response over, and over, and over! The wrong answer I suspect is, "well my profession now requires the doctorate."

■ SUMMARY

After all this analysis, where does the 2006 essentials stand a decade later? I think the answer is—very well. It was a document that did look to the future and while a decade later it is certainly time for an update (as most of the initial DNP curricula have changed and some have changed more than once), the basic curriculum structure is sound. The new white paper on the DNP (AACN, 2015) has expanded some of the discussion and while it provided some additional clarity on nomenclature for the final DNP scholarly outcome, there is more intellectually territory to mine as the profession truly figures out that the domain of knowledge development for the DNP really is. Restrictions on empirically derived nursing knowledge or restrictions in methodology are a nuisance in the academy. At the doctoral level, creative, enthusiastic inquiry needs to be supported and if a student has the zest and interest to pursue an area of clinical problem solving, then it is the student, mentor's and faculty's role to identify those educational experiences. Since the beginning of the modern university, PhD students have been counseled (and often required) to moderate their ideas, narrow their focus, produce a less complicated end product (a typical plea from a dissertation chair), while maintaining a high level of scholarship. The DNP student, at least in this academic dean's view, should similarly be counseled. Still, some DNP faculty proclivities insist on a "Change Project" or some form of "Improvement Science Project," as the basis of every attempt to solve any clinical nursing problem in the scientific method. Instead, faculty insistence that doctoral practice scholarship focus on problem solving that is demanded (and needed) by the market, the Joint Commission Core Measures (2016) for example, could enhance the position of DNP scholarship.

Would I add clinical or organizational ethics as a singular and distinct *Essential*, the answer is yes. Would I find a way to combine advocacy, advocacy for safety, and advances in population health, yes I would (*Essential* V, VI, and VII). The marginalization of more advanced practice skills for the post-master's student needs to be explored. We stopped putting RN/BSN students in all the generic BSN courses decades ago. More skill in motivational interviewing, or more specifically, increased depth in encouraging social behavioral change, is an area of expertise where the master's prepared primary care nursing provider already excels. In those one third states that already have APRNs practicing to their current fullest extent, why cannot they be the innovators and explorers of the next level of doctoral advanced nursing practice? Do those progressive states have to wait for the other two third to catch up before they can expand their practice domain? Also, the burdens of the new DNP in the academy who struggles with the tripartite mission (teaching, practice, and service, whereas practice is not voluntary but required to maintain certification) is real, as reported by Smeltzer, et al. (2015). Hopefully, in the next revision of the AACN's *Essentials of Doctoral Education for Advanced Nursing Practice*, there will a significant number of DNP-prepared clinical scholars who can pave the way for the *next* decade of practice.

■ CRITICAL THINKING QUESTIONS

1. *Do you believe the eight* Essentials of Doctoral Education for Advanced Nursing Practice *indeed guide practice? Defend your answer.*
2. *Why does the debate over the proper delineation of DNP scholarship remain so controversial?*
3. *Discuss some of the survey results that surprised you.*
4. *What gives you optimism and pessimism about DNP education?*
5. *Which essential do you consider the most evidence-based and strongly belongs in DNP education?*
6. *Which essential does your own program emphasize particularly well?*
7. *Which essential is underdeveloped in your current curriculum?*
8. *Discuss your own comfort level with advanced health care technology and your experiences with TIGER initiatives.*
9. *Do you have a better conceptualization of what DNP knowledge development is? Explain.*
10. *Devise four new essentials for the next revision of this document.*

■ NOTES

1. The working definition of "advanced nursing clinicians" includes "NPs, nurse midwives, nurse anesthetists, and clinical nurse specialists" prepared at either the master's or doctoral level. "Doctoral advanced nursing clinicians" have explicit, added, doctoral, DNP preparation.

2. PhD in Nursing/Nursing Science programs are not accredited, nor are there any options for them to be accredited even if they wanted to do so.

■ REFERENCES

Accenture. (2015). *Doctors survey 2015: Six-country report*. Retrieved from https://www.accenture .com/t20160418T023924__w__/no-en/_acnmedia/Accenture/Conversion-Assets/DotCom/ Documents/Global/PDF/Dualpub_9/Accenture-Doctors-Survey-NO-Global.pdf#zoom=50

Almidei, N. (2010). *So you want to make a difference: Advocacy is the key* (16th ed.). Washington, DC: OMB Watch.

American Association of Colleges of Nursing. (2006). *The essentials of doctoral education for advanced practice nursing practice*. Retrieved from http://www.aacn.nche.edu/publications/position/ DNPEssentials.pdf

American Association of Colleges of Nursing. (2011). *The essentials of master's education in nursing*. Retrieved from http://www.aacn.nche.edu/education-resources/MastersEssentials11.pdf

American Association of Colleges of Nursing. (2015). The doctor of nursing practice: Current issues and clarifying recommendations. Report from the task force on the implementation of the DNP. Retrieved from http://www.aacn.nche.edu/aacn-publications/white-papers/DNP -Implementation-TF-Report-8–15.pdf

American Organization of Nurse Executives. (2015). Nurse executive competencies. Retrieved from http://www.aone.org/resources/nec.pdf

Bertka, W. (2011, August 1). Hospitals and patient centered medical homes: A practical pairing. Becker's Hospital Review. Retrieved from http://www.beckershospitalreview.com/hospital-physician -relationships/hospitals-and-patient-centered-medical-homes-a-practical-pairing.html

Brock, D., Abu-Rish, E., Chiu, C. R., Hammer, D., Wilson, S., Vorvick, L., . . . Zierler, B. (2013). Interprofessional education in team communication: Working together to improve patient safety. *BMJ Quality & Safety, 22*(5), 414–423.

Cheeseman, S. E. (2012). Information literacy: Using computers to connect practice to evidence. *Neonatal Network, 31*(4), 253–258.

Columbia University School of Nursing. (2016). DNP curriculum. Retrieved from http://nursing .columbia.edu/academics/academic-programs/doctoral-programs/doctor-nursing-practice/ dnp-curriculum

Dahnke, M. D., & Dreher, H. M. (2010). *Philosophy of science for nursing practice: Concepts and applications* (1st ed.). New York, NY: Springer Publishing.

Dahnke, M. D., & Dreher, H. M. (2016). *Philosophy of science for nursing practice: Concepts and applications* (2nd ed.). New York, NY: Springer Publishing.

Devore, S., & Champion, R. W. (2011). Driving population health through accountable care organizations. *Health Affairs (Project Hope), 30*(1), 41–50.

Dreher, H. M. (2016a). What is a practice discipline? In M. D. Dahnke & H. M. Dreher's (Eds.), *Philosophy of science for nursing practice: Concepts and applications* (2nd ed., pp. 3–30). New York, NY: Springer Publishing.

Dreher, H. M. (2016b). The 100-year path to nursing science, 1910–2010: With epilogue 2010–2015. In M. D. Dahnke & H. M. Dreher's (Eds.), *Philosophy of science for nursing practice: Concepts and applications* (2nd ed., pp. 313–354). New York, NY: Springer Publishing.

Dreher, H. M., & Smith Glasgow, M. E. (2011). Global perspectives on the professional doctorate. *International Journal of Nursing Studies, 48*(4), 403–408.

Doctors of Nursing Practice, Inc. (2015). 2015 DNP practice outcomes survey. Retrieved from http:// www.doctorsofnursingpractice.org/dnp-survey-results

Dolansky, M. A., & Moore, S. M. (2013). Quality and safety education for nurses (QSEN): The key is systems thinking. *The Journal of Online Issues in Nursing, 18*(3), Manuscript 1. Retrieved from http:// www.nursingworld.org/Quality-and-Safety-Education-for-Nurses.html

Fairman, J. A., Rowe, J. W., Hassmiller, S., & Shalala, D. E. (2011). Broadening the scope of nursing practice. *The New England Journal of Medicine, 364*(3), 193–196.

Freudenheim, M. (2012, October 9). The ups and downs of electronic medical records. *New York Times*, D4.

Hain, D., & Fleck, L. (2014). Barriers to nurse practitioner practice that impact healthcare redesign. *The Online Journal of Issues in Nursing, 19*(2), Manuscript 2. Retrieved from http://www.nursingworld .org/MainMenuCategories/ANAMarketplace/ANAPeriodicals/OJIN/TableofContents/Vol-19 -2014/No2-May-2014/Barriers-to-NP-Practice.html

Hebda, T., & Calderone, T. L. (2010). What nurse educators need to know about the TIGER initiative. *Nurse Educator, 35*(2), 56–60.

Institute of Medicine. (2011). *The future of nursing: Leading change, advancing health*. Washington, DC: National Academies Press.

Johns Hopkins Berman Institute of Bioethics. (n.d.). Nursing education domain. Retrieved from http://www.bioethicsinstitute.org/nursing-ethics-summit-report/blueprint-for-the-future/nursing-education

The Joint Commission. (2016). Core measures sets. Retrieved from https://www.jointcommission.org/core_measure_sets.aspx

Journal of Doctoral Nursing Practice. (2016). Journal website. Retrieved from http://www.springerpub.com/journal-of-doctoral-nursing-practice.html

Kalb, K. A., & O'Conner-Von, S. (2007). Ethics education in advanced practice nursing: Respect for human dignity. *Nursing Education Perspectives, 28*(4), 196–202.

Levine, M. (2016). Obamacare's 'wellness' gamble. Retrieved from http://www.politico.com/agenda/agenda/story/2016/05/wellness-obamacare-000114

Lyle-Edrosolo, G., & Waxman, K. T. (2016). Aligning healthcare safety and quality competencies: Quality and safety education for nurses (QSEN), The Joint Commission, and American Nurses Credentialing Center (ANCC) Magnet® Standards Crosswalk. *Nurse Leader, 14*(1), 70–75.

Morse, J. (1999). Who is the ethics expert? The original footnote to plato. *Business Ethics Quarterly, 9*(4), 693–697.

National Organization of Nurse Practitioner Faculties. (2012). Nurse practitioner core competencies. Retrieved from http://c.ymcdn.com/sites/www.nonpf.org/resource/resmgr/competencies/npcorecompetenciesfinal2012.pdf

National Organization of Nurse Practitioner Faculties. (2014). Nurse practitioner core competencies content. Retrieved from http://c.ymcdn.com/sites/nonpf.site-ym.com/resource/resmgr/Competencies/NPCoreCompsContentFinalNov20.pdf

Oklahoma City University. (2016). DNP curriculum. Retrieved from http://www.okcu.edu/nursing/programs/doctor-nursing-practice/curriculum/index

Penn, C. E. (2014). Integrating just culture into nursing student error policy. *The Journal of Nursing Education, 53*(9, Suppl.), S107–S109.

Planetree.org. (2014). Organization website. Retrieved from http://planetree.org

Periyakoil, V. S. (2007). Taming wicked problems in modern health care systems. *Journal of Palliative Medicine, 10*(3), 658–659.

Porter, M. E., & Lee, T. H. (2013). The strategy that will fix health care. *Harvard Business Review, 91*(10), 50–70.

Rizzuti, C. J. (1983). Who should teach ethics? *New Directions for Teaching and Learning, 13*, 53–59.

Smeltzer, S. C., Sharts-Hopko, N. C., Cantrell, M. A., Heverly, M. A., Jenkinson, A., & Nthenge, S. (2015). Work-life balance of nursing faculty in research- and practice-focused doctoral programs. *Nursing Outlook, 63*(6), 621–631.

Sweigart, L. I., Umoren, R. A., Scott, P. J., Carlton, K. H., Jones, J. A., Truman, B., & Gossett, E. J. (2016). Virtual TeamSTEPPS® simulations produce teamwork attitude changes among health professions students. *The Journal of Nursing Education, 55*(1), 31–35.

Thetigerinitiative.org. (2009). The TIGER initiative: Collaborating to integrate evidence and informatics into nursing practice and education: An executive summary. Retrieved from http://s3.amazonaws.com/rdcms-himss/files/production/public/FileDownloads/tiger-report-executive-summary.pdf

Tigersummit.com. (2007). The TIGER initiative: Evidence and informatics transforming nursing: 3-year action steps toward a 10-year vision. Retrieved from http://www.aacn.nche.edu/education-resources/TIGER.pdf

Tomajan, K. (2012). Advocating for nurses and nursing. *The Online Journal of Issues in Nursing, 17*(1), Manuscript 4. Retrieved from http://nursingworld.org/MainMenuCategories/ANAMarketplace/ANAPeriodicals/OJIN/TableofContents/Vol-17-2012/No1-Jan-2012/Advocating-for-Nurses.html

University of Utah. (2016). College of nursing—University of Utah, post-MS to DNP 2016 cohort. Retrieved from http://nursing.utah.edu/students/POS-Current/postms-dnp_feb2016.pdf

Vanderbilt University. (2016). DNP course of study. Retrieved from http://www.nursing.vanderbilt.edu/dnp/study_plan.html

Reflective Response

Joy Elwell

Practicing across the settings of health policy, primary health care, and academia, I find the authors' perspectives on the 2006 *Essentials of Doctoral Education for Advanced Nursing Practice* provocative. The authors outline the eight essentials and in their discussions, imply the question, "Do Doctor of Nursing Practice (DNP)-prepared nurses know their place?" Although this question may offend, it should be asked. Another question implied is, "Why is anyone trying to narrowly define what a DNP-prepared nurse can do after graduation?" Further, the chapter suggests that the essentials may, unintentionally, or otherwise, seek to exclude DNP-prepared nurses from certain specialties for example, research, academia.

■ DISCUSSION

Is practice for the DNP-prepared nurse based on the essentials? Should it be? The authors ask, and we must ask ourselves, why make any attempt to constrain the practice of any doctoral nurse? There is no good reason for this. Doing so is an example of turf-protection and protectionism within nursing and broadens the divide that already exists between the different types of doctoral nurses.

The authors discuss the evolution of DNP programs with regard to standardization and quality. In discussing *Essential III: Clinical Scholarship and Analytical Methods for Evidence-Based Practice*, they present the perspective that time will take care of normalization and standardization. The essentials, as the authors indicate, should guide, and provide a framework for the student, and new graduate, but they should not define, or limit the graduate's practice. Take, for example, research. The authors point out that DNP graduates are discouraged, and perhaps prevented from engaging in research. According to Vincent, Johnson, Velasquez, and Rigney (2010):

> The amount of scientific knowledge is seemingly growing exponentially, and the need for translating this knowledge into clinical practice has never been greater. DNP graduates must be prepared in rigorous doctoral curricula to address this need. As practitioner-researchers, DNP graduates are context experts who will be key to closing the research-to-practice gap and improving health outcomes in the United States. (p. 33)

The emerging need for translational research, to bridge the gap between research and practice, is growing significantly. Yet, many in academia fret that DNP-prepared nurses should be excluded from being involved in research. Nothing could be further from the truth. There is more than enough room for all doctoral nurses to contribute to research.

Observing the hand wringing over how the essentials are addressed in DNP programs is puzzling. Regarding the DNP scholarly project, such great emphasis is placed on the end product, the importance of the content of the courses can appear almost an afterthought. There is no arguing the point that nursing needs all doctoral nurses to disseminate knowledge in writing. There is no arguing the point that DNP students develop important projects with the potential to improve health care, and can do so only by being published. Further, publishing one's scholarly work is an example of Boyer's scholarship of integration, which is essential for those pursuing careers in academia. According to Peterson and Stevens (2013) academics equate acceptable publications solely with the peer-review process creating a dilemma for the advanced practice nurse academician. Therefore, to prepare nurses with practice doctorates to survive in academic settings, DNP programs must support and facilitate students writing for publication. Beyond that need, there is the real need within the profession to disseminate knowledge, as voiced in the chapter. Many within nursing voice the concern that, if nurses themselves do not disseminate knowledge from their practice environments, the only evidence in health care used in practice will be from other disciplines. The authors point out that, in addition to the negative influence on health care, the profession of nursing suffers. Nursing's image, while positive, continues to be one of an assistant in the health care milieu, and it is a false image, with many negative implications for the workforce, including lower salaries, substandard working conditions, and the loss of the "best and brightest" to other "STEM" (science, technology, education, and math) professions. Beyond the negative implications for the individual nurse, and the profession, is the risk that this poses to global health. Limiting opportunities for DNP-prepared primary nursing clinicians, scholars, and clinician–scholars artificially constrains the contributions they can make in improving health care at the local, regional, national, and global levels. Maximizing and optimizing outcomes in health care is dependent on fully using the contributions of all doctoral nurses with, as the co-authors of this chapter so eloquently state, "the synergy of a community of who are uniquely qualified and extraordinarily prepared to bridge the gap between practice and the academy" (p. 539).

■ CONCLUSION

The essentials should serve as a framework and guide for DNP programs. Graduates of DNP programs should not be limited or constrained by the essentials but should use them as a springboard, to launch their careers. Nursing must not fall into the trap other professions have, that of jealously protecting areas of nursing practice to the detriment of the profession. One has only to observe organized medicine's attempts to prevent advanced practice nurses from practicing to the full extent of their education and competency to understand the futility and waste in protectionism. Nursing will best serve its own interests and those of society by celebrating the richness in its diversity.

■ REFERENCES

Peterson, K., & Stevens, J. (2013). Integrating the scholarship of practice into the nurse academician portfolio. *Journal of Nursing Education and Practice, 3*(11), 84–92.

Vincent, D., Johnson, C., Velasquez, D., & Rigney, T. (2010). DNP-prepared nurses as practitioner-researchers: Closing the gap between research and practice. *The American Journal for Nurse Practitioners, 14,* 28–34.

Today, Tomorrow, and in the Future: What Roles Are Next for Nurses Engaged in Doctoral Advanced Nursing Practice?

H. Michael Dreher and Mary Ellen Smith Glasgow

Despite the plethora of still surging numbers of new Doctor of Nursing Practice (DNP) programs, the impact these graduates will ultimately have on the U.S. health care system remains largely unknown. This is perhaps both disconcerting and opportunistic. There is need for more data that examine the health outcomes of aggregate populations from DNP-directed care and administration, if the role of the DNP graduate is to be supported by the free market and by consumers. Beyond the work of Mundinger et al. (2000) that supports this degree's likelihood of having a positive impact on health outcomes, not initially having substantive pilot data for the DNP degree still presents a challenge to the profession. It is up to the now decade-long cadre of DNP graduates and educators to discern the value of this new doctoral degree. We are optimistic that in time work on evaluating the degree's worth will be done, and the innovation of the DNP degree will be affirmed. This concluding chapter takes a summary view of the three primary doctoral advanced practice roles we have delineated in this text—practitioner, clinical executive, and educator. We have purposely included the educator role because probably more DNPs appear to either complete the degree while in current academic roles, or enter academia postgraduation. There is too much of an employment trend to pretend that DNPs are completing the degree specifically to retain or attain an academic position. We have certainly tried to be honest about it in this text, and confront this trend directly. In this chapter, we reflect on what the DNP degree is today and what it will likely look like tomorrow, as programs already in existence are beginning to tweak and modify their curricula after having had many cohorts of graduates entering the workforce. Finally, we look at the future. We make some creative projections about where this degree might lead the new graduate. As we move further into the 21st century and the unfolding first and next decade of health reform ahead of us, our projections evolve out of Toffler's (1971) groundbreaking 1970s' work *Future Shock*, Naisbitt's (1982) *Megatrends* from the 1980s, and from the 1990s to today, with the contemporary work of Harvard Business School professor and innovation guru Clayton Christensen, who first coined the term *disruptive innovation* (Christensen, 1997; Christensen, Grossman, & Hwang, 2008). These futuristic works from over several decades form the footprints for this degree's ultimate future. These luminaries and social critics of society, and our own record of progress and future serve as models for our own predictions about the roles *that are next* perhaps for the DNP graduate. It should be an exciting journey!

■ THE DOCTORAL ADVANCED NURSING PRACTICE "PRACTITIONER"

When *U.S. News and World Report* featured a doctorally prepared RN on the cover of its January 2005 issue with the title "Who needs doctors: Your future physician might not be an MD—and you may be better off!"—indeed a Pandora's Box was opened, and the rush to anoint an alternate supply of primary care providers in the United States was ushered in, but retrospectively in a most controversial way (Fischman, 2005). That was in 2005, and now more than a decade later, we have grown from less than 10 DNP programs in 2005 to some 269 as of 2014 (American Association of Colleges of Nursing [AACN], 2015a). We are certain that the designers of this degree (a dean's task force at the AACN) had no idea this would be the projected growth of this degree. Indeed, in 2015a, the number of DNP programs has far surpassed the number of PhD ($N = 134$) programs in nursing, a degree that has been around since 1934 (Dreher, 2009a). With this large number of DNP programs producing doctorally prepared *practitioners* (referring broadly to nurse practitioners [NPs], nurse midwives, nurse anesthetists, and clinical nurse specialists) for the health care market, two fundamental questions remain. Will they perform differently than if they were instead master's-prepared advanced practice nurses and will doctorally prepared clinicians improve health outcomes beyond those improvements made by master's-prepared advanced practice registered nurses (APRNs)?

In 2009, Dreher and Montgomery proposed the term *doctoral advanced practice registered nursing* (the acronym "DAPRN" is used in this text) to better differentiate the practice of a DNP graduate from the practice of a traditional master's-prepared clinician or practitioner. We think this is critical, because if there are no new, real, identifiable skills that a new doctorally prepared practitioner possesses, then why should APRNs have pursued the doctorate, and why should the market place pay these health care professionals more money? So our challenge to the profession and in particular to the DNP educator and graduate, is to be very clear about what additional skills *beyond the MSN* the DNP graduate is going to acquire. It is our view that the emergence of new roles for the DNP-prepared practitioner will be dependent on a critical mass of graduates presenting new prospective employers with measurable claims of what they have acquired during their doctoral education. For this reason, we do believe there will be both: (a) programs that will produce quality graduates (the programs that are very adept at producing clinicians ready to practice at the doctorally advanced practice level); and, unfortunately, also (b) programs that will do a poor job of this. We are particularly concerned about the impact of programs that poorly differentiate graduates with the master's versus the doctoral degree, and whether graduates hired from weak programs will leave their new employers skeptical of graduates with this new degree.

To combat this, we encourage DNP students, especially new DNP students reading this text early in their curriculum, to challenge the faculty to make sure you are getting more of what *The Essentials of Doctoral Education for Advanced Nursing Practice* (AACN, 2006) refers to in *Essential VIII* as *Advanced Nursing Practice* (p. 16). In other words, for the post-master's DNP student—you already are an *advanced practice nurse* and now matriculating to become a *doctoral advanced practice nurse*—what in your respective curriculum fits specifically into this box? Are you getting additional content in practice? Are you building on what you already know? Is your program leveraging technology to give you additional experience with complex standardized patients (very critical in bachelor of science in nursing [BSN]-to-DNP programs), or informatics skills to track and document patient assessments and outcomes in near real time? We hear that family NP graduates from master's programs indicate that they wish they had more advanced skills at differential diagnosis, and more in-depth, cadaver-based anatomy in which to better support their case presentations during grand rounds with other interprofessional colleagues (often interns, residents, and other medical professionals). Perhaps most importantly, we firmly believe that DAPRNs ought to be the most skilled at implementing social/behavioral interventions for their primary care patients.[1] Do you have a course that focuses on or includes this content? We challenge you *to challenge your faculty* to be clear about what additional skill sets your DNP program offers you and is going to help you achieve. For BSN-to-DNP program students the challenge is similar, but different. Here the question is what didactic curriculum can be clearly differentiated as truly doctoral advanced nursing practice content and what would typically belong to a traditional MSN practitioner's program? Whether you are a post-master's (entering with an earned master's degree) or an entry-level DNP student (entering with a BSN), we know these may be difficult questions for new programs to answer.[2] However, only by creating a different kind of graduate will the degree and the permanence of the DNP graduate in the marketplace take hold and graduates likely be compensated additionally and equitably for the higher education they possess.

In the classic futurist book *Future Shock*, Toffler (1971) coined the term *information overload*. Certainly, this was one of the many reasons given for the formation of the DNP degree. With technological advances in society increasing exponentially, it was often assumed that in order to master more information, the APRN in a typical master's program needed more courses and more credit hours to maintain competency. Even though many master's programs in other disciplines typically are completed in 30 to 36 semester credits, many MSN programs, especially those preparing advanced practitioners, vastly exceeded 30 credits. Thus, one rationale for creating the DNP degree was to avoid any further master's "credit creep" and to recognize that the current length of the MSN degrees was already heading toward common total credits awarded for a doctorate (American Association of Colleges of Nursing, 2006). Therefore, a powerful argument for degree credit parity was made for the creation of this doctoral degree instead of again just adding more additional master's credits and courses (Dracup & Bryan-Brown, 2005). We agree that information overload, possibly a problem for society even pre-Toffler, remains a contemporary issue for the DNP student and graduate. Upon reflection, in some ways the pace of new knowledge has probably not changed since 1970. However, today's DNP student and graduate increasingly faces, perhaps more than ever, the legal burden (not to mention the ethical obligation) to "keep up to date" to maintain expected practice competencies. We would even go as far as to surmise that the DNP graduate, especially the practitioner who may often be working side-by-side in clinic environments with other doctorally prepared clinicians, may have an additional burden to project and demonstrate that their practice skill set is superior to APRN colleagues who have a master's degree.

One of the precepts of another seminal book on futurism, *Megatrends*, from the 1980s, was that "We are moving in the dual direction of high tech/high touch, matching each new technology with a compensatory human response" (Naisbitt, 1982, p. 1). We think the future DNP practitioner is going to be more technology oriented than even today. Indeed, it is the doctorally prepared clinician who is the most adept at knowledge management and who will likely become the most expert clinician (Dreher, 2009b). The question for today's DNP student is what kind of focus on technology does your curriculum include? Are you learning how to manage the massive amount of information input you need, to evaluate and discriminate among in order to stay abreast of your particular field? This means going much further than subscribing to and reading the right journals in your discipline. It is about using technology devices that can comb new articles and findings in one's field electronically, and having them sent directly to one's iPhone or smartphone, or perhaps to the next-generation device that has not even been identified yet. Indeed, one such program (PubMed) does this and was described in Chapter 14. We do not know today what kind of technology competencies will be required for DAPNs to maintain the kind of expert practice required of them in the future. But we already see clinicians in progressive practices walking out of patient rooms with Dictaphones in hand, dictating their notes in real time using DragonFly, probably the leading voice recognition software on the market today in health care practices. What about you? What is your technology quotient? Are you a "techie"? If not, are you at least competent with the latest health care support technology? More importantly, how do you envision your future practice, and how do you plan to "keep up" and be competitive with your other health care professional colleagues? Already it is increasingly recognized that baccalaureate and master's nursing education programs have increased their emphasis on technology in health care, and particularly the use of digital recordings of standardized patients and high-fidelity simulation (Defenbaugh & Chikotas, 2016; Mompoint-Williams, Brooks, Lee, Watts, & Moss, 2014). Similarly, at the doctoral level, we believe this is a prime area where DNP graduates can show a level of technology mastery above and beyond what the other health care practitioners from other disciplines commonly use. Again, look at your own DNP curriculum. Is the technology support you will need for doctoral advanced nursing practice there?

H. M. Dreher, the first author of this chapter, was privileged to attend the Harvard Macy Institute's Program for Leading Innovations in Health care and Education at the Harvard Business School and Harvard Medical School in 2007. The week-long program was led by the guru of innovation, Clayton Christensen, DBA (Doctor of Business Administration, Harvard). With an audience largely comprised of physician educators from medical schools from around the world (but with some nursing faculty and other related disciplines also in attendance), Dr. Christensen startled the attendees one morning by announcing that physicians should stop their turf battles over who should provide primary care. Of course my ears pricked up with this discussion (as I am sure did the ears of the several other nurses in attendance), and he went on to say that there were already nonphysician primary care providers such as NPs and physician assistants who have demonstrated they can provide a high level of primary care effectively. Moreover, he thought many physicians were simply underused for the vast education and expertise they possess. He encouraged physicians to focus less on the less complex diagnosis and treatment of common disorders, which other disciplines could manage more cost effectively, and instead focus on the next horizons of medical specialty practice and science. Dr. Christensen's (2009) book (with Grossman & Hwang), *The Innovator's Prescription: A Disruptive Solution for Health Care*, even states "NPs (and other physician extenders) practicing in retail clinics, should disrupt the precision medicine portion of the physician's practice" (p. 112). I found the discussion absolutely exhilarating, and as a department chair managing a DNP program at the time, I was convinced that my own graduates were absolutely positioning themselves to be this new kind of expert, non-physician, primary care provider he was applauding. So at least the Harvard Business School was sympathetic to the work product of NPs and other advanced practice clinicians; however, we dislike the use of physician extender as we see nurse practitioners as more than an extension of physician's practice. Indeed, even if their opposition has decreased down some, they continue to oppose, in particular, the practice of the DNP graduate and their use of the title *Doctor* (Moore, Judge, & Angelini, 2013; Schreiner, 2014). Furthermore, the stances taken by the AMA in its 2009 policy paper warning about the spread and encroachment of nonphysician primary care providers, is still being proliferated by The Physician's Foundation in its white paper *Accept No Substitute: A Report on Scope of Practice* (Isaacs & Jellenik, 2012). However, one must not assume all physicians are against doctorally prepared advanced practice nurses, and we cannot view medicine as "the enemy." From our perspective, the AMA (at least institutionally), perceives the DNP graduate and practitioner who will call themselves doctor to be a threat to their sphere of influence and to their power and authority as experts on health care, and also, most certainly, as a financial threat.

We continue to be uncertain of the future of the Diplomat in Comprehensive Care examination (the DNP examination or the "ABCC examination" as some prefer). Although we believe it will help better differentiate the clinically oriented DNP graduate from the DNP graduate who pursues a nonclinical or leadership-focused DNP, the numbers of individuals who have passed this examination since its founding in 2008 remains small. The examination does not appear to have made a critical impact on DNP education. Moreover, there was broad opposition to it within the profession at its inception, including the then-president of the American College of Nurse Practitioners (ACNP), Dr. Julie Stanik-Hutt (2008). Initially, some of the opposition came from PhD-prepared NPs who likely felt left out because, without a DNP degree, they could not take the examination. That remains a fair argument, but in the end, a PhD is a research-intensive degree, and its aim has never been to improve the clinical skills of master's-prepared advanced practice nurses. It remains to be seen whether patients and payers will recognize that this subset of DNP graduates (Diplomates of Comprehensive Care) are the "clinical experts of choice" as former Dean Mary Mundinger and the Columbia University School of Nursing faculty suggests ("Ten Years of Progress," 2010, p. 25).

We think it is more prudent for DAPRNs to work from a positive frame of reference and to find ways to explore collaboration with physicians, particularly with those who do respect the practice of highly educated advanced practice nurses. We encourage you to seek out these sympathetic physician partners and to work with them and to establish successful partnerships. One of the first Drexel DNP graduates runs a primary care practice with an MD colleague, and she is a full partner in the joint practice. She did not have that kind of practice arrangement *prior* to having her DrNP degree. This is clear indication of the kind of leverage the new DAPRN may exert today and perhaps more commonly in the future. It is the expert role modeling of today's practice DNP graduates and their demonstration of advanced knowledge, skill, expertise, and ability that will go a long way toward paving the way for future graduates who may themselves secure full partnership primary practice positions with physicians and other health care providers.

Finally, we envision primary care primary practices comprised completely of DNP prepared practitioners. It is not hard to imagine a practice being set up with full partners (founders and highly experienced DAPN) and employing new associate partners as new graduates are hired with an expanding practice. We envision new associate partners working their way up the ladder to full partner and then enjoying the benefits of a jointly managed nursing primary care practice, much like what happens in the legal field. We especially predict that these types of doctoral nursing primary care practices could be competitive for contracts to provide health services, especially to vulnerable populations in medically underserved areas where physicians just do not want to practice. These environments might include prisons, nurse-managed primary community health care centers, inner city and rural health care clinics, and other areas. Banded together, we predict that a practice of DNP graduates (how about a cadre of transdisciplinary NPs, nurse-midwives, and clinical nurse specialists?) could negotiate real autonomy and provide expert primary health care in a diversity of health care agencies and venues. And with certified nurse midwives finally winning 100% reimbursement under Medicare (since 1988 they have only been reimbursed at 65% of the rate paid to a physician for the same services) for disabled and senior women needing reproductive health services and maternity care, maybe even the payment models for advanced practice nursing care are moving in the right direction (Summers, 2010). However, a quirk in the Medicare law still prevents APRNs from "signing home health plans of care and from certifying Medicare patients for the home health benefit" (Conant, 2010, p. 18). Additionally, physicians are still unnecessarily insistent they be leaders of any Medical Home practice (Pho, 2013). Nevertheless, with the 2010 Patient Protection and Affordable Care Act, and real health care reform now in place for 6 years, the future is bright for DAPN's, especially if they creatively and innovatively design efficient models of health care delivery. We are really optimistic about what the DNP practitioner/clinician graduate can contribute to the new American health care system. Are you?

■ THE DOCTORAL ADVANCED NURSING PRACTICE "CLINICAL EXECUTIVE"

Given that fundamental change is still needed in the U.S. health care delivery system to improve quality care, the Institute of Medicine (IOM) has continually published groundbreaking policy papers,[3] including the 2010 report on nursing, *The Future of Nursing: Leading Change, Advancing Health,* in collaboration with the Robert Wood Johnson Foundation. The doctoral advanced nursing practice–educated *clinical executive* (chief nursing officers, vice presidents, and other executive-level nurse leaders) will be called upon to address emergent and challenging issues for nursing practice, as well as to create opportunities that will shape and implement innovative changes in our evolving health care system. But today, the doctoral level clinical nurse executive is in short supply. Future doctoral-level nurse administrators and executive leaders will also be charged to improve health and health care outcomes through evidence-based practice in diverse clinical and health care settings. The clinical executive with doctoral advanced nursing practice education emphasizes evidence-based and practice-based approaches for quality and safety improvement in practice settings, applies research methods to decision making, and translates credible research findings to increase the effectiveness of both direct and indirect nursing practice. Some of the specific competencies outlined in the Essentials documents for the DNP clinical executive include: (a) using sophisticated, conceptual, and analytical skills in evaluating the links between clinical, organizational, fiscal, and policy issues; (b) establishing processes for interorganizational collaboration for the achievement of organizational goals; (c) designing patient-centered care delivery systems or policy-level delivery models; (d) collaborating effectively with legal counsel and financial officers around issues related to legal and regulatory guidelines; and (e) demonstrating advanced levels of clinical judgment, cultural sensitivity, and systems thinking (AACN, 2006). The clinical executive track of the DNP degree[4] offers numerous courses on leadership theories, the process of leadership, and leadership as it pertains to a health care setting. The practicum experiences for the clinical executive student provide an opportunity for the student to apply leadership theories in health care settings. The challenge for the DNP clinical executive may be in the attainment of 1,000 practicum hours (post-BSN) that both the Commission on Collegiate Nursing Education (CCNE) and Council on Graduate Education on Administration in Nursing (CGEAN) require. The 2015b AACN white paper on the DNP states, "All DNP students, including those in post-master's programs, are expected to complete a minimum of 1,000 post-baccalaureate practice hours" (p. 7). Additionally, Council on Graduation Education for Administration in Nursing (CGEAN, 2011), while noting that more than 50% of nurses in leadership-titled positions are estimated to have *less than baccalaureate degree preparation*, recommend:

- Nurse managers should be minimally prepared at the baccalaureate or preferably the master's in nursing level
- Nurse executives are encouraged to seek educational preparation at the doctoral level to enhance their roles and contributions to improving health care outcomes and systems
- CGEAN supports the implementation of the DNP as a post-master's terminal degree option with an aggregate/systems/organizational focus in administration, health care policy, informatics, and population-based specialties as detailed in the DNP Essentials document
- CGEAN embraces the role of nurses prepared through PhD programs to expand knowledge development in relevant leadership and administrative areas to enhance practice effectiveness and outcomes (p. 3)

In 2012, CGEAN announced that "Until substantial research produces evidence for a specified number of practice hours, professional doctoral programs that build on the master's degree are expected to provide a minimum of 400 practice hours" (p. 2). Whether CGEAN guidelines are contradictory to total post-BSN hours required by the AACN/CCNE would then depend on the individual student's program of study at the master's and doctoral level.

The program of study for the DNP clinical executive should allow students to further develop their own leadership through introspection, coursework, clinical work, and mentorship. These types of educational experiences can be elemental, as the clinical executive tries to execute and provide for more quality health care. Furthermore, it will be critical for the DNP curriculum to have a heavy emphasis on business ethics as well as clinical ethics. The clinical executive may be one of a few individuals in senior leadership with a true understanding of the complexity of patient care, nurses' roles/responsibilities, and the requisite human and fiscal resources required for positive clinical outcomes. As the voice of nurses in the organization, the clinical executive needs to have political capital—a good reputation and irreproachable ethics. In order to fulfill one's fiduciary responsibilities, the clinical executive must also be knowledgeable and vigilant with regard to fiscal accountability.

Doctoral level nurse executives will be called upon to bring their respective organizations to a better position than where they found it. Ideally, the doctoral advanced nursing practice-educated clinical executive will: (a) earn the trust of one's organization; (b) be deeply engaged with nursing staff and/or employees; (c) earn legitimacy and mobilize one's own people around a focused agenda; (d) devote considerable efforts to developing one's employees and building the organization's collective leadership capabilities; and (e) strive for high performance in the organization while delicately balancing a high commitment to the institution (Eisenstat, Beer, Foote, Fredberg, & Norrgren, 2008). These requisite leadership skills, coupled with the knowledge to influence health care outcomes, afford doctoral-level clinical executives an opportunity to effect change like no other time in nursing's history.

At the end of the day, it is all about leadership. The clinical executive of tomorrow, with a doctoral advanced nursing practice education, plays a pivotal role in supporting an autonomous and professional nursing practice culture. Successful implementation of an empowered environment rests with the nurse leader's ability to create a constructive atmosphere, which involves the implementation of supportive infrastructures that encompass accountability, pursuit of excellence, and open communication. In this way, clinical nurses are allowed the autonomy to make decisions and foster practices in accordance with professional nursing standards. Thus, a progressive nurse leader can shape an institution through one's value system and passion for nursing. With this model, innovative care models will develop and flourish (Upenieks, 2003).

High-performing organizations and/or those organizations that aspire to become high-performing organizations will closely scrutinize leadership capacity (Wells & Hejna, 2009). Hospitals and health care institutions will be among them. Magnet hospitals, designated facilities that have been certified by the American Nurses Credentialing Center (ANCC) for their excellence in nursing practice, will continue to be recognized as institutions with superior measures of nursing job satisfaction and patient outcomes because of their distinguished organizational characteristics. These institutions will maintain well-qualified nurse executives in an organizational structure that emphasizes open participatory management and will use professional practice models for the delivery of nursing care. Strong leadership and advocacy for nursing offers an autonomous, self-managed, self-governed climate that allows nurses to fully practice their clinical expertise. Additionally, the burgeoning Planetree Model of Care[5] is an important new player in hospital/health care network certification, or recognition wave mostly started by the Magnet® Corporation. Planetree was founded by a patient, Angelica Thieriot, in the 1970s who had a bad experience while being hospitalized (Rovner, 2012). The Planetree Model focuses on patient-centered care that is built on the cultural transformation of an institution, patient activation, staff engagement, leadership development, performance improvement, and design services that support adaptive, healing environments, wellness, and enhancing the safety and nurturing of patients. Magnet, Planetree, and Nurses Improving Care for Healthsystem Elders (NCHE) recognized health care facilities as all institutions where executive nursing leadership is at the core of high-level health care innovation and delivery, and where advanced education can readily make the difference on both an institutional and systems level.

As clinical nurse executives acquire doctoral-level knowledge and competencies in greater numbers and with health care reform expanding every year, nurse leaders will be asked to participate on hospital boards, lead organizations, and provide consultation on various practice models and initiatives. The doctoral-level nurse executive will have the requisite knowledge, experience, and competencies to skillfully manage an array of complex organizational issues. In the future, we will see clinical executives with doctoral advanced nursing practice education in greater numbers as senior health care executives such as chief executive officer, chief operating officer, or chair of the Board of Trustees, as organizations begin to realize their value. As DNP-educated nurse executives improve health and health care outcomes through evidence-based practice, utilize knowledge related to evidence-based approaches for quality and safety improvement, and apply research processes to decision making, we will see innovation like never before.

■ THE DOCTORAL ADVANCED NURSING PRACTICE "EDUCATOR"

To meet current and projected nursing shortages, nursing education programs need to increase their capacity. However, these programs are faced with a *severe shortage of faculty*, particularly doctorally prepared faculty, making it difficult to expand. Furthermore, the already small pool of qualified faculty is rapidly shrinking—almost one third are older than 55 years (Benner, Sutphen, Leonard, & Day, 2009). The current system of doctoral education in nursing does not have the capacity to prepare the number of graduates necessary to replace retiring faculty, and does not have a sufficient number of nurse researchers to generate knowledge for the discipline (Potempa, Redman, & Anderson, 2008). Therefore, in the United States, the nursing profession is at an important crossroads that could determine the direction of nursing education and knowledge development. Equally important, will DNP graduates really be prepared to assume competent nurse educator roles for advanced practice programs? Who will generate the knowledge of the discipline? Furthermore, the current climate does not encourage young men and women to embrace the faculty role or the conduct of research in its broadest sense.

Current expectations of the tripartite nursing faculty role in relation to teaching, scholarship, and service are not realistic in advancing nursing science, clinical practice, or education. Nursing faculty juggle large teaching and service loads while attempting to engage in scholarship. For those nursing faculty who are actively involved in research, the juggling act is even more pronounced. In addition, few nursing faculty have formal practice appointments as part of their faculty role that allows them to stay clinically updated to perform their teaching. For example, many NP, nurse-midwifery, and nurse anesthesia faculty have outside practice obligations to maintain their clinical hours/expertise for specialty certification in addition to their full-time faculty appointments. Many advanced practice nurse faculty opt for this financial arrangement in order to gain additional compensation given the low salaries of nursing faculty. Efforts to recruit future faculty will continue to be futile unless faculty salaries are increased and brought in line with clinical salaries and teaching positions in other disciplines (Benner et al., 2009). Going forward, nursing faculty salaries must be reevaluated in order to compete with nonacademic positions available to doctoral-level nursing professionals. Nursing leaders need to look to their academic colleagues in male-dominated professions, such as business, engineering, and law, to seek solutions related to faculty compensation. Another recommendation is to tie market salaries to accreditation and create formal academic clinical partnerships, and practice arrangements in an effort to increase salaries and inform clinical teaching. In other words, formal faculty practice arrangements need to become the norm beyond academic health centers.

We are also concerned about whether DAPNs with DNPs who have academic appointments will be promoted or tenured in a clinical track or research track? If the faculty NP, for instance, needs to practice to maintain certification as well as conduct research in order to get tenure, how will this occur? We see three unfortunate scenarios. In scenario A, the faculty NP is not allowed on the tenure track because he/she did not complete a clinical dissertation or doctoral thesis. In this case, vast numbers of faculty NPs will be excluded from full membership in the academy or the professoriate. In scenario B, the DNP graduate *is* allowed on the tenure track, but because this faculty NP now has to produce the level of scholarship necessary for tenure *and* practice—not just for recertification, but to be competent and current in the graduate classroom—this faculty member is set up for failure. In scenario C, the DNP is not prepared to engage in the research/scholarship aspects of the role and has a

superficial understanding of the faculty role and responsibilities. There are unfortunately no easy answers for these dilemmas, but they are serious and require thoughtful consideration.

With the introduction of a critical mass of nursing educators with the DNP degree,
the profession has an opportunity to reexamine the various roles of nurse faculty and
create a model that encourages a model that plays to individual faculty's strengths. The
authors suggest three professorial roles: nurse scientist, educator clinician, and clinician educator. Nursing education must redefine the expectations of the nursing faculty
with a primary focus on research, teaching, or clinical. The doctoral advanced nursing practice educator is in a unique position to serve in the clinician educator role, as
they are able to integrate the knowledge they present in the classroom with a clinical
practice context. The question remains, however: Will DNP students obtain the educational theory and didactic content needed in order to be successful in the classroom
(in person and online)? With more than 30% of DNP graduates now going into academia, will DNP programs create options that do not entail extra courses for DAPNs who
want to teach other advanced practice students and require courses in pedagogy as
part of the curriculum (Zungolo, 2009)? Program evaluation, quality improvement, and
epidemiology curricula also need to be added to strengthen DNP program curricula.
These foundational steps are critical and must be expanded to reduce the gap between
research and practice and bring about reliable and sustainable practice improvement.
This preparation will strengthen the nursing profession's response to this national focus
on improving health care through innovation and quality measurement; however, more
engagement in these opportunities is needed (Johnson, Smith Glasgow, & Guimond,
2016). As we move forward, all DNP programs need to be sufficiently academically
rigorous with the appropriate course content to adequately study and address quality
improvement, access issues, and health promotion needs.

As Potempa and Tilden (2004) have identified, the role of the "PhD prepared nurse
scientist" is critical to generating knowledge in our discipline. Nursing deans need to
find ways to better support research-intensive nursing faculty at the DNP and PhD
levels, perhaps with more realistic teaching loads and service obligations in return for
high scholarly productivity. Rather than have research-active faculty engaged in clinical
teaching, for example, research-active faculty would be better served to have reduced
teaching loads and spend their time teaching nursing research at all levels (undergraduate, master's, and doctoral) and mentoring students in the conduct of research.
In doing so, we create an environment that fosters the mission of scholarly productivity and knowledge development for nursing faculty. Having research-focused faculty
teach both undergraduate and graduate students fosters the desire of young students to
obtain a research doctorate and conduct nursing research. The role of the nurse scientist
requires a change in expectations related to workload, faculty investment, research start-
up funds, and a requisite reward system for scholarly productivity. It is our assumption
that the nursing faculty members who are focused on research will be much more productive than faculty members required to participate in traditional tripartite (teaching,
service, and scholarship) roles. With the appropriate education and training on the conduct of research, both DNP and PhD nursing graduates have the potential to contribute
to the empirical evidence base of nursing.

The Carnegie Foundation for the Advancement of Teaching released the results
of the first national nursing education study in 30 years (Benner et al., 2009). The study
Educating Nurses: A Call for Radical Transformation explores the strengths and weaknesses in nursing education, and identifies the most effective practices for teaching
nursing and argues convincingly that nursing education must be reconstructed. Based
on this study, there is a need to address the specific educational demands of teaching

the complex practice of nursing and reconnect with the practice context of the nursing discipline. The DNP-prepared educator with advanced clinical knowledge and educational foundation to address these critical issues noted in the Carnegie Study. Furthermore, the study recommended that nursing educators make four shifts in their thinking about teaching and in their approaches to fostering student learning for the future:

1. *From a focus on covering decontextualized knowledge to an emphasis on teaching for a sense of salience, situated cognition, and action in particular situations*
   Many faculty organize their classes around lists of abstract theory, giving their students little or no indication about how to integrate the knowledge they present into practice. Nursing faculty should help students learn to apply nursing knowledge and science.
2. *From a sharp separation of clinical and classroom teaching to an integration of the two*
   Traditionally, there has been a sharp divide between classroom and clinical teaching. When faculty provide only simple, rudimentary examples or test students on elemental competencies, they may not be helping students to prepare for diverse, complex, real-life, stressful clinical situations.
3. *From an emphasis on critical thinking to an emphasis on clinical reasoning and multiple ways of thinking*
   Critical thinking alone cannot develop students' perceptual acuity or clinical imagination. Clinical imagination, which requires students to grasp the nature of patients' needs as they change over time, is needed, as well as critical, creative, and scientific reasoning.
4. *From an emphasis on professional socialization to an emphasis on formation*
   Experiential learning environments across the nursing curriculum are needed to support formation. Nursing education must focus on the formation of professional identity rather than on socialization (Benner et al.).

When one ponders the radical transformation that will be required for nursing education in the 21st century, the authors assert that the reconstruction of nursing education and a reconnection to practice will only be achieved by a diverse group of doctoral-level faculty, namely the nurse scientist, educator clinician, and clinician educator. The doctoral advanced nursing practice–trained educator is well suited to integrate the classroom content and the practice context. An innovative DNP program curriculum is needed that truly combines the practice emphasis with education-related content and their practical integration. Case Western Reserve University is one exemplar of this combined approach with a specific track in educational leadership for advanced practice nurses. The AACN has not yet endorsed the practice of the educator in the same way it has embraced the practice of the clinical executive within the design of the DNP degree; however, there is a greater recognition of the need for faculty competencies. As academics, we do not appear to value the faculty role when education-related content is elective. We are facing a critical nursing faculty shortage that will impact the profession and health of our nation. It is incumbent on us to let go of time-honored traditions, such as the current nursing education model that separates theory from practice, the need for extensive clinical practice before matriculating in doctoral programs, and the heavy teaching and service requirements of research-intensive doctoral-prepared faculty in order to move the discipline forward (Tilden & Potempa, 2003). Furthermore, the nurse educator role needs to be included in all doctoral programs in order for the nursing profession to meet current and projected nursing shortages. In our opinion, the AACN

Doctoral Essentials needs to embrace faculty/education competencies as a key essential much like the Jonas Foundation is embracing nursing education at the doctoral level.

■ SUMMARY

Clayton Christensen, heralded as the guru of innovation, describes disruptive innovation as a "process by which a product or service takes root initially in simple applications at the bottom of a market and then relentlessly moves 'up market,' eventually displacing established competitors" (2009, p. 1). In 2006, nursing scholars, using this term first coined for the business world, described the new DNP degree as a disruptive innovation (Hathaway, Jacob, Stegbauer, Thompson, & Graff, 2006). Ten years later, this vision for the DNP has not been realized. Although the numbers have increased, the impact is not as quantifiable. Dracup, Cronenwett, Meleis, and Benner (2005) feared the DNP would be a threat to the nursing discipline by diluting doctoral education, reducing the brain trust that pursues the PhD, and negatively impacting high quality nursing science. In 2016, AACN announced that DNP enrollment has increased 19.1% while PhD enrollment has decreased 3.2% (Deborah Trautman, personal communication, March 21, 2016). When one considers the impact of PhD-prepared faculty retirements in the next decade, it appears that, in the future, the academy will have a greater number of DNP-prepared faculty versus PhD-prepared faculty if this trend continues. It appears as though the DNP is taking nurses away from an academic research career. It is not known if these DNP-prepared faculty will seek a PhD, research doctoral degree post-DNP.

The question remains if the nursing profession should create DNP-to—PhD programs for this *cadre of faculty and/or imbed more research content and skills in the DNP degree which are relevant to the practitioner scholar.* There is also the concern about the uneven quality and rigor in DNP programs. We have heard the final scholarly outcome (i.e. capstones, theses, scholarly projects, clinical or practice dissertations) vary from a pretest/posttest with a poster presentation to complex retrospective studies with large data sets and a final defense. As a profession, we need to come to terms with the goal of the degree, the appropriate amount of epidemiology, statistics, and methods courses, as well as rigor. DNP scholarly projects should focus largely on quality improvement, access issues, and health promotion. Doctoral nursing faculty supervising DNP students should encourage scholarly projects directly focusing on the triple aim of Institute of Healthcare Improvement (IHI) to deliver quality care, improve outcomes, and reduce cost are particularly relevant to health care systems. DNP students need to be educated in "basic science, translation, implementation, teaming, writing, collaborating, and leadership capabilities that are based in evidence and suited to the evolving market" (Terhaar, Taylor, & Sylvia, 2016, p. 8). We concur that the DNP degree will be shaped by the outcome data that will emerge as scholars study these graduates and their impact on the health care system; and by the rapidly changing health care consumer marketplace. With 30 million or more individuals entering the U.S. health care system, DNP graduates are particularly positioned to capitalize on this opportunity to provide more high-quality, effective care. The DNP's success and impact in academia is less clear.

Although supportive of the BSN-to-DNP academic progression model, there is a concern that the transition to the entry-level doctorate for advanced practice and possible dissolution of the master's degree over time may create a decline in overall numbers of new NPs entering practice (Bloch, 2007; Dreher & Gardner, 2009; Ford, 2008). In an attempt to increase the number of NPs, the Obama administration has provided: (a) $30 million to begin training an additional 600 NPs including providing incentives for part-time students to become full time and complete their education sooner; and (b) $15 million to establish 10 new NP-led clinics, which assist in the training of NPs, are staffed by NPs, and provide comprehensive primary health care services to populations living in medically underserved communities (HealthReform.Gov, 2010). This is important when NP roles are expected to grow at an extraordinary rate due to the Patient Protection and Affordable Care Act (PPACA; Auerbach, 2012; Van Vleet & Paradise, 2015). As our medical and health system starts to shift more visibly to a preventive care model, the DAPNs have an opportunity to seize the day. The DAPNs of today, tomorrow, and the future will be the primary generator of "practice knowledge" and "practice-based evidence nursing knowledge" that focuses on finding solutions to real clinical or organizational problems in the field (Dreher, 2010, 2013). The recent AACN (2015b) white paper on the DNP has clarified:

> Graduates of both research- and practice-focused doctoral programs are pre-pared to generate new knowledge. However, research-focused graduates are prepared to generate knowledge through rigorous research and statistical methodologies that may be broadly applicable or generalizable; practice-focused graduates are prepared to generate new knowledge through innovation of practice change, the translation of evidence, and the implementation of quality improvement processes in specific practice settings, systems, or with specific populations to improve health or health outcomes. New knowledge generated through practice innovation, for example, could be of value to other practice 2 settings. This new knowledge is considered transferrable but is not considered generalizable. (pp. 2–3)

This clarification from the 2006 essentials document is progress in the recognition that the DNP can contribute new knowledge, even if classified as "practice knowledge: to the discipline. The early days of some DNP students being told "you cannot call it research!" appears to be fading away as the profession better discerns the domain of knowledge development for the DNP degree. The authors foresee DAPNs creating new practice knowledge and practice evidence for the discipline, and then efficiently translating and disseminating it to practice. Nurses engaged in doctoral advanced nursing practice need to be visible, bold, innovative, data driven, and outcome oriented. The ultimate value of this degree will be the evidence that the DAPRN or DAPN improves the health of individuals (Terhaar et al., 2016). In summary, the role of the DAPRN or DAPN, no matter the setting or job description, has the potential to improve health outcomes. It is also equally as critical that the DAPRN or DAPN be a clinical scholar and conduct rigorous practice-based and evidence-based projects and disseminate their work. This requires leadership from deans and faculty to refine curricula to meet the needs of society so the DAPRN or DAPN are educated to deliver quality care, improve outcomes, reduce cost, and be welcome in the academy as full members. This also requires leadership from nurse executives to provide the time and resources for DAPRNs or DAPNs to engage in formal clinical inquiry and contribute to the evidence base in our discipline in their institutions and beyond; as well as, lead system wide change. Health care system and chief nursing officers' support is critical for the advocacy of DAPRN or DAPN's scholarly release time and increased compensation expected with a higher level degree, increased knowledge, and expanded skill set (Melnyk, 2013; Nichols, O'Connor, & Dunn, 2014). Finally, we need to continue to work diligently to implement the Future of Nursing Report:

■ *THE FUTURE OF NURSING: LEADING CHANGE, ADVANCING HEALTH*

Committee on the Robert Wood Johnson Foundation Initiative on the Future of Nursing at the IOM, chaired by Donna E. Shalala, president of the University of Miami, was released. Highlights of this report with relevance for this text include the following:

1. Include a nurse educator role in all master's and doctoral programs;
2. Increase emphasis on global health and knowledge development at all educational levels;
3. Cultivate disciplinary knowledge across all levels of curricula based on an understanding of the science of the discipline and the scientific process;
4. Develop "scientifically aware" nurse clinicians who will collaborate with nurse scientists to move research to the bedside. Focus on "evidence-creating nursing," the direct collaboration between nurse clinicians and nurse scientists.
5. Reengineer the DNP to include the conduct of research in the form of a practice dissertation (Smith Glasgow, Dunphy, & Mainous, 2010, G8–G9).

■ CRITICAL THINKING QUESTIONS

1. *What core competencies differentiate the master's-prepared advanced practice nurse from the doctoral advanced practice nurse?*
2. *How should DNP programs incorporate technology and knowledge management in their respective curricula?*
3. *Christensen, Grossman, and Hwang in* The Innovator's Prescription: A Disruptive Solution for Health Care *(2008) state, "nurse practitioners practicing in retail clinics, should disrupt the precision medicine portion of the physician's practice." Discuss the role of a NP in retail clinics and other forms of disruptive innovation.*
4. *Describe the role of the doctoral advanced nursing practice "clinical executive" of the future. What specific competencies does the doctoral advanced nursing practice clinical executive require?*
5. *How can a progressive doctoral-level nurse leader shape an institution through one's value system and passion for nursing?*
6. *Today, many nursing faculty are divorced from clinical practice. How can the doctoral advanced nursing practice "educator" change the current system and reconnect with the practice context of the nursing discipline?*
7. *What are the benefits and risks of the doctoral advanced nursing practice "educator" in academia? Please cite benefits and risks to the individual DNP educator and to the nursing profession as a whole.*
8. *Describe how the academy can develop the productive nurse scientist of the future.*
9. *What effect will the transition to the entry-level doctorate for advanced practice and the dissolution of the master's degree over time have on the nursing profession?*
10. *What do you see as the role of the DNP-prepared nurse of the future? What added-value will the DNP-prepared nurse bring to health care?*

■ NOTES

1. In the forthcoming new Doctor of Nursing Practice in Advanced Clinical Care at The College of New Rochelle we have a course titled "Psychosocial, Behavioral, and Spiritual Interventions in

Advanced Clinical Care" (NURS 821), which will focus on implementation of these advanced social/behavioral interventions.

2. Some BSN-to-DNP programs are including post-master's DNP students in the same coursework. In some instances this may be appropriate, and other times, this kind of course scheduling does not recognize the advanced skills an experienced APRN already has nor recognize the different content needs a post BSN-to-DNP has. We have heard from very frustrated post-master's DNP students who have experienced this. When this is done simply for cost savings, it seems very inappropriate.

3. To Err is Human, Building a Safer Health System, 1999; *Crossing the Quality Chasm: A New Health System for the 21st century.* 2001; *Keeping Patients Safe: Transforming the Work Environment of Nurses,* 2003, Washington, DC: National Academies Press, 2001.

4. The nonclinical degree DNP is not permitted in New York State, which mandates that the DNP only have a clinical, not organizational, focus.

5. Complete list of 2016 Planetree Certified Partners: http://planetree.org/wp-content/uploads/2015/01/Planetree-Partners.pdf

■ REFERENCES

American Association of Colleges of Nursing. (2006). *Essentials of doctoral education for advanced nursing practice.* Retrieved from http://www.aacn.nche.edu/dnp/Essentials.pdf

American Association of Colleges of Nursing. (2015a). *2015 annual report: Leading excellence and innovation in academic nursing.* Retrieved from http://www.aacn.nche.edu/publications/AnnualReport15.pdf

American Association of Colleges of Nursing. (2015b). *The doctor of nursing practice: Current issues and clarifying recommendations, report from the Task Force on the Implementation of the DNP.* Retrieved from http://www.aacn.nche.edu/aacn-publications/white-papers/DNP-Implementation-TF-Report-8-15.pdf

American Medical Association. (2009). *AMA scope of practice data sets: Nurse practitioners.* Chicago, IL: Author.

Auerbach, D. (2012). Will the NP workforce grow in the future? New forecasts and implications for healthcare. *Medical Care, 50*(7), 606–610.

Benner, P., Sutphen, M., Leonard, V., & Day, L. (2009). *Educating nurses: A call for radical transformation.* Stanford, CA: The Carnegie Foundation for the Advancement of Teaching.

Bloch, J. (2007). *The DNP/DrNP degree as entry into NP practice: Is this nursing's answer to eliminate disparities in health care access for vulnerable populations?* Paper presented at The Practice Doctorate: Where is it Headed? The First National Conference on the Doctor of Nursing Practice: Meanings and Models, Annapolis, MD, March 28–30.

Christensen, C. (1997). *The innovator's dilemma: When new technologies cause great firms to fail.* Cambridge, MA: Harvard Business Press.

Christensen, C. (2009). Clayton Christensen, other key concepts: Disruptive innovation. Retrieved from http://www.claytonchristensen.com/key-concepts

Christensen, C., Grossman, J., & Hwang, J. (2008). *The innovator's prescription: A disruptive solution for health care.* New York, NY: McGraw-Hill Professional.

Conant, R. (2010). Headlines from the hill: Lawmakers need to hear from nurses on home health care. *American Nurse Today, 5*(7), 18.

Council on Graduation Education for Administration in Nursing. (2011). CGEAN position statement on the educational preparation of nurse executives and nurse managers. Retrieved from http://www.cgean.org/assets/docs/cgean_positon_on_educational_preparation.pdf

Council on Graduate Education for Administration in Nursing. (2012). Criteria for practice hours in master's and professional doctoral programs for nurse executives and leaders. Retrieved from http://www .cgean.org/assets/docs/position_statement_on_practice_hours_04-2012.pdf

Defenbaugh, N., & Chikotas, N. E. (2016). The outcome of interprofessional education: Integrating communication studies into a standardized patient experience for advanced practice nursing students. *Nursing Education in Practice, 16*(1), 176–181.

Dracup, K., & Bryan-Brown, C. (2005). Doctor of nursing practice: MRI or total body scan. *American Journal of Critical Care, 14*(4), 278–281.

Dracup, K., Cronenwett, L., Meleis, A. I., & Benner, P. E. (2005). Reflections on the doctorate of nursing practice. *Nursing Outlook, 53,* 177–182.

Dreher, H. M. (2009a). *The doctor of nursing practice degree in the U.S.: History & politics, problems & progress.* Paper presented at the International Conference on Professional Doctorates, London, England, November 9–10.

Dreher, H. M. (2009b). How do RNs today best stay informed? Do we need knowledge management? *Holistic Nursing Practice, 23*(5), 263–266.

Dreher, H. M. (2016). Next steps toward practice knowledge development: An emerging epistemology in nursing. In M. D. Dahnke & H. M. Dreher (Eds.), *Philosophy of science for nursing practice: Concepts and application* (pp. 355–391). New York, NY: Springer Publishing.

Dreher, H. M. (2013). Differentiating clinical evidence and clinical knowledge. *Clinical Scholars Review,* 6(1), 9–12.

Dreher, H. M., & Gardner, M. (2009). *With the rise of the DNP, who will conduct primary care research?* Paper presented at the Second National Conference on the Doctor of Nursing Practice: The Dialogue Continues…, Hilton Head Island, SC, March 24–27.

Dreher, H. M., & Montgomery, K. (2009). Let's call it "doctoral" advanced practice nursing. *The Journal of Continuing Education in Nursing, 40*(12), 1–2.

Eisenstat, R., Beer, M., Foote, N., Fredberg, T., & Norrgren, F. (2008). The uncompromising leader. *Harvard Business Review, 86*(7–8), 50–57.

Fischman, J. (2005). Who will take care of you? *U.S. World News & Report,* January 31/February 7, 46.

Ford, J. (2008). Editorial: DNP a bad idea. *Advanceweb.com.* Retrieved from http://community.advance web.com/blogs/np_1/archive/2008/07/23/editorial-on-dnp.aspx

Hathaway, D., Jacob, S., Stegbauer, C., Thompson, C., & Graff, C. (2006). The practice doctorate: Perspectives of early adopters. *Journal of Nursing Education, 45*(12), 487–496.

HealthReform.Gov. (2010). *Fact sheet: Key features of the Affordable Care Act by year.* U.S. Department of Health & Human Services. Retrieved from https://web.archive.org/web/20121017201051/ http://www.healthreform.gov/newsroom/primarycareworkforce.html

Institute of Medicine. (2010). *The future of nursing: Leading change, advancing health.* Washington, DC: National Academies Press.

Isaacs, S., & Jellinek, P. (2012). Accept no substitute: A report on scope of practice. *The Physician's Foundation: Empowering physicians, improving healthcare.* Retrieved from http://www.physicians foundation.org/uploads/default/A_Report_on_Scope_of_Practice.pdf

Johnson, C., Smith Glasgow, M. E., & Guimond, M. E. (2016). Quality improvement research methods. In J. Bloch, M. Clark, & M. Courtney (Eds.), *Practice-based clinical inquiry in nursing: Looking beyond traditional methods for PhD and DNP research* (pp. 69–89). New York, NY: Springer Publishing.

Melynk, B. M. (2013). Distinguishing the preparation and roles of doctor of philosophy and doctor of nursing practice graduates: National implications for academic curricula and health care systems. *Journal of Nursing Education, 52*(8), 442–448.

Mompoint-Williams, D., Brooks, A., Lee, L., Watts, P., & Moss, J. (2014). Using high fidelity simulation to prepare advanced practice nursing students. *Clinical Simulation in Nursing, 10*(1), e5–e10.

Moore, A., Judge, D., & Angelini, D. (2013). MDs vs. NPs in primary care . . . The conflict continues. *New England Journal of Medicine Journal Watch.* Retrieved from http://www.jwatch.org/ na31192/2013/06/05/mds-vs-nps-primary-care-conflict-continues

Mundinger, M., Kane, R., Lenz, E., Totten, A., Tsai, W., Cleary, P., . . . Shelanski, M. L. (2000). Primary care outcomes in patients treated by nurse practitioners or physicians: A randomized trial. *Journal of the American Medical Association, 283,* 59–68.

Naisbitt, J. (1982). *Megatrends.* New York, NY: Warner Books.

Nichols, C., O'Connor, N., & Dunn, D. (2014). Exploring early and future use of DNP prepared nurses within healthcare organizations. *The Journal of Nursing Administration, 44*(2), 74–78.

Obama, B. (2009). Remarks by the president on the "Education To Innovate" campaign. Retrieved from https://www.whitehouse.gov/the-press-office/remarks-president-education-innovate-campaign

Pho, K. (2013). How I would end the war between nurse practitioners and doctors. *Kevin's Take blog.* Retrieved from http://www.kevinmd.com/blog/2013/05/war-nurse-practitioners-doctors.html

Potempa, K. M., Redman, R. W., & Anderson, C. A. (2008). Capacity for the advancement of nursing science: Issues and challenges. *Journal of Professional Nursing, 24*(6), 329–336.

Potempa, K. M., & Tilden, V. (2004). Building high impact science: The dean as innovator. *Journal of Nursing Education, 43*(11), 502–505.

Rovner, J. (2012). By putting patients first, hospital tries: To make care more personal. *npr.org: shots, health-care news from npr.* Retrieved from http://www.npr.org/sections/health-shots/2012/05/23/153442476/by-putting-patients-first-hospital-tries-to-make-care-more-personal

Schreiner, J. (2014). DNP discussions: Doctor v. doctor. *Advance, advanceweb.com.* Retrieved from http://community.advanceweb.com/blogs/np_7/archive/2014/07/09/doctor-vs-doctor.aspx

Smith Glasgow, M. E., Dunphy, L. M., & Mainous, R. O. (2010). *Innovative nursing educational curriculum for the 21st century: Transformational models of nursing across different settings.* Washington, DC: National Academies Press.

Stanik-Hutt, J. (2008). Debunking the need to certify the DNP degree. *The Journal for Nurse Practitioners, 4*(10), 739.

Summers, L. (2010). How the health care reform law affects APRNs. *The American Nurse, 42*(3), 16.

Ten years of progress: The council for the advancement of comprehensive care. (2010, Spring). *The Academic Nurse: The Journal of Columbia University School of Nursing and its Alumni,* 20–27.

Terhaar, M. F., Taylor, L. A., & Sylvia, M. L. (2016). The doctor of nursing practice: From start-up to impact. *Nursing Education Perspectives, 37*(1), 3–9.

Tilden, V., & Potempa, K. (2003). The impact of nursing science: A litmus test. *Nursing Research, 52*(5), 275.

Toffler, A. (1971). *Future shock.* New York, NY: Bantam Books.

Upenieks, V. V. (2003). What constitutes effective leadership? Perceptions of magnet and nonmagnet nurse leaders. *The Journal of Nursing Administration, 33*(9), 456–467.

Van Vleet, A., & Paradise, J. (2015). Tapping nurse practitioners to meet rising demand for primary care. Retrieved from http://kff.org/medicaid/issue-brief/tapping-nurse-practitioners-to-meet-rising-demand-for-primary-care

Wells, W., & Hejna, W. (2009). Developing leadership talent in healthcare organizations. *Healthcare Financial Management, 63*(1), 66–69.

Zungolo, E. (2009). *The DNP and the faculty role: Issues and challenges.* Paper presented at the Second National Conference on the Doctor of Nursing Practice: The Dialogue Continues…, Hilton Head Island, SC, March 24–27.

Reflective Response 1

Suzanne S. Prevost

This final chapter by Dreher and Smith Glasgow raises several important questions and challenges for faculty, graduates, and employers of Doctor of Nursing Practice (DNP)-prepared advanced practice nurses. The rapid expansion of DNP programs, from less than 10 in 2005 to 269 in 2014 (American Association of Colleges of Nursing, 2015), demonstrates the broad acceptance of this phenomenon by nursing faculty and administrators across the United States. Likewise, the exploding volume of DNP student applications and enrollment provides evidence that this movement is enthusiastically embraced by students and practicing nurses, as well as those in academe. It is both intriguing and challenging to observe such a positive response to a nursing innovation, while there is still minimal evidence to support its effectiveness.

Why are we moving forward with such blind faith? Perhaps this reaction is based on the widespread acceptance of the inadequacies of our existing health care delivery systems and the consensus that we need new models of health care delivery and better-prepared knowledge workers on the front lines. We must, however, instill a sense of urgency among DNP faculty and students to work cohesively and intentionally to build this body of evidence. The authors suggest that the emergence of new DNP roles will depend on graduates presenting employers with measurable claims of what they have acquired in their education. I would challenge these graduates to go beyond measurable claims to the presentation of significant results. In this case, significance is not limited to statistical significance but might be equally compelling in the form of clinical or economic significance.

I applaud Drs. Dreher and Smith Glasgow for their clear delineation of the doctoral advanced practice roles of practitioner, clinical executive, and educator in this text. Although the practitioner and clinical executive roles are becoming widely accepted, some controversy remains regarding the optimal preparation and roles of DNP-prepared nurse educators (Florczak, 2010).

The rapid development of doctoral level advanced practitioner programs across the United States demonstrates the growing national sentiment favoring this level of preparation for advanced practitioners. However, I concur with the authors that the variability in DNP program quality, specifically in relation to the level and intensity of advanced clinical practice experiences, remains a valid concern. Most faculty and administrators of DNP programs have implemented and documented adherence to the minimum clinical hour requirements set forth in the 2006 AACN essentials document as they prepare their graduates for certification examinations and prepare their programs for accreditation visits. However, the specific nature of those clinical experiences, the content within them, and the levels of supervision remain widely divergent. More specific delineation of what constitutes minimal clinical experiences for master's level advanced practice nurses and how doctoral level clinical experiences exceed this standard are needed. The authors of this chapter provide excellent recommendations to guide future applicants and DNP students to critically assess and evaluate the clinical content of DNP programs in this regard.

The value of doctoral preparation for clinical executives seems to be less controversial. A totally new skill set is required to succeed in current and future executive level leadership positions. Our history of promoting the most beloved nurse clinicians into such leadership positions will not serve the profession well in environments of increasing competition to produce clinical and financial outcomes consistent with constantly rising benchmark targets. Dreher and Smith Glasgow advocate for a combined high-tech/high-touch approach in the preparation of practitioners. This combination is equally important for clinical executives. Advanced competencies in emotional intelligence, appreciative inquiry, and motivation must be combined with a high degree of technologic proficiency, financial acumen, and political savvy. Awareness and understanding of, and adaptability to new technologies will be essential because these decisions and applications increasingly influence system efficiencies and the financial bottom line. I agree with the authors that these leaders will not be limited to traditional positions in nursing administration, but will also be well suited for a variety of chief executive and interdisciplinary leadership positions, as well as offices and board positions in professional organizations and community service agencies. DNP faculty should challenge these students to dream big and invest at least a portion of their clinical practicum hours in mentored leadership experiences beyond traditional clinical nursing administration.

Expectations regarding the role of DNP graduates as educators have evolved over the past decade. Early in the development of DNP programs, many opponents expressed the concern that DNP programs would divert potential PhD candidates and therefore contribute to the growing shortage of nursing faculty (Meleis & Dracup, 2005). Of course, this concern was predicated on the assumption that DNP graduates could not or should not be considered for nursing faculty positions. It is important to note that the AACN Essentials document states, "the basic DNP curriculum does not prepare the graduate for a faculty teaching role any more than the PhD curriculum does. Graduates of either program planning a faculty career will need (additional) preparation" (AACN, p. 7).

As DNP programs proliferate, the DNP-prepared advanced nursing practice educator who is actively engaged in practice will be the candidate of choice to fill these DNP faculty positions. Likewise, these practitioners will be better prepared to teach undergraduate nursing students, especially in clinical settings, than many PhD-prepared researchers. In publications, including the 2010 report from the Institute of Medicine (IOM) titled *A Summary of the February 2010 Forum on the Future of Nursing*, some nurse leaders advocate for the recognition of nursing education as a specialized area within advanced nursing practice which could be taught in DNP tracks specifically designed for educators. The authors of this chapter have been leaders in this charge. I agree with their recommendation that the AACN doctoral essentials should reconsider and embrace faculty/education competencies.

Dreher and Smith Glasgow raise important questions regarding workload expectations and compensation for these advanced practitioner educators. Their suggestion of a new differentiated model, including the roles of nurse scientist, educator clinician, and clinician educator, offers an innovative approach to differentiating and clarifying academic role expectations. Colleges of nursing, such as the University of Kentucky, have demonstrated value for DNP-prepared educators as essential leaders in both teaching and practice initiatives, by refining compensation models for these faculty members. In addition to incorporating practice hours into the faculty workload, compensation for practice activities should be consistent with the market salaries for other practitioners in the region.

The role of clinical scholar or nurse scientist is probably the most controversial for doctoral advanced practice nurses. For decades, many nurses have been instrumental members of clinical research teams, especially in teams conducting pharmaceutical and medical device trials. Unfortunately, these study coordinators are rarely given high-level decision-making authority, nor are they usually given substantive credit or compensation in the dissemination of patents or other products of those studies. Formal and specific doctoral preparation will help to legitimize this important nursing role. The role of the DNP-prepared clinical scholar is innovative and fills an important niche in health-oriented research, development, and scholarship.

Dreher and Smith Glasgow raise additional questions that merit discussion. Should the profession create DNP to PhD programs and/or imbed more research content and skills in the DNP degree to better prepare nurse educators? We have recently seen both of these trends evolve in the state of Alabama. My response is not either/or; but yes and yes. The authors also question whether DNP-prepared educators and scholars will achieve tenure in the academy. The answers to these questions may also be embedded in Christensen's notion of "disruptive innovation." Early in the DNP movement, the most common response to these questions was "No." Similarly, 20 years ago, most nursing faculty responded "No," when asked whether nursing courses could be taught effectively online. Time changes things. As Christensen would say, when the disruptive DNP innovation moves up market it will displace the established competitors. Or in this case, it will gain the respect of the new majority rather than be inhibited by those who cling to traditional models of nursing practice, education, and research.

Health care and education are changing rapidly. Nursing educators and practitioners must keep an open mind and search for new solutions to keep pace and succeed in such dynamic environments. The potential for success in education, scholarship, and the tenure process may be influenced more by individual intellect, talent, and persistence than the type of doctoral program, if all candidates are given equal consideration and opportunities. I encourage DNP students and graduates to go forth, select programs that provide optimal preparation for the future, lead clinical innovations, and document the evidence to show the world the important contributions of DNP-prepared nurses. I also challenge established nursing leaders to reframe our traditional definitions of significance, productivity, and effectiveness to embrace and support these "disruptive" yet progressive practitioners, clinical executives, educators, and clinical scholars.

■ REFERENCES

American Association of Colleges of Nursing. (2006). Essentials of doctoral education for advanced nursing practice. Retrieved from http://www.aacn.nche.edu/dnp/Essentials.pdf

American Association of Colleges of Nursing. (2015). *Leading excellence and innovation in academic nursing: 2015 annual report*. Retrieved from http://www.aacn.nche.edu/publications/AnnualReport15.pdf

Florczak, K. L. (2010). Research and the doctor of nursing practice: A cause for consternation. *Nursing Science Quarterly, 23*(1), 13–17.

Institute of Medicine. (2010). *A summary of the February 2010 forum on the future of nursing education*. Washington, DC: National Academies Press.

Meleis, A., & Dracup, K. (2005). The case against the DNP: History, timing, substance, and marginalization. *The Online Journal of Issues in Nursing, 10*(3). Retrieved from http://www.nursingworld.org/MainMenuCategories/ANAMarketplace/ANAPeriodicals/OJIN/TableofContents/Volume102005/No3Sept05/tpc28_216026.aspx

Reflective Response 2

Margaret Slota

Dreher and Smith Glasgow note that although the doctor of nursing practice (DNP) degree was originally considered a *disruptive innovation* and has a significant increase in the number of graduates in recent years, "ten years later, this vision for the DNP has not been realized...the impact is not as quantifiable." Our essential challenge in DNP academic education is to identify and measure outcomes, which differentiate the practice of nurses in advanced nursing roles prepared at the master's degree level compared to those educated at the doctoral level. Exploring the future and unlimited possibilities for innovative DNP roles requires that we quantify the DNP students' or doctorally prepared nurses' impact on practice. The Institute of Medicine (IOM) recommended doubling the number of doctoral prepared nurses in the United States by 2020 (IOM, 2010). Although the number of DNP programs and enrollment has substantially increased, PhD program enrollment has been maintained. (American Association of Colleges of Nurses [AACN], 2015). As nurse scientists/researchers generate knowledge, DNP graduates in their respective roles as practitioners, executives, faculty, and to-be-determined innovative roles are needed as leaders in facilitating the translation of research into "safe, high-quality, and cost-effective care" (Redman, Pressler, Furspan, & Potempa, 2015; Smeltzer et al., 2015). *It is essential that academic faculty facilitate transformative education and continued development of nursing science in order to help students develop creative clinical reasoning to expand the roles and impact of DNP scholars. Transformative learning is key in differentiating doctoral level practice.*

The authors' comment that there is "uneven quality and rigor in DNP programs" is very concerning and, as such, may derail efforts to promote acceptance of the DNP graduate as a scholar, capable of contributing evidence to continued growth and translation of nursing science. DNP academic administrators have a responsibility to ensure that transformative learning occurs during DNP education, so that students develop skill in scholarly activities, and quality and rigor are supported throughout the academic program.

DNP graduates exit doctoral education as scholar-practitioners (McClintock, 2004a, 2004b). Their education needs to be grounded in theory and research evidence to inform their practice and encourage initiative. If they study with a community of scholars and select topics congruent with their own interest and values, they gain the ability to solve problems creatively and to disseminate their findings and innovative solutions. Problem-solving skills needs to be developed and applied not only to course assignments, but also to practice settings. The *Future of Nursing* document (IOM, 2010) included two recommendations specifically germane to this discussion of DNP scholar-practitioners: (a) develop "scientifically aware" nurse clinicians who will collaborate with nurse scientists to move research to the bedside. Focus on "Evidence-Creating Nursing," the direct collaboration between nurse clinicians and nurse scientists and (b) reengineer the DNP to include the conduct of research in the form of a practice dissertation (Smith Glasgow, Dunphy, & Mainous, 2010). In my opinion, these are essential.

For the scholar–practitioner, metacognition is an essential meaning-making activity involving reflection in-action and reflection on-action (Schön, 1983, 1987) as related to professional contexts rich in teachable moments and challenging dilemmas. The initial process occurs through critical reflection about disorienting dilemmas. The concept of reflective practice has generated other tools and methods to analyze and reflect on errors, dissatisfaction, and outcomes in health care practice, resulting in improvements in the quality of care. At the metacognitive level, the scholar-practitioners' analysis of their practice, especially as they consider what decisions they made and what caused them to make those decisions, enables them to access knowledge that often operates at an intuitive level. In assigning meaning to their professional and educational experiences, they acknowledge their significance and inform their developing practice. A clinician who has developed awareness of metacognition is better situated to reflect on the possible consequences of a specific action, and make valuable and practical contributions. Foreseeable consequences can be prevented, or managed and therefore do not result in unintended consequences. Complex organizations or complex systems are often characterized by "unknown unknowns." A DNP who has developed metacognition will be able to bridge the unknown gap and be able to demonstrate that some unknowns are actually known,and therefore can be prevented, or the consequences resulting from an action can be mitigated.

Limited research has been published concerning transformative learning in doctoral students. Transformative learning, discussed by Mezirow (1991, 2000) and others, generally refers to learning experiences resulting in a transformational outcome, a change in worldview or perspective. Taylor (1998, 2007, 2008) conducted systematic reviews of completed studies related to transformative learning in higher education, its relationship to learner-centered teaching, and the impact of context. Stevens-Long, Schapiro, and McClintock (2004a) conducted a study that sought to develop an integrated understanding of transformative learning among graduate students. Participants in their study reported more perceptive and complex thinking, capability for multiple perspectives, ability to appreciate research and theory, more tolerance and confidence, and expanded consciousness. In respect to the impact of graduate education on their behaviors, they described themselves as being continuous learners, more communicative, and resilient. Behavior changes indicated that the students were acting on their changed perspectives, not just thinking about them. Participants identified key factors in their transformative learning –interactive learning, self-reflection and self-direction, interpersonal relationships with faculty and peers, and curricular content that led to a transformation in perspective and worldview. Most importantly, the self-directed study in the program evaluated may have created a disorienting dilemma for the students, as they were not told what to do by faculty. The authors concluded that doctoral students experienced multiple learning outcomes, beyond intellectual development, which they attributed to transformative learning because of the changes in perspective.

We must ensure that DNP curricula and learning processes support transformative outcomes and multidisciplinary/collaborative learning. AACN's practice doctorate statement (2004) focuses on four aspects of scholarship that are salient to academic nursing—discovery, teaching, applications in clinical practice, and integration of ideas from nursing and other disciplines. Students enter doctoral education with varying academic experiences and skills. In particular, some students have experienced a long gap between completion of a bachelor of science in nursing (BSN) or master of science in nursing (MSN) and initiation of doctoral study. Their academic writing skills may not be strong, particularly if their MSN program was practice focused, and they are accustomed to point and click documentation. DNP students are required to *synthesize* a large body of knowledge to gain knowledge in the DNP Essentials (AACN, 2006) and translate evidence into practice. I agree with the authors that we must *"imbed more research content and skills in the DNP degree"* and ensure, with certainty, the rigor that is required to produce quality outcomes with projects that are strong and sustainable.

Even when highly clinically competent, many advanced practice nurses lack the competence and confidence to showcase their expertise, negotiate with strong and challenging stakeholders, analyze big data, develop comprehensive business models, facilitate structured decision making, and impact the delivery of care at the systems level. The skills to do so, gained during DNP study, can assist graduates to practice at a doctoral level, and create new roles and outcomes that are quantifiable and transferable. Our curricula need to be engaging, self-directed with faculty facilitation of learning, transformative, and interdisciplinary, allowing DNP students to critically evaluate their experiential learning, create links between prior knowledge and new information thereby scaffolding learning, apply the new knowledge in a practice setting, and reflect on the outcomes. In this way, we can begin to measure quantifiable outcomes that differentiate doctoral level practice.

■ REFERENCES

American Association of Colleges of Nursing. (2004). *AACN position statement on the practice doctorate in nursing*. Washington, DC: Author. Retrieved from http://www.aacn.nche.edu/publications/position/DNPpositionstatement.pdf

American Association of Colleges of Nursing. (2006). *The essentials of doctoral education for advanced nursing practice*. Retrieved from http://www.aacn.nche.edu/publications/position/DNPEssentials.pdf

American Association of Colleges of Nursing. (2015). *The doctor of nursing practice: Current issues and clarifying recommendations report from the Task Force on the implementation of the DNP*. Retrieved from http://www.aacn.nche.edu/aacn-publications/white-papers/DNP-Implementation-TF-Report-8-15.pdf

Institute of Medicine. (2010). *The future of nursing: Leading change, advancing health*. Washington, DC: National Academies Press.

McClintock, C. (2004a). Scholar practitioner model. In A. DiStefano, K. Rudestam, & R. Silverman (Eds.), *Encyclopedia of Distributed Learning* (pp. 394–397). Retrieved from http://sk.sagepub.com/reference/distributedlearning/n134.xml

McClintock, C. (2004b). The scholar-practitioner model. In A. DiStefano, K. Rudestam, & R. Silverman (Eds.), *Encyclopedia of distributed learning* (pp. 393–405). Thousand Oaks, CA: Sage.

Mezirow, J. (1991). *Transformative dimensions of adult learning*. San Francisco, CA: Jossey-Bass.

Mezirow, J. (Ed.). (2000). *Learning as transformation: Critical perspectives on a theory in progress*. San Francisco, CA: Jossey-Bass.

Redman, R. W., Pressler, S. J., Furspan, P., & Potempa, K. (2015). Nurses in the United States with a practice doctorate: Implications for leading in the current context of health care. *Nursing Outlook, 63*(2), 124–129.

Schön, D. A. (1983). *The reflective practitioner: How professionals think in action*. New York, NY: Basic Books.

Schön, D. A. (1987). *Educating the reflective practitioner.* San Francisco, CA: Jossey-Bass.

Smeltzer, S. C., Sharts-Hopko, N. C., Cantrell, M. A., Heverly, M. A., Nthenge, S., & Jenkinson, A. (2015). A profile of U.S. nursing faculty in research- and practice-focused doctoral education. *Journal of Nursing Scholarship, 47*(2), 178–185.

Smith Glasgow, M. E., Dunphy, L. M., & Mainous, R. O. (2010). Innovative nursing educational curriculum for the 21st century. In *the future of nursing: Leading change, advancing health* (pp. G8–G12). Committee on the Robert Wood Johnson Foundation Initiative on the Future of Nursing at the Institute of Medicine. Washington, DC: National Academy of Sciences. Retrieved from http://www.nap.edu/catalog/12956.html

Stevens-Long, J., Schapiro, S. A., & McClintock, C. (2003) Passionate scholars: Transformative learning in doctoral education. *Adult Education Quarterly, 62*(2), 180–198. doi:10.1177/0741713611402046

Taylor, E. W. (1998). *The theory and practice of transformative learning: A critical review* (Information Series No. 374). Columbus, OH: Eric Clearinghouse on Adult, Vocational and Continuing Education.

Taylor, E. W. (2007). An update of transformative learning theory: A critical review of the empirical research (1999–2005). *International Journal of Lifelong Education, 26,* 173–191.

Taylor, E. W. (2008). Transformative learning theory. In S. Merriam (Ed.), *Third update of adult learning theory: New directions for adult and continuing education no. 119* (pp. 5–15). San Francisco, CA: Jossey-Bass.

Index

AACN. *See* American Association of Colleges of Nursing

AACN-AONE Academic-Practice Partnership Awards, 294

academic administration
preparation for, 509

academic health centers (AHCs), 295

academic interdisciplinary partnerships, 399–401

academic leaders. *See also* leadership; leadership consciousness
preparation for, 508–509
shortage of, 508–509

academic role, 521–526
academic administration. *See* academic administration
academic leaders. *See* academic leaders
advanced education, 517–518
Bellini, perspective from, 511–512
case study, 514–517
clinical track versus research track, 561–562
Denisco, perspective from, 512–514
Lias, perspective from, 524–526
preparation of future nurse leaders, 510
and preparation of nurse educators, 506
preparation path for NPs, 141–142
service classification, 521–522
shortage of faculty, 508–509, 561
supply and demand for faculty, 506–508

Academic-Service Partnership Council (ASPC), 290

academic-service partnerships
creating strong infrastructure to support, 290–292
in the education of DNP, 287–289

access to health care services, 419

accountable care organizations (ACOs), 87, 543

Accreditation Commission for Education in Nursing (ACEN), 182

Accreditation Commission for Midwifery Education (ACME), 82

Accrediting Commission for Education in Nursing (ACEN), 21

ACNP. *See* American College of Nurse Practitioners

action research, engagement in, 222

Active Worlds, 342

ADN degree, 16

advanced nursing practice (ANP), 544–545, 555. *See also* doctoral advanced nursing practice (DANP)
AACN definition, 133
AACN's essentials, 120
contemporary, 90

advanced practice, 257

advanced practice nurses (APNs), 9, 24–25, 28, 34, 77, 86, 217, 220
AACN, 17, 28
to ANP, 24
APRN current and future outcomes, 93
APRN practice outcomes, 92–93
clinical nurse specialists, 26, 61, 87–88, 108–111
clinical scholarship, 217
consensus model and LACE, 89–90
DNP-prepared, 128, 134
doctoral. *See* doctoral advanced practice nurse
education, 20
nurse anesthetist, 83–85
nurse-midwives, 79–83
nurse practitioner, 85–87
primary care settings, 328
programs, 17, 24
roles, 56
from silos to common vision, 94–95
technology, 323
unification of APRN education, regulation, and practice, 88–89
uniqueness of APRN "practice," 90–92

advanced practice registered nurses (APRNs), 3, 10, 17, 25, 88, 113, 121, 141, 143, 229, 288, 502
  behavior, 101
  case study, 122–127
  challenges, 105
  characteristics, 89–90
  and CNS practitioners, 109
  consensus model, 89–90, 479–480, 481, 486
  critical thinking questions, 95
  current and future outcomes, 93
  DNP-prepared, 114, 121, 128–129
  education, regulation, and practice, 88–89
  LACE, 89
  master's-prepared versus doctorally prepared, 470–472
  MSN-prepared, 115, 121
  MSN versus DNP, 485–487, 489–490, 500
  organizations, 26
  outcomes, 115
  practice outcomes, 92–93
  roles, 24, 101, 115, 141–142
  terminal degree for clinicians, 113
  uniqueness, 90–92
advocacy, 103, 542, 543
affiliation agreements, 290–291
affordable care, 206
Agency for Healthcare Research and Quality (AHRQ), 204, 206, 210
  inpatient quality indicators, 208
  patient safety indicators, 208
  quality improvement process, 207
  website, 349
Air Force, nurse-midwifery program started by, 82
ambient intelligence, 335
American Academy of Family Physicians, 542
American Academy of Nurse Practitioners (AANP), 26, 329, 417
American Academy of Nurse Practitioners Certification Board, 86
American Academy of Pediatrics (AAP), 87, 417, 542
American Association of Colleges of Nursing (AACN), 3–4, 9, 13, 20, 24, 25, 28, 114, 141, 143, 161, 181, 183, 219, 242, 257, 285, 324, 328–329, 371, 378, 394, 416, 417, 420, 422, 473, 480, 500, 502, 507, 517, 522
  2015 position, 29–33
  advanced nursing practice, 116–120, 144
  APN, 28
  APRN organizations, 26
  clinical executive, 24, 25, 162
  doctoral education, 116–120, 162–163
  doctorates in the health professions, 29

early developmental work on DNP degree, 26–29
  Essentials, 116–120, 148, 150, 152, 162–163
  hybrid degree, 31
  and NONPF, 27
  nursing issues, 18
  position statement document, 25
American Association of Nurse Anesthetists (AANA), 26, 142, 329, 523
American Association of Nurse Practitioners (AANP), 417, 472
American Board of Comprehensive Care (ABCC), 467, 477, 479, 480
American College of Nurse-Midwives (ACNM), 26, 81, 82, 330, 469
American College of Nurse Practitioners (ACNP), 26, 472, 473
American College of Physicians (ACP), 87, 104, 105, 542
American Medical Association (AMA), 66, 87, 101–102, 104–105, 328, 472, 557
American Nurse Credentialing Center (ANCC), 468
American Nurses Association (ANA), 3, 18, 56, 81, 422, 468
American Nurses Credentialing Center (ANCC), 86, 350, 560
American Organization of Nurse Executives (AONE), 162, 329, 422, 530
  nurse executive competencies, 171–172
American Osteopathic Association, 542
anesthesia care team (ACT), 83, 84
anesthesia delivery, 83
APRN Clinical Training Task Force, 530
APRNs. See advanced practice registered nurses
artificial intelligence, affective computing, robotics, 335
associate degree (AD), 68
  versus BSN, 15
  -level nurses, 56
Association of Faculties of Pediatric Nurse Practitioners (AFPNP), 473
Association of Social Work Boards (ASWB), 102
Atlas, 328
augmented reality technology, 342

bachelor of science in nursing (BSN), 10, 21, 56, 147, 286, 287, 477
  to DNP, 16, 17, 39, 87, 242, 536, 555, 564
  to PhD, 32
  for professional nursing, 22
behavior under stress, awareness of, 304
Bellevue School of Midwifery, 80

bibliographic databases, 334
Bill and Melinda Gates Foundation, 401, 402
bioelectronics, human-machine symbiosis, neuroelectronics, 335
biometrics, impact of, 336
blame, 366, 367
Bolton Act, 77
Boston-Bedford Veterans Administration (VA) hospital system, 295
Boston Medical Society, 79
Boyer's Model of Scholarship, 509
Breckinridge, Mary, 80
Brewster, Mary, 64
"Bridges to the Doctorate for Minority Nursing Students," 385

capstone project, 163
Carnegie Foundation for the Advancement of Teaching, 562
Carnegie Study, 563
Carter Center, 401, 402
Case Western Reserve University (CWRU), 22, 464–465, 563
Centers for Medicaid & Medicare Service, 205
certification examination. *See* DNP certification examination
certified clinical nurse specialist, 89
certified nurse anesthetist, 89
certified nurse educator (CNE), 128, 189–190
certified nurse-midwife (CNM), 89, 468, 469, 486
certified nurse practitioner (CNP), 89, 468, 486
certified registered nurse anesthetist (CRNA), 10, 83, 84, 329, 468, 486, 523
chief clinical information officer (CCIO), 350
chief executive officer (CEO), 169
chief financial officer (CFO), 169
chief information officer (CIO), 350
chief medical officer (CMO), 169
chief nursing informatics officer (CNIO), 350
chief nursing officer (CNO), 165, 237, 371
Christel House International, 401, 402
Christensen, Clayton, 556–557
CINAHL database, 327
CiteULike, 327
clinical decision support (CDS), 349
clinical dissertation model, 12, 29, 31
clinical doctorate, 9, 12–13, 22–24, 26, 27, 33–34, 113, 128, 282, 351
clinical executive, 161, 553, 558–560, 571
    AACN essentials, 162–163
    AONE nurse executive competencies, 171–172
    competencies, 558–559
    definition of, 162
    DNP, 163–165, 173

future perspectives, 172–173
    importance, 161–162
    master's versus doctoral education, 165–170
    nurse executive preparation, 170–171
    supply, demand, and preparation of, 161–162
clinical knowledge, importance of, 435, 440
clinical nurse specialist (CNS), 11, 24, 77, 468, 486. *See also* advanced practice nurses; advanced practice registered nurses
    role, 87–88
    scope of practice, 87
    specialization taxonomy, 108
clinical practice, 24, 26, 32, 41, 113, 143–144, 218–219
    dissertation, 32
clinical prevention, 542–544
clinical role, 499–501, 502–503
    description, 484–485
    dissemination and implementation science, 491–494
    evolution of, 499
    of NPs, 490
    pathways to potential roles, 489–490
    and practice doctorate, 487–488
    tips, 495–496
clinical scholarship, 217, 538–539, 549, 572
    definition, 217–220
    demonstrated in DNP graduates, 220–221
    engagement in action research, 222
    evidence-based practice, use of, 221–222
    future of, 223–224
    role in dissemination, 222–223
clinical scientist, 331
clinician educator. *See* educator
closing MS-level NP programs, 147–148
cloud computing, 342
CNE. *See* certified nurse educator
Coalition for Patients' Rights (CPR), 104
collaboration, effective, 290
collaborative learning software applications, 334
collaborative teams, 541
Commission for Nursing Education Accreditation (CNEA), 121
Commission on Collegiate Nursing Education (CCNE), 21, 37, 114, 143, 182, 477, 486, 559
Committee for the Study of Nursing Education, 67
common sense, and successful negotiation, 363
Community-Based Nurse Midwifery Program (CNEP), 82
community service learning, 409
competencies, 399–400

complexity, uncertainty, volatility, and ambiguity (CUVA), 251
comprehensive library training, 331
confidence, and negotiation, 362
conflict resolution, 357
Connotea, 327
consensus model, 479–480, 481, 486
and LACE. *See* LACE
contemporary practice doctorate movement, 23–25
contempt, 366, 367
content knowledge, for successful negotiation, 363
cost, of health care, 419–420
cost-benefit analyses, 210
Council for the Advancement of Comprehensive Care (CACC), 151, 467, 468, 470
Council on Accreditation of Nurse Anesthesia Educational Programs (COA), 523
Council on Graduate Education on Administration in Nursing (CGEAN), 559
County Health Improvement Program, 81
Crile, George W., 83
criticism, 366, 367
CRR Global system, 358, 359–360
Crystal Reports, 328
cultural transformation, 354
Cumulative Index to Nursing and Allied Health Literature (CINAHL), 333
cybersecurity, 342

DAPRN. *See* doctoral advanced practice registered nurse
Dartmouth Hitchcock Medical Center in Lebanon, New Hampshire, 163
database resource list, 333
data collection and analysis, 244
tools for, 327, 328
defensiveness, 366, 367
degree credit parity, 555
diplomate in comprehensive care (DCC), 467
exam, 557
disciplinary amnesia, 281
disciplinary stewardship, 280–281
disruptive innovation. *See* innovation
dissemination and implementation science, 491–494
dissemination process, engagement in, 222–223
DNAP. *See* doctor of nurse anesthesia practice
DNP. *See* doctoral of nursing practice
DNP certification examination, 477–478, 479–481
arguments against, 472–473

arguments for, 468–472
eligibility criteria, 468
future directions, 473–474
outline, 467–468
doctoral advanced nursing practice (DANP), 217
clinical executive, 553, 558–560, 571
educator, 553, 561–564, 571
practitioner, 553, 554–558, 571
doctoral advanced practice, 28
doctoral advanced practice nurse (DAPN), 6, 55, 57, 58, 59, 60, 75
evolving and emerging trends to enhance, 338–340
expectations, 324
factors influencing expectations of, 330
informatics competencies for, 325–326
knowledge management competencies for, 326–327
necessity of additional certification to indicate, 151–152
negotiation skills for, 357, 358–367
professional organizations and informatics expectations of, 328–330
role and relevance of, 331
technological tools that can support, 327–328
technology for leadership roles and responsibilities of, 337–338
doctoral advanced practice registered nurse (DAPRN), 28, 35, 204, 237, 238, 239, 244, 247, 542–543, 554, 555, 557, 565
DNP clinical executive, 239–240
DNP educator, 240–241
practice, 239
doctoral degree in nursing, 4
doctorally prepared advanced practice nurse, 237
doctorally prepared NP, arrival of, 144–146
doctoral nursing faculty, national study of, 255
background, 256–259
comparative results, 265
data analyses, 261, 265
doctoral education in nursing, 266–268
nursing faculty in doctoral education, 269
professional growth and work satisfaction, 269
professional profile of doctoral faculty participants, 265
salary analyses, 269–272
sampling, 260–265
study design, 260
succession planning and future vision, 273
survey questionnaire, 260–261, 262–264
doctoral nursing program exchange, 21

doctoral of nursing practice (DNP), 5, 9, 10, 20, 55, 142–144, 161, 173, 182–183, 237, 285, 417–418
  AACN's early developmental work on, 26–29
  academic-service partnerships in the education of, 287–289
  advanced practice registered nurses (APRNs), 128–129
  changes in practice, 534
  changing and evolutionary context and environment of, 245–246
  clinical executive, 239–240
  clinical executive practica, 163–165
  clinical scholarship, 220–221, 222–223
  competencies, 165
  creating strong infrastructure to support academic service partnerships, 290–292
  curriculum, 487, 536, 575
  degree and tenure, 191–193
  and DrNP, 23–25
  educator, 186, 240–241
  emergence of, 114–115
  emerging feelings of confidence and respect in the role as, 246
  Essentials. *See Essentials of Doctoral Education for Advanced Nursing Practice*
  experiences of, 241–242
  faculty, 257
  finding a settled place in the perceived role of, 246–247
  future, 223–224
  graduate from, 173
  graduates, 185, 247, 248
  informant recruitment and informed consent, 243–244
  international implications for, 40–41
  leadership role, 226
  moving from affiliation to partnership, 285–287
  nurse educator focus, 187–188
  versus other degree options, 170–171
  to PhD, 564
  and PhD program, 257–258, 266–268, 277
  -prepared advanced practice registered nurses (APRNs), 121
  -prepared faculty, 259
  -prepared nurse-midwife, 192–193
  -prepared practitioner, 239
  program evaluation, 164–165
  research design and procedures, 243
  role descriptions, 238
  role in negotiation. *See* negotiation
  role in quality improvement, 203–212
  as scholar, 490–491
  scholar-practitioners, 574

doctoral-prepared nurse from miniscule pool, 15–18
doctorates, need for nurses with, 17
doctor of business administration (DBA) degree, 11
doctor of education (EdD), 113
doctor of medicine (MD), 11, 22
doctor of nurse anesthesia practice (DNAP), 85, 570–571
doctor of nursing practice (DNP)-prepared nurse, 219
doctor of nursing practice (DNP/DrNP) program, 3, 9, 23–25, 26, 294
  variability among, 148–150
doctor of nursing science (DNS/DNSc), 9, 25
doctor of pharmacy (PharmD), 11
doctor of philosophy (PhD), 4, 5, 11–12, 20–22, 37–40
doctor of physical therapy (DPT), 11
doctor of psychology degree (PsyD), 12
doctor of science in nursing (DSN), 12, 22, 25
Doctors of Nursing Practice, Inc., 531
Drexel DrNP program's international study-abroad program, 29, 38
  accompanying doctoral faculty abroad, funding for, 447–448
  doctoral students studying abroad, funding for, 446–447
  Dublin program, doctoral student's perspective (case study), 453–454
  Dublin program, faculty perspective, 452–453
  funding, 446–448
  idea of, 445
  lessons learned, 454–455
  London program, doctoral student's perspective (case study), 450–451
  London program, faculty perspective, 448–450
  reasons for mandating, 445–446
Dual Concerns Model, 372
Duquesne DNP-in-Rome study-abroad opportunity
  faculty perspective, 457–458
  student's perspective (case study), 459–460
DynaMed, 337

ecologic educational framework, 488–489
EdD degree, 4, 9, 11, 12, 14
education and training, simulation for, 338–339
Education Program Association, 82
Education Resources Information Center (ERIC), 333

educator, 144, 181, 506, 553, 561–564, 571
  certification for, 189–190
  DNP degree and tenure, 191–193
  educating, 184–185
  nursing education research, 190–191
  nursing practice curricula today, 185–189
  qualifications, 181–182
  shortage, 181–184
educator clinician, 562
effectiveness/outcome evaluation, 210
electronic health records (EHRs), 324
e-mail notifications, 336
e-mentoring, 378, 396
Emergency Maternity and Infant Care
    Program, 80
emotional intelligence, awareness of, 304–305
Endnote®, 328
episteme, 431
essential skills, 152–153, 331, 332
  emerging technologies impacting health
    care, 334, 335–336
  information literacy skills, 325
  keeping skills up-to-date, 334, 336–337
  library search skills, 331, 333–334
*Essentials of Doctoral Education for Advanced
    Nursing Practice*, 221, 287, 545–546
  advanced practice/clinician perspective,
    527–528, 549–550
  Essential I, 535–537
  Essential II, 537–538
  Essential III, 538–539, 549
  Essential IV, 539–542
  Essential V, 416, 418, 419, 423, 427, 542–544
  Essential VI, 420, 542–544
  Essential VII, 402, 542–544
  Essential VIII, 544–545, 555
  exploration of practice after graduation, 528
  guidance for practice, 529–531
  incorporation of, 532
  and outcome improvements, 531–533
  perspective from an academic dean, 535–545
  practice based on, 528–529
evidence-based practice (EBP), 219, 221–222,
    226–227, 330, 440, 538–539, 549
  education about, 281–282
e-visits, 354
executive coaching, 297, 307
  behavior under stress, awareness of, 304
  case example, 309–313
  effectiveness, 307–308
  emotional intelligence, awareness of,
    304–305
  inner critic awareness, 305–306
  leadership and leadership consciousness,
    302–303
    leadership roles, transitions into, 301–302
    mindfulness, awareness as, 306
    personal styles and strengths,
      awareness of, 303–304
    professional development. *See* professional
      development
    self-awareness and leadership
      consciousness, 303
exploration of practice after graduation, 528

Federal Division of Nursing, 81
federal reclassification of nursing, 66
  emergence of recognized professionalism
    of nursing, 66–68
  nursing's status post-World War II—
    the 1960s, 68–69
Federal Trade Commission (FTC), 87
Federation of State Board of Physical
    Therapy (FSBPT), 102
Federation of State Medical Board (FSMB), 102
first practice doctorate, 22
Fisher's Exact test, 261
Flexner Report, 15
Foundation for International Education
    (FIE), 447
Four Horsemen of the Apocalypse, 357, 366
"The Four Horsemen of the
    Apocalypse," 366–367
Frank, Louis, 83
Frontier Nursing Service (FNS), 80
future Internet, 335
future nurse leaders, preparation of, 510

gender, and negotiation, 360–361, 362
genetics and genomics, impact of, 336
Goldmark, Josephine, 67
graduate nursing education (GNE) site, 288
grants, 491
Great Recession, 16
Gregory, Samuel, 79

health care
  cost of, 419–420
  providers, 331
  reformers, 203
  societal forces, 158
Healthcare Information and Management
    Systems Society (HIMSS), 540
health information system (HIS), 326
health information technologies
    (HITs), 289, 326
health insurance, 419
health policy, 418–419, 427–428, 542–544
  access to health care services, 419
  competence, 421–422, 428

didactic, and residency courses, 401
and organizations, 422–423
population health, 419, 420
quality of care, 421, 423
health-system informatics nurses, 292
healthy people/ healthy communities, 206
High Fidelity, 342
high-performing organizations, 560
Hill-Burton Act, 68
holographic images, 335
home monitoring, 354
Hong Kong University (HKU), 463
Hospital Consumer Assessment of Health-care
     Providers and Systems (HCAHPS), 172
human frame, of organizations, 359
human patient simulator, 339
human science approach, 436
hybrid professional doctorates, 29, 31
hybrid simulation, 339

impression management, 137
i-net Clear Reports, 328
informants, 241, 243, 247–248
     findings, 244
     interview, 244
     themes, 245
informatics competencies, 325–326, 332
information
     literacy skills, 325
     mastery, 326–327
     and negotiation, 364
     overload, 555
information systems/technology, 338, 539–542
inner critic awareness, 305–306
innovation, 5
     disruptive, 354, 554, 564, 572, 573
     regulatory authority, 88
     technological, 327, 334, 341–342
inpatient quality indicators, 207, 208
inside-out knowledge, 431
Institute for Healthcare Improvement (IHI),
     212, 564
Institute of Medicine (IOM), 113, 203, 223, 354,
     371, 397, 399, 418, 420, 480–481, 558
     intense scrutiny, 323
     timeline leading, 114
internal resources for scholarship, 276
international higher education, 444
international implications for DNP
     degree, 40–41
Internet, use of, 342
interprofessional and interdisciplinary
     practice, 397, 398, 403–404, 406–410,
     412–414
     academic, 399–401

barriers to, 408
and clinical research, 412–413
collaborative research, 402–403
communication misunderstanding, 408
coordination and collaboration, 400
difference between, 406–407
evidence appraisal, 413
governmental, 401
guidelines development, 413
nongovernmental organizations, 401–402
scholarly project, 403
service learning, 408–409
interprofessional collaboration, 119,
     542–544
interprofessional courses, 400
interprofessional education
     (IPE), 397, 407, 543
interprofessional teams (IPT), 229–230

JabRef, 327
Johnson, Lyndon, 81
Johnson & Johnson Foundation, 401, 402
Johns's model of structured
     reflection, 434, 439
Journal of Online Issues in Nursing, 29
*Journal of the American Medical Association
     (JAMA)*, 23
Just Culture, 543

Kellogg Foundation, 205
knowledge management
     competencies, 326–327
     DNP degree graduate's role in, 35
Kolb's learning cycle, 430

LACE (licensure, accreditation,
     certification, and education), 89–90,
     146, 486
leadership, 302–303, 560
     transitions into, 301–302
leadership consciousness, 302–303
     behavior under stress, awareness of, 304
     emotional intelligence, awareness of,
     304–305
     inner critic awareness, 305–306
     mindfulness, 306
     personal styles and strengths, awareness of,
     303–304
leadership theory, 163
learning experiences, 223
LexisNexis, 333
library search skills, 331, 333–334
lifelong learning, 334
Logical Observation Identifiers Names and
     Codes (LOINC), 348

Magnet Corporation, 560
magnet recognition program, 288
mandatory study-abroad program. *See* study-
    abroad program, mandatory
market competition, 419, 420
master of science in nursing (MSN), 165, 170,
    183, 252, 287, 417, 483
    advanced practice nurse, 115–121
    degree programs, 220
    versus DNP, 485–487, 489–490, 500
master's-level practitioner, 324
Maternity Center Association (MCA), 80, 81
Medicaid, 419
medical errors, eliminating, 209
Medical Home practice, 558
Medicare, 419, 420, 558
MEDLINE, 334
men, and negotiation, 360
mentees, 376
    models of, 378–379
    tips for, 386–387
mentorship, 6, 191, 223, 391–392, 394–396
    for academic roles, 517
    case studies, 382–383
    early history, 377
    e-mentoring, 378, 396
    future directions and recommendations,
        387–388
    group mentoring, 378
    models of, 378–379
    multifaceted mentoring model, 379
    multiple mentoring model, 379
    organizational and system
        support for, 381
    overview, 375–376
    process, 379–380
    in professional nursing, 378
    professional role development, 394–395
    tips for mentees, 386–387
    tips for mentors, 385–386
    traditional, 376, 378
    transformational, 376
    of underrepresented groups, 383–385, 395
    using technology, 395
    value and support for, 376–377
    and willingness, 391, 392, 395
Merit-based Incentive Payment System
    (MIPS), 87
metacognition, 574
mindfulness, 306, 432, 436, 439
minority culture, nurses from, 383–384
mobile devices, 340, 342
mobile health (mHealth), 354
mode 1 knowledge. *See* theoretical
    knowledge

mode 2 knowledge. *See* practice knowledge
multifaceted mentoring model, 379
multiple mentoring model, 379
Myers-Briggs Type Inventory (MBTI), 304, 310

National Academy of Sciences (NAS), 33
National Association of Boards of Pharmacy
    (NABP), 102
National Association of Clinical Nurse
    Specialists (NACNS), 26, 110, 142, 285
National Association of Nurse Practitioners in
    Women's Health (NPWH), 473
National Association of Pediatric Nurse
    Practitioners (NAPNAP), 417, 473
National Board of Certification on
    Occupational Therapy (NBCOT), 102
National Board of Medical Examiners
    (NBME), 467, 468, 470
National Certification Board for Pediatric
    Nurse Practitioners and Nurses, 86
National Certification Corporation (NCC), 86
National Conference of Gerontological Nurse
    Practitioners (NCGNP), 473
National Council Licensure Examination
    (NCLEX), 190, 477
National Council of State Boards of Nursing
    (NCSBN), 86, 88, 89, 102
National Health Service Corps, 81
National Institutes of Health (NIH), 31, 76, 522
National League for Nursing (NLN), 20, 81,
    181, 189, 190, 194, 422, 473, 506, 507, 517
    Core Competencies for Nurse
        Educators, 506
National League for Nursing Accrediting
    Commission (NLNAC), 34, 121, 486
National Organization of Nurse
    Practitioner, 194
National Organization of Nurse Practitioner
    Faculties (NONPF), 3, 17, 28, 39, 142, 285,
    417, 473, 480, 507, 525, 530, 535
National Organization of Public Health
    Nurses (NOPHN), 64, 68
National Research Council of the National
    Academies (NRCNA), 142
National Strategy for Quality Improvement in
    Health Care (NQS), 206
National Task Force, 89
natural science approach, 436
ND degree, 22–23
negotiation, 357, 371–374
    barriers to, 365–367
    definition of, 357
    effectiveness, fundamentals for, 373
    elements, 364–365
    essentiality, 372

gender effects in, 360–361, 362
and information, 364
methodologies to improve, 374
mistakes, 367
political frame, 360
and power, 364
process steps, 365
rank and privilege effect on, 361–362
strategic role of DNP, 358–362
symbolic frame, 360
and systems theory, 358–359
tactical role of DNP, 362–367
and time, 364
traits of, 363–364
NERVANA, 295–296
New Careers in Nursing (NCIN)
    program, 379
New Mexico program, 81
Nightingale, Florence, 61–63, 377, 378, 383
NLN. *See* National League for Nursing
non-BSN-prepared nurses, 56
NONPF. *See* National Organization of Nurse
    Practitioner Faculties
non-tenure track (NTT) faculty, 273, 275
nurse administrators, 143, 289
nurse anesthetists, 11, 24, 77, 83–85
    Mayo training program for, 83
    scope of practice, 84
nurse executive
    competencies, 171–172
    preparation, 170–171
Nurse Executive, Advanced Board
    Certification (NEA-BC), 350
nurse informaticists, 350
nurse leaders, 221, 222, 223
nurse-led clinics, 398, 400
nurse-midwives, 11, 24, 77, 79
    educational program for, 79–83
    history, 79
    modular curriculum for, 81
    pivotal events, 79–80
nurse practitioner (NP), 11, 24, 77, 85–87, 288,
    564–565
    academic preparation for, 141–142
    certification, 479–480
    controversies, 141, 151
    with DNP degrees, 490–491
    as frontline care providers, 143
    future role of, 146
    movement, 85, 86
    MS-level NP prógrams pitfalls, 147–148
    shortage of, 147–148
nurse scientist, 37, 562, 572
Nurse Scientist Program, 415
Nurse-Scientist Training Program, 14

Nurses Improving Care for Healthsystem
    Elders (NCHE), 560
Nurse Training Act (NTA), 68, 86
nursing
    academic leaders, 259
    administration, 17, 38, 173, 178, 277,
        362, 530
    doctorate, 10, 13, 40, 41, 58
    educator. *See* educator
    faculty, 181–184, 269
    future of, 566
    knowledge, 231
    leadership, 487
    paradigm in, 436
    praxis, 435
    research, 190–191
nursing practice curricula, 185–189
NVivo, 328

Obama, Barack, 565
occupational therapy, 29, 31
opinion leaders, 204
organizational leadership, 537–538
organizational learning, 210
organizations, frames of, 359–360
outside-in knowledge, 431

Pandora's box for DNP programs, 21
patient care technology, 539–542
Patient Protection and Affordable Care Act
    (2010), 3, 94, 113, 203, 251, 288, 419,
        558, 565
patient safety, 209–212
    composites and descriptions, 211
    indicators, 207, 208
pedagogical skills, 185
pediatric care providers, 85
Pediatric Nursing Certification Board
    (PNCB), 86, 186
performance measurement and reporting,
        208–209
personal integrity, for successful
    negotiation, 363
personal knowledge, 435
personal learning environment (PLE), 337
personal learning spaces, 337
personal physician, 542
personal styles and strengths, awareness of,
        303–304
PhD degree, 9, 11, 12, 14, 25, 39, 280
    and DNP programs, 257–258, 266–268, 277
    dwindling supply of nursing faculty
        with, 18–22
    graduates, 185
    in nursing, 4

phronesis, 431
physician leadership, 542
Physician Practice Patient Safety
    Assessment, 212
physicians emerged dominant over nurses in
    public health role, 65
Planetree Model of Care, 541, 560
planning skills, for successful negotiation, 363
political activism, 542
political frame, of organizations, 360
population health, 419, 420, 542–544
positive deviance, 503
post-World War II advancements, 68
power, and negotiation, 363, 364
practice-based evidence, 435
practice doctorate, 4, 13, 22, 24, 32, 115, 133,
    500. See also DNP
  clinical role, 487–488
  ecologic educational framework, 488–489
  evolution of, 415–417
practice-focused doctorates, 193, 194, 219,
    232, 258
practice knowledge, 32, 36, 325, 354, 431, 435
practice-theory-practice gap, 434
practitioner, 141, 553, 554–558, 571
  closing MS-level NP programs, 147–148
  DNP, 142–144
  DNP, variability among, 148–150
  doctorally prepared NP, arrival of, 144–146
  essentials, 152–153
  evolving academic preparation for, 141–142
  necessity of additional certification, 151–152
  scholarship and DNP essentials, concept of,
    150–151
Predictive Analytics Software (PASW), 328
Preston Retreat Hospital, 80
principal investigator (PI), 127, 134
privilege, effect on negotiation, 361–362
problematization of practice, 430
process/implementation evaluation, 210
professional development
  boundary challenge, 299
  competency challenge, 300
  confidence challenge, 300
  identity challenge, 300–301
  loneliness challenge, 299–300
  transitions in, 298–299
professional doctorate, 4, 22, 31, 40
professional growth and work satisfaction, 269
professionalizers, 10
professional registered nurse, 56
professional roles of nursing, 55
  "Americanized" Nightingale nursing
    model, 62–63
  emergence of, 61–63

emergence of the recognized
    professionalism, 66–68
  federal reclassification of nursing, 66–69
  meaning for new DNP graduates, 58
  Nightingale influence, 61–62
  nursing's role in the public's health, 63–65
  nursing's status post-World War II, 68–69
  physicians emerged dominant over nurses
    in public health role, 65
  public health nurse, 66
  sociology, 59–61
  toil and contribution of public health nurses
    to nursing, 63–66
program evaluation, 208–209
  types, 210
propositional knowledge, 435
public health nurse, 61, 63–65, 66, 68, 85

Quality and Safety Education for Nurses
    (QSEN), 330, 399, 543
quality health care, 205
quality improvement (QI), 204, 205, 206,
    537–538
  process, 207
  program evaluation, 208–209
quality of care, 421, 423
quantum computing, 335

rank, effect on negotiation, 361–362
really simple syndication (RSS), 336
recognized professionalism of nursing,
    emergence of, 66–68
reference alerts, 336
reference management tools, 327
reflective practice, 439–440, 574
  bother to reflect, 431–432
  defined, 429–431
  methods, 433–434
  and nursing knowledge, 434–435
  overview, 436–437
  paradigm in nursing, 436
  reflection-for-action, 433
  reflection-in-action, 432–433
  reflection-on-action, 432–433
  and self-awareness, 432, 436, 439
RefWorks, 328
Registered Nurse, 28
relationships
  system of, 359
  two-way nature of, 409
research-active faculty, 562
research-based practice, 435
research-based support, interfacing with
    libraries for, 338
research doctorate, 488, 489

research-focused and practice-focused scholarship, distinguishing between, 392, 490
research-focused doctorate, 30, 258
research knowledge, 431
Re-visioning PhD Education Project, 416
Robert Wood Johnson Foundation (RWJF), 82, 205, 330, 371, 416, 558
Executive Nurse Fellows Program, 518
Rockefeller Foundation, 67
roles, 57. *See also* academic role; clinical role
ambiguity, 237, 238
conflict, 237, 238
defined, 58
new DNP graduates, role and its meaning for, 58
sociology, 59–61
role strain, 238
role stress, 237–238
role-taking, 60
role theory, 6, 57–61
RWJF. *See* Robert Wood Johnson Foundation

salary analyses, 269–272
scholarship
defined, 232
and DNP essentials, concept of, 150–151
scientific underpinnings for practice, 535–537
Scope of Practice Partnership (SOPP), 101, 104
second generation clinical doctorate, 22
Second Life, 342
second professional doctorate in nursing, 22–23
Selected Dissemination of Information (SDIs), 334
self-assurance, and negotiation, 362
self-awareness, 432, 436, 439
self-awareness, and leadership consciousness, 303
behavior under stress, awareness of, 304
emotional intelligence, awareness of, 304–305
inner critic awareness, 305–306
mindfulness, awareness as, 306
personal styles and strengths, awareness of, 303–304
self-talk, 305, 306
service learning, 408–409
Shippen, William, 79
Sigma Theta Tau International Leadership Institute, 217, 220, 517

simulation
for education and training, 338–339
for research, 339–340
Smarter Internet, 341
SNOMED Clinical Terms, 348
social determinants of health (SDOH), 427
social exchange theory, 375
sociological schools of thought on roles, 59–61
software as a service (SAAS), 336
solution versus compromise, 357–358
spirit of inquiry, 184
standardized patient, 339
"state-of-the-art" health care, 161
Statistical Analysis System (SAS), 328
Statistical Package in the Social Sciences (SPSS), 261, 328
stonewalling, 366, 367
strategic role of DNP, in negotiation, 358
structural frame, of organizations, 359
study-abroad program, mandatory, 463–465
Drexel DrNP program. *See* Drexel DrNP program's international study-abroad program
Duquesne University. *See* Duquesne DNP-in-Rome study-abroad opportunity, faculty perspective
overview, 443, 455–456
rationale for, 444
subpar skills, 374
succession planning, 174, 260, 273
supervisor/manager expectations and actions, 210
sustainability, integrated model of, 398
symbolic frame, of organizations, 360
Synthesis Science, 440
systems leadership, 537–538
systems theory, and negotiation, 358–359
systems thinking, 537–538

task trainers, 339
Taussig, Fred, 79
team building, 29
Team Strategies and Tools to Enhance Performance and Patient Safety (TeamSTEPPS), 399–400, 543
teamwork within units, 210
techne, 431
technical rationality, 434, 440
technological innovations, 327, 334, 341
cloud computing, 342
data collection, 342
smarter web, 341

technology, 323, 556
  for communication and information access, 340
  current APN technology expectations, 323
  doctoral APN. *See* doctoral advanced practice nurse
  emerging technologies, 334, 335–336
  essential skills, developing and maintaining, 331, 332
  expectations for master's-level practitioner, 324
  horizon, 341–342
  keeping skills up-to-date, 334, 336–337
  library search skills, 331, 333–334
  virtual worlds for education and research, 340–341
Technology Informatics Guiding Educational Reform (TIGER), 325–326, 330
tenure, 191
The Joint Commission, Core Measure Sets, 538, 546
theoretical knowledge, 33, 36
theory-practice gap, 434, 439–440
thinking clearly under stress, for successful negotiation, 363
3D bio printing, 335
3D laser scan, 335
360-feedback, 304, 317
TIGER initiative, 540–541
time, and negotiation, 364
toxic behaviors, 366–367
traditionalists, 10
transformative learning, 574–575
translational research, 39–40, 227
Tri-Council for Nursing, 25, 422, 423
Twitter, 336–337

underrepresented groups, mentoring, 383–385
United States Medical Licensing Examination (USMLE), 468, 469
universal agreement, 291
University College Cork in Cork (UCC), 464–465
University of Pittsburgh Medical Center (UPMC), 286, 290, 291
University of Texas MD Anderson Cancer Center in Houston, Texas, 163
unlearning, 430–431, 439
User Comparative Database Report, 210
U.S. National Quality Strategy (NQS), 204
U.S. Public Health Service (USPHS), 63

values-driven health care model, 544
verbal ability, for successful negotiation, 363
virtual/augmented reality, 335
virtual reality simulation, 339
virtual visits (e-visits), 354
virtual worlds, 340–341
visiting nurses, 64, 65
VP of Clinical Informatics, 350

Wald, Lillian, 64
waste reduction policy, 419–420
Web 2.0, 336
Web 3.0, 336
web resource list, 336
whole person orientation, 542
Winslow, C.-E. A., 65
win-win approach, 357
wise action, 435
women, and negotiation, 360–361
Wonderland, 342
Work Progress Administration (WPA), 67

Printed in the United States
By Bookmasters